Modern Dentistry

Modern Dentistry

Edited by April Hilbert

hayle medical
New York

Hayle Medical,
750 Third Avenue, 9th Floor,
New York, NY 10017, USA

Visit us on the World Wide Web at:
www.haylemedical.com

ISBN: 978-1-63241-571-4

The publisher's policy is to use permanent paper from mills that operate a sustainable forestry policy. Furthermore, the publisher ensures that the text paper and cover boards used have met acceptable environmental accreditation standards.

Printed in China.

Cataloging-in-Publication Data

Modern dentistry / edited by April Hilbert.
p. cm.
Includes bibliographical references and index.
ISBN 978-1-63241-571-4
1. Dentistry. 2. Oral medicine. 3. Teeth. I. Hilbert, April.
RK51 .M63 2019
617.6--dc23

Table of Contents

Preface

It is often said that books are a boon to mankind. They document every progress and pass on the knowledge from one generation to the other. They play a crucial role in our lives. Thus I was both excited and nervous while editing this book. I was pleased by the thought of being able to make a mark but I was also nervous to do it right because the future of students depends upon it. Hence, I took a few months to research further into the discipline, revise my knowledge and also explore some more aspects. Post this process, I begun with the editing of this book.

The branch of medicine concerned with oral health and the diagnosis and management of diseases of the dentition, oral mucosa and related structures and tissues in the maxillofacial area is known as dentistry. Some of the specializations in the science of dentistry are endodontics, geriodontics, oral implantology, periodontology, prosthodontics, oral and maxillofacial surgery, pathology and radiology, etc. Some of the common procedures used in the treatment of oral diseases are the surgical extraction of tooth, root canal treatment, scaling and root planing, restoration of teeth, etc. Complex treatments like bone grafting, gingival grafts, dental implants and sinus lifts as well as highly invasive oral and maxillofacial surgical procedures may be required for the treatment and management of dental conditions. This book is compiled in such a manner, that it will provide in-depth knowledge about modern dentistry. Different approaches, evaluations, methodologies and advanced studies have been included herein. For all readers who are interested in dentistry, the case studies included herein will serve as an excellent guide to develop a comprehensive understanding.

I thank my publisher with all my heart for considering me worthy of this unparalleled opportunity and for showing unwavering faith in my skills. I would also like to thank the editorial team who worked closely with me at every step and contributed immensely towards the successful completion of this book. Last but not the least, I wish to thank my friends and colleagues for their support.

Editor

1

Assessment of Elementary School Teachers' Level of Knowledge and Attitude regarding Traumatic Dental Injuries in the United Arab Emirates

Manal A. Awad,[1] Eman AlHammadi,[2] Mariam Malalla,[1] Zainab Maklai,[1] Aisha Tariq,[1] Badria Al-Ali,[1] Alaa Al Jameel,[3] and Hisham El Batawi[1]

[1]*Department of Preventive and Restorative Dentistry, College of Dental Medicine, University of Sharjah, Sharjah, UAE*
[2]*Dubai Health Authority, Dubai, UAE*
[3]*Princess Nourah Bint Abdulrahman University, Riyadh, Saudi Arabia*

Correspondence should be addressed to Manal A. Awad; awad@sharjah.ac.ae

Academic Editor: Louis M. Lin

Introduction. In this cross-sectional study, the level of knowledge and attitude of elementary school teachers regarding traumatic dental injuries (TDI) were assessed. *Materials and Methods.* A questionnaire was distributed to 330 elementary school teachers in 30 randomly selected schools in the Emirates of Sharjah and Dubai. The questionnaire collected information on participants' demographic characteristics, first aid training, and attitude about emergency management of TDI. *Results.* 292 teachers (88%) completed the questionnaires; of these, 95% were females, and 50% of the participants had first aid training. Knowledge about tooth avulsion was inadequate, and first aid training was not associated with correct responses to management of avulsed teeth ($p > 0.05$). A significantly higher percentage of younger teachers ($p < 0.05$) expressed the need for future education on TDI management. A significantly higher percentage of participants who had an educational position (95%) indicated that they did not have enough knowledge regarding TDI compared to physical education teachers (79%) and administrators (87%) ($p < 0.05$). *Conclusions.* Elementary school teachers in the UAE have a low level of knowledge regarding the management of dental trauma. Educational programs that address TDI are needed and could improve the elementary school teachers' level of knowledge in emergency management of TDI.

1. Introduction

Traumatic dental injuries (TDI) among children are considered a public health concern [1] Dental injuries can lead to tooth loss; subsequently it can have a negative impact on children's psychological well-being [2–4]. A study from Brazil showed that adolescents with severe untreated TDI were 2.4 times more likely to report worse oral-health-related quality of life than adolescents without untreated TDI [4]. Accordingly, the prognosis of injured teeth depends on immediate and appropriate management by those present at the site where the trauma took place; this includes schoolteachers and staff [4, 5].

Studies have demonstrated that TDI are sometimes not properly treated, one of the reasons for this problem being the time between the trauma episode and seeking dental treatment, which can sometimes be years [6].

The main cause of TDI among school-age children are unpreventable falls in schools. It has been previously reported that approximately 50% of schoolchildren have experienced a TDI prior to graduation [7]. Therefore, it is highly likely that first aid would be provided by teachers and other school staff. Accordingly, teachers' knowledge of the management of TDI is essential to improve prognosis. Although many studies have been conducted in different countries to assess schoolteachers' knowledge of TDI [1, 2, 6–11], only one has previously been conducted in the UAE [12], and this included only Arabic-speaking teachers in the Emirate of Ajman.

The main objective of this study is to evaluate the level of knowledge and attitudes of elementary schoolteachers in two Emirates in the UAE, Dubai and Sharjah, regarding TDI among school-age children.

2. Material and Methods

In this cross-sectional study, a self-administered questionnaire was distributed to 330 elementary school teachers in the Emirates of Sharjah and Dubai. Permission to conduct the study was obtained from the educational authorities of the participating schools. Schools principals approved participation of the school teachers in the study and all participating teachers signed consent forms. The questionnaire used in this study is based on those previously used in Jordan [6] Saudi Arabia [8], Australia [13], and Iran [9]. This questionnaire consisted of four parts. Part 1 included questions related to the demographic characteristics of the study participants, including gender, age, position, first aid training, and experience with dental trauma. Part 2 included questions related to participants' attitude towards emergency management of dental trauma. These attitude questions included 10 items with five possible answers for each (strongly agree, agree, disagree, neither agree nor disagree, agree, and strongly disagree). Part 3 provided participants with two case scenarios of dental injuries. The first concerned a fractured tooth in a nine year old, and the second was a case of a 13-year-old child with an avulsed tooth. These two scenarios had previously been used to assess schoolteachers' knowledge about dental injuries in other studies [5, 12]. For each scenario, participants were given several options to choose from. Part 4 of the questionnaire was related to self-assessment, in which participants were asked the following three questions: (a) "Is your knowledge on dental emergency management enough?" (b) "Do you need future education in this regard?" (c) "Are you able to provide proper action when needed?" For each question, participants gave a yes or no answer.

The questionnaire was translated to Arabic and backward and forward translation was used to establish equivalency. Because some teachers were not Arabic-speaking, participants were given the option of responding either to the English or the Arabic version of the questionnaire.

2.1. Statistical Analysis. Data were analyzed using the statistical analysis package SPSS (Version 20, Chicago, IL). Results were analyzed by frequency distribution. Chi-square tests were also utilized to assess the effect of first aid training on knowledge of management of presented cases. In addition, Chi-square tests were also used to evaluate the relationship between self-assessments of knowledge, need for additional education, and proper action according to gender, position, school, age, and first aid training. For all assessments, level of significance was set at alpha 0.05, two-tailed.

3. Results

Of the 330 teachers who were approached from 30 randomly selected schools in Sharjah and Dubai, 88% ($N = 292$) responded to the questionnaire. The majority of participants were females ($N = 278$; 95%) and approximately half of school teachers had first aid training ($n = 146$; 51%) (Table 1). In this study, 36% of the participants indicated that teachers are not responsible for traumatic dental injuries, and the majority (89%) believed that time is an important factor in the prognosis of dental trauma. In addition, 81% indicated that educational experience can assist in the management of TDI (Table 2).

Table 1: Characteristics of study participants.

Variable	N (%)
Gender	
Males	14 (4.8)
Females	278 (95.2)
Age group	
<35	148 (51)
36–45	102 (35)
>45	42 (14)
Education	
High school/diploma	58 (20)
Bachelor, masters	227 (80)
Position	
Educational	246 (87)
Health/physical education	14 (5)
Administration	24 (9)
First aid	
Yes	146 (51)
No	49 (49)
Dental emergency training	
Yes	13 (5)
No	249 (95)
Witness	
Yes	84 (29)
no	201 (71)

Table 3 depicts the participants' responses to the two cases presented to them. Only 58% knew that the damaged tooth was permanent. More than half of the participants ($n = 165$; 57%) responded that the immediate action would be to contact the parents and advise them to send the child to the dentist. Only 33% knew that the correct immediate action is to look for the broken tooth and send the child to the dentist.

Table 3 also summarizes the responses to questions regarding tooth avulsion. Only 6% selected the option to wash the tooth and put it back in its place in the mouth, while the majority ($n = 174$; 61%) thought that stopping the bleeding by compressing a cloth over the injury was the correct immediate action. Of all the participants, 12% indicated that they would go to a general dentist. When asked about tetanus vaccination, more than half ($n = 163$; 59%) responded correctly; 31% did not know what to do if the tooth fell on dirty ground, and 32% gave the correct answer that the tooth should be rinsed under tap water and put back into the socket. Forty-six percent of the participants thought that the tooth should be wrapped in a handkerchief or paper tissue to be transported to the dentist. The highest percentage (41%) thought that the liquid that the tooth should be stored in is

Table 2: Participants attitude towards traumatic dental injuries.

Questions	Strongly agree/agree N (%)
A teacher is not responsible for posttraumatic dental injuries	104 (36)
Time consciousness for emergency management of dental trauma can play a vital role in improving tooth prognosis	282 (89)
A tooth after avulsion will be lost definitely, so there is no need for treatment	35 (12)
Dental trauma emergency management must become one of the educational priorities for teachers	177 (61)
Dental trauma emergency is not an emergency situation	41 (14)
Teacher intervention in school dental injuries may play a key role in traumatized tooth	212 (73)
Emergency management of dental trauma requires special education and therefore there is no need for teacher intervention	114 (40)
Wearing a mouth guard should be compulsory in all contact sports	186 (65)
Due to legal considerations, it is advisable that a teacher refrains from intervening in such scenarios	102 (35)
Having some short pertinent educational experiences, educators can provide better assistance in traumatic dental scenarios	232 (81)

tap water. Only 23% indicated that the best time for the tooth to be replaced in its socket was immediately after the accident.

Table 4 shows that first aid training did not make a significant difference to the correctness of participants' responses.

A significantly higher percentage of younger participants (<35) acknowledged that they needed future education on dental emergency management compared to other groups ($p < 0.05$) (Table 5). In addition, 94% of those with an educational position did not have enough knowledge of management of dental emergencies compared to other groups ($p < 0.05$). In addition, a significantly higher percentage of teachers from government schools (93%) believed that they could benefit from further education on TDI compared to those in private schools (78%). First aid training was not related to self-assessment regarding dental emergency management.

4. Discussion

This study included teachers from randomly selected schools in the Emirates of Sharjah and Dubai. Similar to previous reports from Iran [12], Jordan [6], and Brazil [2], approximately half of the teachers (51%) in this study had first aid training. However, this percentage is higher than previously reported in the UAE [12], in which only 32% of school teachers in the Emirate of Ajman had first aid training and in Saudi Arabia, in which only 18% of primary school teachers had first aid training [8]. As previously reported [9], this training did not contribute to providing correct answer to the case scenarios provided. These findings highlight the importance of continuing education programs that are specifically directed towards management of TDI. Moreover, in this study, 81% of the school teachers indicated that short educational programs could assist them in the management of TDI. More than half of the teachers agreed that they are responsible for the management of dental trauma when it occurs in schools. These findings emphasis the need for tailored educational activities.

Consistent with a previous study in the UAE [12], more than half of the participants (58%) in this study did not know that the broken tooth in the nine-year-old child was a permanent tooth. Lack of knowledge about the eruption timing of teeth suggests that teachers may take actions that could have future negative consequences. For example, it is important that teachers and school staff are aware that an avulsed primary tooth should not be reimplanted to avoid/reduce damage to succeeding permanent tooth, while an avulsed permanent tooth should be immediately reimplanted to keep periodontal cells viable [14, 15].

In case 2, few (23%) participants responded that an avulsed tooth must be replanted immediately and the highest percentage of teachers (43%) did not know what to do. Similar results were observed in studies in Iran [7] and the UAE [12], in which 39% and 19%, respectively, of participating teachers indicated that they did not know what to do regarding the appropriate time to replant an avulsed tooth. Although immediate implantation of an avulsed tooth is necessary for long-term prognosis and reduction of possible complications, an obstacle for immediate action is the lack of parental consent [12, 16].

The lack of knowledge among elementary school teachers about TDI calls for action to improve education about the types of teeth that are likely to suffer from TDI and the proper manipulation and handling of teeth to maintain vitality of cells. Moreover, our findings show that 30% of teachers had witnessed TDI; this indicates that TDI are not uncommon and that schools in collaboration with health authorities should take action to educate teachers about proper management of TDI. Furthermore, reports from previous studies [17–20] showed that providing teachers with information that specifically addressed teeth avulsion had enhanced their knowledge about TDI. For example, Pujita et al. [17] examined primary school teachers' knowledge on TDI before and after an intervention, in which a promotion program was implemented on TDI. The authors reported that teachers' knowledge significantly improved as a result of providing them with the promotion sessions. In another study, Lieger

Table 3: Teachers responses to two scenarios on traumatic dental injuries.

Scenario	N (%)
Case 1	
During school hours, a 9-year-old child is hit in the face with softball. Her upper front tooth is broken. Otherwise, she is healthy, unhurt, and conscious	
The broken tooth is likely to be	
(i) Temporary	73 (25)
(ii) Permanent	166 (58)
(iii) Do not know	49 (17)
Your immediate emergency management of the case is	
(i) Calm down the child and send her back to class	6 (17)
(ii) Contact parents and advise them to send child to the dentist immediately	165 (57)
(iii) Look for broken tooth piece and send child to the dentists with it	96 (33)
(iv) Do not know what to do	10 (4)
Case 2	
A 13-year-old boy is hit in the face and his upper front tooth is missing and there is blood in his mouth. Otherwise, he is unhurt, healthy, and he did not lose consciousness	
The immediate emergency action you would take is	
(i) Stop the bleeding by compressing a cloth over the injury	174 (61)
(ii) Look for the tooth, wash it, and put it back in its place	17 (6)
(iii) Save the tooth in child's mouth and look for professional help	53 (18)
(iv) Place the tooth in a paper and send the child to dentist after the school time	26 (9)
(v) Do not know what to do	14 (5)
What type of health services would you seek first?	
(i) General physician	34 (11)
(ii) Pediatric physician	13 (5)
(iii) Hospital	27 (10)
(iv) Dental School University	11 (4)
(v) General dentists	97 (33)
(vi) Pediatric dentist	96 (33)
(vii) Endodontist	7 (2)
Would you investigate if the child had tetanus?	
(i) Yes	163 (59)
(ii) No	113 (41)
If the tooth has fallen on the dirty ground what would you do?	
(i) Rinse the tooth under tap water and put it back into its socket	90 (32)
(ii) Rub away the dirt by a sponge and soap and put it back	17 (6)
(iii) Put it back into the socket immediately without cleaning	5 (2)
(iv) Discard the tooth	81 (29)
(v) Do not know what to do	87 (31)
How would you transport the tooth on the way to the dentist if you cannot put the tooth back into its socket?	
(i) Put the tooth in ice	58 (20)
(ii) Put the tooth in liquid	76 (27)
(iii) Place the tooth in the child's mouth	19 (7)
(iv) Place the tooth in the child's hand	2 (1)
(v) Wrap the tooth in a handkerchief or paper tissue	130 (46)

TABLE 3: Continued.

Scenario	N (%)
Mark desirable liquids for storing a tooth that has been knocked out while you are on your way to the dentist	
(i) Tap water	100 (37)
(ii) Fresh milk	23 (9)
(iii) Child's saliva	29 (11)
(iv) Alcohol	9 (3)
(v) Saline solution	65 (24)
(vi) Disinfecting solution	44 (16)
(vii) Chicken egg white	0 (0)
Which is the best time for putting back a tooth in if it is knocked out of the mouth?	
(i) Immediately after the accident?	66 (23)
(ii) Within 30 min after the bleeding has stopped	55 (19)
(iii) Within the same day	18 (6)
(iv) This is not a crucial factor	23 (8)
(v) Do not know what to do	122 (43)

TABLE 4: Relationship between first aid training and teachers responses to the case scenarios[a].

Questions	First aid course		p value
	Yes	No	
(1) Emergency management			$p = 0.2$
Correct	89 (62)	77 (55)	
Other responses	55 (38)	64 (45)	
(2) The best health services			
Correct	51 (35)	45 (32)	$p = 0.50$
Other responses	92 (65)	97 (68)	
(3) Tetanus vaccine			$p = 0.83$
Correct	9 (6)	8 (6)	
Other responses	133 (94)	131 (94)	
(4) Cleaning before replantation of a dirty tooth	53 (38)	42 (30)	$p = 0.37$
	87 (62)	98 (70)	
(5) Transportation vehicle	48 (35)	42 (30)	$p = 0.37$
	89 (65)	98 (70)	
(6) Storage media			
Correct	116 (81)	106 (76)	$p = 0.31$
Incorrect	27 (19)	33 (24)	
(7) Time to replant avulsed tooth			$p = 0.11$
Correct	39 (51)	103 (48)	
Incorrect	27 (41)	113 (52)	

[a]Based on Chi-square test.

et al. [19] tested the effect of posters displayed in schools on teachers' management of TDI. Findings from this study showed that, five years after the poster campaign, teachers who worked in the areas where the posters were displayed had significantly better knowledge in management of TDI compared to teachers who worked in other areas. These findings are encouraging and could be easily adopted, and their effects could be examined in elementary schools in the UAE as well.

Approximately 37% of the teachers in this study reported that they could provide proper action in case of TDI, and compared to other groups, a significantly higher percentage of younger teachers (<35 years old) indicated that they were not able to provide proper action in this regard. These findings suggest that teachers in general may have overestimated their knowledge, which may lead to mismanagement of broken or avulsed teeth in children. However, younger teachers are more likely to admit to their lack of ability to handle TDI.

Recently, Al-Musawi et al. [21] demonstrated that providing information on the management of TDI through the use

Table 5: Relationship between self-assessment and sociodemographic factors and first aid training[a].

Variables	Knowledge		Need future education		Proper action	
	Enough	Not enough	Yes	No	Yes	No
	N (%)	*N* (%)	*N* (%)	*N* (%)	*N* (%)	*N* (%)
Gender						
Male	3 (21)	11 (79)[b]	11 (79)	3 (21)	5 (36)	9 (64)
Female	19 (7)	254 (93)	218 (80)	53 (20)	100 (37)	166 (63)
Age						
<35	10 (7)	136 (93)	111 (77)	34 (23)	46 (32)	97 (68)[b]
36–45	6 (6)	95 (94)	86 (85)	15 (15)	39 (39)	60 (61)
>45	69 (15)	34 (85)	32 (82)	7 (18)	20 (19)	18 (11)
Position						
Educator	14 (6)	228 (94)[b]	193 (80)	47 (20)	84 (36)	152 (64)
Health teacher	3 (21)	11 (79)	14 (100)	0 (0)	7 (54)	6 (46)
Administration	3 (13)	21 (87)	20 (83)	4 (17)	9 (38)	15 (63)
First aid						
Yes	11 (8)	131 (92)	116 (82)	26 (18)	51 (37)	88 (63)
No	11 (8)	131 (92)	111 (79)	29 (21)	53 (38)	85 (62)

[a]Based on Chi-square test, [b]$p < 0.05$.

of smartphone applications among a group of 28 schoolteachers was significantly more effective than providing lectures only ($N = 32$) on management of avulsed teeth. The use of such a device is worth exploring in a more pragmatic situation in which stress is an important factor that should also be taken into consideration.

5. Conclusion

The results of this study show that there is a need for education about TDI among school teachers in the UAE. Our findings also highlight the fact that more than one-third of the teachers and staff did not think that handling TDI was their responsibility. These disturbing findings should be addressed and teachers should be informed about the important role that they could play in handling TDI, as well as the negative consequences of poor management or neglect of TDI.

Educational programs and training are needed to improve proper management of traumatic injuries by schoolteachers and avoid unnecessary negative consequences. Guidelines on the management of TDI in schoolteachers' training curriculum should also be given serious consideration.

Disclosure

This study was presented at the AADR/CADR Annual Meeting, Los Angeles, CA, March 16–19, 2016. This project was self-funded.

References

[1] T. S. Borges, F. Vargas-Ferreira, P. F. Kramer, C. A. Feldens, and P. M. Milgrom, "Impact of traumatic dental injuries on oral health-related quality of life of preschool children: A systematic review and meta-analysis," *PLoS One*, vol. 12, no. 2, Article ID e0172235, 2017.

[2] J. Traebert, M. A. Peres, V. Blank, R. Da Silva Böell, and J. A. Pietruza, "Prevalence of traumatic dental injury and associated factors among 12-year-old school children in Florianópolis, Brazil," *Dental Traumatology*, vol. 19, no. 1, pp. 15–18, 2003.

[3] E. B. Bastone, T. J. Freer, and J. R. McNamara, "Epidemiology of dental trauma: a review of the literature," *Australian Dental Journal*, vol. 45, no. 1, pp. 2–9, 2000.

[4] C. B. Bendo, S. M. Paiva, J. W. Varni, and M. P. Vale, "Oral health-related quality of life and traumatic dental injuries in Brazilian adolescents," *Community Dentistry and Oral Epidemiology*, vol. 42, no. 3, pp. 216–223, 2014.

[5] M. Nirwan, A. A. Syed, S. Chaturvedi, P. Goenka, S. Sharma, and N. Marwah, "Awareness in primary school teachers regarding traumatic dental injuries in children and their emergency management: a survey in south jaipur," *International Journal of Clinical Pediatric Dentistry*, vol. 9, no. 1, pp. 62–66, 2016.

[6] S. H. Al-Jundi, H. Al-Waeili, and K. Khairalah, "Knowledge and attitude of Jordanian school health teachers with regards to emergency management of dental trauma," *Dental Traumatology*, vol. 21, no. 4, pp. 183–187, 2005.

[7] J. J. Ravn, "Dental injuries in Copenhagen schoolchildren, school years 1967-1972," *Community Dentistry and Oral Epidemiology*, vol. 2, no. 5, pp. 231–245, 1974.

[8] M. Al-Obaida, "Knowledge and management of traumatic dental injuries in a group of Saudi primary schools teachers," *Dental Traumatology*, vol. 26, no. 4, pp. 338–341, 2010.

[9] M. Raoof, F. Zaherara, N. Shokouhinejad, and S. Mohammadalizadeh, "Elementary school staff knowledge and attitude with regard to first-aid management of dental trauma in Iran: A basic premise for developing future intervention," *Dental Traumatology*, vol. 28, no. 6, pp. 441–447, 2012.

[10] M. I. De Souza Cortes, W. Marcenes, and A. Sheiham, "Impact of traumatic injuries to the permanent teeth on the oral health-related quality of life in 12-14-year-old children," *Community*

Dentistry and Oral Epidemiology, vol. 30, no. 3, pp. 193–198, 2002.

[11] D. Chandukutty, "Awareness of Dental Trauma Management among School Teachers of Kannur, Kerala, India," *Journal of Clinical and Diagnostic Research*, vol. 11, no. 2, pp. ZC08–ZC12, 2017.

[12] R. Hashim, "Dental trauma management awareness among primary school teachers in the Emirate of Ajman, United Arab Emirates," *European Journal of Paediatric Dentistry*, vol. 12, no. 2, pp. 99–102, 2010.

[13] S. L. Raphael and P. J. Gregory, "Parental awareness of the emergency management of avulsed teeth in children," *Australian Dental Journal*, vol. 35, no. 2, pp. 130–133, 1990.

[14] E. L. Zamon and D. J. Kenny, "Replantation of avulsed primary incisors: a risk benefit assessment," *Journal (Canadian Dental Association)*, vol. 67, no. 7, p. 386, 2001.

[15] CF. Wilson, "Management of trauma to primary and developing teeth," *Dent Clin North Am*, vol. 39, no. 1, pp. 133–167, 1995.

[16] M. Singh, P. Yadav, N. Ingle, and N. Kaur, "Evaluation of knowledge and attitude of school teachers about emergency management of traumatic dental injury," *Journal of International Society of Preventive and Community Dentistry*, vol. 5, no. 2, pp. 108–113, 2015.

[17] C. Pujita, S. Nuvvula, G. Shilpa, S. V. S. G. Nirmala, and V. Yamini, "Informative promotional outcome on school teachers' knowledge about emergency management of dental trauma," *Journal of Conservative Dentistry*, vol. 16, no. 1, pp. 21–27, 2013.

[18] F. K. Kahabuka, W. Willemsen, M. van't Hof, and R. Burgersdijk, "The effect of a single educational input given to school teachers on patient's correct handling after dental trauma," *SADJ : journal of the South African Dental Association = tydskrif van die Suid-Afrikaanse Tandheelkundige Vereniging*, vol. 56, no. 6, pp. 284–287, 2001.

[19] O. Lieger, C. Graf, M. El-Maaytah, and V. Arx, "Impact of educational posters on the lay knowledge of school teachers regarding emergency management of dental injuries," *Dental Traumatology*, vol. 25, no. 4, pp. 406–412, 2009.

[20] S. Ghadimi, B. Seraj, H. Keshavarz, AR. Shamshiri, and R. Abiri, "The effect of using an educational poster on elementary school health teachers' knowledge of emergency management of traumatic dental injuries," *Journal of Dentistry of Tehran University of Medical Sciences (JDT)*, vol. 11, no. 6, pp. 620–628, 2014.

[21] A. Al-Musawi, M. Al-Sane, and L. Andersson, "Smartphone App as an aid in the emergency management of avulsed teeth," *Dental Traumatology*, vol. 33, no. 1, pp. 13–18, 2017.

2

Estimation of Antioxidant Levels in Saliva and Serum of Chronic Periodontitis Patients with and without Ischemic Heart Disease

Anahita Punj,[1] Santhosh Shenoy,[1] N. Suchetha Kumari,[2] and Priyanka Pampani[1]

[1]*Department of Periodontics, A.B. Shetty Memorial Institute of Dental Sciences, Nitte University, Deralakatte, Mangalore, Karnataka 575018, India*
[2]*Department of Biochemistry, K.S. Hegde Medical Academy, Nitte University, Deralakatte, Mangalore, Karnataka 575018, India*

Correspondence should be addressed to Anahita Punj; anahitapunj@gmail.com

Academic Editor: Gilberto Sammartino

Objective. To investigate whether there is a relationship between periodontitis and ischemic heart disease by estimation of total antioxidant status in saliva and serum. *Materials and Methods.* A total of 80 samples were collected and divided equally into 4 groups of healthy controls, chronic periodontitis patients, ischemic heart disease patients with periodontitis, and ischemic heart disease patients without periodontitis. Saliva and venous blood samples were collected and analyzed for levels of total antioxidant capacity, superoxide dismutase, glutathione peroxidase, and catalase. *Results.* There were significant ($p < 0.05$) differences in the mean serum levels of total antioxidant capacity ($p < 0.001$), superoxide dismutase ($p < 0.001$), glutathione peroxidase ($p < 0.006$), and catalase ($p < 0.001$) within the 4 groups, whereas the mean salivary levels were significant only for glutathione peroxidase ($p = 0.001$). Both of these serum and salivary antioxidant levels were lower in disease groups of IHD + CP, IHD + H, and CP as compared to healthy controls, with different patterns. *Conclusion.* Antioxidant capacity is significantly hampered in chronic periodontitis and ischemic heart disease patients with or without periodontitis as compared to healthy controls. The salivary and serum antioxidants may not follow the same increase or decrease as a result of increased oxidant stress due to disease.

1. Introduction

The periodontium is a specialized connective tissue that includes the gingiva, periodontal ligament, cementum, and alveolar bone. All these collectively act as a single unit that supports the tooth in its socket [1].

Chronic periodontitis is an infectious disease set off by Gram-negative bacteria residing in the subgingival biofilm, leading to the destruction of soft and hard tissues surrounding the teeth, and is responsible for causing tooth loss [1].

Periodontal pathogens and their products activate the host defense mechanisms and induce the formation of reactive oxygen species (ROS) or free radicals. Free radicals like O_2^-, H_2O_2, HOCL, and OH^- have unpaired electrons making them highly reactive. These are released by the activated PMNs and cause oxidative killing of bacteria in biofilms [2, 3]. This creates an immune response to the microorganism, which results in further release of cytokines and proinflammatory mediators (IL-1α, IL-1β, IL-6, IL-8, and TNF-α) causing amplification of the inflammatory process. Prolonged exposure to ROS leads to a wide spectrum of pathologic reactions in host tissue (lysis of cell membrane, DNA fragmentation, inactivation of enzymes, and activation of proteolytic enzymes resulting in degradation of specific extracellular matrix components of hyaluronic acid and proteoglycan) [4–6].

However, the release of these species outside of phagocytes is detrimental for the surrounding tissues and contributes to the pathogenesis of various inflammatory diseases, through harmful oxidative reactions [2, 3]. Cells and tissues under physiological conditions also generate ROS, which not only have an important role in the process of cell signaling and metabolic processes (Bogdan et al., 2000) [7] but also are believed to play a role in the pathogenesis of various inflammatory disorders (Davies, 1995; McCord, 2000) [8, 9] which range from periodontal diseases to systemic diseases such as diabetes mellitus and cardiovascular diseases (ischemic heart disease) [7–10].

The human body has a range of antioxidant defense mechanisms (nonenzymatic and enzymatic antioxidants) to eliminate reactive oxygen species and prevent their harmful consequences on the host [2, 3]. Antioxidant enzymes protect tissues against oxidative injury by scavenging free oxygen radicals generated by various metabolic processes, modulating the extent of inflammatory response. Antioxidant molecules are present in all body fluids and tissues. The most important intracellular enzymes which protect cells and tissues from the oxygen-derived free radicals are superoxide dismutase (SOD), which rapidly causes dismutation of the superoxide anion to hydrogen peroxide, glutathione peroxidase (GPx), which reduces hydrogen peroxide (a precursor of more potent radical species) and/or lipid hydrogen peroxides by the oxidation of reduced glutathione or S-nitrosoglutathione, and catalase (CAT), which scavenges hydrogen peroxide by converting it to oxygen and water [3].

A deficiency or decrease in antioxidant capacity increases susceptibility to oxidative stress, and the resulting damage is thought to be involved in the pathogenesis of various diseases. Previous studies have reported that periodontal disease was associated with a reduced salivary antioxidant capacity and increased oxidative damage within the oral cavity. There is increasing evidence that oxidative stress is an important contributing factor in the pathogenesis of cardiovascular disease and periodontal disease [3].

Existing evidence suggests that untreated periodontal disease increases the risk of systemic disease by inducing a prolonged systemic inflammatory response. Current literature evidence has demonstrated a modest but statistically significant association between periodontal disease and cardiovascular disease. In atherogenesis, events such as endothelial cell expression of adhesion molecules and development of fatty streaks have been postulated to be regulated, in addition to other factors, by chronic systemic inflammation [11]. Oxidative stress can result in endothelial dysfunction which is observed in atherosclerotic heart disease [12, 13].

Recently, the advances in our understanding regarding the etiology, risk factors, and progression of periodontal diseases have led to research for specific risk factors such as the antioxidant capacity [14].

Thus, the aim of this study was to investigate the total antioxidant capacity and levels of superoxide dismutase, glutathione peroxidase, and catalase in serum and saliva in chronic periodontitis patients with and without ischemic heart disease and to correlate the salivary and serum levels.

2. Materials and Methods

The research protocol was submitted and approved by the Ethical Committee of Nitte University, dated 06-03-2015 (Cert. number: ABSM/EC/22/2015) and was conducted in accordance with the ethical regulations of the Declaration of Helsinki.

2.1. Study Population. Patients from the Outpatient Department of Periodontics and Department of Cardiology were screened based on selection criteria and a sample of 80 patients were selected. Prior to the study, written informed consent was acquired from all the participants.

Patients between the ages of 25–65 years and with minimum complement of 20 teeth were included in the study. The detailed case history and medical history were recorded for all selected patients.

All the patients were screened to assess their periodontal status. The periodontal examination consisted of Loe and Silness (1963) [15] Gingival Index (GI), Probing Pocket Depth (PPD), and Clinical Attachment Level (CAL). PPD, defined as the distance between the gingival margin and the base of the pocket, was measured on six sites of the tooth (mesial, median, and distal points on the buccal and palatal aspect). Based on the level of gingival margin from the cementoenamel junction (CEJ), Clinical Attachment Level (CAL) is calculated, which is the distance from the CEJ to the base of the gingival sulcus or pocket which is measured using a Michigan "O" probe with William's markings.

Then, patients were categorized into the following four groups with 20 patients each (H: healthy group; CP: chronic periodontitis group; IHD: ischemic heart disease group without periodontitis; IHD + CP: ischemic heart disease group with periodontitis) based on the inclusion criteria mentioned below.

Patients who had no systemic diseases and were periodontally healthy with no attachment loss and probing depth <3 mm were considered as healthy controls. Patients who were diagnosed with ischemic heart disease based on clinical presentation and ECG changes by a cardiologist were included. The duration from the date of diagnosis till sample collection ranged from 6 months to 2 years for ischemic heart disease patients. Patients showing the presence of more than 30% of sites with clinical attachment loss ≥3 mm and probing depth ≥4 mm [16] measured with Michigan "O" probe with William's markings were diagnosed as having a moderate to severe form of chronic periodontitis.

Patients with a history of any antibiotic/anti-inflammatory therapy for 6 months prior to study, any known systemic disease or conditions apart from ischemic heart disease, history of smoking, tobacco consumption, and vitamin/minerals or antioxidants supplements intake during the last 3 months, and periodontal therapy 6 months prior to study and pregnant/lactating women were excluded from the study.

2.1.1. Sample Collection. Participants were instructed not to eat, drink, chew gum, or brush teeth for at least 30 min before sampling. Ischemic heart disease patients were instructed to refrain from taking any medication 24 hours before sampling based on the physician's consent. Unstimulated saliva was collected from patients between 9 and 11 a.m. The patients were asked to sit comfortably and were instructed to allow the saliva to pool in the bottom of their mouth and drain it into plastic containers. After 20 minutes of rest, about 5 mL of venous blood was drawn by venepuncture from the median cubital vein and collected in plain and ethylenediaminetetraacetic acid (EDTA) blood collection plastic tubes. The collected samples were sent for biochemical analysis for estimation of total antioxidants level, superoxide dismutase, catalase, and glutathione peroxidase.

2.1.2. Biochemical Analysis. The levels of superoxide dismutase (SOD), glutathione peroxidase (GPx), catalase (CAT), and total antioxidant capacity (TAC) were estimated by NBT reduction method, Rotruck method, Luck method, and phosphomolybdenum method using a spectrophotometer (Systronics Spectrophotometer 106) at wavelengths of 560 nm, 412 nm, 240 nm, and 695 nm, respectively.

2.2. Statistical Analysis. The data collected was compiled in an Excel sheet and analyzed using SPSS version 22 software. Mean and standard deviation (descriptive statistics) were calculated and presented in tables. Level of significance for this study was 5% with a p value of <0.05. Since the data did not follow normal distribution, Kruskal–Wallis test was used to compare the antioxidant levels between the four groups (healthy patients, patients with chronic periodontitis, and IHD patients with and without periodontitis). To correlate antioxidant levels in saliva and serum, Spearman's correlation coefficient was used. Bar diagrams and scatter plots were used to represent the results of the statistical analysis.

3. Results

Out of the 80 patients included in the study, 25 were females, while 55 were male patients. The mean age of the patients included in the study was 47.3 years. There were no menopausal women in the study.

The mean antioxidant levels in serum and saliva of healthy subjects, chronic periodontitis patients, ischemic heart disease patients, and ischemic heart disease patients with chronic periodontitis are given in all figures and tables.

The results revealed that there were differences in the mean levels of total antioxidant capacity (TAC), superoxide dismutase (SOD), glutathione peroxidase (GPx), and catalase (CAT) within the 4 groups in both serum and saliva (Figures 1 and 2, Tables 1–4).

Results of the serum estimation (Table 1) indicated that the levels of antioxidants (TAC, CAT, and GPx) were comparatively higher in the healthy group as compared to the other 3 groups with the least values observed in the ischemic heart disease group with and without periodontitis. Serum SOD levels depicted higher levels in ischemic heart disease groups and the lowest levels in chronic periodontitis groups. All the values were significant with $p < 0.05$. Pairwise comparison of the serum levels of total antioxidant capacity (TAC), superoxide dismutase (SOD), glutathione peroxidase (GPx), and catalase (CAT) among the four groups (Table 2) further confirmed the differences present among the four groups for each of the antioxidants studied.

The mean salivary levels of the antioxidants (Table 3) showed that the antioxidants values of glutathione peroxidase were higher in the disease groups IHD + CP, CP, and IHD + H as compared to the healthy controls. The difference observed was significant with $p < 0.05$, while the values of total antioxidant capacity, superoxide dismutase, and catalase were nonsignificant. Pairwise comparison of the salivary glutathione peroxidase (GPx) levels among the four groups (Table 4) showed significant differences between CP and IHD + H, IHD + H and H, IHD + H and IHD + CP, and H and IHD + CP for GPx.

Correlation between Serum and Salivary Antioxidants (Table 5, Figure 3). In the ischemic heart disease group without periodontitis, a positive correlation was seen between serum and salivary SOD levels. In the healthy group, a positive correlation was seen between serum and salivary SOD, serum and salivary GPx, and serum and salivary catalase levels. On the other hand, a negative correlation was observed

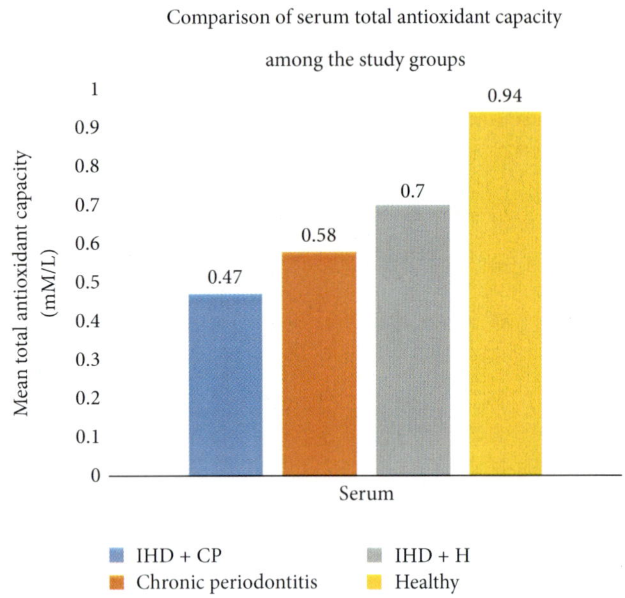

FIGURE 1

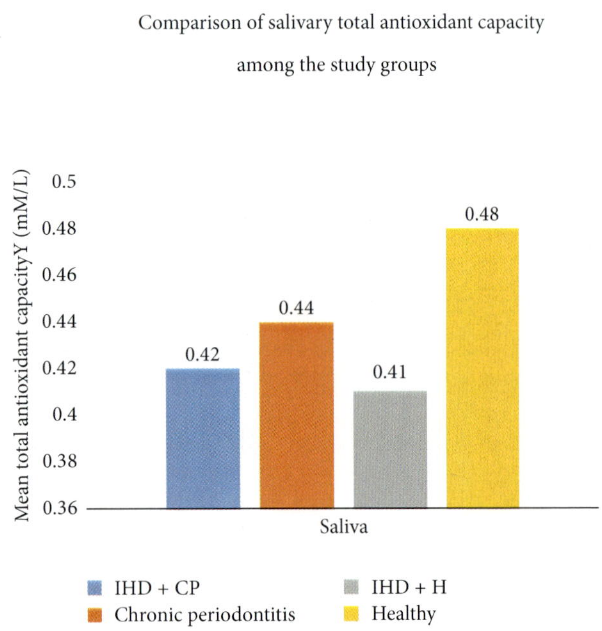

FIGURE 2

TABLE 1: Comparison of serum levels.

Antioxidant	Group	N	Mean (SD)	Median (Q1–Q3)	H-value[#] (df)	p value
Serum TAC (mM/L)	IHD + CP	20	0.47 (0.17)	0.42 (0.37–0.51)	37.33 (3)	<0.001*
	CP	20	0.58 (0.13)	0.57 (0.48–0.72)		
	IHD + H	20	0.70 (0.05)	0.70 (0.66–0.73)		
	H	20	0.94 (0.36)	0.83 (0.66–1.19)		
Serum SOD (U/mg Hb)	IHD + CP	20	28.17 (2.62)	28.15 (26.28–30.35)	33.27 (3)	<0.001*
	CP	20	27.72 (4.20)	26.63 (24.65–30.79)		
	IHD + H	20	35.70 (3.72)	36.59 (32.62–38.95)		
	H	20	30.34 (3.93)	30.51 (28.71–33.84)		
Serum GPx (U/mg Hb)	IHD + CP	20	125.10 (59.63)	129.00 (62.00–173.50)	12.280 (3)	0.006*
	CP	20	156.20 (84.40)	143.00 (75.00–219.50)		
	IHD + H	20	96.50 (53.37)	70.00 (68.00–86.00)		
	H	20	167.70 (56.21)	174.00 (140.00–199.25)		
Serum CAT (U/mg Hb)	IHD + CP	20	25.02 (4.76)	25.47 (24.11–27.53)	18.292 (3)	<0.001*
	CP	20	25.58 (6.73)	26.11 (22.17–30.03)		
	IHD + H	20	22.01 (1.69)	21.9 (21.08–23.60)		
	H	20	26.71 (4.16)	26.80 (23.65–27.81)		

[#]Kruskal–Wallis test; * $p < 0.05$, statistically significant.

TABLE 2: Pairwise comparison using Mann–Whitney U test (serum).

Dependent variable	(I) condition	(J) condition	Mean difference ($I - J$)	95% confidence interval Lower	Upper	U statistic[#]	p value
Serum TAC (mM/L)	CP	IHD + CP	0.10	−0.07	0.29	99.50	0.007*
		IHD + H	−0.12	−0.30	0.06	103.00	0.009*
		H	−0.35	−0.54	−0.17	61.50	<0.001*
	IHD + H	IHD + CP	0.23	0.04	0.41	27.00	<0.001*
		H	−0.23	−0.41	−0.05	130.00	0.058 (NS)
	H	IHD + CP	0.46	0.28	0.65	27.00	<0.001*
Serum SOD (U/mg Hb)	CP	IHD + CP	−0.45	−3.59	2.69	163.00	0.317 (NS)
		IHD + H	−7.97	−11.12	−4.83	36.00	<0.001*
		H	−2.61	−5.76	0.52	118.0	0.027*
	IHD + H	IHD + CP	7.52	4.37	10.66	23.00	<0.001*
		H	5.36	2.21	8.50	59.50	<0.001*
	H	IHD + CP	2.16	−0.98	5.30	123.00	0.037*
Serum GPx (U/mg Hb)	CP	IHD + CP	31.10	−24.23	86.43	164.50	0.337 (NS)
		IHD + H	59.70	4.36	115.03	120.50	0.031*
		H	−11.50	−66.83	43.83	171.00	0.433 (NS)
	IHD + H	IHD + CP	−28.60	−83.93	26.73	165.00	0.343 (NS)
		H	−71.20	−126.53	−15.86	68.50	<0.001*
	H	IHD + CP	42.60	−12.73	97.93	119.50	0.029*
Serum CAT (U/mg Hb)	CP	IHD + CP	0.56	−3.45	4.59	180.50	0.598 (NS)
		IHD + H	3.57	−0.45	7.59	91.50	0.003*
		H	−1.12	−5.15	2.89	187.50	0.735 (NS)
	IHD + H	IHD + CP	−3.00	−7.03	1.01	71.50	0.001*
		H	−4.70	−8.72	−0.67	59.00	<0.001*
	H	IHD + CP	1.69	−2.33	5.71	164.00	0.330 (NS)

[#]Mann–Whitney U test; * $p < 0.05$, statistically significant; $p > 0.05$, nonsignificant (NS).

Table 3: Comparison of salivary levels.

Antioxidant	Group	N	Mean (SD)	Median (Q1–Q3)	H-value# (df)	p value
Saliva TAC (mM/L)	IHD + CP	20	0.42 (0.17)	0.37 (0.26–0.60)	3.921 (3)	0.270 (NS)
	CP	20	0.44 (0.14)	0.40 (0.33–0.50)		
	IHD + H	20	0.41 (0.18)	0.34 (0.32–0.38)		
	H	20	0.48 (0.18)	0.53 (0.36–0.56)		
Saliva SOD (U/mg protein)	IHD + CP	20	27.60 (8.37)	25.60 (20.70–32.03)	4.939 (3)	0.176 (NS)
	CP	20	26.34 (9.08)	24.61 (18.72–33.47)		
	IHD + H	20	30.10 (6.25)	31.51 (30.58–32.89)		
	H	20	32.78 (11.76)	33.15 (22.48–44.33)		
Saliva GPx (μg/g protein)	IHD + CP	20	0.39 (0.10)	0.37 (0.29–0.46)	17.230 (3)	0.001*
	CP	20	0.38 (0.09)	0.38 (0.30–0.46)		
	IHD + H	20	0.44 (0.05)	0.46 (0.40–0.47)		
	H	20	0.34 (0.06)	0.35 (0.30–0.35)		
Saliva CAT (U/mg protein)	IHD + CP	20	20.34 (3.92)	20.02 (17.72–22.82)	7.449 (3)	0.059 (NS)
	CP	20	21.11 (5.71)	21.49 (15.71–25.50)		
	IHD + H	20	23.74 (3.71)	25.48 (20.00–26.51)		
	H	20	21.91 (5.24)	23.75 (16.98–26.24)		

#Kruskal–Wallis test; * $p < 0.05$, statistically significant; $p > 0.05$, nonsignificant (NS).

Table 4: Pairwise comparison using Mann–Whitney U test.

Dependent variable	(I) condition	(J) condition	Mean difference ($I - J$)	Std. error	95% confidence interval Lower	Upper	U statistic#	p value
Saliva GPx (μg/g protein)	CP	IHD + CP	−0.01	0.02	−0.08	0.05	194.50	0.882 (NS)
		IHD + H	−0.06	0.02	−0.13	0.01	123.00	0.037*
		H	0.04	0.02	−0.02	0.11	144.0	0.128 (NS)
	IHD + H	IHD + CP	0.05	0.02	−0.01	0.12	121.5	0.03*
		H	0.10	0.02	0.03	0.17	39.50	<0.001*
	H	IHD + CP	−0.05	0.02	−0.12	0.01	124.50	0.04*

#Mann–Whitney U test; * $p < 0.05$, statistically significant; $p > 0.05$, nonsignificant (NS).

Table 5: Correlation between serum and salivary levels of TAC, SOD, GPx, and CAT.

Parameters	Condition IHD + CP	CP	IHD + H	H
TAC				
Correlation coefficient	−0.399	0.203	0.261	0.374
p value	0.081 (NS)	0.390 (NS)	0.266 (NS)	0.104 (NS)
SOD				
Correlation coefficient	−0.487	−0.403	0.680	0.568
p value	0.030*	0.078 (NS)	0.001*	0.009*
GPx				
Correlation coefficient	−0.042	−0.196	−0.341	0.467
p value	0.860 (NS)	0.409 (NS)	0.141 (NS)	0.038*
CAT				
Correlation coefficient	−0.114	0.232	−0.026	0.475
p value	0.631 (NS)	0.326 (NS)	0.912 (NS)	0.034*

Spearman's correlation test; * $p < 0.05$, statistically significant; $p > 0.05$, nonsignificant (NS).

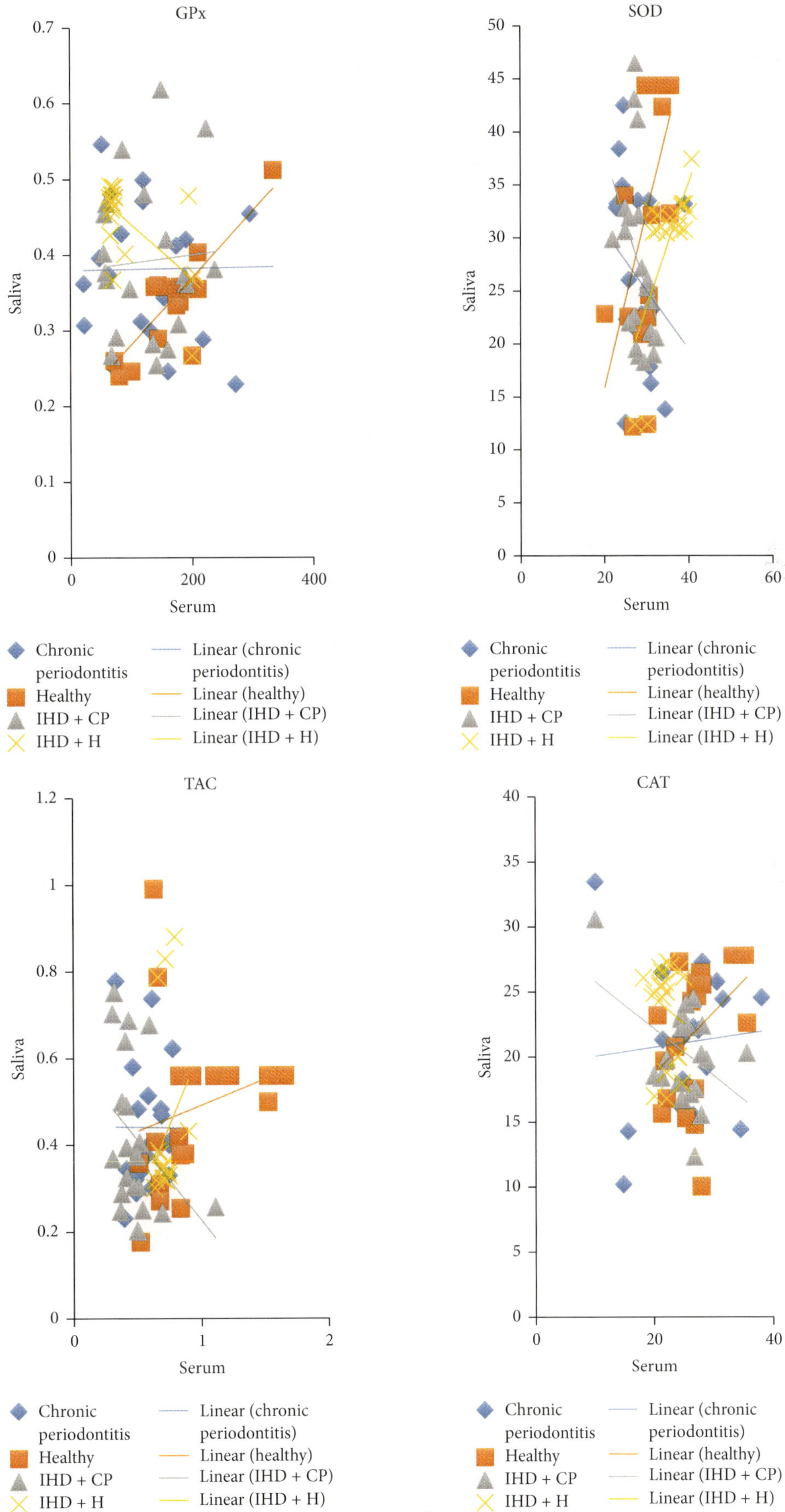
GPx
Saliva
Serum
0.7
0.6
0.5
0.4
0.3
0.2
0.1
0
200
400
Chronic periodontitis
Healthy
IHD + CP
IHD + H
Linear (chronic periodontitis)
Linear (healthy)
Linear (IHD + CP)
Linear (IHD + H)
SOD
Saliva
Serum
50
45
40
35
30
25
20
15
10
5
0
20
40
60
Chronic periodontitis
Healthy
IHD + CP
IHD + H
Linear (chronic periodontitis)
Linear (healthy)
Linear (IHD + CP)
Linear (IHD + H)
TAC
Saliva
Serum
1.2
1
0.8
0.6
0.4
0.2
0
1
2
Chronic periodontitis
Healthy
IHD + CP
IHD + H
Linear (chronic periodontitis)
Linear (healthy)
Linear (IHD + CP)
Linear (IHD + H)
CAT
Saliva
Serum
40
35
30
25
20
15
10
5
0
20
40
Chronic periodontitis
Healthy
IHD + CP
IHD + H
Linear (chronic periodontitis)
Linear (healthy)
Linear (IHD + CP)
Linear (IHD + H)

FIGURE 3

between serum and salivary SOD levels in the ischemic heart disease group with chronic periodontitis. The serum and salivary antioxidants in chronic periodontitis showed no correlation.

4. Discussion

Antioxidants like free radical scavenging enzymes (SOD) and H_2O_2 degrading enzyme (catalase) are of importance in providing protection to normal cells and matrix components from oxidation and have a protective role to play in our body against oxidant stress. Previous studies [2–4, 10, 17] suggested that an imbalance in antioxidant-oxidant stress makes patients more susceptible to periodontal disease as the oxygen-derived species like hydrogen peroxide (H_2O_2) and hydroxyl radical (OH^-) cause cell injury, are involved in degenerative changes, and are often associated with increased peroxidative processes and linked to low antioxidant concentrations. This imbalance in the antioxidant-oxidant stress is also implicated in the pathophysiology of atherosclerotic disease process resulting in ischemic heart disease [18].

The present study showed statistically significant differences in the levels of the estimated antioxidants within the 4 groups. Comparatively higher levels of antioxidants were observed in the healthy group, which indicated that the oxidant related stress in the body is effectively balanced by the antioxidants. Lower levels of antioxidants in diseased states of chronic periodontitis and ischemic heart disease point towards the conclusion that the disease process is a result of a balance tipped in favor of the oxidants, with failure of antioxidants to balance the oxidant levels. The higher levels of SOD in IHD + H as compared to healthy controls (Table 1) probably reflect an effort of SOD to counteract the excessive oxidant stress present in IHD + H. Similarly, the higher salivary GPx levels in disease groups of IHD + CP, IHD + H, and CP as compared to the healthy controls (Table 3) could probably be a result of a compensatory increase of GPx to the oxidant stress in diseased states. The lower salivary GPx level could be due to either the increased consumption of GPx or the decreased oxidant levels in healthy saliva.

There were significant differences in the salivary TAC levels between healthy and chronic periodontitis patients (Figure 2). These findings are in accord with a study done by Diab-Ladki et al. (2003), who evaluated total antioxidant activity of saliva in periodontitis patients, which revealed that there was a significant decrease in total antioxidant activity of saliva in patients with periodontitis when compared to healthy individuals [3].

A study done by Sculley and Langley-Evans (2003) also reported similar findings and concluded that the decrease in salivary TAC could be explained by the destruction caused by the imbalance between antioxidants and ROS [2].

The results of this study for serum TAC (Figure 1) are in broad agreement with observations of Chapple et al. and Brock et al. wherein the TAC levels are decreased in the periodontitis group as compared to healthy controls [17, 19].

Kusano and Ferrari (2008) conducted a study which revealed that there was an inverse relation association between total antioxidant capacity and the number of damaged vessels and increased risk of coronary artery disease [20].

Significant differences in serum catalase were also observed between the healthy and ischemic heart disease groups which are supported by the study done by Noichri et al. (2013) [21].

Studies done by Ogunro et al. (2009) and Kumar et al. (2012) in ischemic heart disease patients revealed a significant decrease in total antioxidant levels and serum antioxidant levels (SOD and CAT), respectively, in comparison with control groups [22, 23].

Intracellular SOD (the most prominent antioxidant in mammalian tissues) is predominantly localized in the periodontal ligament in association with collagen fibrils and fibroblasts. A study by Ellis et al. [24] reported a decrease in SOD levels with the increase in probing depth; the decrease in SOD levels caused an increase in leukocytes and an increase in ROS. Depressed levels of serum antioxidants in chronic periodontitis in comparison to the healthy group can be explained by the hyperactivity of neutrophils (in chronic periodontitis) producing ROS in response to Fc γ receptor stimulation [7].

Catalase guards the cells from hydrogen peroxide generated within them. It plays a role in tolerance acquisition to oxidative stress in the adaptive response of cells. Lower catalase levels are seen in periodontitis [7, 10, 25].

Glutathione peroxidase is a selenium containing peroxidase and shares substrate (H_2O_2) with catalase. It alone can react effectively with lipid and other organic hydroperoxidases. Glutathione peroxidase provides protection against low levels of oxidant stress, whereas catalase becomes more significant in defending against severe oxidant stress [7, 10, 26, 27].

Panjamurthy et al. [28] reported that the enzymatic antioxidant activity (SOD, CAT, and GPx) in plasma, erythrocytes, erythrocyte membrane, and gingival tissue of periodontitis patients was significantly higher in the chronic periodontitis group relative to parameters found in healthy patients.

Positive correlation between serum and salivary SOD levels in the ischemic heart disease group and healthy group is in accordance with the study by Al-Rawi et al. (2008) where the salivary SOD followed serum SOD [29].

The results of this study are in contrast to studies done by Moore et al. [30] and Chapple et al. [17], which showed no significant differences in the levels of antioxidants in periodontitis patients in comparison with control groups.

Tsai et al. [31] found that there was no difference in the salivary GPx activity in periodontitis patients relative to controls. This is in contrast to the present study, where the salivary GPx levels are significantly higher in disease groups to compensate the oxidant stress. Kim et al. [4] in their research found that the salivary total antioxidant level was higher in severe chronic periodontitis patients than in the healthy or gingivitis controls before scaling and root planning, whereas SOD activity of the periodontitis patients was lower than of the controls at each time [20].

Wei et al. measured the levels of superoxide dismutase in serum, saliva, and GCF in chronic periodontitis patients before and after periodontal therapy and found that the levels of superoxide dismutase (SOD) were significantly higher in the chronic periodontitis group than in the healthy control group. After periodontal therapy, SOD levels significantly decreased compared to basal levels ($p < 0.05$) in serum, saliva, and GCF [32].

This study is the first to compare the serum and salivary levels of the antioxidants (TAC, SOD, catalase, and glutathione levels) within the groups of healthy subjects, chronic periodontitis patients, and ischemic heart disease patients with or without periodontitis.

5. Limitations

This study had a small sample size. A larger sample size and better selection criteria with the use of adjusted models for confounding factors could have been used. All these limitations warrant further studies of prospective, interventional, and experimental study designs.

6. Conclusion

The present study showed a statistically significant reduction in total antioxidant capacity, superoxide dismutase, catalase, and glutathione peroxidase in patients with chronic periodontitis and ischemic heart disease with or without periodontitis when compared to healthy patients.

Overall, there was a significant correlation between the salivary and serum levels of SOD in the four antioxidant parameters between the four groups, although few parameters showed negative or no correlation. This indicates that probably saliva may not serve as a substitute to serum as a diagnostic sample for antioxidant estimation, as there is no uniformity in the correlation of serum and salivary antioxidant levels observed in this study.

Thus, the antioxidant capacity is significantly hampered in chronic periodontitis and ischemic heart disease patients with or without periodontitis.

However, the oxidant stress in chronic periodontitis generated by free radicals may result in endothelial dysfunction of the blood vasculature, predisposing to atherosclerotic plaque formation and increasing predisposition to ischemic heart disease. It is difficult to conclude to what extent chronic periodontitis has an effect on ischemic heart disease, as depicted by the levels of antioxidants in the human body. However, it is important to note that the reduced antioxidant capacity may result either from an increase in oxidative stress or from lower antioxidant defence status.

Long-term studies are required to justify whether antioxidant levels can be used as a prognostic or diagnostic marker to predict the association between chronic periodontitis and ischemic heart disease.

Acknowledgments

This study was supported by research funding from Nitte University. The grant for the study was provided as a part of Nitte Student Research Project, University Research Grant no. NURG/STU/01/7-2015. The authors would like to acknowledge the work done by Harshini Ullal for the biochemical estimation and by Dr. Vinayak Kamath for providing the statistical analysis.

References

[1] M. G. Newman, H. H. Takei, P. R. Klokkevold, and F. A. Carranza, *Carranza's Clinical Periodontology, A South Asia Edition*, Elsevier, Philadelphia, Pa, USA, 11th edition, 2012.

[2] D. V. Sculley and S. C. Langley-Evans, "Periodontal disease is associated with lower antioxidant capacity in whole saliva and evidence of increased protein oxidation," *Clinical Science*, vol. 105, no. 2, pp. 167–172, 2003.

[3] R. Diab-Ladki, B. Pellat, and R. Chahine, "Decrease in the total antioxidant activity of saliva in patients with periodontal diseases," *Clinical Oral Investigations*, vol. 7, no. 2, pp. 103–107, 2003.

[4] S.-C. Kim, O.-S. Kim, O.-J. Kim, Y.-J. Kim, and H.-J. Chung, "Antioxidant profile of whole saliva after scaling and root planing in periodontal disease," *Journal of Periodontal and Implant Science*, vol. 40, no. 4, pp. 164–171, 2010.

[5] P. M. Bartold, O. W. Wiebkin and, and J. C. Thonard, "The effect of oxygen-derived free radicals on gingival proteoglycans and hyaluronic acid," *Journal of Periodontal Research*, vol. 19, no. 4, pp. 390–400, 1984.

[6] J. Varani, S. E. G. Fligiel, G. O. Till, R. G. Kunkel, U. S. Ryan, and P. A. Ward, "Pulmonary endothelial cell killing by human neutrophils: possible involvement of hydroxyl radical," *Laboratory Investigation*, vol. 53, no. 6, pp. 656–663, 1985.

[7] C. Bogdan, M. Röllinghoff, and A. Diefenbach, "Reactive oxygen and reactive nitrogen intermediates in innate and specific immunity," *Current Opinion in Immunology*, vol. 12, no. 5, p. 604, 2000.

[8] K. J. Davies, "Oxidative stress: the paradox of aerobic life," *Biochemical Society Symposium*, vol. 61, pp. 1–31, 1995.

[9] J. M. McCord, "The evolution of free radicals and oxidative stress," *The American Journal of Medicine*, vol. 108, no. 8, pp. 652–659, 2000.

[10] I. L. C. Chapple and J. B. Matthews, "The role of reactive oxygen and antioxidant species in periodontal tissue destruction," *Periodontology 2000*, vol. 43, no. 1, pp. 160–232, 2007.

[11] P.-Ö. Söder, B. Söder, J. Nowak, and T. Jogestrand, "Early carotid atherosclerosis in subjects with periodontal diseases," *Stroke*, vol. 36, no. 6, pp. 1195–1200, 2005.

[12] R. Jay Widmer and A. Lerman, "Endothelial dysfunction and cardiovascular disease," *Global Cardiology Science and Practice*, vol. 2014, no. 3, p. 43, 2014.

[13] D. Harrison, K. K. Griendling, U. Landmesser, B. Hornig, and H. Drexler, "Role of oxidative stress in atherosclerosis," *The American Journal of Cardiology*, vol. 91, no. 3, pp. 7A–11A, 2003.

[14] R. J. Genco, "Current view of risk factors for periodontal diseases," *Journal of Periodontology*, vol. 67, no. 10, supplement, pp. 1041–1049, 1996.

[15] H. Loe and J. Silness, "Periodontal disease in pregnancy. I. Prevalence and severity," *Acta Odontologica Scandinavica*, vol. 21, pp. 533–551, 1963.

[16] G. C. Armitage, "Periodontal diagnoses and classification of periodontal diseases," *Periodontology 2000*, vol. 34, pp. 9–21, 2004.

[17] I. L. C. Chapple, G. R. Brock, M. R. Milward, N. Ling, and J. B. Matthews, "Compromised GCF total antioxidant capacity in periodontitis: cause or effect?" *Journal of Clinical Periodontology*, vol. 34, no. 2, pp. 103–110, 2007.

[18] S. V. V. Lakshmi, G. Padmaja, P. Kuppusamy, and V. K. Kutala, "Oxidative stress in cardiovascular disease," *Indian Journal of Biochemistry and Biophysics*, vol. 46, no. 6, pp. 421–440, 2009.

[19] G. R. Brock, C. J. Butterworth, J. B. Matthews, and I. L. C. Chapple, "Local and systemic total antioxidant capacity in periodontitis and health," *Journal of Clinical Periodontology*, vol. 31, no. 7, pp. 515–521, 2004.

[20] C. Kusano and B. Ferrari, "Total antioxidant capacity: a biomarker in biomedical and nutritional studies," *Journal of Cell and Molecular Biology*, vol. 7, no. 1, pp. 1–15, 2008.

[21] Y. Noichri, A. Chalghoum, L. Chkioua et al., "Low erythrocyte catalase enzyme activity is correlated with high serum total homocysteine levels in tunisian patients with acute myocardial infarction," *Diagnostic Pathology*, vol. 8, article 68, 2013.

[22] P. S. Ogunro, W. O. Balogun, F. F. Fadero et al., "Plasma lipid peroxidation and total antioxidant status among dyslipidaemic and hypertensive Nigerians with high risk of coronary heart disease," *West African Journal of Medicine*, vol. 28, no. 2, pp. 87–91, 2009.

[23] E. P. Kumar, R. Mukherjee, R. Senthil, S. Parasuraman, and B. Suresh, "Evaluation of oxidative stress and antioxidant status in patients with cardiovascular disease in rural populations of the Nilgiris, South India," *ISRN Pharmacology*, vol. 2012, Article ID 941068, 6 pages, 2012.

[24] S. D. Ellis, M. A. Tucci, F. G. Serio, and R. B. Johnson, "Factors for progression of periodontal diseases," *Journal of Oral Pathology & Medicine*, vol. 27, no. 3, pp. 101–105, 1998.

[25] C. R. Hunt, J. E. Sim, S. J. Sullivan et al., "Genomic instability and catalase gene amplification induced by chronic exposure to oxidative stress," *Cancer Research*, vol. 58, no. 17, pp. 3986–3992, 1998.

[26] C. O. Enwonwu and C. S. Ritchie, "Nutrition and inflammatory markers," *The Journal of the American Dental Association*, vol. 138, no. 1, pp. 70–73, 2007.

[27] N. Novakovic, T. Todorovic, M. Rakic et al., "Salivary antioxidants as periodontal biomarkers in evaluation of tissue status and treatment outcome," *Journal of Periodontal Research*, vol. 49, no. 1, pp. 129–136, 2014.

[28] K. Panjamurthy, S. Manoharan, and C. R. Ramachandran, "Lipid peroxidation and antioxidant status in patients with periodontitis," *Cellular and Molecular Biology Letters*, vol. 10, pp. 255–264, 2005.

[29] N. Al-Rawi, F. Jaber, and K. Atiyah, "Assessment of salivary and serum oxidative stress and antioxidants as plausible parameters in prediction of ischemic stroke among Iraqi Samples," *The Internet Journal of Third World Medicine*, vol. 7, no. 2, 2008.

[30] S. Moore, K. A. C. Calder, N. J. Miller, and C. A. Rice-Evans, "Antioxidant activity of saliva and periodontal disease," *Free Radical Research*, vol. 21, no. 6, pp. 417–425, 1994.

[31] C. C. Tsai, H. S. Chen, S. L. Chen et al., "Lipid peroxidation: a possible role in the induction and progression of chronic periodontitis," *Journal of Periodontal Research*, vol. 40, no. 5, pp. 378–384, 2005.

[32] D. Wei, X.-L. Zhang, Y.-Z. Wang, C.-X. Yang, and G. Chen, "Lipid peroxidation levels, total oxidant status and superoxide dismutase in serum, saliva and gingival crevicular fluid in chronic periodontitis patients before and after periodontal therapy," *Australian Dental Journal*, vol. 55, no. 1, pp. 70–78, 2010.

3

Efficacy and Safety of Topical Corticosteroids for Management of Oral Chronic Graft versus Host Disease

Basma Abdelaleem Elsaadany,[1] Eman Magdy Ahmed,[2] and Sana Maher Hasan Aghbary[3]

[1]*Faculty of Dentistry, Cairo University, Giza, Egypt*
[2]*Faculty of Oral and Dental Medicine, Beni Suef University, Beni Suef, Egypt*
[3]*Faculty of Dentistry, Aden University, Aden, Yemen*

Correspondence should be addressed to Basma Abdelaleem Elsaadany; basma.abdelalim@dentistry.cu.edu.eg

Academic Editor: Yoshitaka Hara

Background. Oral chronic graft versus host disease (cGVHD) is a major complication in transplantation community, a problem that can be addressed with topical intervention. Topical corticosteroids are the first line of treatment although the choice remains challenging as none of the available treatments is supported by strong clinical evidence. *Objective.* This systematic review aims to determine the clinical efficacy and safety of topical corticosteroids for the management of the mucosal alterations of oral cGVHD. *Data Sources.* Electronic search of different databases was conducted: PubMed, Cochrane library, Grey literature, WHO, and clinical trials.gov for clinical trial registration as well as hand search in the references of relevant articles up to November 2016. *Data Extraction.* Extracted pieces of information were intervention, population, sample sizes, and outcomes. *Data Synthesis.* Six studies were included: 2 randomized clinical trials (RCTs), 3 cohort studies, and 1 pre-post clinical trial. *Results.* There is a limited evidence concerning clinical efficacy of topical corticosteroids. Clobetasol, dexamethasone, and budesonide were the topical corticosteroid of choice. The highest level of evidence score was given to clobetasol followed by budesonide with a lower evidence level. *Conclusion.* All three topical corticosteroid preparations are effective for management of oral chronic GVHD with minimal easily avoided side effects.

1. Introduction

Graft versus host disease (GVHD) is a multisystem immunologically mediated disease that has been accused as major complication in allogeneic transplantation process. The disease affects up to half of all hematopoietic stem cell transplant (HSCT) patients [1]. GVHD usually affects the skin, mouth, eyes, gastrointestinal tract (GIT), and liver but other systems such as the lungs, joints, and genitourinary tract may also be involved with the oral cavity being the second most commonly involved organ system, after skin [2]. Oral chronic GVHD (oral cGVHD) is presented as generalized mucosal erythema, erosions, ulcerations, white striae, or papules resembling oral lichen planus and can also develop oral mucoceles. Patients may complain as well from xerostomia and pain [1, 3]. The oral involvement may be the only presentation of the condition or a part of multisystem involvement. Symptomatic management with systemic therapy and topical treatment alone or in combination are the choices to provide local palliation. However, clinically oral cGVHD develops during reduction of systemically administered immunosuppressant after HSCT [3]. Topical agents in oral cGVHD reduce doses or accelerate healing when used with systemic immunosuppressant therapy minimizing their side effects [4].

Usually topical steroids are used to treat oral cGVHD; although they are not specifically approved for oral cGVHD, they have been adopted for use in oral cGVHD based on their well accepted use for other oral mucosal conditions, particularly for oral lichen planus [1].

Budesonide is a synthetic glucocorticoid. Recently it has been used with high efficiency both as local and systemic treatment. The drug has renowned safety profile and has

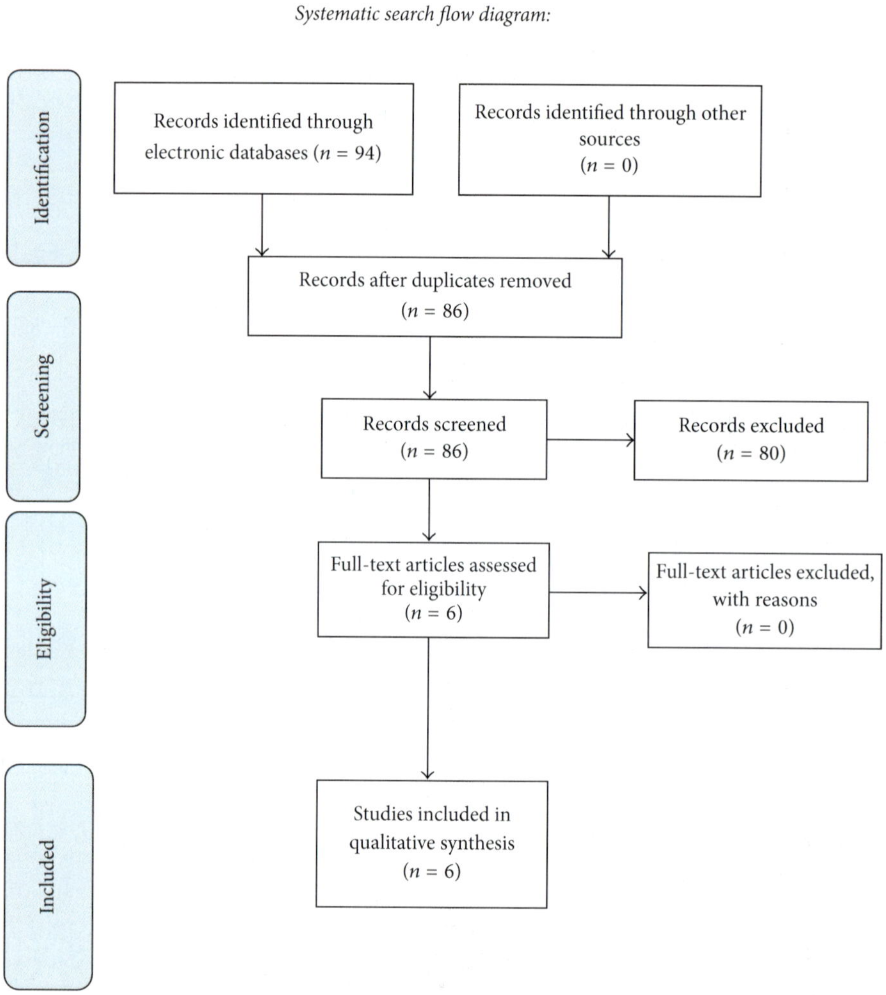

FIGURE 1: Flow diagram of article selection.

successfully been used topically to treat different oral lesions of cGVHD [5].

Clobetasol is a super potent topical corticosteroid with remarkable results in management of mucocutaneous lesions of cGVHD. The drug has a limited bioavailability providing less systemic effect [6].

Dexamethasone is a prednisolone analogue 25 times more potent with longer duration of action compared to hydrocortisone [13]. Oral lesions due to cCVHD respond dramatically to topical dexamethasone application [10].

This systematic review aims to determine the clinical efficacy and safety of topical corticosteroids for the management of the mucosal manifestations of oral cGVHD.

2. Methodology

We conducted an electronic search of the following databases PubMed, Cochrane Central Register of controlled clinical trials, WHO clinical trial registration, and Grey literature up to November 2016, based on the search strategy developed for PubMed using the key words "oral", "chronic", "graft versus host disease", and "topical corticosteroids" but revised appropriately for each database and manual searching through the central library of Cairo University, library of Faculty of Dentistry, and the central library of the Egyptian National Institute of Cancer. Also, the bibliographies of included papers and relevant review articles were checked for studies not identified by the search strategies above (see Figure 1).

We included all clinical trials using any form, dose, or concentration of topical corticosteroid preparation for management of symptomatic mucosal lesion of oral cGVHD. We excluded any article with additional systemic therapy other than anti-GVHD medications or treatment with another concomitant topical preparation during the 12 weeks before the trial except for prophylaxis against infections (e.g., antifungal and antiviral agents). Critical outcomes measured are subjective symptoms (pain), clinical improvement (in term of mucositis scale), time to maximum improvement, relapse, and side effects. The authors independently evaluated each included study using the Cochrane risk of bias assessment tool for RCT [5] and SIGN checklist for cohort study [6]. The evidence level of the included studies was assessed using the Oxford CEBM "levels of evidence" [13].

TABLE 1: Study reports on the use of topical steroids in management of oral cGVHD.

Study	Author's name	Study	Design
1	Noce et al. [7]	Randomized double-blind clinical trial comparing clobetasol and dexamethasone for the topical treatment of symptomatic oral chronic graft versus host disease	Randomized clinical trial
2	Park et al. [8]	Comparison of budesonide and dexamethasone for local treatment of oral chronic graft versus host disease	Cohort (prospective)
3	Sari et al. [9]	The effect of budesonide mouthwash on oral chronic graft versus host disease	Cohort (retrospective)
4	Elad et al. [10]	Improvement in oral chronic graft versus host disease with the administration of effervescent tablets of topical budesonide—an open, randomized, multicenter study	Randomized clinical study (pilot study)
5	Wolff et al. [11]	Oral PUVA and topical steroids for treatment of oral manifestations of chronic graft versus host disease	Cohort (prospective)
6	Elad et al. [12]	Budesonide: a novel treatment for oral chronic graft versus host disease	Before and after clinical trial

Data extraction form has been generated by the authors to collect all the data items specified in the review synthesis strategy to address the review questions. Any conflict between authors was solved by a methodological expert. Extracted information about the studies (i.e., intervention, population, context, sample sizes, outcomes, and study quality) will be tabulated in a manner consistent with the review question.

3. Results

The electronic literature search produced 94 articles; after removal of duplicates 84 underwent screening for title and abstract and 6 met the inclusion criteria (Table 1). No more eligible studies were identified by hand search. The evidence table includes study design, interventions, outcomes (pain reduction, clinical score, time to maximum improvement, relapse, and adverse effects), level of evidence, and grade of recommendation (see Table 2). From the 6 included studies in (Table 1), budesonide, dexamethasone, and clobetasol were the topical steroid agents evaluated in included studies. Of the reviewed studies, there were 2 RCTs [7, 10], 3 cohort studies [8, 9, 11], and 1 pre-post clinical trial [12].

4. Dexamethasone

In 2004 there was a retrospective cohort study [11] in which 16 patients with oral cGVHD were enrolled, using 0.01% of dexamethasone sol. as oral rinse for 28 days. The daily dose however was not clearly reported. With a level of evidence evaluated as 4 and Grade C, the results showed that 68.7% of patients reported symptomatic improvement. Median pain visual analogue scale (VAS) difference and side effects of the treatment were not reported.

The authors did not also report the severity of the oral cGVHD at the beginning of the study.

In 2013, a prospective cohort study [8] used the same drug form and concentration also, for 28 days on 24 patients given as 5–10 mL oral rinse 3–6 times per day. The level of evidence of their study was evaluated as 2b graded B. According to severity of oral involvement at baseline 20.8% of patients presented with mild symptoms, 70.8% with moderate symptoms, and 8.3% with severe symptoms. The results of their study showed 27.2% average reduction in modified oral mucositis rating scale (mOMRS), 29.1% of patients reported symptomatic improvement with the topical treatment, and average VAS reduction was 28.5%. The study reported 16.6% of patients complained from side effects, two cases with burning sensation, one with taste alteration, and one with fungal infection. In consistence in 2014 a randomized clinical trial [7] used the same drug, same form and concentration, on 18 patients for 28 days. The level of evidence was 1b graded A. the results showed 50% average reduction in mOMRS, 33% of patients reported symptomatic improvement with the topical treatment, and average VAS reduction was 29.7%. However, the study did not report the severity of the condition at the baseline. Concurrent prophylactic antifungal treatment was prescribed. The study reported 5.5% of patients complaining from possible side effects presented as one case with burning sensation and no reported fungal infections.

5. Clobetasol

Only one randomized controlled clinical trial [7] reported the use of 0.05% clobetasol oral rinse, level of evidence evaluated as 1b graded A. The study was conducted on 14 patients with a daily dose of 5 mL three times for 28 days. The results showed 50% average reduction in mOMRS, 85% of patients reported symptomatic improvement with the topical treatment, and average VAS reduction was 44.6%. One case (7% of patients) with burning mouth was reported as possible side effect. Concurrent prophylactic antifungal treatment was prescribed.

6. Budesonide

In 2003, a pre-post treatment clinical trial [12] was conducted using 0.06% budesonide oral rinse on 12 patients for 1 to 6 months. The evidence level was evaluated as 4 graded C. The study reported mean time for maximum improvement to be

TABLE 2: The evidence table including study design, interventions, outcomes, level of evidence, and grade of recommendation.

Study	Quality assessment		Number of patients	Drug properties				Clinical response (efficacy)				Safety %
	Level	Grade		Drug	Conc.	Dose mL	Dose t/d	Average time for best results (D)	Average mOMRS reduction (%)	Patients with mOMRS improvement (%)	VAS red. (%)	Side effects %
Clobetasol												
Noce et al. [7]	1b	A	14	Oral rinse	0.5	5	3	28	50	85	44.6	7
Dexamethasone												
Noce et al. [7]	1b	A	18	Oral rinse	0.01	5	3	28	50	33	29.7	5.5
Park et al. [8]	2b	B	24	Oral rinse	0.01	10	3-4	28	27.2	29.1	28.5	16.6
Wolff et al. [9]	4	C	16	Oral rinse	0.01	NR	NR	28	NR	68.7	NR	NR
Budesonide												
Park et al. [8]	2b	B	26	Oral rinse	0.03	5–10	3–6	28	50	53.8	37.5	19
Elad et al. [10]	2b	B	18	Oral rinse	0.03	10	2-3	45.5	70	70	70	50
Sari et al. [9]	4	C	12	Oral rinse	0.03	10	3	28	66.6	83.3	54.4	16.6
Elad et al. [12]	4	C	12	Oral rinse	0.06	5	2-3	54	UC	100	UC	8

RCT: randomized clinical trial, *pro-cohort*: prospective cohort, *Retro. Cohort*: retrospective cohort, *UC*: unclear, and *NR*: not reported.

54 days. With unclear results of mOMRS, the study reported that 100% of patients showed clinical improvement. One case (8%) complained from burning mouth.

In 2007, a retrospective cohort study [9] evaluated topical budesonide along with systemic treatment. They used 0.03% budesonide sol. as oral rinse for 28 days; evidence level was evaluated as 4 graded B. The results showed 66.5% average reduction in mOMRS, 83.3% of patients reported symptomatic improvement with the topical treatment, and average VAS reduction was 54.4%. The study reported one case with burning mouth and one with HSV infection representing 16.6% of patients. The severity of oral involvement at baseline was 25% mild symptoms, 41.6% moderate symptoms, and 33.3% severe symptoms. No concurrent antifungal prophylaxis was used.

Budesonide was investigated again in 2013, but in a prospective cohort study [8] with evidence level 2b graded B, in which they used 0.03% budesonide sol. as oral rinse on 26 patients with oral cGVHD for 28 days. The results of their study showed 50% average reduction in mOMRS, 53.8% of patients reported symptomatic improvement with the topical treatment, and average VAS reduction was 37.5%. The study reported 19% of patients complaining from side effects presented as one case with taste alteration and four with fungal infection. The severity of oral involvement at baseline was 30.8% mild symptoms, 53.8% moderate symptoms, and 15.4% severe symptoms. No antifungal prophylaxis was used throughout the study time.

A pilot randomized clinical trial [10] used the same form and concentration of budesonide different daily doses on 18 patients for 60 days and up to 6 months. The evidence level of this study was 2b graded B, mean time for maximum improvement was 45.5 days, average reduction in mOMRS was 70%, 70% of patients reported symptomatic improvement, and average VAS reduction was 70%. Also, 50% of patients complained from a possible side effects including cheilitis, esophagitis, fungal infection, and taste alteration. A concurrent prophylactic antifungal, antibacterial, and antiviral drug were prescribed.

Regarding the clinical results and concerning the level of evidence and grading, the highest level of evidence score was given to Noce et al. [7] for their RCT stating efficient clinical results for topical clobetasol. This is followed by Park et al. [8] in the good quality prospective cohort study and the pilot RCT of Elad et al. [10] both reporting a promising clinical results of budesonide; the results of those studies enforced the week evidence from Sari et al. [9] and Elad et al. [12].

7. Discussion

Six clinical trials were included in this systematic review of evidence evaluating the efficacy and safety of three different topical corticosteroids in the management of oral cGVHD. There was a heterogeneity regarding the trial outcomes and outcome assessment and the mixed study design hindered gathering the studies for statistical analysis. It is acknowledged for most practitioners that topical corticosteroids are the first line of treatment for oral cGVHD [1, 4, 14]. Upon evaluation of the available evidence we agree on the net benefit of topical corticosteroids with a recommendation to "probably" the use of topical steroid is effective in management of signs and symptoms of oral mucosal GVHD with minimal easily avoided side effects. That is because of uncertainty about the quality of the available evidence.

Considering safety of topical corticosteroids, the results demonstrated that oral fungal infection is the most common side effect. However, this problem is strictly governed by the use of antifungal prophylaxis during treatment. Treatment regimen with concurrent prophylactic treatment ended up with no fungal infection [7, 10]. On the other hand oral fungal infection was reported in treatment regimen where no antifungal prophylaxis was added [8, 9].

Uncertainty about the quality of the available evidence is mainly attributed to shortage of high quality RCTs, small sample size, methodological limitations, and inconsistency across studies.

Inconsistency refers to the dissimilarity of estimates of effect across studies.

Lack of randomized clinical trial is a major limitation concerning judging the efficacy and safety of a defined intervention. The low number of clinical trials on this topic and the small sample size notably found in all studies could be attributed to the nature of the disease and practical difficulties concerning patients with oral cGVHD, which can raise both ethical and logistical concerns. Based on our search up to this date there are two ongoing randomized clinical trials registered on centre and clinical trials.gov: Identifier: NCT01557517 and Identifier: NCT00887263. We expect the results of these trials likely to have an important impact on our confidence in the estimate of topical steroid effect.

The methodological limitations and inconsistency of the included clinical trials were adjudicated based on the following. (a) Three studies did not state the severity of the disease for participants at baseline [7, 11, 12]. (b) Two studies did not clearly report pain reduction which is very important outcome regarding the efficacy of the intervention [11, 12]. (c) All but one study [11] did not report the occurrence of relapse. (d) The sample size calculation was unclear for all but one study [7] and due to lack of clinical trials on chronic oGVHD, the sample size of this study was calculated based on studies of OLP. (e) Follow-up period was variant between studies and three studies [7, 10, 12] did not report clearly the follow-up. (f) For randomized clinical trials, randomization and allocation concealment were unclear [10] and blinding was unclear neither for the participant patients nor for outcome assessor [10]. Based on these findings one clinical trial was judged as high risk of bias [10] and one judged as low risk of bias [7].

In accordance was the review [4] which reported a shortage in clinical trials and low quality of the available evidence referring to the nature of the disease and ethical issues concerning the patients' condition. The review could not make recommendations regarding any topical intervention in oral cGVHD. Another study [14], a clinical survey, was conducted assessing clinical interventions for diagnosis and management of oral cGVHD. They reported that topical corticosteroids were the first line of treatment chosen by oral specialists.

Moreover, report from the International Consensus Conference on clinical practice in cGVHD stated that "current treatment recommendations rely on clinical experience of respected authorities or very small controlled trials rather than rigorously controlled trials." In addition they denoted that topical treatment is of a special clinical value [1].

8. Conclusion

Based on the available evidence we concluded that there is moderate evidence supporting use of topical corticosteroid for management of oral cGVHD with minimal easily avoided side effects. According to level of evidence clobetasol followed by budesonide reported a promising clinical efficacy. Further research is likely to have an important impact on our confidence in the estimate of effect.

References

[1] J. W. Mays, H. Fassil, D. A. Edwards, S. Z. Pavletic, and C. W. Bassim, "Oral chronic graft-versus-host disease: Current pathogenesis, therapy, and research," *Oral Diseases*, vol. 19, no. 4, pp. 327–346, 2013.

[2] M. M. Schubert and M. E. P. Correa, "Oral graft-versus-host disease," *Dental Clinics of North America*, vol. 52, no. 1, pp. 79–109, 2008.

[3] M. M. Imanguli, I. Alevizos, R. Brown, S. Z. Pavletic, and J. C. Atkinson, "Oral graft-versus-host disease," *Oral Diseases*, vol. 14, no. 5, pp. 396–412, 2008.

[4] R. Albuquerque, Z. Khan, A. Poveda et al., "Management of oral graft versus host disease with topical agents: A systematic review," *Medicina Oral, Patologia Oral y Cirugia Bucal*, vol. 21, no. 1, pp. e72–e81, 2016.

[5] J. P. Higgins and S. Green, *Cochrane Handbook for Systematic Reviews of [Internet], Version 5.1.0*, 2008, http://onlinelibrary.wiley.com/doi/10.1002/9780470712184.fmatter/summary.

[6] Sign, "Critical appraisal: Notes and checklists [Internet]," 2014, http://www.sign.ac.uk/methodology/checklists.html#.

[7] C. W. Noce, A. Gomes, V. Shcaira et al., "Randomized double-blind clinical trial comparing clobetasol and dexamethasone for the topical treatment of symptomatic oral chronic graft-versus-host disease," *Biology of Blood and Marrow Transplantation*, vol. 20, no. 8, pp. 1163–1168, 2014.

[8] A. R. Park, H. O. La, B. S. Cho et al., "Comparison of budesonide and dexamethasone for local treatment of oral chronic graft-versus-host disease," *American Journal of Health-System Pharmacy*, vol. 70, no. 16, pp. 1383–1391, 2013.

[9] I. Sari, F. Altuntas, I. Kocyigit et al., "The effect of budesonide mouthwash on oral chronic graft versus host disease," *American Journal of Hematology*, vol. 82, no. 5, pp. 349–356, 2007.

[10] S. Elad, I. Zeevi, J. Finke et al., "Improvement in oral chronic graft-versus-host disease with the administration of effervescent tablets of topical budesonide-an open, randomized, multicenter study," *Biology of Blood and Marrow Transplantation*, vol. 18, no. 1, pp. 134–140, 2012.

[11] D. Wolff, V. Anders, R. Corio et al., "Oral PUVA and topical steroids for treatment of oral manifestation of chronic graft-vs.-host disease," *Photodermatology Photoimmunology and Photomedicine*, vol. 20, no. 4, pp. 184–190, 2004.

[12] S. Elad, R. Or, A. A. Garfunkel, and M. Y. Shapira, "Budesonide: A novel treatment for oral chronic graft versus host disease," *Oral Surgery, Oral Medicine, Oral Pathology, Oral Radiology, and Endodontics*, vol. 95, no. 3, pp. 308–311, 2003.

[13] B. Phillips, C. Ball, D. Sackett, D. Badenoch, S. Straus, and B. D. M. Haynes, "Oxford Centre for Evidence-Based Medicine Levels of Evidence [Internet]," 2001, http://www.cebm.net/index.aspx?o=1025.

[14] S. Elad, S. B. Jensen, J. E. Raber-durlacher, N. Mouradian, and M. T. Brennan, "Clinical approach in the management of oral chronic graft-versus-host disease (cGVHD) in a series of specialized medical centers," *Support Care Cancer*, vol. 23, no. 6, pp. 15–22, 2014.

4

Sox Genes Show Spatiotemporal Expression during Murine Tongue and Eyelid Development

Ryuichi Ishikawa,[1] Maiko Kawasaki,[1] Katsushige Kawasaki,[1,2] Akane Yamada,[1] Supaluk Trakanant,[1] Fumiya Meguro,[1] Atsushi Kitamura,[1] Takehisa Kudo,[1] Takeyasu Maeda,[2] and Atsushi Ohazama[1]

[1]*Division of Oral Anatomy, Department of Oral Life Science, Niigata University Graduate School of Medical and Dental Sciences, Niigata, Japan*
[2]*Research Center for Advanced Oral Science, Department of Oral Life Science, Niigata University Graduate School of Medical and Dental Sciences, Niigata, Japan*

Correspondence should be addressed to Atsushi Ohazama; atsushiohazama@dent.niigata-u.ac.jp

Academic Editor: Tommaso Lombardi

The tongue is a critical organ, involved in functions such as speaking, swallowing, mastication, and degustation. Although *Sox* genes are known to play critical roles in many biological processes, including organogenesis, the expression of the *Sox* family members during tongue development remains unclear. We therefore performed a comparative *in situ* hybridization analysis of 17 *Sox* genes (*Sox1–14, 17, 18,* and *21*) during murine tongue development. *Sox2, 4, 6, 8, 9, 10, 11, 12,* and *21* were found to be expressed in the tongue epithelium, whereas *Sox2, 4–6, 8–11, 13,* and *21* showed expression in the mesenchyme of the developing tongue. Expression of *Sox1, 4, 6, 8–12,* and *21* were observed in the developing tongue muscle. *Sox5* and *13* showed expression only at E12, while *Sox1* expression was observed only on E18. *Sox6, 8, 9,* and *12* showed expression at several stages. Although the expression of *Sox2, 4, 10, 11,* and *21* was detected during all the four stages of tongue development, their expression patterns differed among the stages. We thus identified a dynamic spatiotemporal expression pattern of the *Sox* genes during murine tongue development. To understand whether *Sox* genes are involved in the development of other craniofacial organs through similar roles to those in tongue development, we also examined the expression of *Sox* genes in eyelid primordia, which also contain epithelium, mesenchyme, and muscle. However, expression patterns and timing of *Sox* genes differed between tongue and eyelid development. *Sox* genes are thus related to organogenesis through different functions in each craniofacial organ.

1. Introduction

The tongue plays a critical role in speaking, swallowing, mastication, and degustation. Malformations of the tongue, including macroglossia, hypoglossia, and aglossia, are seen as congenital defects. Therefore, it is crucial to understand the molecular mechanisms involved in tongue development; however, these mechanisms remain unclear.

The mammalian tongue is composed of the epithelium, connective tissue, and striated muscle. The connective tissue and vasculature of the tongue are derived from the cranial neural crest, whereas most tongue muscles are formed by myoblasts that migrate from the occipital somites [1]. It is believed that there is an interaction between neural crest-derived and myogenic cells during tongue development [2, 3].

In mice, tongue development begins at embryonic day (E) 10.5–11.0 with the formation of medial lingual swelling from the first branchial arch. Next, lateral lingual swellings are formed on each side of the median tongue bud. They overgrow the medial lingual swelling and eventually fuse to form the anterior two-thirds of the tongue. The medial lingual swelling does not form any identifiable part of the adult tongue. The third branchial arch gives rise to the copula and the hypopharyngeal eminence. Subsequently, the hypopharyngeal eminence overgrows the copula, which in turn disappears progressively. Consequently, the rostral part of the hypopharyngeal eminence develops into the posterior third of the tongue [2, 3, 4]. Thus, the embryonic origin in the anterior two-thirds and posterior third of the tongue differs. In addition, the anterior two-thirds of the tongue is mobile, whereas the posterior third is relatively immobile.

Tongue muscles are classified as either intrinsic or extrinsic. They are bilateral and separated by the lingual septum, which consists of fibrous connective tissue. Four different types of tongue papillae can be distinguished: fungiform, circumvallate, foliate, and filiform. They are known to develop through epithelial-mesenchymal interactions. Although the lingual epithelium is histologically homogeneous during the early stages of tongue development, the papillae become distinct and protrude from the dorsum of the tongue on approximately E12. A single circumvallate papilla is located at the center of the terminal sulcus. Fungiform papillae are present on the anterior part of the tongue in a pattern of longitudinal rows bracketing the median furrow. Unlike the other three types of papillae, filiform papillae cover the entire dorsal surface of the tongue.

Sox proteins are characterized by a highly conserved DNA-binding motif called high-mobility group domain. To date, 20 *Sox* genes have been identified in mice. Members of the *Sox* gene family show dynamic and diverse expression patterns during development, and they play multiple roles during development, as evidenced by mutation analyses in mice [5, 6]. Spatiotemporal expression patterns of *Sox* genes have been reported in tooth and pancreas development [7, 8]. In the trunk and limb region, it has been reported that *Sox6* is involved in skeletal muscle formation, while *Sox7, 15, 17,* and *18* have been shown to be related to function of satellite cells [9–13]. Although *Sox2* has been reported to be involved in the development of tongue papillae [14], the expression pattern of other *Sox* genes during the entire development of the tongue remains unclear. Therefore, we performed a comparative *in situ* hybridization analysis of 17 *Sox* genes (*Sox1–14, 17, 18,* and *21*) during murine tongue development and identified their dynamic spatiotemporal expression.

2. Materials and Methods

2.1. Production and Analysis of Mice. CD-1 strain mice were used in this study. The noon time of the day on which the plugs were detected was considered as E0.5. To accurately assess the age of the embryos, somite pairs were counted, and the stage was confirmed using morphological criteria, e.g., relative sizes of maxillary and mandibular primordia, extent of nasal placode invagination, and size of limb buds.

2.2. In Situ Hybridization. Embryo heads were fixed in 4% buffered paraformaldehyde, wax embedded, and serially sectioned at 7 μm. Decalcification using 0.5 M EDTA (ethylenediaminetetraacetic acid, pH 7.6) was performed after fixation of the newborn mice. Sections were split over three to ten slides and prepared for histology or radioactive *in situ* hybridization. *In situ* hybridization with [^{35}S]UTP-labeled riboprobes (Table 1) was performed as previously described [15]. Briefly, the slides were pretreated with proteinase K and acetic anhydride to reduce the background. Hybridization was carried out overnight in a humidified chamber at 55°C. The slides were then washed and treated with RNAse A for 30 min at 37°C to remove any nonspecifically bound probe. The high stringency washes were repeated, and the sections were then dehydrated. The slides were air-dried and dipped in Ilford K-5 photographic emulsion. Autoradiography was performed by exposing the sections in a light-tight box at 4°C for 10–14 days. Slides were developed using Kodak D19, fixed in Kodak Unifix, and counterstained with malachite green or hematoxylin.

3. Results

The expression of *Sox3* and *14* was not detected in the developing tongue (data not shown).

3.1. E11. The tongue primordium is firstly recognizable on the mandibular processes as a small protrusion (Figure 1(a)). To identify muscle progenitor cells, *Myf5* expression was examined in the developing tongue. Two domains of *Myf5* expression were observed in the center of the tongue primordium, which was found to be further divided into four domains in the caudal region (Figure 1(b)). *Sox4, 11,* and *21* were ubiquitously expressed in the developing tongue (Figures 1(d), 1(f), and 1(g)). *Sox2* and *10* expressions were observed in the mesenchyme at the lateral side of the tongue primordium, whereas *Sox2* also showed the expression in the epithelium (Figures 1(c) and 1(e)). *Sox1, 5, 6, 8, 9,* and *12–14* showed no expression in the developing tongue at E11 (data not shown).

Since distinct morphological structures are present in the developing tongue along the anterior-posterior axis, it is likely that the expression patterns differ among the various regions of the developing tongue. Therefore, we examined the expression patterns of the *Sox* gene family members in the anterior, middle, and posterior regions of the tongue.

3.2. E12. At E12, condensation of mesenchymal cells was observed in the spatulate tongue (Figures 2(a)–2(a″)). A primitive muscle was identified only in the middle and posterior regions of the developing tongue (Figures 2(a)–2(a″)). *Myf5* was expressed in primitive vertical and transverse (vt), genioglossus (gg), hyoglossus (hg), superior and inferior longitudinal (sil), geniohyoid (gh), and mylohyoid (mm) muscle regions (Figures 2(b)–2(b″)). *Sox2* was expressed in the mesenchyme between the sil and gg muscles in the middle and posterior regions of the tongue as well as in the epithelium throughout the tongue (Figures 2(c)–2(c″)). The expression of

Table 1: Probe information.

	Size of fragment of cDNA	Exon
Sox1	255 bp	1
Sox2	700 bp	1
Sox3	900 bp	1
Sox4	2.9 kb	1
Sox5	1.5 kb	1–11
Sox6	5.0 kb	2–16
Sox7	867 bp	2
Sox8	780 bp	1–3
Sox9	510 bp	3
Sox10	2.5 kb	1–4
Sox11	3 kb	1
Sox12	900 bp	1
Sox13	3.3 kb	2–11
Sox14	1.9 kb	1
Sox17	960 bp	4,5
Sox18	856 bp	2
Sox21	714 bp	1

Sox4 was found in the septum of the posterior region of the tongue (Figures 2(d)–2(d″)). *Sox5* was weakly expressed in the mesenchyme between the sil and gg muscles in the middle and posterior regions of the tongue (Figures 2(e)–2(e″)). Weak expression of *Sox6* was observed in the epithelium and vt and gg muscles (Figures 2(f)–2(f″)). *Sox9* expression was observed in vt muscles, mesenchyme between vt muscles, and epithelium of the entire tongue (Figures 2(g)–2(g″)). *Sox10* expression was detected in the mesenchyme between the sil and gg muscles in the middle and posterior regions of the tongue as well as in the hg muscle region (Figures 2(h)–2(h″)). *Sox11* was ubiquitously expressed in the developing tongue (Figures 2(i)–2(i″)). Weak expression of *Sox13* was observed in the mesenchyme between the sil and gg muscles in the middle and posterior regions of the tongue (Figures 2(j)–2(j″)). *Sox21* was expressed in the lingual septum of the posterior developing tongue (Figures 2(k)–2(k‴)). *Sox1*, *8*, and *12* showed no expression in the developing tongue at E12 (data not shown). *Sox5*, *6*, and *9* also showed strong expressions in the presumptive Meckel's cartilage region.

3.3. E13. The vt, gg, and hg muscles were histologically identifiable at E13 (Figures 3(a)–3(a″)). *Myf5* expression in the anterior and middle regions of the tongue was comparable to that at E12, while it was divided into two expression domains in the gg muscles (Figures 3(b)–3(b″)). *Sox2* was expressed in the mesenchyme between the vt and sil muscles and epithelium of the entire tongue (Figures 3(c)–3(c″)). The expression of *Sox4* was observed in the mesenchyme surrounding the vt muscles, including the lingual septum throughout the tongue (Figures 3(d)–3(d″)). *Sox6* was expressed in the epithelium and the vt, gg, hg, and sil muscles of the entire developing tongue (Figures 3(e)–3(e″)). *Sox8* was weakly expressed in the septum of the entire tongue, the sil muscle in the anterior and middle tongue, and the gg muscle in the posterior regions of the tongue (Figures 3(f)–3(f″)). Expression of *Sox9* was detected in the lingual septum in the entire tongue, while it was also weakly expressed in the sil muscle of the entire tongue (Figures 3(g)–3(g′). Weak expression of *Sox9* was also found in the gg muscle region of the posterior tongue (Figures 3(g″)). *Sox10* was expressed in the mesenchyme between the vt and sil muscles in the entire tongue, as well as in the gg muscle in the posterior region of the tongue (Figures 3(h)–3(h″)). *Sox11* showed ubiquitous expression in the entire developing tongue (Figures 3(i)–3(i″)). *Sox12* was expressed in the epithelium of the entire tongue, and the vt and gg muscles in the posterior region of the tongue (Figures 3(j)–3(j″)). *Sox21* expression was observed in the vt muscle in the anterior and middle tongue, while it was found in the septum in the middle and posterior tongue (Figures 3(k)–3(k‴)). *Sox1, 5,* and *13* showed no expression in the developing tongue at E13 (data not shown).

3.4. E14. Each muscle was found to be more morphologically obvious at E14 (Figures 4(a)-4(b″)). *Myf5* was also expressed in the gg muscle in the anterior tongue (Figures 4(b)). *Myf5* expression was divided into several domains in the vt muscle region of the entire developing tongue (Figures 4(b) and 4(b′)). *Sox2* showed expression in the epithelium of the entire tongue (Figures 4(c)–4(c″)). Expression of *Sox4* was observed in the mesenchyme surrounding the vt muscles, including the septum throughout the tongue, as well as in the epithelium (Figures 4(d)–4(d″)). *Sox6* showed expression in the vt, hg, and gg muscles in the entire tongue, as well as in the epithelium (Figures 4(e)–4(e″)). *Sox8* showed weak and ubiquitous expression in the entire tongue (Figures 4(f)–4(f″)). In the anterior and middle regions of the tongue, *Sox9* was strongly expressed in the gg muscles, and weakly expressed in the sil muscle (Figures 4(g)–4(g″)). Expression of *Sox10* was observed in the mesenchyme underneath the vt muscles in the anterior and middle regions of the tongue, and in the gg muscle in the posterior region (Figures 4(h)–4(h″)). Weak expression of *Sox11* was detected in the epithelium of the entire tongue and gg muscles in the anterior region of the tongue (Figures 4(i)–4(i″)). *Sox12* showed weak expression in the epithelium of the entire tongue and the gg muscles in the posterior part of the tongue (Figures 4(j)–4(j″)). *Sox21* showed ubiquitous expression in the entire developing tongue (Figures 4(k)–4(k″)). *Sox1, 5,* and *13* showed no expression in the developing tongue at E14 (data not shown).

3.5. E18. Most tongue muscle progenitor cells had already been differentiated into myoblasts by E18. Therefore, only weak expression of *Myf5* could be observed in the tongue at E18 (data not shown). *Sox1* showed weak expression in the sil, vt, gg, and gh muscles in the middle and posterior regions of the tongue (Figures 5(b)–5(b″)). *Sox2* has been shown to be expressed in the epithelium at this developmental stage [14]. *Sox4* showed weak expression in the epithelium and vt muscles in the middle and posterior regions of the tongue (Figures 5(c)–5(c″)). *Sox6* showed ubiquitous expression in the entire tongue (Figures 5(d)–5(d″)). Expression of *Sox8* was

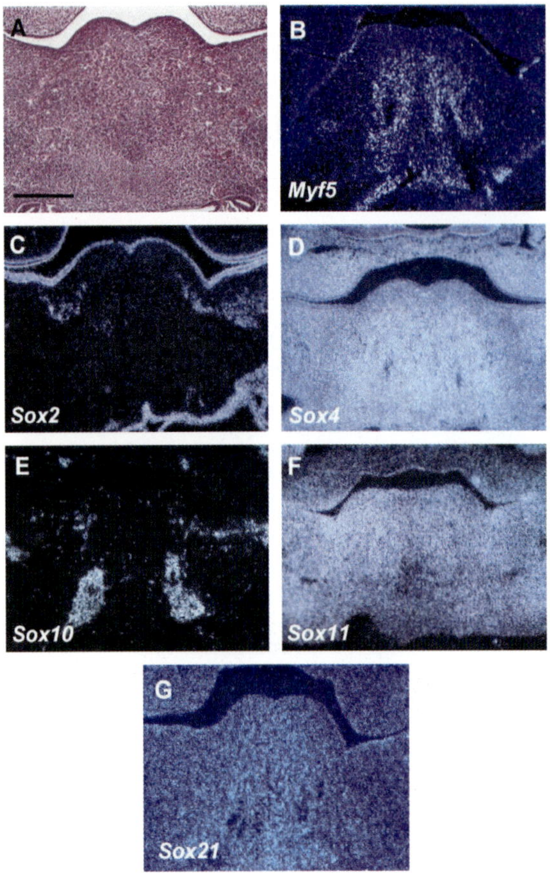

Figure 1: Expression of *Sox* genes in tongue development at E11. Frontal sections showing histology (a) and *in situ* hybridization (b–g) in wild-type tongue at E11. Scale bar: 300 μm for (a–g).

detected in the mesial part of the vt muscles in the anterior region of the tongue, as well as in both the mesial part of the vt muscles and the rostral part of the gg muscle in the posterior region of the tongue (Figures 5(e)–5(e″)). Weak expression of *Sox10* was found in the vt muscles in the middle and posterior regions of the tongue, as well as in the epithelium in the posterior region of the tongue (Figures 5(f)–5(f″)). *Sox11* was weakly expressed in the dorsum epithelium in the anterior region of the tongue (Figures 5(g)–5(g″)). *Sox12* expression was detected in the vt muscles in the middle region of the tongue, as well as in the vt and sil muscles in the posterior region of the tongue (Figures 5(h)–5(h″)). *Sox21* showed ubiquitous expression in the entire developing tongue (Figures 5(i)–5(i″)). *Sox2, 5, 9,* and *13* showed no expression in the developing tongue at E18 (data not shown).

Sox7, 17, and *18* belong to group F of the *Sox* gene family (SoxF). Members of SoxF have been shown to regulate blood and lymphatic vascular development [16–18]. A punctate expression pattern of *Sox7, 17,* and *18* was seen throughout the developing tongue, and it probably represents vascularization of the tissue (data not shown).

3.6. Sox Genes in Eyelid Development. Among the craniofacial organs, the eyelid shows some similarities with the tongue: Both are mobile organs and develop through epithelium, neural crest-derived mesenchyme, and mesoderm [2, 3, 19, 20]. In addition, it has been shown that the lack of Shh signaling pathway and microRNAs result in developmental defects of both the eyelid and the tongue [21–25]. These features suggest the possibility that tongue and eyelid development are under similar molecular mechanisms. To understand whether *Sox* genes are also involved in other craniofacial organs through similar roles as those in tongue development, we examined the expression of *Sox* genes in eyelid development. Murine eyelid initiates by groove formation at approximately E11, and the protrusion of the eyelid primordia occurs from E12 (Figures 6(a), 6(f), 6(k), and 6(p)) [20]. Fusion of eyelid is observed at approximately E16, since the mammalian eyes require temporary fusion and re-opening between the upper and lower eyelids during their development and growth (Figure 6(u)). *Myf5* expression was observed in the eyelid primordia only at E14 and E18 (Figures 6(a′), 6(f′), 6(k′), 6(p′), and 6(u′)). At E11, *Sox4, 11,* and *21* showed ubiquitous expressions in the developing eyelid, whereas *Sox6* was only expressed in

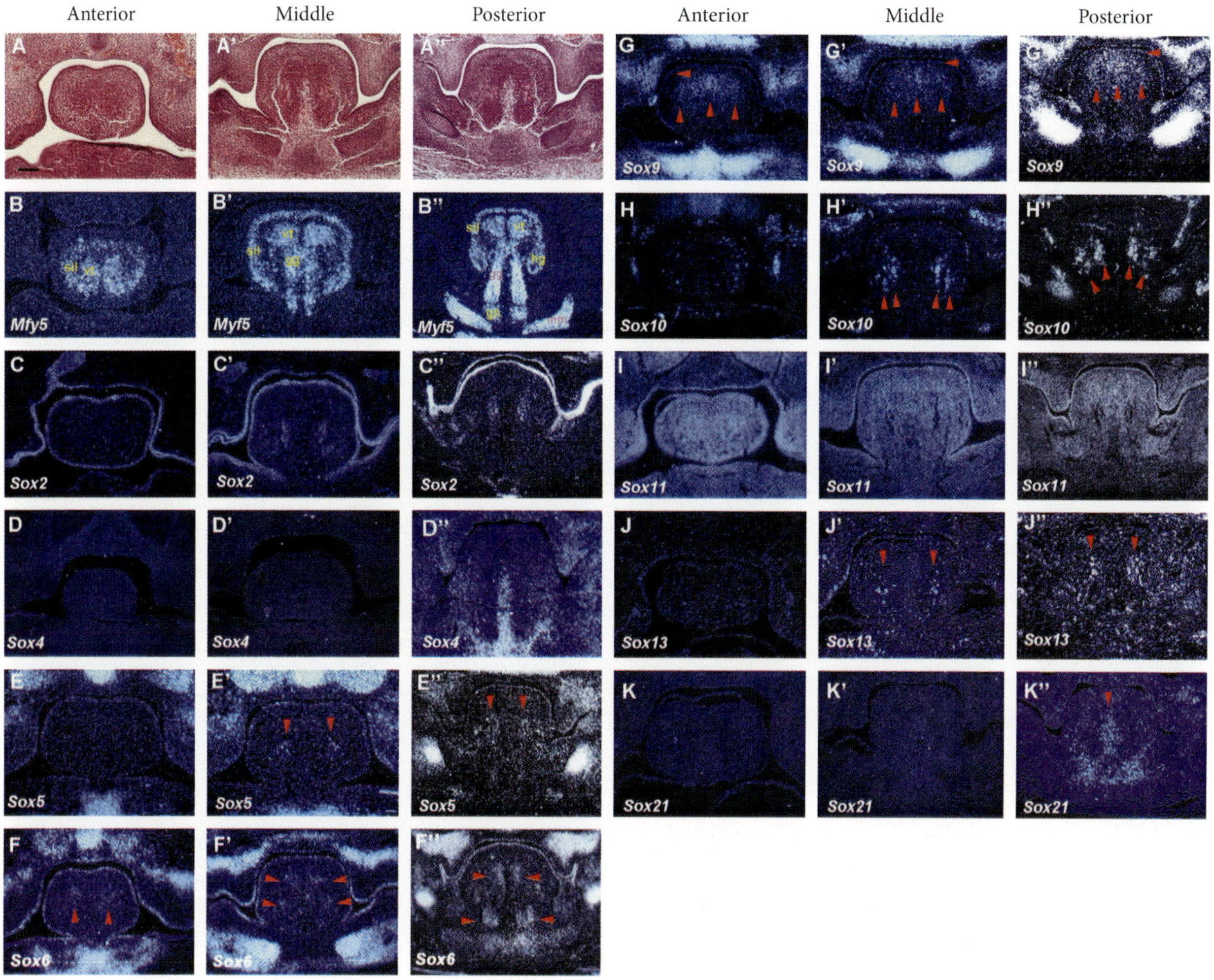

FIGURE 2: Expression of Sox genes in tongue development at E12. Frontal sections showing histology ((a)–(a″)) and *in situ* hybridization ((b)–(k″)) at the anterior, middle, and posterior regions of mandible in wild-type at E12. Vertical and transverse muscle (vt), genioglossus muscle (gg), superior and inferior longitudinal muscle (sil), geniohyoid muscle (gh), mylohyoid (mm), and hyoglossus muscle (hg). Arrowheads indicate weak expression. Scale bar: 125 μm for (a)–(k″).

the eyelid epithelium (Figures 6(b)–6(e)). At E12 and E13, *Sox4* and *11* expressions were observed in both the epithelium and mesenchyme, whereas *Sox6* and *9* were only expressed in the epithelium (Figures 6(g)–6(j) and 6(l)–6(o)). At E14, *Sox4* was ubiquitously expressed in the developing eyelid, with a slightly stronger expression in the muscles (Figure 6(q)). *Sox6, 9,* and *12* were expressed in the epithelium of eyelid primordia, whereas *Sox11* expression was observed in both the epithelium and mesenchyme (Figures 6(r)–6(t)), data not shown). At E18, *Sox21* was ubiquitously expressed in the developing eyelid, with a slightly stronger expression in the muscles (Figure 6(y)). Expressions of *Sox4* and *6* could be observed in the muscle of eyelid primordia, whereas *Sox11* was expressed in the epithelium (Figures 6(v)–6(x)). *Sox4, 6,* and *11* were also expressed in the extraocular muscle region. Expressions of *Sox1-3, 5, 8, 10, 13,* and *14* could not be detected in the developing eyelid (data not shown).

4. Discussion

The mammalian tongue is composed of the epithelium, connective tissue, and striated muscle. Our comparative *in situ* hybridization analysis demonstrated a dynamic spatiotemporal expression pattern of *Sox* genes during murine tongue development. *Sox2* and *11* were expressed in the tongue epithelium during all five stages investigated in this study, whereas *Sox8* and *9* were expressed in the tongue epithelium only at E14 and E12, respectively. *Sox4, 6, 12,* and *21* showed expressions in the epithelium at several stages (Table 2). *Sox4* and *21* were expressed in the mesenchyme at all stages, whereas *Sox5, 6,* and *13* were only detected in the mesenchyme at E12 (*Sox5, 13*) and E18 (*Sox6*). *Sox2, 8, 9, 10,* and *11* showed detectable expressions in the mesenchyme at several stages (Table 2). Unlike the epithelium and mesenchyme, none of the *Sox* genes were expressed in the tongue muscle during all five stages. *Sox1* was expressed in

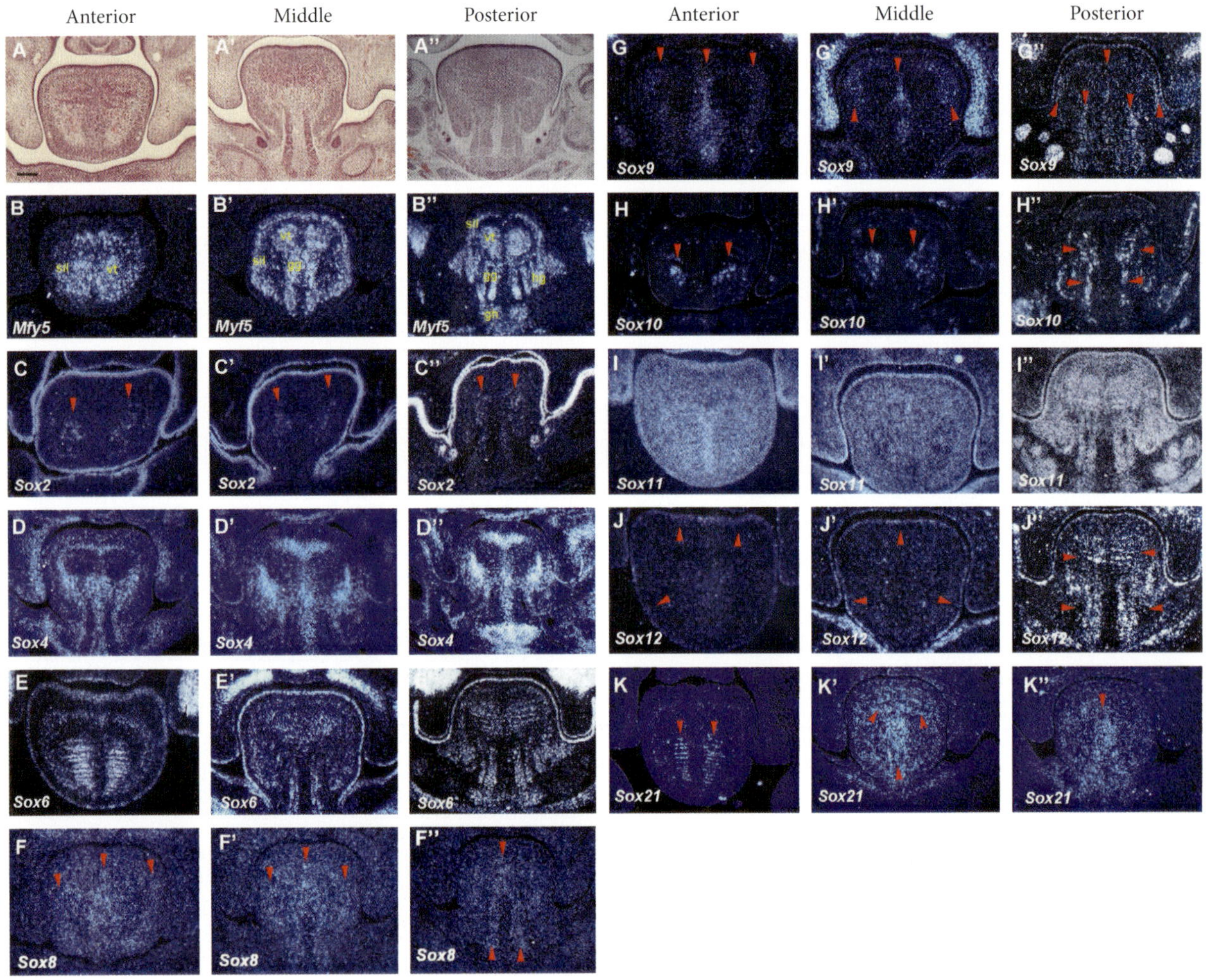

FIGURE 3: Expression of *Sox* genes in tongue development at E13. Frontal sections showing histology ((a)–(a″)) and *in situ* hybridization ((b)–(k″)) at the anterior, middle and posterior regions of mandible in wild-type at E13. Vertical and transverse muscle (vt), genioglossus muscle (gg), superior and inferior longitudinal muscle (sil), geniohyoid muscle (gh), hyoglossus muscle (hg). Arrowheads indicate weak expression. Scale bar: 125 μm for (a)–(k″).

the tongue muscle only at E18. *Sox6* and *10* were not detected in the muscle at E11 but were expressed during the other four developmental stages (E12–E18). Additionally, *Sox11* was not expressed in the muscle at E18 but was expressed during the other four developmental stages (E11–E14). *Sox4, 8, 9, 12,* and *21* showed detectable expressions in the muscle at several stages (Table 2). *Sox1* was only expressed in the muscle, whereas *Sox5* and *13* were expressed only in the mesenchyme. *Sox2* could not be detected in the muscle at any stage, whereas *Sox12* showed no expression in the mesenchyme at any stage. Although the expressions of *Sox2, 4, 10, 11,* and *21* were detected in the developing tongue during all five stages investigated in this study, their expression patterns differed among the stages. Our results also revealed a different expression pattern of *Sox* genes between the anterior, middle, and posterior region of the developing tongue (Figure 7). *Sox* genes thus showed a dynamic spatiotemporal expression pattern during murine tongue development.

Fungiform, circumvallate, and foliate papillae contain taste buds and are referred to as taste (or gustatory) papillae, whereas filiform papillae do not contain taste buds and are thus regarded nongustatory. Although *Sox2* has been shown to play a critical role in regulating the formation of gustatory papillae, its expression has also been detected in the nongustatory tongue epithelium [14]. Our results revealed that *Sox2, 4, 6, 8, 9, 10, 11, 12,* and *21* were expressed in the epithelium of the entire tongue. Although none of these genes showed a restricted expression pattern in the tongue papillae, it is possible that they are involved in regulating the formation of all papillae types.

Skeletal muscle fibers are classified as "slow-twitch fiber" (type I) and "fast-twitch fiber" (type II), which display marked differences in contraction strength, metabolic strategies, and susceptibility to fatigue. Slow-twitch fibers are rich in mitochondria, have increased contraction endurance with lesser strength potential, and use predominantly oxidative phosphorylation for energy production. Fast-twitch fibers contain comparatively less numbers of mitochondria and rely more heavily on anaerobic glycolysis for energy production, which allows considerable strength and contraction speed, but only for short anaerobic bursts of activity

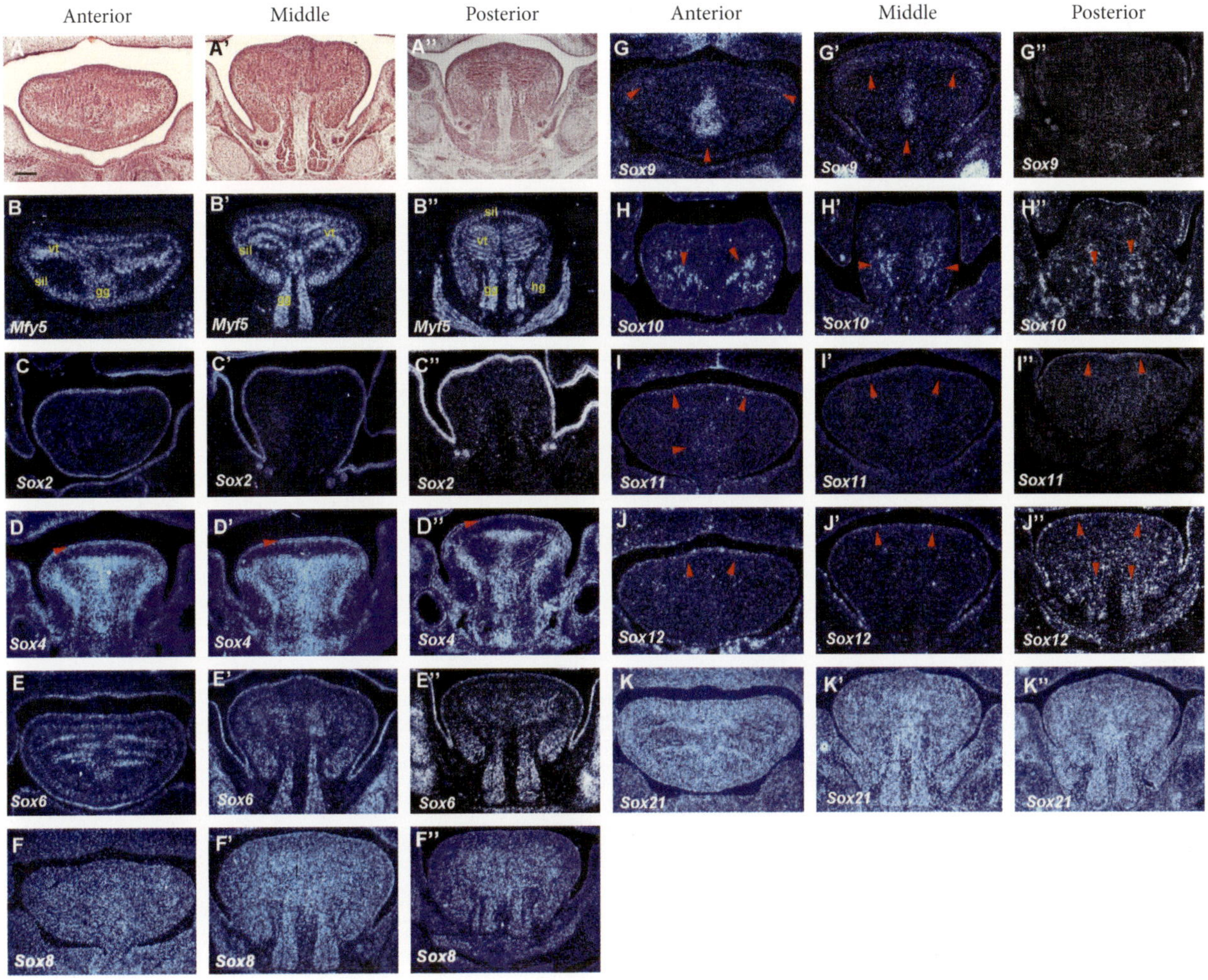

FIGURE 4: Expression of *Sox* genes in tongue development at E14. Frontal sections showing histology ((a)–(a″)) and *in situ* hybridization ((b)–(k″)) at the anterior, middle and posterior regions of mandible in wild-type at E14. Vertical and transverse muscle (vt), genioglossus muscle (gg), superior and inferior longitudinal muscle (sil), geniohyoid muscle (gh), hyoglossus muscle (hg). Arrowheads indicate weak expression. Scale bar: 300 μm for (a)–(k″).

before the muscles fatigue. It has been reported that *Sox6* is involved in fast-twitch muscle fiber differentiation in the trunk region [9, 10]. It is known that rodent tongue is composed of only fast-twitch fiber, and we also found *Sox6* expression in the muscles of the developing tongue [26, 27]. These suggest that *Sox6* is likely to be involved in fast-twitch muscle fiber differentiation during tongue development. *Sox8, 9, 10, 12,* and *21* were observed in the tongue muscles where *Sox6* was expressed, suggesting the possibility that these *Sox* genes also regulate fast-twitch muscle fiber differentiation. On the other hand, unlike the mouse tongue, the human tongue shows high proportion of slow-twitch fibers, suggesting that the role of *Sox* genes differs between the human and mouse tongue [28].

The developmental origin of the masticatory muscles is the cardiopharyngeal mesoderm, while the tongue and other muscles, including the trunk and limb muscles, are derived from the somites [29]. Although the embryonic origins are the same in the tongue, limb, and trunk muscle, it has been shown that the program controlling tongue myogenesis, including the specification and migration of muscle progenitor cells, differs from those of the trunk and limb myogenesis [2, 3, 30]. Therefore, we could not exclude the possibility that the role of *Sox* genes expressing in developing tongue muscle differ from that in trunk and limb muscle development.

The tongue consists of many types of muscles, including vt, sil, and gg muscles [2, 30, 31]. Although our results indicated that many *Sox* genes were expressed in these tongue muscles, there was no specific *Sox* gene expressing in the particular muscles (Figure 7). *Sox* genes are therefore unlikely to play a critical role in tongue muscle specification. Different expression patterns between *Sox* genes in each tongue muscle type suggested that each muscle type is controlled by different molecular mechanisms during development.

Skeletal myogenesis consists of six phases: specification, migration, proliferation, determination, differentiation, and

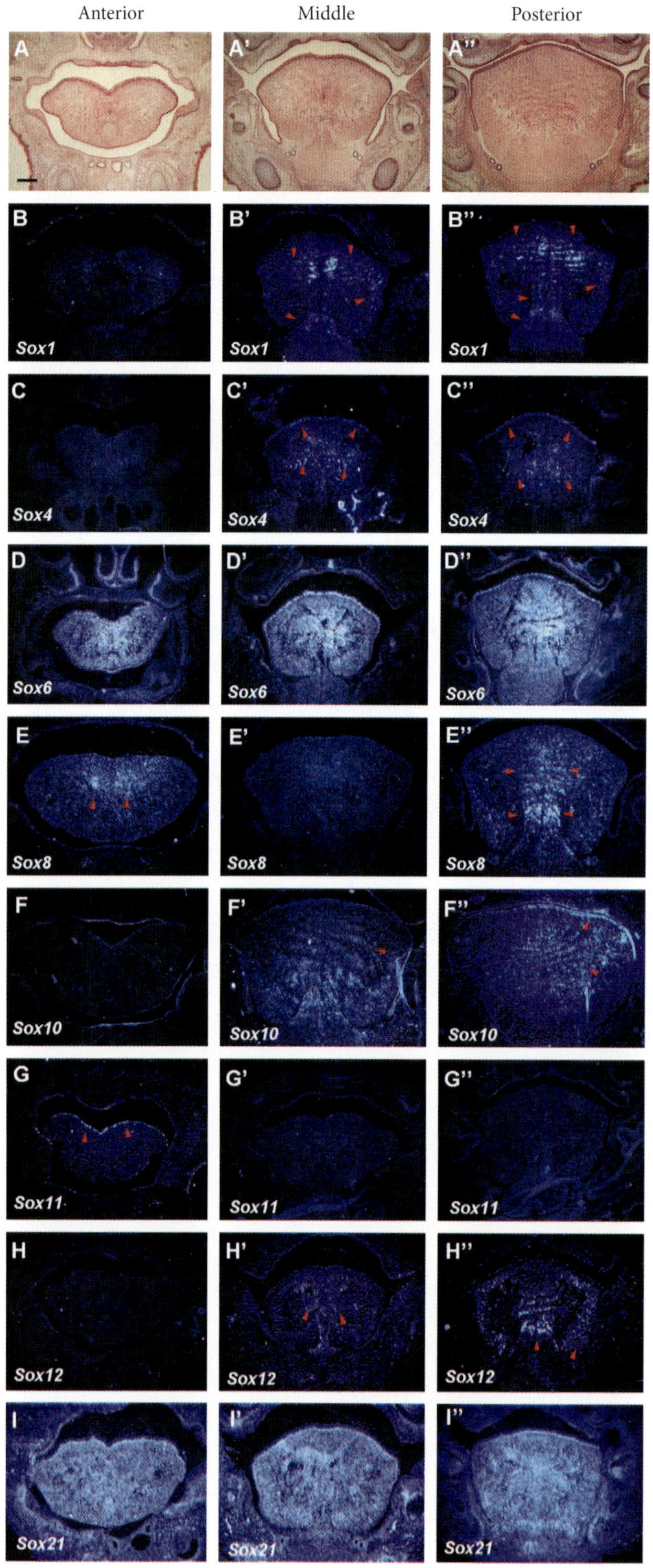

FIGURE 5: Expression of *Sox* genes in tongue development at E18. Frontal sections showing histology ((a)–(a″)) and *in situ* hybridization ((b)–(i″)) at the anterior, middle, and posterior regions of mandible in wild-type at E18. Arrowheads indicate weak expression. Scale bar: 700 μm for (a)–(i″).

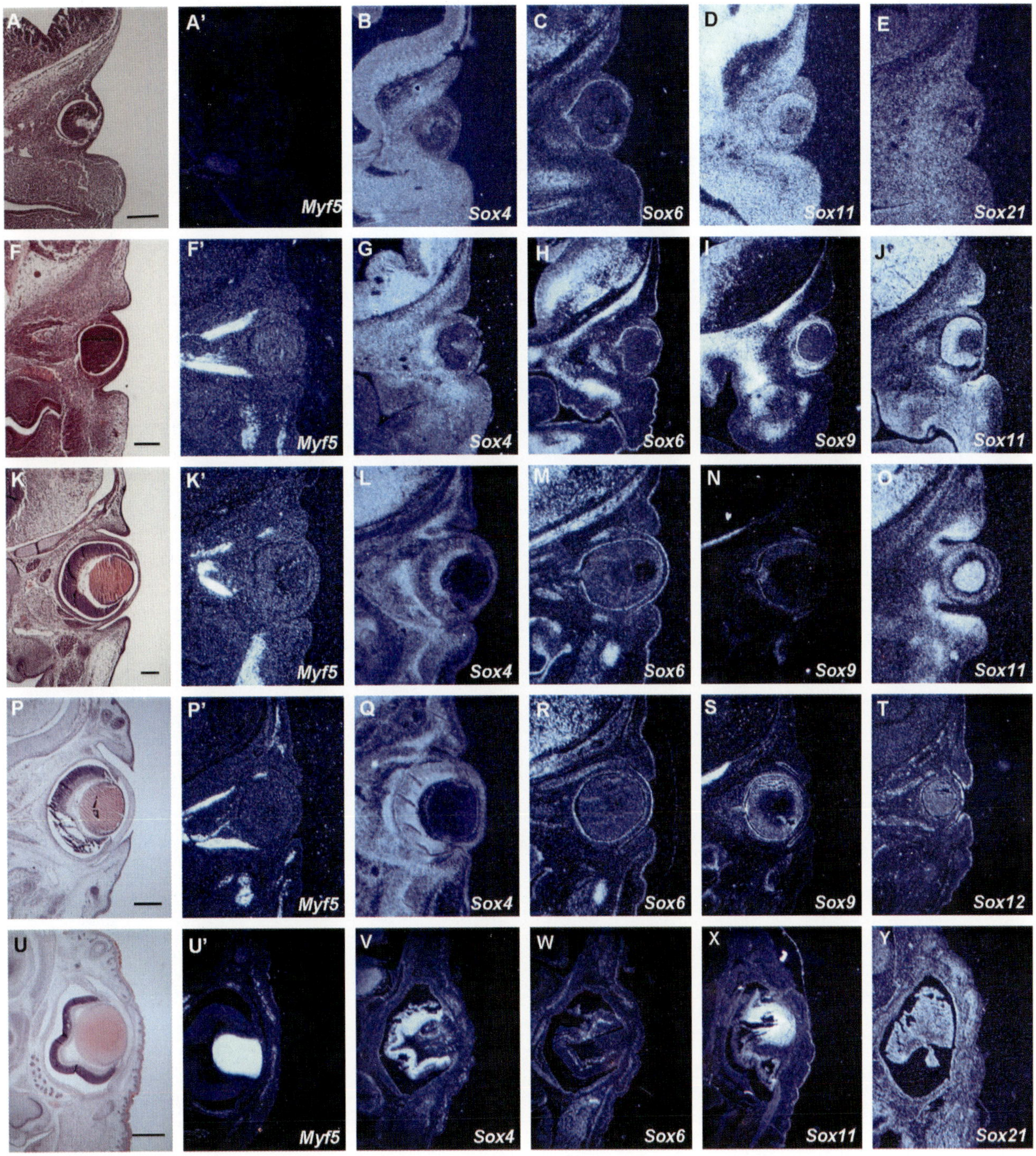

FIGURE 6: Expression of *Sox* genes in eyelid development. Frontal sections showing histology (a), (f), (k), (p), (u) and *in situ* hybridization ((a′)–(e), (f′)–(j), (k′)–(o), (p′)–(t), and (u′)–(y)) in wild type at E11 ((a)–(e)), E12 ((f)–(j)), E13 ((k)–(o)), E14 ((p)–(t)), and E18 ((u)–(y)). Scale bar: 150 μm for (a)–(e), 125 μm for (f)–(j), 125 μm for (k)–(o), 300 μm for (p)–(t), 700 μm for (u)–(y).

maturation [1, 2, 29–31]. It is unlikely that each phase of myogenesis proceeds at the same time in all types of tongue muscle since the timing of appearance differs between muscle types in the tongue [1, 2, 29–32]. It is possible that the different expression patterns of *Sox* genes in tongue muscles could be correlated with the onset of these stages, although the molecular mechanisms regulating the initiation of each phase during tongue development remain unclear. It has been shown that *Sox7, 15, 17* and *18* are involved in the function of satellite cells after birth, although these are not exerted at embryonic stages [11–13]. Therefore, a punctate expression pattern of *Sox7, 17,* and *18* observed in the embryonic tongue are likely to represent vascularization of the tissue. Furthermore, these also indicated that function of

Table 2: Summary of expression of *Sox* genes in developing tongue and eyelid.

Tongue epithelium												
E11	—	*Sox2*	*Sox4**	—	—	—	—	—	*Sox11**	—	—	*Sox21**
E12	—	*Sox2*	—	—	*Sox6*	—	*Sox9*	—	*Sox11**	—	—	—
E13	—	*Sox2*	—	—	*Sox6*	—	—	—	*Sox11**	*Sox12*	—	—
E14	—	*Sox2*	*Sox4*	—	*Sox6*	*Sox8**	—	—	*Sox11*	*Sox12*	—	*Sox21**
E18	—	*Sox2*	*Sox4*	—	*Sox6**	—	—	*Sox10*	*Sox11*	—	—	*Sox21**
Tongue mesenchyme												
E11	—	*Sox2*	*Sox4**	—	—	—	—	*Sox10*	*Sox11**	—	—	*Sox21**
E12	—	*Sox2*	*Sox4*	*Sox5*	—	—	*Sox9*	*Sox10*	*Sox11**	—	*Sox13*	*Sox21*
E13	—	*Sox2*	*Sox4*	—	—	*Sox8*	*Sox9*	*Sox10*	*Sox11**	—	—	*Sox21*
E14	—	—	*Sox4*	—	—	*Sox8**	—	*Sox10*	—	—	—	*Sox21**
E18	—	—	*Sox4*	—	*Sox6**	—	—	—	—	—	—	*Sox21**
Tongue muscle												
E11	—	—	*Sox4**	—	—	—	—	—	*Sox11**	—	—	*Sox21**
E12	—	—	—	—	*Sox6*	—	*Sox9*	*Sox10*	*Sox11**	—	—	—
E13	—	—	—	—	*Sox6*	*Sox8*	*Sox9*	*Sox10*	*Sox11**	*Sox12*	—	*Sox21*
E14	—	—	—	—	*Sox6*	*Sox8**	*Sox9*	*Sox10*	*Sox11*	*Sox12*	—	*Sox21**
E18	*Sox1*	—	*Sox4*	—	*Sox6**	*Sox8*	—	*Sox10*	—	*Sox12*	—	*Sox21**
Eyelid mesenchyme												
E11	—	—	*Sox4**	—	—	—	—	—	*Sox11**	—	—	*Sox21**
E12	—	—	*Sox4*	—	—	—	—	—	*Sox11*	—	—	—
E13	—	—	*Sox4*	—	—	—	—	—	*Sox11*	—	—	—
E14	—	—	*Sox4**	—	—	—	—	—	*Sox11*	—	—	—
E18	—	—	—	—	—	—	—	—	—	—	—	*Sox21**
Eyelid muscle												
E14	—	—	*Sox4**	—	—	—	—	—	—	—	—	—
E18	—	—	*Sox4*	—	*Sox6*	—	—	—	—	—	—	*Sox21*

*Ubiquitous expression.

Sox genes differ between embryonic and postnatal stages in tongue formation.

Previous studies have reported that neural crest-derived cells give rise to tissues surrounding the skeletal muscles, including the perimysium, epimysium, endomysium, and tendon, during tongue development [33, 34]. *Sox* genes have been shown to regulate the functions of neural crest-derived cells including their differentiation, collagen synthesis, and melanocyte formation [35, 36, 37]. In our study, *Sox9* displayed a restricted expression pattern in the lingual septum, which is composed of neural crest-derived cells [2, 3]. It has been reported that *Scleraxis* is expressed in a similar pattern to that of *Sox9* during tongue development [2, 32]. Interestingly, *Sox9* shows coordinated expression with *Scleraxis* during digital tendon development [38]. Therefore, it is possible that *Sox9/Scleraxis*-expressing cells are involved in the formation of tongue muscle tendons.

The origin of the tongue is known to be hybrid, neural crest-derived cells, the mesoderm, and endoderm. It has been shown that there is an interaction between neural crest-derived and myogenic cells during tongue development [2, 3]. We detected the expressions of *Sox1, 4, 6, 8, 9, 10, 11, 12, 13,* and *21* in the muscles of the developing tongue and of *Sox2, 4, 5, 6, 8, 9, 10, 11,* and *21* in the mesenchyme. It is possible that these genes are involved in the interaction between neural crest-derived and myogenic cells during tongue development. In fact, some *Sox* genes have been proven to be involved in the interaction between the epithelium and mesenchyme in digestive tract development [39, 40].

Members of the *Sox* gene family play multiple roles during development [5, 6]. The dynamic spatiotemporal expression pattern of *Sox* genes discovered in this study indicates their critical role during murine tongue development. We also examined the expression of *Sox* genes in eyelid development (Table 2). Both organs consist of connective tissue, muscle, and epithelium, and there is an interaction between these tissues during their development [2, 3, 19, 20]. In addition, both tongue and eyelid are mobile organs. Although there are thus numerous similarities between the eyelid and tongue, our results showed that the expression patterns and timing of *Sox* genes significantly differed between tongue and eyelid development. *Sox* genes are thus likely to be involved in organogenesis through different functions in each organ.

5. Conclusion

Sox genes show a dynamic spatiotemporal expression pattern during murine tongue development.

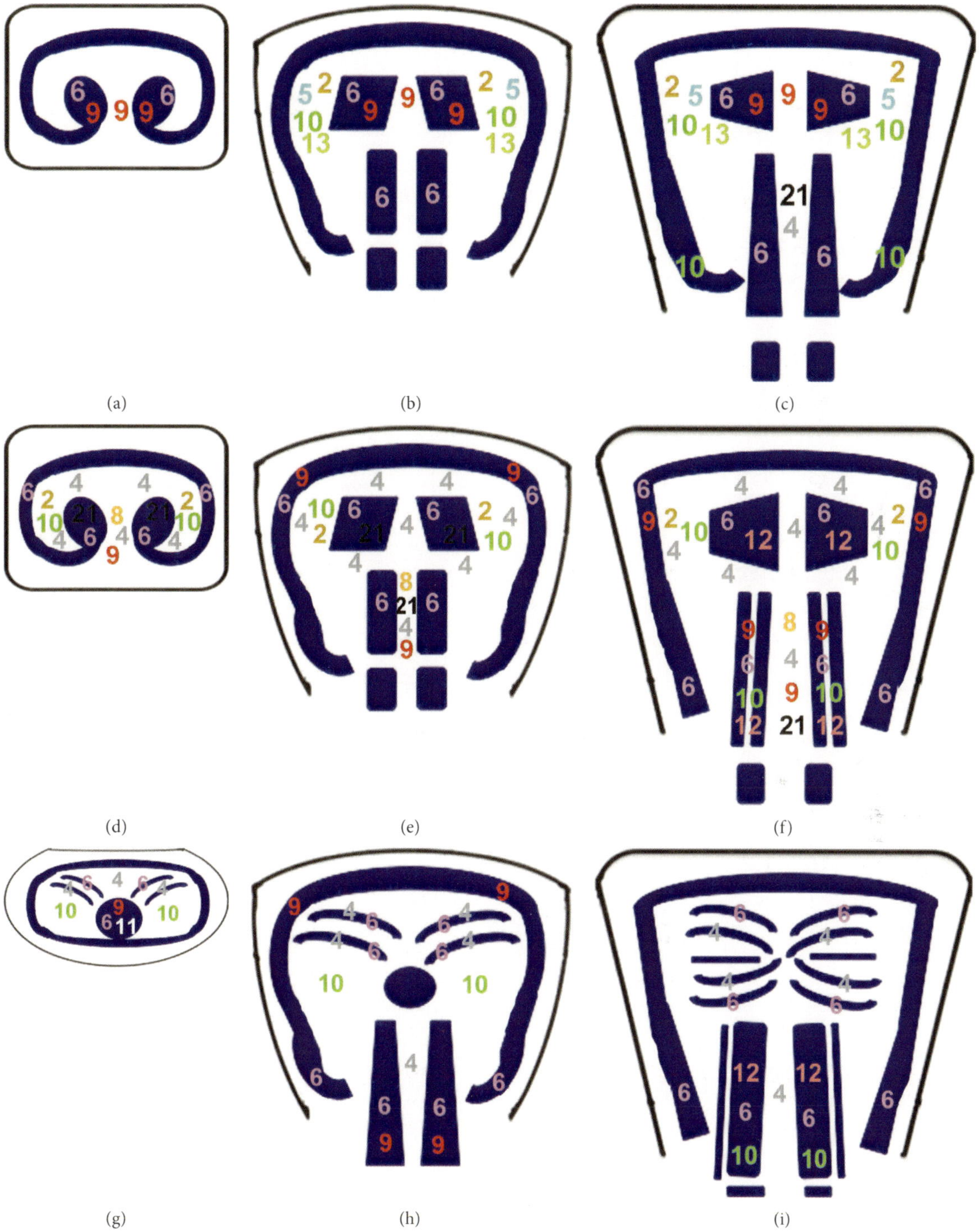

FIGURE 7: Summary of expression of *Sox* genes in tongue mesenchyme and muscle during development. Diagrammatic representation of developing tongue of the anterior (a), (d), (g); middle (b), (e), (h); and posterior region (c), (f), (i) at E12 (a–c), E13 (d–f), and E14 (g–i). The muscle is shown in blue. The numbers represent each *Sox* gene. *Sox* genes showing ubiquitous expression are excluded.

Acknowledgments

This research was funded by the Japan Society for the Promotion of Science (JSPS; 17H01601).

References

[1] D. M. Noden and P. Francis-West, "The differentiation and morphogenesis of craniofacial muscles," *Developmetal Dynamics*, vol. 235, no. 5, pp. 1194–1218, 2006.

[2] C. Parada, D. Han, and Y. Chai, "Molecular and cellular regulatory mechanisms of tongue myogenesis," *Journal of Dental Research*, vol. 91, no. 6, pp. 528–535, 2012.

[3] C. Parada and Y. Chai, "Mandible and Tongue Development," *Current Topics in Developmental Biology*, vol. 115, pp. 31–58, 2015.

[4] M. T. Cobourne, S. Iseki, A. A. Birjandi et al., "How to make a tongue: Cellular and molecular regulation of muscle and connective tissue formation during mammalian tongue development," *Seminars Cell and Developmental Biology*, 2018, In press.

[5] L. H. Pevny and R. Lovell-Badge, "Sox genes find their feet," *Current Opinion in Genetics and Development*, vol. 7, no. 3, pp. 338–344, 1997.

[6] Z. Y. She and W. X. Yang, "SOX family transcription factors involved in diverse cellular events during development," *European Journal of Cell Biology*, vol. 94, no. 12, pp. 547–563, 2015.

[7] K. Kawasaki, M. Kawasaki, M. Watanabe et al., "Expression of Sox genes in tooth development," *International Journal of Developmental Biology*, vol. 59, no. 10-12, pp. 471–478, 2015.

[8] O. Lioubinski, M. Müller, M. Wegner, and M. Sander, "Expression of Sox transcription factors in the developing mouse pancreas," *Developmental Dynamics*, vol. 227, no. 3, pp. 402–408, 2003.

[9] H. E. Jackson and P. W. Ingham, "Control of muscle fibre-type diversity during embryonic development: the zebrafish paradigm," *Mechanisms of Devevelopment*, vol. 130, no. 9-10, pp. 447–457, 2013.

[10] S. Lin, X. Lin, Z. Zhang et al., "Copy number variation in *Sox6* contributes to chicken muscle development," *Genes*, vol. 17, no. 9, p. 42, 2018.

[11] S. Alonso-Martin, F. Aurade, D. Mademtzoglou, A. Rochat, P. S. Zammit, and F. Relaix, "SOXF factors regulate murine satellite cell self-renewal and function through inhibition of β-catenin activity," *Elife*, vol. 8, p. 7, 2018.

[12] A.P. Meeson, X. Shi, M.S. Alexander et al., "Sox15 and Fhl3 transcriptionally coactivate Foxk1 and regulate myogenic progenitor cells," *EMBO Journal*, vol. 26, no. 7, pp. 1902–1912, 2007.

[13] R.F. Rajgara, N. Lala-Tabbert, F. Marchildon et al., "SOX7 Is Required for Muscle Satellite Cell Development and Maintenance," *Stem Cell Reports*, vol. 9, no. 4, pp. 1139–1151, 2017.

[14] T. Okubo, L. H. Pevny, and B. L. Hogan, "Sox2 is required for development of taste bud sensory cells," *Genes and Development*, vol. 20, no. 19, pp. 2654–2659, 2006.

[15] A. Ohazama, E. B. Johnson, M. S. Ota et al., "Lrp4 modulates extracellular integration of cell signaling pathways in development," *PLoS One*, vol. 3, no. 12, Article ID e4092, 2008.

[16] M. Francois, P. Koopman, and M. Beltrame, "SoxF genes: key players in the development of the cardio-vascular system," *International Journal of Biochemistry and Cell Biology*, vol. 42, no. 3, pp. 445–448, 2010.

[17] M. Francois, N. L. Harvey, and B. M. Hogan, "The transcriptional control of lymphatic vascular development," *Physiology*, vol. 26, no. 3, pp. 146–155, 2011.

[18] M. F. Morini and E. Dejana, "Transcriptional regulation of arterial differentiation via Wnt, Sox, and Notch," *Current Opinion in Hematology*, vol. 21, no. 3, pp. 229–234, 2014.

[19] S. Creuzet, C. Vincent, and G. Couly, "Neural crest derivatives in ocular and periocular structures," *International Journal of Developmental Biology*, vol. 49, no. 2-3, pp. 161–171, 2005.

[20] H. Ohuchi, "Wakayama Symposium: Epithelial-mesenchymal interactions in eyelid development," *Ocular Surface*, vol. 10, no. 4, pp. 212–216, 2012.

[21] Y. Lan and R. Jiang, "Sonic hedgehog signaling regulates reciprocal epithelial-mesenchymal interactions controlling palatal outgrowth," *Development*, vol. 136, no. 8, pp. 1387–1396, 2009.

[22] J. Jeong, J. Mao, T. Tenzen, A. H. Kottmann, and A. P. McMahon, "Hedgehog signaling in the neural crest cells regulates the patterning and growth of facial primordial," *Genes and Development*, vol. 18, no. 8, pp. 937–951, 2004.

[23] A. Zehir, L. L. Hu, E. L. Maska, Y. Morikawa, and P. Cserjesi, "Dicer is required for survival of differentiating neural crest cells," *Developmental Biology*, vol. 340, no. 2, pp. 459–467, 2010.

[24] T. Huang, Y. Liu, M. Huang, X. Zhao, and L. Cheng, "Wnt1-cre-mediated conditional loss of Dicer results in malformation of the midbrain and cerebellum and failure of neural crest and dopaminergic differentiation in mice," *Journal of Molelular Cell Biology*, vol. 2, no. 3, pp. 152–163, 2010.

[25] X. Nie, Q. Wang, and K. Jiao, "Dicer activity in neural crest cells is essential for craniofacial organogenesis and pharyngeal arch artery morphogenesis," *Mechanisms of Development*, vol. 128, no. 3-4, pp. 200–207, 2011.

[26] T.I. Prigozy, K. Dalrymple, C. Shuler, and L. Kedes, "Differential expression of troponin C genes during tongue myogenesis," *Developmental Dynamics*, vol. 209, no. 1, pp. 36–44, 1997.

[27] A. J. Sokoloff, "Localization and contractile properties of intrinsic longitudinal motor units of the rat tongue," *Journal of Neurophysiology*, vol. 84, no. 2, pp. 827–835, 2000.

[28] I. Sanders, L. Mu, A. Amirali, H. Su, and S. Sobotka, "The human tongue slows down to speak: muscle fibers of the human tongue," *Anatomical Record*, vol. 296, no. 10, pp. 1615–1627, 2013.

[29] R. Diogo, R.G. Kelly, L. Christiaen et al., "A new heart for a new head in vertebrate cardiopharyngeal evolution," *Nature*, vol. 520, no. 7548, pp. 466–473, 2015.

[30] A. Yamane, "Embryonic and postnatal development of masticatory and tongue muscles," *Cell and Tissue Research*, vol. 322, no. 2, pp. 183–189, 2005.

[31] H. Aoyagi, S. Iwasaki, and T. Asami, "Three-Dimensional Architecture of the Mouse Tongue Muscles Using Micro-CT with a Focus on the Transverse, Vertical, and Genioglossus Muscles," *Surgical Science*, vol. 6, no. 8, pp. 358–368, 2015.

[32] R. Hosokawa, K. Oka, T. Yamaza et al., "TGF-beta mediated FGF10 signaling in cranial neural crest cells controls development of myogenic progenitor cells through tissue-tissue interactions during tongue morphogenesis," *Developmental Biology*, vol. 341, no. 1, pp. 186–195, 2010.

[33] G. F. Couly, P. M. Coltey, and N. M. Le Douarin, "The developmental fate of the cephalic mesoderm in quail-chick chimeras," *Development*, vol. 114, no. 1, pp. 1–15, 1992.

[34] D. J. Evans and D. M. Noden, "Spatial relations between avian craniofacial neural crest and paraxial mesoderm cells," *Developmental Dynamics*, vol. 235, no. 5, pp. 1310–1325, 2006.

[35] Y. Aoki, N. Saint-Germain, M. Gyda et al., "Sox10 regulates the development of neural crest-derived melanocytes in Xenopus," *Developmental Biolology*, vol. 259, no. 1, pp. 19–33, 2003.

[36] T. Suzuki, D. Sakai, N. Osumi, H. Wada, and Y. Wakamatsu, "Sox genes regulate type 2 collagen expression in avian neural crest cells," *Development, Growth and Differentiation*, vol. 48, no. 8, pp. 477–486, 2006.

[37] M. Cheung and J. Briscoe, "Neural crest development is regulated by the transcription factor Sox9," *Development*, vol. 130, no. 23, pp. 5681–5693, 2003.

[38] Y. Asou, A. Nifuji, K. Tsuji et al., "Coordinated expression of scleraxis and Sox9 genes during embryonic development of tendons and cartilage," *Journal Orthopaedic Research*, vol. 20, no. 4, pp. 827–833, 2002.

[39] L. Le Guen, S. Marchal, S. Faure, and P. de Santa Barbara, "Mesenchymal-epithelial interactions during digestive tract development and epithelial stem cell regeneration," *Cellular and Molecular Life Science*, vol. 72, no. 20, pp. 3883–3896, 2015.

[40] S. Yasugi and K. Fukuda, "The mesenchymal factors regulating epithelial morphogenesis and differentiation of the chicken stomach," *Zoological Science*, vol. 17, no. 1, pp. 1–9, 2000.

5

Prevalence of Anterior Dental Trauma and Its Associated Factors among Preschool Children Aged 3–5 Years in Khartoum City, Sudan

Alaa Gamaleldin Sulieman and Elhadi Mohieldin Awooda

Department of Endodontics, Faculty of Dentistry, University of Medical Sciences and Technology, Khartoum, Sudan

Correspondence should be addressed to Elhadi Mohieldin Awooda; sowaraldahb@gmail.com

Academic Editor: Andrea Scribante

Background. Traumatic dental injury (TDI) is a challenging public health problem. Its incidence and prevalence vary within countries, states, and different social groups. *Aim.* The purpose of this study was to determine the prevalence of traumatic dental injuries in primary incisors among 3–5-year-old Sudanese preschool children and associated factors such as age, sex, and size of overjet and anterior open bite. *Materials and Methods.* Descriptive cross-sectional study was carried out among 600 preschool children (3–5 years old) selected by multistage cluster technique from preschools located in Khartoum city, Sudan. The data regarding age, sex, causes, and treatment of TDI were collected from the mothers through structured interview questionnaire. Children were examined in an upright position, using mouth mirror and torch. A single examiner assessed the type of trauma, the tooth involved, and overbite/overjet. The data were analyzed statistically through descriptive analysis, and the chi-square test was used to compare between different variables with $P < 0.05$. *Results.* The prevalence of traumatic dental injuries (TDIs) was 18.5%. Enamel fractures were the most common type (74.8%), followed by enamel and dentin (11.7%). The maxillary central incisors were the most commonly affected teeth, and the home was most common place for TDI. The prevalence rate was 45% in boys and 55% in girls with a statistically significant difference ($P = 0.02$). *Conclusions.* The prevalence of traumatic dental injuries to the primary anterior teeth among the Sudanese preschool children was relatively high (18.5%). Factors such as overjet size, overbite size, and lip competency were not significantly correlated with dental trauma among the studied population.

1. Introduction

Traumatic dental injury (TDI) is a challenging public health problem to professionals, and it has been seriously neglected [1]. The incidence of dental trauma among the primary school children is an emerging dental health problem. Epidemiological data showed a wide variation in the prevalence of dental injuries in preschool children [2–4]. Several studies revealed that the prevalence of traumatic injuries in children has increased during the last few decades [5, 6]. Dental trauma can result in displacement, fracture, or loss of tooth [4]. The consequence of traumatic injuries to primary teeth includes alteration in physical appearance, speech defects, and emotional impacts, thus affecting the child's quality of life [7, 8]. TDI to primary teeth may eventually create problems to the underlying permanent teeth, such as hypoplasia, discoloration, delay eruption time, and tooth malformation [9, 10]. Preschool children are more prone to TDI due to their poor stability, passive reflexes, and indefinite movements [3, 10]. Predisposing factors to TDI include physical features such as increased incisal overjet, open bite, protrusion, and lip incompetence [8].

In many countries, high cost, low standard of living, and lack of knowledge regarding urgent treatment of dental trauma may result in delaying the treatment [8, 11]. Studies of TDIs among the preschool children are of paramount importance, as individuals with previous trauma in the primary dentition are prone to further trauma in the permanent dentition [12].

A recent meta-analysis study on February 2018 through literature search (publication years 1996–2016 of the prevalence of TDIs) aimed at covering as many countries, communities, and ethnic groups as possible. They showed that more than one billion living people have had TDI [13]. Research studies on TDIs among the Sudanese population are not well documented to be part of the global frequency, so data from the Sudan are needed to achieve high generalizability. The objectives of this study were to determine the prevalence of TDI among the Sudanese preschool children aged 3–5 years and to assess the relation among associated factors such as overbite, overjet, age, gender, and site to the severity of TDI.

2. Materials and Methods

A cross-sectional study was carried out on children aged 3–5 years, of both sexes, living in Khartoum city. The inclusion criteria were the child being healthy and of Sudanese nationality attending a public or private preschools. The exclusion criteria included children who experienced significant dental anxiety and those who were identified by the preschool authority to have medical or intellectual problems. Data collection began on November 2016 over a period of two months. The sample size was determined after obtaining the total number of preschools in Khartoum locality, the number of public preschools was 13, and the number of private preschools was 507 with a total number of children within these schools compromising 23,000. We estimated that a minimum sample size of 585 children was required to achieve the level of precision with a standard error of 4% or less and the 95% confidence interval level and a prevalence of dental trauma of 50% used for the calculation. The decision to use a prevalence of 50% was due to the lack of information of the actual published prevalence of TDI among preschool children in Sudan. However, any calculation using a different figure than 50% would require a smaller sample size to achieve the same precision [14]. The number was rounded to 600.

Ethical clearance was obtained from the Ethical Committee of the University of Medical Science and Technology. Local authorities (Ministry of Health and Ministry of Education in Khartoum state) provided the necessary information for the construction of a sample frame including names, locations of preschools in Khartoum, their addresses, contact information, and the total number of children in the locality. Permission to examine the children was obtained from the school authorities concerned. A letter was handed to all parents explaining the objectives of the study and requesting the acceptance of voluntary participation themselves to answer the questionnaire and their children to be examined for the presence of TDI. Those who agreed to participate were signed informed written consent.

Data were collected through intraoral examination of eligible children and their mother's response to a self-administered closed-ended questionnaire including demographic data, etiology, localization, place, time elapsed between injury and treatment, and the treatment provided. The data were collected in the classrooms, and a single examiner, who is the first author, performed the clinical examination. The examined child was seated in classroom chair in the upright position; mouth mirror and torch were used to enhance visualization. One of the parents or schoolteachers sometimes helped to carry very young children. A sample of 15 children was used to train and to calibrate the examiner and test the feasibility of the intraoral visual examination, diagnosis of TDI, and the interview procedures. Training was performed with the help of an experienced endodontist and paedodontist from the University of Medical Sciences and Technology. No changes were made on the methods previously proposed, and the first author carried out all the procedure.

The criteria for the diagnosis of anterior dental trauma were assessed according to the method used by Andreasen et al. [15]. The number of injured teeth, type of trauma, type of tooth, and location in the upper or lower jaw were recorded. The presence of anterior open bite was assessed based on the criterion of lack of vertical overlap of the incisors in the occlusal position [9]. The overjet size was measured in millimeters by a metal ruler. Root fracture was not recorded, and no intraoral radiographs were taken. The data were subjected to simple descriptive analysis, and the statistical analysis was performed by SPSS version 21 (SPSS Inc., Chicago, USA). Statistical significance for the association between the occurrence of dental trauma and the distribution of dental injuries by age, gender, children's incisal overjet size, and overbite size was determined using the chi-square test with the level of statistical significance set at $P < 0.05$.

3. Results

A total of 600 children aged 3–5 years and all attending preschools in Khartoum locality, Sudan, were included in this study; the overall children affected by TDI were 111 with the prevalence of 18.5%. The prevalence rate was 45% in boys and 55% in girls, and a statistical significant difference was found between them ($P = 0.02$).

The maxillary central incisors were the most common teeth affected by trauma (54.9%), the right maxillary central incisor accounted for 35.1% of the injuries, and the left maxillary central incisor accounted for 19.8% followed by the maxillary lateral incisors (32.4%); meanwhile, the percentage of mandibular incisors was 6.3%, and the least affected tooth was found to be the canine (Table 1).

Enamel fracture accounted for 74.8% and was the most common type of TDI in maxillary and mandibular teeth, followed by fractures involving both enamel and dentin, while complete avulsion affected only 9.9% as displayed in Table 2. TDIs occurred at home accounted for 71.2%. Tripping and falling were the most common causes of TDI with a percentage of 63.1% (Table 3). Regardless of the dental injuries, we found that 95.5% of the subjects did not receive any dental treatment or control of the problem. There is no statistical significant difference between the size of overjet and overbite with occurrence of TDI as seen in Tables 4 and 5.

4. Discussion

The most common type of facial injuries is traumatic dental injury accounting for as high as 18% of the all facial injuries [16]. This cross-sectional survey identified the prevalence of dental trauma to the primary anterior teeth in 3–5-year-old

Table 1: Distribution of the study sample according to the type of the traumatized tooth.

	N	%
Right maxillary central incisor	39	35.1
Right maxillary lateral incisor	24	21.6
Right maxillary canine	3	2.7
Left maxillary central incisor	22	19.8
Left maxillary lateral incisor	12	10.8
Left maxillary canine	1	0.9
Left mandibular central incisor	4	3.6
Left mandibular lateral incisor	1	0.9
Left mandibular canine	3	2.7
Right mandibular central incisor	2	1.8
Total	111	100.0

Table 2: Distribution of the study sample according to the type of dental trauma to the anterior teeth.

	Code	*N*	%
1	No injury seen	1	0.9
2	Treated dental injury	1	0.95
3	Enamel fracture only	83	74.8
4	Enamel/dentin fracture	13	11.7
5	Enamel/dentin and pulp injury	2	1.8
6	Missing tooth due to trauma	11	9.9
7	Excluded tooth	0	0
	Total	111	100

Table 3: Distribution of the study sample according to the cause of anterior dental trauma.

Type	*N*	%
Trips and falls	70	63.1
Collision with objects or person	15	13.55
Bicycles	0	0
Road traffic accident	0	0
Violence or fights	2	1.8
Do not remember	24	21.6
Other (specify)	0	0
Total	111	100.0

Table 4: The relationship between traumatic dental injury and overbite size among the studied preschool children.

Overbite		TDI		Total	*P* value
		Yes	No		
Normal	Count	107	459	566	0.681* Pearson's *R* (0.017)
	% of total	17.8%	76.5%	94.3%	
Open bite	Count	4	30	34	
	% of total	0.7%	5.0%	5.7%	
Cross bite	Count	0	0	0	
	% of total	0	0	0	
Total	Count	111	489	600	
	% of total	18.5%	81.5%	100.0%	

TDI: traumatic dental injury, $^*P > 0.05$ indicates no significant relation between TDI and overbite.

Table 5: The relation between traumatic dental injury and overjet size among the studied preschool children.

Size of overjet		TDI		Total	*P* value
		Yes	No		
0–3 mm	Count	109	477	586	0.298* Pearson's *R* (0.043)
	% of total	18.2%	79.5%	97.7%	
3–6 mm	Count	2	12	14	
	% of total	0.3%	2.0%	2.3%	
More than 6 mm	Count	0	0	0	
	% of total	0%	0%	0%	
Total	Count	111	489	600	
	% of total	18.5%	81.5%	100.0%	

$^*P$ value ≥ 0.05 indicates no significant difference between TDI and overjet size.

preschool children in Khartoum city. In this city, there are no clear variations in socioeconomic status; the city is a melting pool of different ethnic groups coming from other states and regions in the Sudan, so with some cautions, we can generalize the results to the whole Sudan. The prevalence of TDI was higher when compared to another study [17] and lower when compared to most studies of trauma to primary teeth [18]. However, it is difficult to compare the prevalence figures found in different studies due to lack of uniformity in selected population, dental examination procedure, diagnostic criteria, and age groups [19].

Contradicting the majority of previous studies [20–22], which reported a higher frequency of dental trauma among boys than among girls, our study results are consistent with the results of the study done by Rai et al. [23] and Vuletić et al. [5] that girls tend to experience more dental injuries than boys, while the results of other studies revealed no statistically significant differences [3, 17]. However, some studies showed that there is an increase in TDI among girls and this increasing trend of dental trauma among girls is probably because of their increasing participation in sports or physical activities formerly practiced by boys only [24].

Majority of them have enamel fracture; this finding corresponds with previous research studies carried out on different populations [3, 18, 25, 26]. Other studies have reported different results; one such study, which surveyed Turkish children, found that avulsion and crown fractures were the most common injuries [27]. Others reported subluxation and avulsions as the most frequent types of dental trauma [28, 29]. The difference in the findings of these different studies may be due to the population being examined.

Similar to the results of other studies [4, 18], traumatic dental injuries occur more in the maxilla than in the mandible. This may be due to relative prominence of the maxillary anterior teeth. The maxillary central incisors are the teeth most commonly affected, similar to what was obtained by previous studies [3, 4]. The reason may be due to its central position which is more prone to direct assault. In addition, the upper central incisors are generally more proclined than the lower centrals and tend to be the first to receive a direct blow [3]. Also, the upper jaw is fixed to the skull which makes it rigid, while the lower jaw, being a flexible part, tends to reduce the impact forces directed on the lower anterior teeth by movement [30].

The majority of TDIs occurred at home and at school during a physical activity that lead to fall, as demonstrated in this study; 63.1% of dental trauma occurred due to a fall followed by a collision with an object or person. Our results were consistent with the literature that reported the most common cause of injury was a fall and the home being the commonest place [18, 31]; however, some studies concluded that TDIs occur most common in a field/playground or outdoors [27, 32].

Different studies have found an association between an overjet >3 mm and inadequate lip coverage and the occurrence of dental trauma in permanent teeth [3, 8, 11, 18, 31]. A few studies have shown a relationship in deciduous teeth [26, 33, 34]. Our results reveal that there is no significant relation between increased overjet and overbite with TDI among preschoolers. The reason behind this inconsistency cannot be justified, and further studies are needed to prove otherwise.

Relatively high prevalence of TDIs in our study could be due to the increased number of private schools when compared to government schools. This increases the risk of subjecting children to more trauma. As most of the private schools do not follow the standard of an ideal school environment and they build or rent small area in floor building, the space is limited for the children to play free, which leads to crashes with each other. However, this assumption contradicted the result made by Singh et al., where the prevalence of TDIs among preschool children was low (4.10%) and they interpreted due to the relative lack of outdoor activities and more emphasis on education [19].

Majority of traumatized subjects (95.5%) did not seek or receive any dental treatment, and similar result obtained by others [35, 36]. It revealed a poor perception of parents and caregivers toward child's oral health and a lack of awareness regarding TDI to primary teeth. A further study is needed to verify failure of seeking dental trauma treatment to primary teeth.

The prevention of trauma and the need for treatment following TDIs are very important to avoid possible unfavorable consequences that may precipitate [10, 37]. More interestingly and importantly, the report of the study by Awad et al. revealed a low level of knowledge among primary schoolteachers regarding the management of TDIs [38]. As our results showed, most of the trauma happened at home and school; public health care services, as well as primary and preschools, could be the target of educational campaigns directed at parents/teachers to increase their knowledge and practice in emergency management of TDIs.

5. Conclusion

The prevalence of traumatic dental injuries to the primary anterior teeth among Sudanese preschool children was relatively high (18.5%). Girls being more affected than boys, enamel fracture was the most common type, and maxillary central incisors were the most affected; no association was found between TDI, overbite size, and overjet size.

Acknowledgments

This study was supported by the University of Medical Sciences and Technology, Sudan.

References

[1] A. F. Granville-Garcia, I. T. Vieira, M. J. Siqueira, V. A. de Menezes, and A. L. Cavalcanti, "Traumatic dental injuries and associated factors among Brazilian preschool children aged 1–5 year," *Acta Odontológica Latinoamericana*, vol. 23, no. 1, pp. 47–52, 2010.

[2] T. S. Ain, R. L. Telgi, S. Sultan et al., "Prevalence of traumatic dental injuries to anterior teeth of 12-year-old school children in Kashmir," *Archives of Trauma Research*, vol. 5, no. 1, p. e24596, 2016.

[3] K. P. Bharath, "The reverberations of traumatized primary dentition: a practitioner's perspective," *Journal of Contemporary Dental Practice*, vol. 12, pp. 511–515, 2011.

[4] R. Lam, "Epidemiology and outcomes of traumatic dental injuries: a review of the literature," *Australian Dental Journal*, vol. 61, no. 1, pp. 4–20, 2016.

[5] M. Vuletić, J. Škaričić, G. Batinjan, Z. Trampuš, I. Bagić, and H. Hrvoje Jurić, "A retrospective study on traumatic dental and soft-tissue injuries in preschool children in Zagreb," *Bosnian Journal of Basic Medical Sciences*, vol. 14, no. 1, pp. 12–15, 2014.

[6] H. C. Gungor, "Management of crown-related fractures in children: an update review," *Dental Traumatology*, vol. 30, no. 2, pp. 88–99, 2013.

[7] M. B. Siqueira, M. C. Gomes, A. C. Oliveira, C. C. Martins, A. F. Granville-Garcia, and S. M. Paiva, "Predisposing factors for traumatic dental injury in primary teeth and seeking of post-trauma care," *Brazilian Dental Journal*, vol. 24, no. 6, pp. 647–654, 2013.

[8] K. Garg, N. Kalra, R. Tyagi, A. Khatri, and G. Panwar, "An appraisal of the prevalence and attributes of traumatic dental injuries in the permanent anterior teeth among 7–14-year-old schoolchildren of North East Delhi," *Contemporary Clinical Dentistry*, vol. 8, no. 2, pp. 218–224, 2017.

[9] M. Ranka, H. Dhaliwal, S. Albadri, and C. Brown, "Trauma to the primary dentition and its sequelae," *Dental Update*, vol. 40, no. 7, pp. 534–543, 2013.

[10] M. Fontenele, M. Macedo, P. Reboucas et al., "Sequelae in primary teeth after traumatic injury," *Brazilian Dental Science*, vol. 20, no. 2, pp. 70–75, 2017.

[11] R. R. Kalaskar, A. R. Kalaskar, R. M. Wankhade, and J. D. Mehta, "Evaluation of prevalence, etiological and risk factors of traumatic dental injury in 12–14 years old school going children of central India," *SRM Journal of Research in Dental Sciences*, vol. 5, no. 2, pp. 73–77, 2014.

[12] M. L. Goettems, L. C. Brancher, C. T. Costa, M. L. Bonow, and A. R. Romano, "Does dental trauma in the primary dentition increases the likelihood of trauma in the permanent dentition? A longitudinal study," *Clinical Oral Investigations*, vol. 21, no. 8, pp. 2415–2420, 2017.

[13] S. Petti, U. Glendor, and L. Andersson, "World traumatic dental injury prevalence and incidence, a meta-analysis–one billion living people have had traumatic dental injuries," *Dental Traumatology*, vol. 34, no. 2, pp. 71–86, 2018.

[14] B. R. Kirkwood and J. A. C. Sterne, *Essentials of Medical Statistics*, John Wiley & Sons, Hoboken, NJ, USA, 2010.

[15] J. O. Andreasen, E. Lauridsen, T. A. Gerds, and S. S. Ahrensburg, "Dental trauma guide: a source of evidence based treatment guidelines for dental trauma," *Dental Traumatology*, vol. 28, no. 5, pp. 345–350, 2012.

[16] J. O. Andreasen, F. Andreasen, and L. Andersson, *Textbook and Color Atlas of Traumatic Injuries to the Teeth*, Blackwell, Oxford, UK, 4th edition, 2007.

[17] M. Shekhar and R. Mohan, "Traumatic dental injuries to primary incisors and the terminal or occlusal plane relationship in Indian preschool children," *Community Dental Health Journal*, vol. 28, no. 1, pp. 104–106, 2011.

[18] L. A. Antunes, I. F. Gomes, M. H. Almeida, E. A. Silva, J. D. Calasans-Maia, and L. S. Antunes, "Increased overjet is a risk factor for dental trauma in preschool children," *Indian Journal of Dental Research*, vol. 26, no. 4, pp. 356–360, 2015.

[19] N. Singh, A. Singh, and M. S. Jolly, "Prevalence of traumatic dental injuries in school going children of Lucknow, India," *International Journal of Oral Health and Medical Research*, vol. 2, no. 2, pp. 39–42, 2015.

[20] G. N. Chowdary, R. Hemalatha, R. Vijayakumar, R. Ganesh, H. Selvakumar, and S. Mangaiyarkarasi, "Prevalence of traumatic dental injuries in primary teeth: a retrospective study," *SRM Journal of Research in Dental Sciences*, vol. 5, no. 1, pp. 11–13, 2014.

[21] B. Carvalho, C. Franca, M. Heimer, S. Vieira, and V. Colares, "Prevalence of dental trauma among 6-7-yearold children in the city of recife, PE, Brazil," *Brazilian Journal of Oral Sciences*, vol. 11, no. 1, pp. 72–75, 2012.

[22] M. A. De Jesus, L. A. A. Antunes, P. A. Risso, M. V. Freire, and L. C. Maia, "Epidemiologic survey of traumatic dental injuries in children seen at the Federal University of Rio de Janeiro, Brazil," *Brazilian Oral Research*, vol. 24, no. 1, pp. 89–94, 2010.

[23] B. Rai, M. Madan, R. Jain, and S. C. Anand, "Traumatic teeth in 2 to 10 years: in tertiary dental care centre," *Internet Journal of Dental Science*, vol. 4, no. 2, 2007.

[24] M. J. C. Rocha and M. Cardoso, "Traumatized permanent teeth in Brazilian children assisted at the Federal University of Santa Catarina, Brazil," *Dental Traumatology*, vol. 17, no. 6, pp. 245–249, 2001.

[25] V. P. Chalissery, N. Marwah, M. Jafer, E. P. Chalisserry, T. Bhatt, and S. Anil, "Prevalence of anterior dental trauma and its associated factors among children aged 3–5 years in Jaipur City, India-a cross sectional study," *Journal of International Society of Preventive and Community Dentistry*, vol. 6, no. 7, pp. S35–S40, 2016.

[26] A. Rouhani, T. Movahhed, J. Ghoddusi, Y. Mohiti, E. Banihashemi, and M. Akbari, "Anterior traumatic dental injuries in east Iranian school children: prevalence and risk factors," *Iranian Endodontic Journal*, vol. 10, no. 1, pp. 35–38, 2015.

[27] M. E. Sari, B. Ozmen, A. E. Koyuturk, U. Tokay, P. Kasap, and D. Guler, "A retrospective evaluation of traumatic dental injury in children who applied to the dental hospital, Turkey," *Nigerian Journal of Clinical Practice*, vol. 17, no. 5, p. 644, 2014.

[28] J. A. Díaz, L. Bustos, A. C. Brandt, and B. E. Fernández, "Dental injuries among children and adolescents aged 1–15 years attending to public hospital in Temuco, Chile," *Dental Traumatology*, vol. 26, no. 3, pp. 254–261, 2010.

[29] L. R. da Silva Assunção, A. Ferelle, M. L. Iwakura, L. S. do Nascimento, and R. F. Cunha, "Luxation injuries in primary teeth: a retrospective study in children assisted at an emergency service," *Brazilian Oral Research*, vol. 25, no. 2, pp. 150–156, 2011.

[30] V. S. Baghdady, L. J. Ghose, and H. Enke, "Traumatic anterior teeth in Iraqi and Sudanese children–a comparative study," *Journal of Dental Research*, vol. 60, no. 3, pp. 677–680, 1981.

[31] J. Vejdani, S. fathollah, and E. Leyli, "Prevalence of traumatic injuries to the anterior primary teeth in preschool children in Rasht, Guilan, 2012," *Journal of Dentomaxillofacial Radiology, Pathology and Surgery*, vol. 2, no. 4, pp. 23–28, 2014.

[32] D. Lexomboon, C. Carlson, R. Andersson, I. Bultzingslowen, and T. Mensah, "Incidence and causes of dental trauma in children living in the county of Varmland, Sweden," *Dental Traumatology*, vol. 32, no. 1, pp. 58–64, 2016.

[33] B. Agostini, L. Pinto, M. Koehler, B. Emmanulli, C. Piovesan, and T. Ardenghi, "Trend of traumatic crown injuries and associated factors in preschool children," *Brazilian Oral Research*, vol. 30, no. 1, p. e112, 2016.

[34] M. C. Patel and S. G. Sujan, "The prevalence of traumatic dental injuries to permanent anterior teeth and its relation with predisposing risk factors among 8–13 years' school children of Vadodara city: an epidemiological study," *Journal of Indian Society of Pedodontics and Preventive Dentistry*, vol. 30, no. 2, pp. 151–157, 2012.

[35] R. Firmino, M. Siqueira, R. Vieira-Andrade et al., "Prediction factors for failure to seek treatment following traumatic dental injuries to primary teeth," *Brazilian Oral Research*, vol. 28, no. 1, pp. 1–7, 2014.

[36] N. De Paiva, C. Paiva, J. De Paula Silva et al., "Is there an association between traumatic dental injury and social capital, being drinking and socioeconomic indicators among schoolchildren?," *PLoS One*, vol. 10, article e0118484, 2015.

[37] P. F. Kramer, J. Onetto, M. T. Flores, T. S. Borges, and C. A. Feldens, "Traumatic dental injuries in the primary dentition: a 15-year bibliometric analysis of dental traumatology," *Dental Traumatology*, vol. 32, no. 5, pp. 341–346, 2016.

[38] M. A. Awad, E. AlHammadi, M. Malalla et al., "Assessment of elementary school teachers' level of knowledge and attitude regarding traumatic dental injuries in the United Arab Emirates," *International Journal of Dentistry*, vol. 2017, Article ID 1025324, 7 pages, 2017.

6

Fracture Resistance of Ceramic Laminate Veneers Bonded to Teeth with Class V Composite Fillings after Cyclic Loading

Leyla Sadighpour,[1] Farideh Geramipanah,[2] Vanya Rasaei,[1] and Mohammad J. Kharazi Fard[3]

[1]*Department of Prosthodontics, Faculty of Dentistry, Tehran University of Medical Sciences, Tehran, Iran*
[2]*Dental Implant Research Center, Faculty of Dentistry, Tehran University of Medical Sciences, Tehran, Iran*
[3]*Dental Research Center, Faculty of Dentistry, Tehran University of Medical Sciences, Tehran, Iran*

Correspondence should be addressed to Farideh Geramipanah; geramipa@tums.ac.ir

Academic Editor: Ali I. Abdalla

Purpose. Porcelain laminate veneers (PLVs) are sometimes required to be used for teeth with composite fillings. This study examined the fracture strength of PLVs bonded to the teeth restored with different sizes of class V composite fillings. *Materials and Methods.* Thirty-six maxillary central incisors were divided into three groups ($n = 12$): intact teeth (control) and teeth with class V composite fillings of one-third or two-thirds of the crown height (small or large group, resp.). PLVs were made by using IPS e.max and bonded with a resin cement (RelyX Unicem). Fracture resistance (N) was measured after cyclic loading (1×10^6 cycles, 1.2 Hz). For statistical analyses, one-way ANOVA and Tukey test were used ($\alpha = 0.05$). *Results.* There was a significant difference between the mean failure loads of the test groups ($P = 0.004$), with the Tukey-HSD test showing lower failure loads in the large-composite group compared to the control ($P = 0.02$) or small group ($P = 0.05$). The control and small-composite groups achieved comparable results ($P > 0.05$). *Conclusions.* Failure loads of PLVs bonded to intact teeth and to teeth with small class V composite fillings were not significantly different. However, extensive composite fillings could compromise the bonding of PLVs.

1. Introduction

Porcelain laminate veneers (PLVs) represent an excellent treatment option for restoring aesthetics while preserving the integrity of the remaining tooth structure. Its clinical acceptance is mainly due to minimal preparation, successful clinical outcomes, and high patient satisfaction [1]. The estimated survival rate of PLVs has been reported to be 94.4% after five years and 93.8% after 10 years [2]. The most frequent causes of failure, including microleakage, debonding, and fracture, are related to the quality of the bonding surface and the choice of the luting agent [3, 4]. Because the retention of PLVs relies solely on the bond to the tooth structure, the availability of sufficient enamel has been considered as a critical factor for its long-term success [5]. For a predictable result, it is recommended that at least 50% of the labial enamel or intraenamel margins be present [6, 7]. The amount of enamel may be compromised by several factors, such as fracture, wear, and preparation of various types of restorations, including composite fillings [8–10]. Even standard preparations for PLVs could result in serious enamel damage. Various preparation techniques could compromise 30% to 50% of the labial surface enamel, leading to dentin exposure [11, 12].

Patients commonly seek esthetic treatment for discoloured or aged composite fillings [7, 13]. One study on the clinical performance of PLVs showed that 70% of patients had previous composite fillings [2]. Under such circumstances, some clinicians believe that the preparation margins should be extended to sound enamel, far to the interproximal or even to the lingual enamel, to create intraenamel margins [7, 8]. Findings from several clinical studies support this approach. For example, higher failure rates were observed when laminate veneers were bonded to large-composite fillings [2, 3]. A reliable bonding could be achieved with greater quantities of enamel surface and margins.

However, this process compromises excess dental hard tissue [13, 14].

An alternative approach is to bond PLV onto an acceptable composite filling [15, 16]. Gurel et al. [12] found no relation between the existing restorations and PLV failure. Similarly, Gresnigt et al. [17] found no significant difference in the 40-month clinical performances of PLVs bonded to teeth with and without existing composite fillings. Moreover, the overall survival rate remained high, at 94.6%. Although the available literature suggests that the size, age, and location of composite fillings are among the factors that may influence the failure rate of PLVs bonded to existing restorations, these factors have not been clearly identified over literature. Quantifying the amount of enamel that can be replaced by composite fillings without affecting the fracture resistance may improve our clinical decision-making. Few investigations have been conducted with a focus on the performance of PLVs when bonded to composite fillings with defined dimensions [16–18]. In an in vitro study, Sadighpour et al. [18] found that fracture resistance of PLVs bonded to intact teeth or teeth with a classic class III composite filling was similar. In addition, fracture resistance decreased and microleakage of PLVs increased when the composite fillings were removed and replaced by veneers. Class V composite fillings could differ from class III fillings in location, size, and stress patterns [19]. Furthermore, a typical class V cavity could compromise a greater amount of labial enamel than either a class III or IV cavity that has not been investigated.

In the light of this background, the aim of the present study was to examine the fracture strength of PLVs bonded to teeth restored with different sizes of class V composite fillings. The null hypothesis was that the fracture strength of teeth restored with PLVs would not be affected by the presence of class V composite fillings of different sizes.

2. Materials and Method

The sample for this study included 36 human maxillary central incisors that had been extracted from adults within the past three months due to periodontal problems. All patients provided informed consent for extraction and subsequent use of their teeth for experimental study, according to the protocol of the Clinical Research Ethics Board at Tehran University of Medical Sciences. Only teeth with no caries, cracks, or excessive wear were included in the study.

Teeth were cleaned of tissue tags and debris by using a hand instrument and were stored in 1% chloramine for two weeks and then in distilled water until use. The teeth fell into three groups based on the labial surface area (65 ± 5 mm, 75 ± 5 mm, and 85 ± 5 mm).

Teeth from each size group were randomly assigned to three groups: control (NC) (intact with no composite fillings), small-composite (SC), and large-composite (LC) ($n = 12$).

In the NC group, the incisal edges were reduced by 1 mm. Three orientation grooves were made on the labial surface by a 0.3 mm cutting-depth diamond bur (868B.314.018, Komet

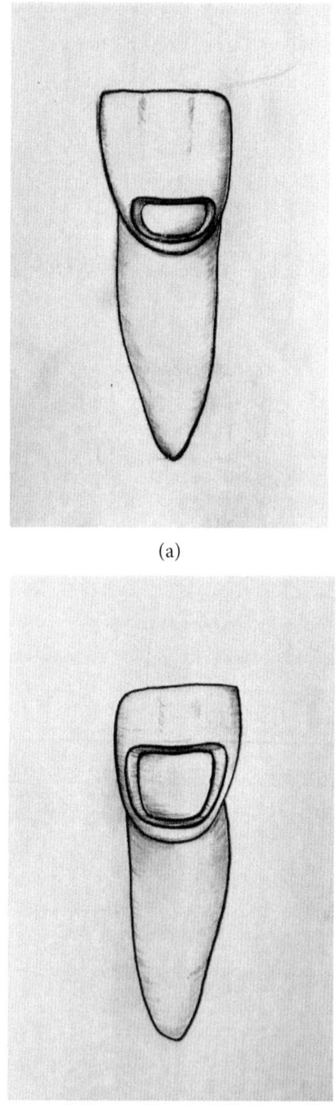

(a)

(b)

FIGURE 1: (a) Representative of a small class V cavity (b) and large class V cavity.

Dental, Lemgo, Germany) and were joined together by a round-end diamond bur (868.018, Komet Dental). Cervical finish lines were ended 1 mm above the cementoenamel junction (CEJ) to ensure intraenamel margins. Proximally, the reduction was extended by 1 mm toward the lingual surface. All line angles were rounded, and the margins were finished.

In SC and LC groups, a class V cavity at one-third or two-thirds of the crown height, respectively, was prepared for composite filling. Each cavity was 1 mm short of the proximal finish line and 2 mm short of the CEJ, Figure 1. Autopolymerised acrylic resin (GC Pattern Resin, GC America Inc., Alsip, IL, USA) was used in one cavity each from the SC and LC groups to fabricate a template for the remaining teeth, Figure 2. Cavities were etched for 15 s with 38% phosphoric acid (Etching Gel, Faghihi Dental Co., Tehran, Iran), rinsed for 15 s, and then gently air dried.

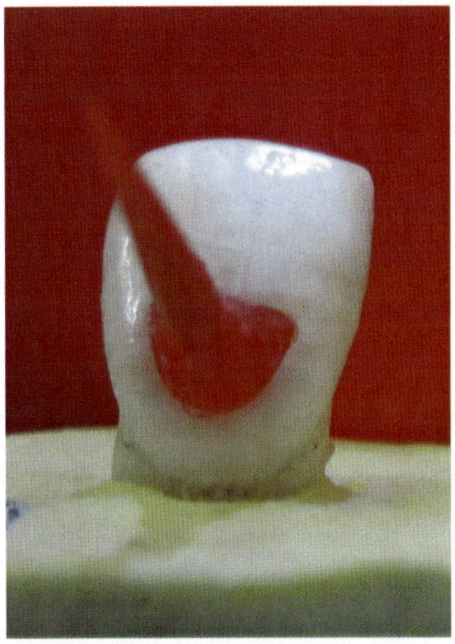

FIGURE 2: Resin template for guiding the cavity preparation.

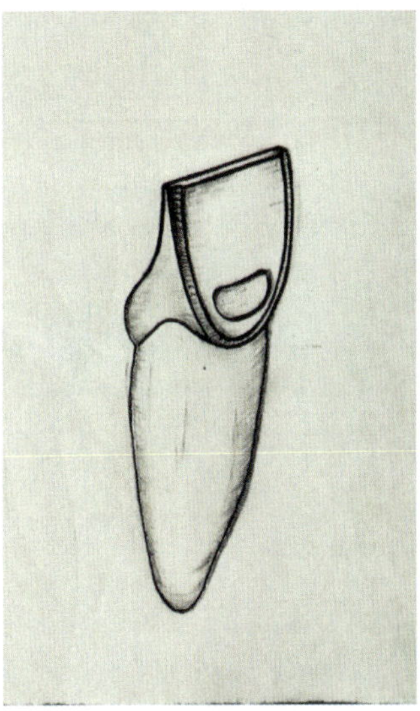

FIGURE 3: Schematic representation of final preparation.

An etch-and-rinse dentin bonding agent (Single Bond, 3M ESPE, MN, USA) was applied for 30s and light polymerised (Bluephase 16i, Ivoclar/Vivadent, Schaan, Liechtenstein) with a 5 s burst at 1100 mW/cm^2. Cavities were restored by using a universal microhybrid composite resin (Filtek Z250, 3M ESPE), which was inserted in two layers and light polymerised with an LED light unit (Bluphase 16i). Teeth were prepared for PLV in a similar way as in the NC group, Figure 3. Specimens were stored in water at room temperature of 25°C for three weeks before receiving veneers. A custom tray was fabricated with autopolymerising acrylic resin (Tray Material, Major, Moncalieri, Italy) for each specimen. Impressions were made by a polyvinyl siloxane material (Monopren, Kettenbach GmbH, Eschenburg, Germany) and poured with type IV dental stones (Fuji Rock, GC Corp., Tokyo, Japan). PLVs were fabricated with a lithium disilicate ceramic (IPS e.max Press, Ivoclar/Vivadent) using the lost-wax technique. Wax patterns were fabricated at a uniform thickness of 0.7 mm, sprued with four patterns per cylinder, invested with a phosphate-bound investment (IPS Pres/Vest, Vivadent/Ivoclar), and burned out in a conventional porcelain-firing furnace (Vaccumat 300, Vita, Zahnfabrik H. Rauter GmbH, Bad Sackingen, Germany) at 850°C. Low-translucency ceramic ingots in shade A2 were pressed in a Programat furnace (Ivoclar/Vivadent) at 1050°C. Molds were divested by using 50 μm aluminium oxide air particles at 0.4 MPa and a distance of 10 mm for 5 s and then cleaned in an ultrasonic cleaner (Prosonic 300, Sultan Health Care, Englewood, NJ, USA).

PLVs on teeth were investigated for any cracks or flaws under 5x magnification, and the fit was examined on the corresponding dies. PLVs were glazed (IPS e.max Ceram Glaze, Vivadent/Ivoclar) in a conventional porcelain-firing furnace (Vacumat 300) at 750°C. PLVs were etched with 9.5% hydrofluoric acid (Porcelain Etchant, Bisco Inc., Schaumburg, IL, USA) for 90s, cleaned under water for 30 s and then silanized (Monobond S, Vivadent/Ivoclar). Enamel surfaces and margins were etched by 37% phosphoric acid (Etching Gel) for 15 s and washed for 15 s. A self-adhesive resin cement (RelyX Unicem, Automix, 3M/ESPE, St Paul, MN, USA) was applied on the bonding surface of veneers and then seated on the tooth surface and held in place with finger pressure for 10 s. The excess cement was removed by a scalpel blade. Light polymerisation (Bluephase 16i, Vivadent/Ivoclar) was performed for 10 s. The specimens were stored for 24 h in water at room temperature before being subjected to thermal cycling (2000 thermal cycles between 5°C and 55°C, with a dwell time of 30 s in each bath and a transfer time of 10 s). The periodontal ligament was simulated with polyether elastomer (Impergum F, 3M/ESPE) on the roots of the teeth before being mounted on a chewing simulator. Specimens were mounted at 135° with the contact point on the cingulum. To simulate three years of service, specimens were subjected to 1.2×10^6 cycles of 50 N loads at a frequency of 2 Hz.

Fracture resistance was measured by applying a static load to the specimens until fracture using a universal testing machine (Zwick Roell Z050, Ulm, Germany). A compressive load was applied at 1 mm/min to the incisal edge of the specimens with a stainless-steel sphere, 8 mm in diameter, and a thin sheet in between the contact points. The fracture load was automatically recorded as the fracture resistance of each PLV.

The failure mode was examined with a stereomicroscope (Zeiss OPM1, Carl Zeiss, Oberkochen, Germany) at a magnification of ×20. The failure mode was categorised as adhesive (failure between the tooth and laminate), cohesive (failure within the laminate or tooth), or mixed. The homogeneity of variances and normal distribution of data were verified by Levene's test and the Kolmogorov–Smirnov test, respectively. Then, the mean values of fracture resistance were statistically analysed by one-way ANOVA and Tukey-HSD post hoc using SPSS (SPSS Inc., Chicago, IL, USA) at a significance level of 95% ($\alpha = 0.05$).

3. Results

During cyclic loading, one specimen each in the NC and SC groups and two specimens in the LC group were lost due to

Table 1: The descriptive data for failure load values of test groups.

Test group	Number	Mean (N)	Standard deviation (N)	Min. (N)	Max. (N)	95% confidence interval	
						Lower bound	Upper bound
NC	11	364.28[a]	114.88	219.30	616.50	−296.46	432.10
SC	11	324.57[a]	89.25	220.10	471.4	−271.88	377.53
LC	10	207.26[b]	90.62	110.10	369.00	−151.05	263.47

Items in the rows with dissimilar letters are significantly different at 95% level of confidence; [a]values are nonsignificantly different at $P = 0.81$; [b]value is significantly different at $P = 0.004$.

Table 2: Failure modes of broken specimens.

Group	Cohesive fracture in tooth	Cohesive fracture in laminate	Adhesive	Mixed cohesive and adhesive
Control	5	1	0	5
SC	4	0	3	4
LC	1	0	5	4
Total	10	1	8	13

fracture. Fracture value for the lost specimens was set to zero.

The descriptive data of fracture resistance are summarised in Table 1. The mean failure loads were significantly different among the test groups ($P = 0.004$ by one-way ANOVA). Tukey-HSD revealed that the failure load in the LC group was lower than the failure load in the NC or SC group ($P = 0.02$ and 0.05, resp., by Tukey's test). Adhesive failure mode was dominant in the LC group, and cohesive failure occurred more often in the NC and SC groups (Table 2).

4. Discussion

The mean fracture resistance of the PLV-restored teeth with class V composite fillings was examined after cyclic loading. No difference in fracture resistance was found between teeth with composite filling to one-third of the crown height (small-composite group) compared to teeth with an intact labial surface (control). However, the mean fracture resistance was significantly lower in the large-composite group compared to the small-composite or control group. Therefore, the null hypothesis should be partially accepted.

In this study, teeth with 33% of the original enamel remaining (one-third) on the labial surface showed the lowest fracture strength among the groups. Gurel et al. [12] have also emphasised on the role of the remaining enamel on the failure rates of PLVs. They found that PLVs bonded to the dentin had 10 times greater risk of failure than PLVs bonded to the enamel. In contrast, the presence of composite fillings was not correlated with an increased risk of failure, and PLVs bonded to composite fillings had outcomes that were more favourable. However, excessive dentinal exposure, dentinal margins, and the size of composite fillings were not quantified by the authors. Therefore, a direct comparison could not be performed with our study. Contrary to the findings of our study, Gresnigt et al. [17] found that the size of composite fillings did not affect the survival rate of PLVs over a period of 40 months. The size categories in their study were close to those in the small- and large-composite groups of our study. The chairside application of surface silica coating on the resin composite surface before PLV bonding may explain the discrepancy between the studies. Furthermore, the overall follow-up time of their study was short, and most failures occur after years of service [3, 7]. In the present study, fatigue ageing was performed by applying cyclic loading in an attempt to simulate a three-year clinical service.

The luting agent is another contributing factor to the longevity of adhesive restorations [4]. We used a self-adhesive cement, which allows bonding to a range of substrates without pretreatment. The multiple steps of etching, rinsing, and adhesive application are omitted with self-adhesive cement, thereby overcoming the technique and handling errors [20]. Moreover, the setting mechanism of RelyX Unicem self-adhesive cement permits setting with low shrinkage [21]. Contraction during the setting of the resin cement could produce stress within the cement layer, which might induce debonding or cracks in the ceramic over time [22]. However, self-adhesive cement also has some disadvantages, such as lower bond strengths compared to the cement that utilises the etch-and-rinse bonding system. [23]. Nevertheless, in the present study, it was attempted to simulate the worst-case scenario, in that the bond of resin cement to tooth structure was low. Furthermore, for ceramic surface treatment, a protocol was followed that provided a strong bond to ensure no failure from ceramic/cement interface. Therefore, veneers were etched with a 9.5% HF for 90 seconds that has been showed to increase the bond strength of lithium disilicate ceramic to resin cements [24–26].

Regardless of the polymerisation mode, the bonding of resin cement to another resin occurs through a mechanism of free-radical polymerisation and covalent bonding to the organic matrix. However, when a PLV is indicated on a tooth with an old composite filling, the bonding between the resin cement and composite may be compromised due to reduced unreacted monomer because of several degradation processes such as water sorption/solubility, pH action, and mechanical breakdown [27]. The greatest amount of free monomer is present on the surface of a composite filling during the first 24 h after polymerisation and decreases dramatically after one month [15]. In the present study, PLVs were bonded after storage in water for three weeks. Accordingly, minor or no free monomer could be expected on the surface of composite fillings. Unicem contains special methacrylate monomers with bonded phosphoric acid groups with at least two carbon double bonds. It is suggested that the acidic functional monomer in Unicem may ease penetration into the polymeric structure of a composite resin and mediate the acid-base setting reaction with the organic fillers available in the polymer matrix [22]. Simultaneously, radical polymerisation of methacrylate monomers through reactive carbon double bonds promotes copolymerisation with another polymer material [21].

Various surface treatments have been incorporated to improve the bond of new composite resin with an old one including sillicoating, chemical and mechanical roughening, and application of adhesive layers [28, 29]. However, the findings were not consistent. Furthermore, it was shown that the result is highly material-dependent [30]. Therefore, in the present study, the surface of composite fillings was ground using diamond burs, and no further treatment was applied to avoid extra confounding parameters. Surface treatments (e.g., airborne-particle abrasion, acid etching, silanization, and application of a low-viscosity adhesive) might improve the bonding of resin cement to old composites; therewith more favourable outcomes may be expected that could be investigated in future studies.

In the present study, we designed the intraenamel margins to simplify the research parameters. In the clinic, dentinal exposure is inevitable in most PLV preparations, particularly in the cervical area where the enamel is thin (<0.5 mm) [1, 12]. Thus, the effect of the dentinal margin in class V composite fillings should be tested in future studies.

In our study, laminate fracture was rare, and tooth fracture and mixed failure were the two most occurring failure modes in the NC and SC groups (Table 2). It could be argued that in teeth with larger-composite filling (LC), more enamel has been removed, and a decrease in the elastic modulus of the tooth could result in more distortion under loading and an increased rate of debonding. Early debonding may save the LC group from fracture and increase the frequency of adhesive and mixed failure [4, 31]. On the other hand, in the NC and SC groups, adhesive failure was rare. Higher fracture resistance in these groups may imply that the bond strength was high enough to withstand cyclic loading and eventually failure would occur cohesively within the cement layer and/or the tooth itself [4, 13, 14].

This was an in vitro study, and the findings cannot be directly extrapolated to the clinical situation. Nonetheless, several conditions were applied to fit the clinical situation. Thermal cycling and load cycles were applied to simulate certain conditions of real-life restorations. Natural teeth were selected because they have unique properties, such as elasticity, enamel, and dentin bonding properties, as well as a complex geometry of preparation, which may influence the findings of the study. However, we faced obstacles in terms of tooth availability and the standardisation of the tooth size and age. Nevertheless, the results should be regarded with caution as a perfect simulation was not possible. Finally, only one cement type was used in the present study. Further studies involving diverse types of resin cement and composite surface treatments should be performed.

5. Conclusion

Within the limitation of the present study, significantly stronger bonds were achieved in the control and small-composite groups compared to the large-composite group. This result was supported by the prevalence of cohesive failures in the control and small-composite groups. Adhesive failure was predominant in the large-composite group, confirming the weaker bond strength in this group.

Acknowledgments

This research has been supported by the grant no. 21162 from Tehran University of Medical Sciences. The authors are also grateful to Mr. Hassanzadeh for his technical assistance in PLV fabrication.

References

[1] E. Ozturk and S. Bolay, "Survival of porcelain laminate veneers with different degrees of dentin exposure: 2-year clinical results," *Journal of Adhesive Dentistry*, vol. 16, no. 5, pp. 481–489, 2014.

[2] M. Peumans, J. De Munck, S. Fieuws, P. Lambrechts, G. Vanherle, and B. Van Meerbeek, "A prospective ten-year clinical trial of porcelain veneers," *Journal of Adhesive Dentistry*, vol. 6, no. 1, pp. 65–76, 2004.

[3] U. S. Beier, I. Kapferer, D. Burtscher, and H. Dumfahrt, "Clinical performance of porcelain laminate veneers for up to 20 years," *International Journal of Prosthodontics*, vol. 25, no. 1, pp. 79–85, 2012.

[4] H. S. Cotert, M. Dundar, and B. Ozturk, "The effect of various preparation design on the survival of porcelain laminate veneers," *Journal of Adhesive Dentistry*, vol. 11, no. 5, pp. 405–411, 2009.

[5] G. Ibarra, G. H. Johnson, W. Geurtsen, and M. A. Vargas, "Microleakage of porcelain veneer restorations bonded to enamel and dentin with a new self-adhesive resin based dental cement," *Dental Materials*, vol. 23, no. 2, pp. 218–225, 2007.

[6] F. J. T. Burke, "Survival rates for porcelain laminate veneers with special reference to the effect of preparation in dentine: a literature review," *Journal of Esthetic and Restorative Dentistry*, vol. 22, no. 4, pp. 257–265, 2012.

[7] M. Fradeani, M. Redemagni, and M. Corrado, "Porcelain laminate veneers: 6- to 12-year clinical evaluation—a retrospective study," *International Journal of Periodontics and Restorative Dentistry*, vol. 25, no. 1, pp. 9–17, 2005.

[8] A. C. Kasaz, C. E. Pena, R. S. de Alexandre et al., "Effects of a peripheral enamel margin on the long-term bond strength and nano leakage of a composite/dentin interface produced by self-adhesive and conventional resin cements," *Journal of Adhesive Dentistry*, vol. 14, no. 3, pp. 251–263, 2012.

[9] K. K. Schmidt, Y. Chiayabutr, K. M. Phillips, and J. C. Kois, "Influence of preparation design and existing condition of tooth structure on load to failure of ceramic laminate veneers," *Journal of Prosthetic Dentistry*, vol. 105, no. 6, pp. 374–382, 2011.

[10] G. Batalocco, H. Lee, C. Ercoli, C. Feng, and H. Malmstrom, "Fracture resistance of composite resin restorations and

porcelain veneers in relation to residual tooth structure in fractured incisors," *Dental Traumatology*, vol. 28, no. 1, pp. 75–80, 2012.

[11] G. P. Cherukara, G. R. Davis, K. G. Seymour, L. Zou, and D. Y. Samarawichrama, "Dentin exposure in tooth preparation for porcelain veneers: a pilot study," *Journal of Prosthetic Dentistry*, vol. 94, no. 5, pp. 414–420, 2005.

[12] G. Gurel, N. Sesma, M. A. Calamita, C. Coachman, and S. Morimoto, "Influence of enamel preservation on failure rates of porcelain laminate veneers," *International Journal of Periodontics and Restorative Dentistry*, vol. 33, no. 1, pp. 31–39, 2013.

[13] Y. P. Chun, C. Raffelt, H. Pfeiffer et al., "Restoring strength of incisors with veneers and full ceramic crowns," *Journal of Adhesive Dentistry*, vol. 12, no. 1, pp. 45–54, 2010.

[14] M. Ozcan and A. Mese, "Fracture strength of indirect resin composite laminates to teeth with existing restorations: an evaluation of conditioning protocols," *Journal of Adhesive Dentistry*, vol. 11, no. 5, pp. 391–397, 2009.

[15] C. Maneenut, R. Sakoolnamarka, and J. M. J. Tyas, "The repair potential of resin composite materials," *Dental Materials*, vol. 27, no. 2, pp. e20–e27, 2011.

[16] M. M. Grestnigt, M. Ozcan, W. Kalk, and G. Galhano, "Effect of static and cyclic loading on ceramic laminate veneers adhered to teeth with and without aged composite restorations," *Journal of Adhesive Dentistry*, vol. 13, no. 6, pp. 567–579, 2011.

[17] M. M. Gresnigt, W. Kalk, and M. Ozcan, "Clinical longevity of ceramic laminate veneers bonded to teeth with and without existing composite restorations up to 40 months," *Clinical Oral Investigations*, vol. 17, no. 3, pp. 823–832, 2012.

[18] L. Sadighpour, F. Geramipanah, S. Allahyari, B. Fallahi Sichani, and M. J. Kharazi Fard, "In vitro evaluation of the fracture resistance and microleakage of porcelain laminate veneers bonded to teeth with composite fillings after cyclic loading," *Journal of Advanced Prosthodontics*, vol. 6, no. 4, pp. 278–294, 2014.

[19] J. S. Rees and P. H. Jacobsen, "The effect of interfacial failure around a class V composite restoration analyzed by the finite element method," *Journal of Oral Rehabilitation*, vol. 27, no. 2, pp. 111–116, 2000.

[20] E. Ozturk, S. Bolay, R. Hickel, and N. Ilie, "Shear bond strength of porcelain laminate veneers to enamel, dentin and enamel-dentin complex bonded with different adhesive luting systems," *Journal of Dentistry*, vol. 41, no. 2, pp. 97–105, 2013.

[21] J. L. Ferracane, J. W. Stansbury, and F. J. Burke, "Self-adhesive resin cements: chemistry, properties and clinical considerations," *Journal of Oral Rehabilitation*, vol. 38, no. 4, pp. 295–314, 2011.

[22] H. U. V. Gerth, T. Dammaschke, H. Zuchner, and E. Schafer, "Chemical analysis and bonding reaction of RelyX Unicem and Bifix composites- a comparative study," *Dental Materials*, vol. 22, no. 10, pp. 934–941, 2006.

[23] C. Holderegger, I. Sailer, C. Schumacher, R. Schlapfer, C. Hammerle, and J. Fischer, "Shear bond strength of resin cements to human dentin," *Dental Materials*, vol. 24, no. 7, pp. 944–950, 2008.

[24] J. Puppin-Ronrni, D. Sundfeld, A. R. Costa et al., "Effect of hydrofluoric acid concentration and etching time on bond strength of lithium disilicate glass ceramic," *Operative Dentistry*, vol. 42, no. 6, pp. 606–615, 2017.

[25] D. Sundfel Neto, L. Z. Naves, A. R. Costa et al., "The effect of hydrofluoric acid concentration on the bond strength and morphology of the surface and interface of glass ceramics to a resin cement," *Operative Dentistry*, vol. 40, no. 5, pp. 470–479, 2015.

[26] V. K. Kalavacharla, N. C. Lawson, L. C. Ramp, and J. O. Burgess, "Influence of etching protocol and silane treatment with a universal adhesive on lithium disilicate bond strength," *Operative Dentistry*, vol. 40, no. 4, pp. 372–378, 2015.

[27] J. Brendeke and M. Ozcan, "Effect of physiochemical aging conditions on the composite-composite repair bond strength," *Journal of Adhesive Dentistry*, vol. 9, no. 4, pp. 399–408, 2007.

[28] C. Cotes, M. Cardoso, R. M. Melo, L. F. Valandro, and M. A. Bottino, "Effect of composite surface treatment and aging on the bond strength between a core build-up composite and a luting agent," *Journal of Applied Oral Science*, vol. 23, no. 1, pp. 71–78, 2015.

[29] M. Ozcan and G. Pekkan, "Effect of different adhesion strategies on bond strength of resin composite to composite-dentin complex," *Operative Dentistry*, vol. 38, no. 1, pp. 63–72, 2013.

[30] M. Rinastiti, M. Ozcan, W. Siswomihardjo, and H. J. Busscher, "Effect of surface conditioning on repair bond strengths of non-aged and aged microhybrid, nanohybrid, and nanofilled composite resins," *Clinical Oral Investigations*, vol. 15, no. 5, pp. 625–633, 2011.

[31] K. J. Chun, H. H. Choi, and J. Y. Lee, "Comparison of mechanical property and role between enamel and dentin in the human teeth," *Journal of Dental Biomechanics*, vol. 5, pp. 1–7, 2014.

7

Comparison of Oral Microbe Quantities from Tongue Samples and Subgingival Pockets

André Göhler,[1,2] **Stefanie Samietz**,[3] **Carsten Oliver Schmidt**,[4] **Thomas Kocher**,[5] **Ivo Steinmetz**,[1,2] **and Birte Holtfreter**[5]

[1]*Friedrich Loeffler Institute of Medical Microbiology, University Medicine Greifswald, Greifswald, Germany*
[2]*Institute for Hygiene, Microbiology and Environmental Medicine, Medical University of Graz, Graz, Austria*
[3]*Department of Prosthodontics, Gerostomatology and Biomaterials, University Medicine Greifswald, Greifswald, Germany*
[4]*SHIP-Clinical-Epidemiological Research, Institute for Community Medicine, University Medicine Greifswald, Greifswald, Germany*
[5]*Department of Restorative Dentistry, Periodontology, Endodontology, and Preventive and Pediatric Dentistry, University Medicine Greifswald, Greifswald, Germany*

Correspondence should be addressed to Birte Holtfreter; birte.holtfreter@uni-greifswald.de

Academic Editor: Izzet Yavuz

Objectives. To improve understanding of periodontitis pathology, we need more profound knowledge of relative abundances of single prokaryotic species and colonization dynamics between habitats. Thus, we quantified oral microbes from two oral habitats to gain insights into colonization variability and correlation to the clinical periodontal status. *Methods.* We analyzed tongue scrapings and subgingival pocket samples from 237 subjects (35–54 years) with at least 10 teeth and no recent periodontal treatment from the 11-year follow-up of the Study of Health in Pomerania. Relative abundances of *Porphyromonas gingivalis*, *Aggregatibacter actinomycetemcomitans*, *Fusobacterium nucleatum*, *Streptococcus sanguinis*, total bacteria, and *Archaea* were correlated to clinically assessed pocket depths (PD) and clinical attachment levels (CAL). *Results.* Increased relative abundances of *P. gingivalis*, *A. actinomycetemcomitans*, and *F. nucleatum* were linked to increased levels of PD and CAL (i) on the subject level (mean PD, mean CAL) and (ii) in subgingival pockets. Relative abundances of *Archaea* from tongue samples correlated negatively with mean PD or mean CAL. Detection and quantity of bacterial species correlated weakly to moderately between the tongue and subgingival pocket, except for *Archaea*. *Conclusions.* Relative abundances of specific oral species correlated weakly to moderately between habitats. Single species, total bacteria, and *Archaea* were linked to clinically assessed severity of periodontitis in a habitat-dependent manner.

1. Introduction

Various microorganisms colonize oral habitats [1–4]. Each habitat appears to be preferentially populated by different and somewhat unique sets of microbes, whereas in periodontal disease the microbial profile in the subgingival pocket seems to narrow [5]. Periodontitis-associated microorganisms colonize not only subgingival pockets but also other habitats like the tongue dorsum. It harbors species such as *Fusobacterium* and *Porphyromonas* [6, 7] and further acts as a reservoir for recolonization of periodontal pockets after periodontal therapy [8, 9]. This raises the question whether the occurrence and proportion (relative abundance) of different taxa might affect the microbial interplay in the oral cavity. However, comparing the distribution and quantity of single prokaryotic species is complicated because of various detection and quantification methods [9–13]. In a recent study, we used qPCR for quantification of a single species [7], serving as representatives for different stages of oral biofilm formation [9, 14, 15].

Information about *Archaea* in context with periodontitis is rare. According to the published literature, they were detected in periodontally diseased but not in healthy gingival sulci [16–20]. In contrast, we detected archaeal 16S rRNA sequences from tongue scrapings in healthy and periodontally diseased subjects in a previous study [7]. However, other recent studies showed that methanogens were enriched in chronic periodontitis and drive periodontitis due to their metabolic capacity [21, 22].

While our previous study clearly demonstrated the advantage of using bacterial relative abundance levels, it did not compare bacterial colonization patterns between the tongue and the subgingival pocket habitat, considering also the clinical periodontal status [7]. Therefore, we aimed at describing the relation between the relative abundance of four oral microbes (*P. gingivalis*, *A.* actinomycetemcomitans, *F. nucleatum*, and *S. sanguinis*), total bacteria, and *Archaea* in two oral habitats (the tongue dorsum and subgingival pocket) and clinically assessed periodontitis measures in well-characterized study subjects from the 11-year follow-up of the population-based Study of Health in Pomerania (SHIP-2).

2. Materials and Methods

2.1. Study Population. The Study of Health in Pomerania (SHIP) is an ongoing longitudinal cohort study in North-East Germany. Baseline examinations (SHIP-0) were conducted between 1997 and 2001 with 4308 participants [23]. The 11-year follow-up (SHIP-2) included 2333 subjects (2008–2012).

For this study, we considered data of 1560 subjects, for whom data were available until the end of March 2011. Out of this collective, we selected individuals according to the following criteria: 35–54 years of age ($N = 402$ excluded), no periodontal treatment within the last five years ($N = 116$ excluded), complete dental status ($N = 31$ excluded), at least 10 teeth ($N = 309$ excluded), and complete information on further exclusion criteria. Pregnant women ($N = 1$), subjects with diabetes mellitus and increased hemoglobin levels (HbA1c $\geq 6.5\%$) ($N = 14$), and current smokers ($N = 115$) were excluded, leaving 266 individuals. Of those, 237 individuals provided both tongue scrapings and subgingival pocket samples. The study protocol was a priori approved by the local Ethics Committee of the University of Greifswald (Registration Number BB 39/08a). This study was performed in accordance with "Strengthening the Reporting of Observational Studies in Epidemiology" guidelines for human research investigations.

2.2. Covariates. Sociodemographic and behavioral variables were assessed by computer-assisted personal interviews. School education was categorized as <10, 10, and >10 years. Smoking status was defined as never, former, and current smoking. We defined diabetes mellitus as a self-reported physician's diagnosis or intake of antidiabetic medication (Anatomical Therapeutic Chemical (ATC) A10). Body height and weight were determined using calibrated scales. The body mass index (BMI) was calculated and categorized as <25, 25–<30, and $\geq 30\,kg/m^2$.

2.3. Dental Examination. Periodontal examinations comprised probing depths (PD) and clinical attachment levels (CAL). Measurements were assessed at four sites per tooth (disto/mid/mesiobuccal and midlingual) according to the half-mouth method, alternating on the left or right side, excluding third molars and using a periodontal probe (PCP-2, Hu-Friedy, USA). CAL was not measured if the determination of the cementoenamel junction was not clear. Teeth were counted excluding third molars. Five certified and licensed dentists conducted examinations. Calibration exercises were performed before and every 6–12 months during the course of the study. Intrarater correlations for CAL measurements were 0.67–0.89, and interrater correlation was 0.70.

2.4. Sample Collection and DNA Isolation. Tongue biofilm was taken from the middle third of the tongue dorsum with a sterile spatula [7]. The spatula was transferred into 2.0 ml of phosphate-buffered saline (PBS). After shaking vigorously for 30 s, the spatula was removed. Microbial suspensions in PBS were kept at −80°C until further processing. After supragingival plaque was removed with a cotton roll, subgingival plaque was collected from the mesiobuccal pocket of the most distally located, clinically examined, upper tooth in the periodontally examined quadrants. Paper points (ISO 35; Roeka, Langenau, Germany) were inserted until the pocket base for 10 seconds. To avoid cross contamination, the sampling site was confined with cotton rolls. Paper points were stored at −80°C. Before DNA extraction, 230 μl of lysis buffer and 20 μl of proteinase K (both MagNA Pure LC DNA Isolation Kit III, Roche, Mannheim, Germany) were added and samples were incubated at 65°C for 10 min and then at 95°C for 10 min. DNA was extracted as described elsewhere [7] and stored at −20°C.

2.5. Oligonucleotides, Plasmid Standards, and Quantitative PCR. Species- and domain-specific primers and probes (MWG-Eurofins, Ebersberg, Germany) applied in the qPCR assays are listed in Supplemental Table 1 and described in detail elsewhere [7]. Plasmid standards contained respective target sequences in a pSC-B-amp/kan vector backbone (Stratagene, La Jolla, USA). The terms "total bacteria" and "*Archaea*" describe the total number of detected bacterial species by using the primers/probes listed in Supplemental Table 1.

The selected oral microbes were quantified using an established qPCR assay [7]. All samples were analyzed in triplicates using a LightCycler 480-II, and C_t was calculated by $\Delta\Delta C_t$ algorithm of the LightCycler 480 Software version 1.5.0 (Roche, Mannheim, Germany). Efficiencies between 1.9 and 2.1 ensured efficient qPCR amplification in all qPCR runs.

2.6. Statistical Analyses. Continuous data are shown as mean ± standard deviation (SD) if normally distributed (assessed by QQ plots) or median (25% quantile, 75% quantile) if nonnormally distributed. Categorical data are presented as numbers (percentages).

We calculated relative abundances for *P. gingivalis*, *F. nucleatum*, *A. actinomycetemcomitans*, and *S. sanguinis* by dividing the single species count by the number of 16S rRNA gene copies per sample. We knew that this method could possibly lead to an underestimation of single species relative abundances, because the estimation models for species counts within a sample are still controversially discussed [24, 25]. The sum score equals the sum of relative abundances for three (putatively) periodontal pathogens (*P. gingivalis*, *A. actinomycetemcomitans*, and *F. nucleatum*).

Relative abundance values were shifted by 1 and then log transformed (retaining distribution values of 0). To compare relative abundances from tongue scrapings across categories of mean PD/CAL, clinical variables were categorized (1st, 2nd + 3rd, and 4th quartile).

To show coherence between relative abundances and periodontal status, bacterial data from tongue samples and subgingival pocket samples were correlated to subject-level periodontal data (mean PD, mean CAL) and to site-specific levels of PD and CAL of the mesiobuccal pocket. To compare relative abundances across quartile-derived categories of mean PD and mean CAL, we applied Mann–Whitney *U* tests.

We used McNemar's test to determine differences in detection rates in tongue and subgingival pocket samples. To assess the magnitude to which reliability estimates might be biased, the Prevalence index (PI; $(a-d)/N$; range −1 to 1) and the Bias index (BI; $(b-c)/N$; range 0 to 1) were calculated. To circumvent problems associated with the use of kappa, the Prevalence and Bias Adjusted Kappa (PABAK) ($2 \cdot p_o - 1$; p_o, observed agreement; range −1 to +1) was calculated [26] to determine the accordance in detection profiles between tongue scraping and the corresponding subgingival pocket sample (gold standard). Moreover, sensitivity and specificity with 95% confidence intervals were calculated. Relative abundances derived from tongue and subgingival pocket samples were correlated using Spearman's correlation coefficient (r_{SP}; 95% confidence interval). All data analyses were performed using Stata/SE 12.0 [27].

3. Results

3.1. Study Population. Participants were 44.1 (SD 5.5) years old, and 42.2% were male (Table 1). Mean PD and mean CAL were 2.41 and 1.92 mm, respectively. The subgingival pocket sample originated from the second molar in 84.0%.

Table 1: Characteristics of study subjects ($N = 237$).

	Mean ± SD or number (%)
Age, years	44.1 ± 5.5
Males	100 (42.2%)
School education	
<10 years	5 (2.1%)
10 years	169 (71.3%)
>10 years	63 (26.6%)
Smoking status	
Never smokers	128 (54.0%)
Former smokers	109 (46.0%)
Body mass index, kg/m^2	
<25	90 (38.0%)
25–<30	97 (40.9%)
≥30	50 (21.1%)
Information on periodontal status on the subject level	
Bleeding on probing, %	20.5 ± 18.1
Mean PD, mm	2.41 ± 0.36
Percentage of sites with PD ≥ 4 mm, %	8.0 ± 10.4
Mean CAL, mm	1.92 ± 0.91
Percentage of sites with CAL ≥ 4 mm, %	11.3 ± 16.3
Tooth count (excluding third molars)	24.8 ± 3.2
Information on-site level	
Tooth position	
3	2 (0.8%)
4	4 (1.7%)
5	10 (4.2%)
6	22 (9.3%)
7	199 (84.0%)
PD, mm ($N = 232$)	
1-2	46 (19.8%)
3	130 (56.0%)
≥4	56 (24.2%)
CAL, mm ($N = 186$)	
0–2	100 (53.8%)
3	38 (20.4%)
≥4	48 (25.8%)

Data are presented as mean ± standard deviation (SD) or numbers (percentages); PD, probing depth; CAL, clinical attachment level.

3.2. Correlation of Relative Abundances on the Tongue with Clinical Periodontal Status. Overall, correlations between relative abundances from tongue samples and clinical variables were weak (Table 2). Relative abundances of *P. gingivalis, A. actinomycetemcomitans, F. nucleatum*, and total bacteria were significantly related to mean CAL with Spearman's correlation coefficients ranging from $r_{sp} = -0.17$ (95% CI: −0.29 to −0.04; $p = 0.009$) for total bacteria to $r_{sp} = 0.26$ (95% CI: 0.14 to 0.38; $p < 0.001$) for *P. gingivalis*. Mean PD levels were weakly correlated to *P. gingivalis* ($r_{sp} = 0.15$; 95% CI: 0.03 to 0.28; $p = 0.02$), *A. actinomycetemcomitans* ($r_{sp} = 0.23$; 95% CI: 0.11 to 0.35; $p < 0.001$), and *F. nucleatum* ($r_{sp} = 0.25$; 95% CI: 0.13 to 0.37; $p < 0.001$).

Relative abundances from tongue samples were unequally distributed across categories of mean PD and mean CAL (Table 3). Relative abundances of *P. gingivalis* ($p = 0.02$), *A. actinomycetemcomitans* ($p = 0.0005$), *F. nucleatum* ($p = 0.0002$), and *Archaea* ($p = 0.04$), % *Archaea* ($p = 0.006$), and the sum score ($p = 0.001$) differed significantly between the 1st and the 4th quartiles of mean PD. Relative abundances of *P. gingivalis* ($p = 0.0001$), *A. actinomycetemcomitans* ($p = 0.005$), *F. nucleatum* ($p = 0.005$), and total bacteria ($p = 0.04$) and the sum score ($p = 0.0001$) differed significantly between the 1st and the 4th quartiles of mean CAL.

3.3. Correlation of Relative Abundances in Pocket Samples with Clinical Periodontal Status. For subgingival pocket samples, relative abundances correlated weakly to CAL and PD levels of respective mesiobuccal sites (Table 4). Except for *S. sanguinis*, all relative abundances showed weak, though

TABLE 2: Spearman's correlation coefficients (r_{SP}; 95% confidence intervals) between clinical periodontal variables and relative abundances from tongue scrapings (on the subject level).

r_{SP} (95% CI)	Tongue scraping	
	Mean CAL (N = 237)	Mean PD (N = 237)
P. gingivalis	0.26 (0.14, 0.38)	0.15 (0.03, 0.28)
A. actinomycetemcomitans	0.24 (0.12, 0.36)	0.23 (0.11, 0.35)
F. nucleatum	0.23 (0.11, 0.35)	0.25 (0.13, 0.37)
S. sanguinis	−0.01 (−0.14, 0.11)	−0.001 (−0.13, 0.13)
Archaea	−0.11 (−0.24, 0.01)	−0.11 (−0.23, 0.02)
% *Archaea*	−0.10 (−0.23, 0.03)	−0.15 (−0.27,−0.02)
Total bacteria	−0.17 (−0.29, −0.04)	−0.08 (−0.20, 0.05)

PD, probing depth; CAL, clinical attachment level; r_{SP}, Spearman's correlation coefficient; 95% CI, 95% confidence interval.

significant, correlations above 0.1 with the mesiobuccal CAL (range 0.15–0.26). Mesiobuccal PD was weakly correlated to *P. gingivalis* relative abundance (r_{sp} = 0.18; 95% CI: 0.05 to 0.30; p = 0.006).

Consistently, the sum score differed significantly comparing pockets with a mesiobuccal PD of ≤2 mm with those with a mesiobuccal PD of ≥4 mm (p = 0.03; Figure 1). Similar findings were found for detections rates (p = 0.046; Supplemental Figure 1) and relative abundances of *P. gingivalis* (p = 0.01) with highest levels found in pockets with a mesiobuccal PD ≥ 4 mm (median relative abundance 6.3×10^{-6} (0; 1.3×10^{-3}); Supplemental Table 3). Across categories of mesiobuccal CAL, significant differences in detection rates were found for *P. gingivalis* (p = 0.03) and *A. actinomycetemcomitans* (p = 0.046). Accordingly, differences in relative abundances were detected for all single species ($p < 0.05$) except *S. sanguinis*, *Archaea*, total bacteria, and the sum score (Supplemental Table 3).

3.4. Detection of Microorganisms in Tongue and Subgingival Pocket Samples. For *P. gingivalis* agreement between the tongue sample and the subgingival pocket sample was 78.5% with a moderate PABAK of 0.570 (Table 5). Among subjects with *P. gingivalis* negative subgingival pocket samples, 89.6% had a negative tongue sample (specificity). Among subjects with *P. gingivalis* positive subgingival pocket samples, 61.3% had a positive tongue sample (sensitivity). *F. nucleatum* was detected three times less often in tongue samples (N = 53) compared to subgingival pocket samples (N = 168). *S. sanguinis* was detected similarly often in both habitats with a high agreement rate (78.5%) and a high specificity (77.7%) and sensitivity (80.9%). For *Archaea*, agreement was 32.1% and PABAK was low (−0.359). Archaeal sequences were found four times more often in tongue samples (N = 173) compared to subgingival pocket samples (N = 40).

It must be mentioned that the PI and the BI were strongly deviating from the Null for *A. actinomycetemcomitans* (PI = 0.565), *F. nucleatum* (BI = 0.485), and *Archaea* (BI = −0.561), indicating some degree of bias, that would have distracted the kappa. Here, the PABAK provides an unbiased estimate of reliability.

Altogether, 16.1% of tongue scrapings but 43.1% of subgingival pocket samples contained at least two of the three (putative) periodontal pathogens (*P. gingivalis*, *A. actinomycetemcomitans*, or *F. nucleatum*). Accordingly, the number of detected pathogens from tongue and subgingival pocket samples correlated weakly (r_{sp} = 0.35; 95% CI: 0.24 to 0.46).

3.5. Correlation between Relative Abundances from Tongue and Subgingival Pocket Samples. Single species and total bacterial relative abundances demonstrated weak to moderate correlations between both habitats (Table 6). Correlations were moderate for relative abundances of *P. gingivalis* (r_{sp} = 0.63; 95% CI: 0.55 to 0.70; $p < 0.001$) and *S. sanguinis* (r_{sp} = 0.56; 95% CI: 0.46 to 0.64; $p < 0.001$) and weak for relative abundances of *A. actinomycetemcomitans* (r_{sp} = 0.16; 95% CI: 0.03 to 0.28; p = 0.02), *F. nucleatum* (r_{sp} = 0.21; 95% CI: 0.09 to 0.33; p = 0.001), and total bacteria (r_{sp} = −0.14; 95% CI: −0.26 to 0.01; p = 0.03). For illustration purposes, we present untransformed relative abundances in Supplemental Table 2. Restricting samples to those with positive relative abundances from tongue scrapings and subgingival pocket samples lead to more than halved correlation coefficients for single species (Supplemental Table 2).

4. Discussion

To elucidate the interplay of prokaryotic colonization in two habitats, we analyzed tongue and subgingival pocket samples from 237 participants of the 11-year follow-up of the population-based SHIP by qPCR. Relative abundances of *P. gingivalis*, *A. actinomycetemcomitans*, and *F. nucleatum* from subgingival pocket samples and tongue samples were linked to corresponding levels of PD and CAL. Quantitative inspection of oral microbes showed weak to moderate correlations in detection and quantity of oral prokaryotes between the tongue and subgingival pocket, though to different degrees depending on the species.

P. gingivalis is commonly regarded as periodontitis related [28, 29]. Forty-six percent of our participants were *P. gingivalis* positive on the tongue and/or in the subgingival pocket, with a significantly higher detection rate (p = 0.003) in the periodontal pocket (39.2%) compared to the tongue (30.4%). For the tongue, this rate was lower than previously described (56.7%) [7]. Furthermore, relative abundances of *P. gingivalis* were significantly higher in subgingival pocket samples compared to tongue samples (Table 6). Further, relative abundances of *P. gingivalis* increased with increasing periodontal breakdown (Supplemental Table 3). In our

Table 3: Levels (median with Q25% and Q75%) of bacterial relative abundances (log10 transformed) from tongue scrapings across categories of mean probing depths (PD) or mean clinical attachment levels (CAL).

	Mean PD			Mean CAL		
	1.56–2.18 mm (n = 59)	2.18–2.61 mm (n = 120)	2.61–3.91 mm (n = 58)	0.13–1.23 mm (n = 60)	1.23–2.54 mm (n = 118)	2.54–4.45 mm (n = 59)
P. gingivalis	0 (0, $5.1 \cdot 10^{-6}$)	0 (0, $8.6 \cdot 10^{-7}$)	0 (0, $2.7 \cdot 10^{-5}$)**	0 (0, 0)	0 (0, $5.8 \cdot 10^{-6}$)*	0 (0, $3.3 \cdot 10^{-5}$)*,**
A. actinomycetemcomitans	0 (0, 0)	0 (0, 0)*	0 (0, $1.3 \cdot 10^{-7}$)*,**	0 (0, 0)	0 (0, 0)	0 (0, $1.5 \cdot 10^{-8}$)*,**
F. nucleatum	0 (0, 0)	0 (0, 0)*	0 (0, $1.6 \cdot 10^{-5}$)*	0 (0, 0)	0 (0, 0)	0 (0, $1.4 \cdot 10^{-5}$)*,**
S. sanguinis	0 (0, $5.2 \cdot 10^{-7}$)	0 (0, $2.3 \cdot 10^{-6}$)	0 (0, $1.6 \cdot 10^{-6}$)	0 (0, $1.5 \cdot 10^{-6}$)	0 (0, $1.7 \cdot 10^{-6}$)	0 (0, $2.1 \cdot 10^{-6}$)
Archaea	2.67 (2.52, 2.80)	2.70 (1.09, 2.84)	2.42 (0.00, 2.79)*,**	2.71 (2.54, 2.83)	2.61 (0.00, 2.80)	2.59 (0.00, 2.87)
% *Archaea*	0.015 (0.008, 0.024)	0.012 (0.002, 0.029)	0.007 (0, 0.019)*,**	0.015 (0.008, 0.027)	0.010 (0, 0.023)	0.010 (0, 0.035)
Total bacteria	6.41 (6.24, 6.63)	6.48 (6.16, 6.74)	6.32 (6.10, 6.70)	6.48 (6.25, 6.66)	6.41 (6.19, 6.72)	6.30 (6.02, 6.66)*
Sum score	0 (0, $7.0 \cdot 10^{-6}$)	0 (0, $9.6 \cdot 10^{-6}$)	$1.0 \cdot 10^{-5}$ (0, $5.5 \cdot 10^{-5}$)*,**	0 (0, $7.0 \cdot 10^{-7}$)	$1.2 \cdot 10^{-7}$ (0, $1.3 \cdot 10^{-5}$)*	$1.3 \cdot 10^{-5}$ (0, $5.9 \cdot 10^{-5}$)*,**

The sum score was defined as the sum of relative abundances for *P. gingivalis* + *A. actinomycetemcomitans* + *F. nucleatum*; groups were determined as follows: 1st quartile, 2nd + 3rd quartile, and 4th quartile; $^{*}p < 0.05$ in Mann–Whitney U tests versus 1st quartile; $^{**}p < 0.05$ in Mann–Whitney U tests versus (2nd + 3rd) quartile.

Table 4: Spearman's correlation coefficients (r_{SP}; 95% confidence intervals) between clinical periodontal variables at the mesiobuccal site and relative abundances from subgingival pockets (site level).

r_{SP} (95% CI)	Subgingival plaque	
	Mesiobuccal CAL (N = 186)	Mesiobuccal PD (N = 232)
P. gingivalis	0.26 (0.12, 0.39)	0.18 (0.05, 0.30)
A. actinomycetemcomitans	0.18 (0.03, 0.31)	0.10 (−0.03, 0.22)
F. nucleatum	0.23 (0.09, 0.36)	0.07 (−0.06, 0.20)
S. sanguinis	0.07 (−0.08, 0.21)	−0.07 (−0.19, 0.06)
Archaea	0.18 (0.04, 0.31)	0.05 (−0.08, 0.18)
% *Archaea*	0.17 (0.02, 0.30)	0.04 (−0.09, 0.17)
Total bacteria	0.15 (0.01, 0.29)	0.12 (−0.01, 0.24)

PD, probing depth; CAL, clinical attachment level; r_{SP}, Spearman's correlation coefficient; 95% CI, 95% confidence interval.

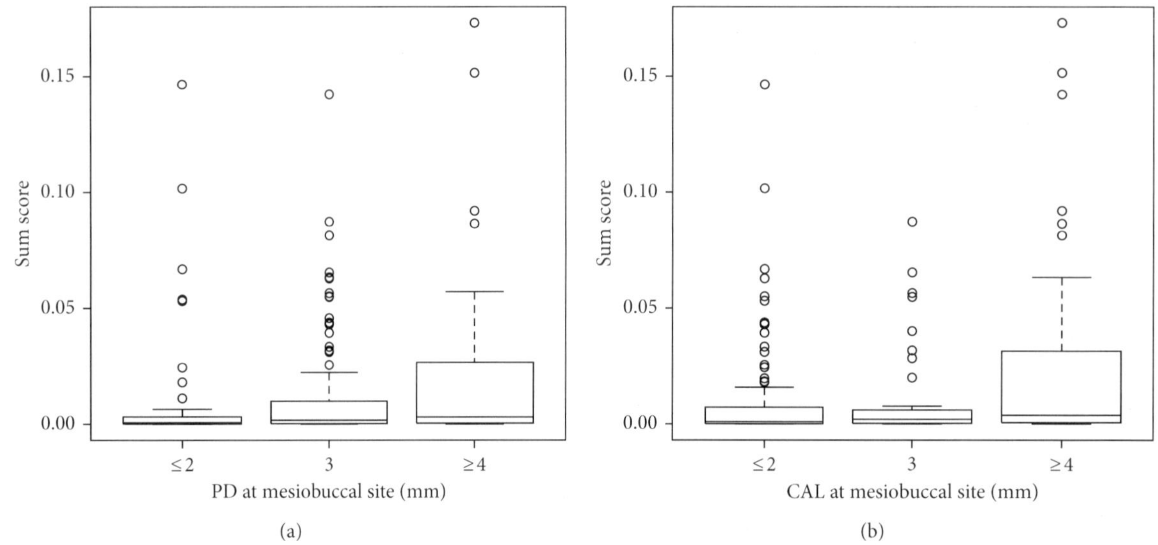

Figure 1: Distribution of the sum score (summed relative abundances of *P. gingivalis*, *A. actinomycetemcomitans*, and *F. nucleatum*) according to probing depth (PD (a)) or clinical attachment level (CAL (b)) at the same mesiobuccal sites.

study, *P. gingivalis* made up to 0.071% of total bacteria (relative abundance) in the subgingival plaque of *P. gingivalis* positive samples (N = 108). In addition, the strong correlation of the relative abundance between tongue and subgingival samples (r_{SP} = 0.63; 95% CI: 0.55 to 0.70) confirms an interaction of these two habitats [30]. Overall, the effect of *P. gingivalis* alone was not prominent; this suggests that an ensemble of different bacteria in the respective oral habitat may determine the periodontal disease severity. However, it is possible that some taxonomic entities (sometimes referred to as "keystone pathogens") at a specific metabolic state play a more prominent role in promoting inflammation [22, 31].

A. actinomycetemcomitans is often found in association with periodontitis. Compared to our previous study (46.2%) [7], the overall detection rate of *A. actinomycetemcomitans* was lower (37.1%). One explanation may be the selection process: instead of selecting healthy and periodontally diseased pairs, we selected all subjects fulfilling the inclusion criteria. Thus, we might have selected more subjects with mild or moderate periodontitis compared to the previous study. Furthermore, the tongue was significantly ($p < 0.001$) less often colonized with *A. actinomycetemcomitans* (14%) compared to the subgingival pocket (29.1%). In Swiss adolescents, this bacterium was detected with similar rates on the tongue (approximately 20%) and with lower rates for shallow pockets (approximately 15–17%) [30]. In a Swedish study, similar detection rates of 30% were found in subgingival plaques of periodontitis patients [32]. In this study, relative abundances on the tongue were only weakly associated with the periodontal status, which is in contrast to findings from the previous study [7]. Taken together, these observations strengthen the hypothesis that tongue levels of *A. actinomycetemcomitans* are only weakly associated with severity of chronic periodontitis.

F. nucleatum, which bridges early-colonizing with late-colonizing pathogens, was found in 74.7% of all tested subjects. The detection rate was approximately three times lower in tongue samples compared to subgingival pocket samples. In line with this, we found higher relative abundances in the later ones. Relative abundances of *F. nucleatum* on the tongue and in the subgingival pocket correlated weakly with corresponding levels of PD and CAL. However, we might assume that members of the genus *Fusobacterium* belong to the core oral human microbiome [10, 33]. The sum score was a useful marker of chronic periodontitis since

Table 5: Cross table for the detection (no/yes) of the microorganisms in tongue scrapings and subgingival samples. Additionally, percentages of agreement, Prevalence and Bias Adjusted Kappa (PABAK), specificities, and sensitivities are given.

Tongue scraping	Subgingival sample No detection	Subgingival sample Detection	Sum	P*	Agreement	PABAK	Specificity (95% CI)	Sensitivity (95% CI)
P. gingivalis								
No detection	129 (89.6%)	36 (38.7%)	165					
Detection	15 (10.4%)	57 (61.3%)	72	<0.001	78.5%	0.570	89.6% (83.4 to 94.1%)	61.3% (50.6 to 71.2%)
Sum	144	93	237					
A. actinomycetemcomitans								
No detection	149 (88.7%)	54 (78.3%)	203					
Detection	19 (11.3%)	15 (21.7%)	34	0.04	69.2%	0.384	88.7% (82.9 to 93.1%)	21.7% (12.7 to 33.3%)
Sum	168	69	237					
F. nucleatum								
No detection	60 (87.0%)	124 (73.8%)	184					
Detection	9 (13.0%)	44 (26.2%)	53	0.03	43.9%	−0.122	87.0% (76.7 to 93.9%)	26.2% (19.7 to 33.5%)
Sum	69	168	237					
S. sanguinis								
No detection	114 (77.0%)	17 (19.1%)	131					
Detection	34 (23.0%)	72 (80.9%)	106	<0.001	78.5%	0.570	77.7% (69.4 to 83.5%)	80.9% (71.2 to 88.5%)
Sum	148	89	237					
Archaea								
No detection	50 (25.4%)	14 (35.0%)	64					
Detection	147 (74.6%)	26 (65.0%)	173	0.21	32.1%	−0.359	25.4% (19.5 to 32.1%)	65.0% (48.3 to 79.4%)
Sum	197	40	237					

*McNemar test; 95% CI, 95% confidence interval; PABAK, Prevalence and Bias Adjusted Kappa.

Table 6: Overview on relative abundances (log10 transformed) for tongue scrapings and subgingival samples and respective Spearman's correlation coefficients (with 95% confidence intervals).

	Relative abundances: Tongue scraping	Relative abundances: Subgingival sample	r_{SP} (95% CI)
P. gingivalis	0 (0, $6.3 \cdot 10^{-6}$)	0 (0, $8.1 \cdot 10^{-5}$)	0.63 (0.55, 0.70)
A. actinomycetemcomitans	0 (0, 0)	0 (0, $3.7 \cdot 10^{-5}$)	0.16 (0.03, 0.28)
F. nucleatum	0 (0, 0)	$8.6 \cdot 10^{-4}$ (0, $5.8 \cdot 10^{-3}$)	0.21 (0.09, 0.33)
S. sanguinis	0 (0, $1.6 \cdot 10^{-6}$)	0 (0, $8.9 \cdot 10^{-4}$)	0.56 (0.46, 0.64)
Archaea	2.63 (0, 2.82)	0 (0, 0)	−0.10 (−0.23, 0.03)
% *Archaea*	0.011 (0, 0.025)	0 (0, 0)	−0.01 (−0.14, 0.12)
Total bacteria	6.41 (6.16, 6.69)	4.22 (3.99, 4.47)	−0.14 (−0.26, 0.01)

Relative abundances are given as median (Q25%, Q75%); r_{SP}, Spearman's correlation coefficient; 95% CI, 95% confidence interval.

higher levels correlated with higher levels of PD and CAL in both habitats (Figure 1).

S. sanguinis frequently colonizes in the healthy human mouth [34, 35]. In contrast to another study in which *S. sanguinis* was not detected on the tongue dorsum of any of the five examined healthy subjects [3], we detected *S. sanguinis* on the middle third of the tongue dorsum in 44.7% of subjects. However, this rate was lower compared to the detection rate of 57.4% in our previous study [7]. In subgingival pocket samples, we detected *S. sanguinis* in 37.5% of samples. This value was between the reported carriage percentages of 25% (periodontally diseased) and 40% (healthy) of a Japanese study [33]. Moreover, the proportion of *S. sanguinis* in positive subgingival plaques was 0.37%, which was in line with a previous study reporting a proportion of 0.33% ± 0.57 for *S. sanguinis* in healthy subjects [33].

Members of the *Archaea* also colonize the oral cavity, especially within subgingival plaques and on tooth surfaces [21, 36–38], while the diversity seems to be very narrow. We detected archaeal sequences in 73.0% of tongue samples, but only 16.9% of subgingival pocket samples. The latter proportion was lower than the so far reported detection range for subgingival pocket samples of 36% [39] to 96.4% [36]. However, the archaeal abundance is probably higher in periodontal pockets with >5 mm pocket depth [21], linking the archaeal abundance to more severe periodontal disease. In this study, we did evaluate a relation between archaeal load and severe probing depths, because the number of subjects with mesiobuccal PD > 5 mm was only seven, precluding further analyses.

Further, Matarazzo et al. found strong correlations between *P. gingivalis* and the archaeal count ($r = 0.75$) in subjects with chronic periodontitis [40]. We found moderate correlations between total bacterial and archaeal load on the tongue ($r_{sp} = 0.53$; 95% CI: 0.44 to 0.62) and within the subgingival plaque ($r_{sp} = 0.41$; 95% CI: 0.30 to 0.51). The relative abundance of *F. nucleatum* was only weakly related to the archaeal relative abundance in subgingival plaque ($r_{sp} = 0.14$; 95% CI: 0.02 to 0.27). Thus, our study only slightly supports the hypothesis of Matarazzo et al. that *Archaea* may favor the settlement of some anaerobic bacterial species such as *P. gingivalis*, *F. nucleatum*, or *Prevotella intermedia* [21, 40]. Very weak and nonsignificant correlations were found between relative abundances of *P. gingivalis* or *A. actinomycetemcomitans* and archaeal load in both habitats ($-0.08 < r_{SP} < 0.09$) showing that not all virulent species are related to the archaeal load. Additionally, archaeal relative abundances on the dorsal tip of the tongue and the subgingival pocket did not correlate ($r_{SP} = -0.10$; 95% CI: −0.23 to 0.03). This, together with the previous observation that low archaeal relative abundances correlate with health-associated effects [7] indicates a more complex picture. Further, metagenome analysis might reveal distinct bacterial/archaeal patterns, which dominate in each habitat depending on the periodontal condition.

For this study a well-defined, homogenous, and periodontally untreated subgroup was a priori selected to ensure that associations seen between tongue scrapings, pocket samples, and clinical periodontal status are more likely to be unbiased by subject-related factors. Specifically, with regard to disease severity, study subjects cover the range from periodontally healthy to moderately diseased subjects, reflecting the general population in contrast to clinical patient cohorts. Some limitations deserve consideration. First, periodontal examinations were taken according to the half-mouth method at four sites per tooth, which might have led to an underestimation of periodontal disease severity on the subject level [41]. Second, an aspect common to most sampling methods applied in oral habitats is that cross contamination of samples cannot be completely excluded.

5. Conclusions

In this study, relative abundances of specific periopathogenic bacteria sampled from subgingival pocket samples and tongue samples correlated significantly to corresponding levels of PD and CAL. Further, we indicated relevant correlations for four periodontal bacteria and *Archaea* between a global oral habitat (the tongue) and a local site (the subgingival pocket sample). This strengthens the hypothesis that the tongue could serve as a reservoir for oral bacteria. In consequence, considering the relation between both habitats might be helpful during/after dental cleaning-events or reinfections. Moreover, the detection and quantification of tongue microbes might help to determine the risk of recolonization of debrided sites after periodontal treatment. Further, the strong correlations between *P. gingivalis* and periodontal parameter variables point to its usage as an indicator for periodontal disease severity.

Ethical Approval

All procedures performed in studies involving human participants were in accordance with the ethical standards of the institutional and/or national research committee and with the 1964 Helsinki Declaration and its later amendments or comparable ethical standards.

Acknowledgments

SHIP is part of the Community Medicine Research net (CMR) of the University of Greifswald, Germany, which is funded by the Federal Ministry of Education and Research under Grant nos. ZZ9603, 01ZZ0103, and 01ZZ0701 and the Ministry of Cultural Affairs as well as the Social Ministry of the Federal State of Mecklenburg-West Pomerania (http://www.community-medicine.de). Microbial analysis and André Göhler were supported by the Federal Ministry of Education and Research under Grant no. 03138010. The authors acknowledge the SHIP data collection team, which comprises dental and medical examiners, technicians, interviewers, and assistants. The authors also thank Anne Kohler and Claudia Wiede for their technical assistance.

References

[1] B. J. Keijser, E. Zaura, S. M. Huse et al., "Pyrosequencing analysis of the oral microflora of healthy adults," *Journal of Dental Research*, vol. 87, no. 11, pp. 1016–1020, 2008.

[2] C. Huttenhower, D. Gevers, R. Knight et al., "Structure, function and diversity of the healthy human microbiome," *Nature*, vol. 486, no. 7402, pp. 207–214, 2012.

[3] J. A. Aas, B. J. Paster, L. N. Stokes, I. Olsen, and F. E. Dewhirst, "Defining the normal bacterial flora of the oral cavity," *Journal of Clinical Microbiology*, vol. 43, no. 11, pp. 5721–5732, 2005.

[4] D. L. Mager, L. A. Ximenez-Fyvie, A. D. Haffajee, and S. S. Socransky, "Distribution of selected bacterial species on intraoral surfaces," *Journal of Clinical Periodontology*, vol. 30, no. 7, pp. 644–654, 2003.

[5] B. Liu, L. L. Faller, N. Klitgord et al., "Deep sequencing of the oral microbiome reveals signatures of periodontal disease," *PLoS One*, vol. 7, no. 6, p. e37919, 2012.

[6] A. M. Eren, G. G. Borisy, S. M. Huse, and J. L. Mark Welch, "Oligotyping analysis of the human oral microbiome," *Proceedings of the National Academy of Sciences*, vol. 111, no. 28, pp. E2875–E2884, 2014.

[7] A. Gohler, A. Hetzer, B. Holtfreter et al., "Quantitative molecular detection of putative periodontal pathogens in clinically healthy and periodontally diseased subjects," *PLoS One*, vol. 9, no. 7, p. e99244, 2014.

[8] A. C. R. Tanner, B. J. Paster, S. C. Lu et al., "Subgingival and tongue microbiota during early periodontitis," *Journal of Dental Research*, vol. 85, no. 4, pp. 318–323, 2006.

[9] C. Do Nascimento, J. P. M. Issa, E. Watanabe, and I. Y. Ito, "DNA checkerboard method for bacterial detection of microbiota from teeth and tongue biofilms. A preliminary study," *Minerva Stomatologica*, vol. 57, no. 11-12, pp. 561–567, 2008.

[10] K. Boutaga, A. J. van Winkelhoff, C. M. J. E. Vandenbroucke-Grauls, and P. H. M. Savelkoul, "The additional value of real-time PCR in the quantitative detection of periodontal pathogens," *Journal of Clinical Periodontology*, vol. 33, no. 6, pp. 427–433, 2006.

[11] B. J. Paster, I. Olsen, J. A. Aas, and F. E. Dewhirst, "The breadth of bacterial diversity in the human periodontal pocket and other oral sites," *Periodontology 2000*, vol. 42, no. 1, pp. 80–87, 2006.

[12] S. Yang, S. Lin, G. D. Kelen et al., "Quantitative multiprobe PCR assay for simultaneous detection and identification to species level of bacterial pathogens," *Journal of Clinical Microbiology*, vol. 40, no. 9, pp. 3449–3454, 2002.

[13] H. J. Lee, J. K. Kim, J. Y. Cho, J. M. Lee, and S. H. Hong, "Quantification of subgingival bacterial pathogens at different stages of periodontal diseases," *Current Microbiology*, vol. 65, no. 1, pp. 22–27, 2012.

[14] P. E. Kolenbrander, R. N. Andersen, D. S. Blehert, P. G. Egland, J. S. Foster, and R. J. Palmer, "Communication among oral bacteria," *Microbiology and Molecular Biology Reviews*, vol. 66, no. 3, pp. 486–505, 2002.

[15] J. M. ten Cate, "Biofilms, a new approach to the microbiology of dental plaque," *Odontology*, vol. 94, no. 1, pp. 1–9, 2006.

[16] N. Belay, B. S. Rajagopal, and L. Daniels, "Methanogenic bacteria from human dental plaque," *Applied and Environmental Microbiology*, vol. 54, no. 2, pp. 600–603, 1988.

[17] C. L. Li, D. L. Liu, Y. T. Jiang et al., "Prevalence and molecular diversity of *Archaea* in subgingival pockets of periodontitis patients," *Oral Microbiology and Immunology*, vol. 24, no. 4, pp. 343–346, 2009.

[18] E. M. Kulik, "Identification of archaeal rDNA from subgingival dental plaque by PCR amplification and sequence analysis," *FEMS Microbiology Letters*, vol. 196, no. 2, pp. 129–133, 2001.

[19] P. B. Eckburg, P. W. Lepp, and D. A. Relman, "*Archaea* and their potential role in human disease," *Infection and Immunity*, vol. 71, no. 2, pp. 591–596, 2003.

[20] K. Yamabe, H. Maeda, S. Kokeguchi et al., "Distribution of *Archaea* in Japanese patients with periodontitis and humoral immune response to the components," *FEMS Microbiology Letters*, vol. 287, no. 1, pp. 69–75, 2008.

[21] H. P. Horz, N. Robertz, M. E. Vianna, K. Henne, and G. Conrads, "Relationship between methanogenic archaea and subgingival microbial complexes in human periodontitis," *Anaerobe*, vol. 35, pp. 10–12, 2015.

[22] Z. L. Deng, S. P. Szafrański, M. Jarek, S. Bhuju, and I. Wagner-Döbler, "Dysbiosis in chronic periodontitis: key microbial players and interactions with the human host," *Scientific Reports*, vol. 7, no. 1, p. 3703, 2017.

[23] U. John, E. Hensel, J. Lüdemann et al., "Study of Health in Pomerania (SHIP): a health examination survey in an east German region: objectives and design," *Sozial- und Praventivmedizin*, vol. 46, no. 3, pp. 186–194, 2001.

[24] J. Bunge, S. S. Epstein, and D. G. Peterson, "Comment on "Computational improvements reveal great bacterial diversity and high metal toxicity in soil"," *Science*, vol. 313, no. 5789, p. 918, 2006.

[25] I. Volkov, J. R. Banavar, and A. Maritan, "Comment on "Computational improvements reveal great bacterial diversity and high metal toxicity in soil"," *Science*, vol. 313, no. 5789, p. 918, 2006.

[26] T. Byrt, J. Bishop, and J. B. Carlin, "Bias, prevalence and kappa," *Journal of Clinical Epidemiology*, vol. 46, no. 5, pp. 423–429, 1993.

[27] StataCorp, *Stata Statistical Software: Release 12*, StataCorp LP, College Station, TX, USA, 2011.

[28] B. J. Paster, S. K. Boches, J. L. Galvin et al., "Bacterial diversity in human subgingival plaque," *Journal of Bacteriology*, vol. 183, no. 12, pp. 3770–3783, 2001.

[29] J. Slots, "Subgingival microflora and periodontal disease," *Journal of Clinical Periodontology*, vol. 6, no. 5, pp. 351–382, 1979.

[30] S. Eick, M. Pietkiewicz, and A. Sculean, "Oral microbiota in Swiss adolescents," *Clinical Oral Investigations*, vol. 17, no. 1, pp. 79–86, 2013.

[31] G. Hajishengallis, R. P. Darveau, and M. A. Curtis, "The keystone-pathogen hypothesis," *Nature Reviews Microbiology*, vol. 10, no. 10, pp. 717–725, 2012.

[32] R. Claesson, C. Höglund-Åberg, D. Haubek, and A. Johansson, "Age-related prevalence and characteristics of *Aggregatibacter actinomycetemcomitans* in periodontitis patients living in Sweden," *Journal of Oral Microbiology*, vol. 9, no. 1, p. 1334504, 2017.

[33] Y. Abiko, T. Sato, G. Mayanagi, and N. Takahashi, "Profiling of subgingival plaque biofilm microflora from periodontally healthy subjects and from subjects with periodontitis using quantitative real-time PCR," *Journal of Periodontal Research*, vol. 45, no. 3, pp. 389–395, 2010.

[34] P. Belda-Ferre, L. D. Alcaraz, R. Cabrera-Rubio et al., "The oral metagenome in health and disease," *ISME Journal*, vol. 6, no. 1, pp. 46–56, 2012.

[35] J. Kreth, R. A. Giacaman, R. Raghavan, and J. Merritt, "The road less traveled-defining molecular commensalism with *Streptococcus sanguinis*," *Molecular Oral Microbiology*, vol. 32, no. 3, pp. 181–196, 2017.

[36] F. Matarazzo, A. C. Ribeiro, M. Feres, M. Faveri, and M. P. Alves Mayer, "Diversity and quantitative analysis of *Archaea* in aggressive periodontitis and periodontally healthy subjects," *Journal of Clinical Periodontology*, vol. 38, no. 7, pp. 621–627, 2011.

[37] B. Dridi, D. Raoult, and M. Drancourt, "*Archaea* as emerging organisms in complex human microbiomes," *Anaerobe*, vol. 17, no. 2, pp. 56–63, 2011.

[38] M. Efenberger, J. Agier, E. Pawłowska, and E. Brzezińska-Błaszczyk, "*Archaea* prevalence in inflamed pulp tissues," *Central European Journal of Immunology*, vol. 40, no. 2, pp. 194–200, 2015.

[39] P. W. Lepp, M. M. Brinig, C. C. Ouverney, K. Palm, G. C. Armitage, and D. A. Relman, "Methanogenic *Archaea* and human periodontal disease," *Proceedings of the National Academy of Sciences of the United States of America*, vol. 101, no. 16, pp. 6176–6181, 2004.

[40] F. Matarazzo, A. C. Ribeiro, M. Faveri, C. Taddei, M. B. Martinez, and M. P. A. Mayer, "The domain *Archaea* in human mucosal surfaces," *Clinical Microbiology and Infection*, vol. 18, no. 9, pp. 834–840, 2012.

[41] A. Kingman, C. Susin, and J. M. Albandar, "Effect of partial recording protocols on severity estimates of periodontal disease," *Journal of Clinical Periodontology*, vol. 35, no. 8, pp. 659–667, 2008.

8

Relationship between the Apical Preparation Diameter and the Apical Seal: An In Vitro Study

Kaoutar Laslami,[1] Sara Dhoum,[1] Amine El Harchi,[2] and Iman Benkiran[1]

[1]*Department of Conservative Dentistry and Endodontics, School of Dentistry of Casablanca, Casablanca, Morocco*
[2]*Private Practice, Casablanca, Morocco*

Correspondence should be addressed to Sara Dhoum; saradhoum@hotmail.com

Academic Editor: Izzet Yavuz

Objectives. The aim of the study is to define the relationship between the apical preparation diameter and the apical sealing ability to highlight the importance of the preservation of the diameter and the original position of the apical foramen. *Materials and Methods.* 50 extracted maxillary incisors were randomly allocated into three groups of 15 teeth each (n = 15) according to the apical preparation size: Group 1: finishing file F1 corresponding to size 20 reached the working length (ProTaper Universal system Dentsply®); Group 2: prepared up to size 30 corresponding to finishing file F30; Group 3: prepared up to size 50 corresponding to finishing file F5. Five teeth were assigned to positive and negative control groups. After the filling of the root canals, the teeth were isolated and immersed in a dye solution, then cut longitudinally, photographed, and the dye penetration were calculated using a computer software. *Results.* Comparison of the three different apical preparation sizes showed no statistically significant differences regarding the apical microleakage. *Conclusion.* The most important value of the dye penetration was observed in the group with the largest apical diameter.

1. Introduction

The root canal filling achieves three significant objectives:

(i) Elimination of residual bacteria from the root canal system

(ii) Prevent the entry of fluid from the periapical tissues

(iii) Prevent coronal microleakage [1, 2].

Three-dimensional and hermetical seal increases the tooth longevity [3]. However, the root canal filling cannot compensate a lack of canal preparation. Thus, it is important to understand that preparation and root canal filling complement one another [4].

It has been shown that 63% of the endodontic treatment failures are related to apical percolation due to an insufficient sealing [5]. It thus appears that the shaping and disinfection of the apical third takes a paramount importance in the success of the endodontic treatment [6].

Two questions arise here: Which apical limit and which apical diameter size should we choose?

For the apical limit, the current recommendations require ideally that instrumentation and obturation should not exceed the root canal space [6, 7]. The shaping of the last apical millimeters should respect mechanical and biological objectives: conicity, respect of the apical diameter and the original position of the foramen are important for the adjustment of the master cone in the apical third [3].

On the other hand, if the main objective of endodontic therapy is to create a favorable environment in the apical healing process, all instrumentation beyond the foramen causes damages to the periapical tissues due to extrusion of the debris and the irrigation solutions and impairs the adequate seal of the apical foramen [7, 8].

As for the apical preparation diameter, one of the main mechanical imperatives in the apical third preparation is to preserve the apical foramen in its initial position and in its narrowest diameter in order to avoid any complication such as tearing, zipping, or transport of the foramen [9, 10].

However, we should not forget that bacteria penetrate deeply in the dentinal tubules, especially when the teeth are infected, and that some authors support the necessity of an apical enlargement in order to reduce as much as we can the bacterial growth in the apical third [11–13].

All things considered, the diameter preparation of the foramen is a very controversial topic in endodontics.

The aim of our study is to compare the apical leakage after the preparation following different apical diameters.

2. Materials and Methods

Freshly extracted 50 central incisors were selected and stored in a physiological serum. All the teeth were free of cracks and had single root canals and mature apices.

The teeth were randomly allocated into 3 experimental groups of 15 teeth each and 2 control groups:

Group 1: Canals were prepared up to size 20 corresponding to finishing file F1 of the ProTaper system (Dentsply).

Group 2: Canals were prepared up to size 30 corresponding to F3.

Group 3: Canals were prepared up to size 50 corresponding to F5.

Group 4: The positive control group contained 3 roots that were not filled and covered with nail polish except for their apical 2 mm.

Group 5: The negative control group included 2 roots that were not filled, and the entire root surface was coated with nail polish, and canal orifices were sealed with cyanoacrylate glue.

2.1. Root Canal Preparation. Endodontic access cavities were realized using high-speed burs under water spray, and all root canals were instrumented by the same operator. Patency of each canal was established by gently passing a 08 k-file, and the working length was determined using a 10 k-file (Dentsply Maillefer) into the canal until it becomes visible through the apical foramen, then subtracting 1 mm.

The canals were instrumented using the crown-down technique with rotary ProTaper nickel-titanium files (Dentsply Maillefer) up to the apical size of the F1 finishing file, and F3 or F5 in order to increase the apical diameter depending on the desired final apical diameter for each group. The canals were irrigated between files with 2 ml of 5.25% sodium hypochlorite (NaOCl). Following instrumentation, the smear layer was removed with 17% EDTA, followed by irrigation with NaOCl at 5.25%. Then, they were dried with sterile paper points. The master-cone adjustment is done thanks to the tug-back test. Then, the root canal filling was performed using the cold lateral condensation technique.

2.2. Sectioning and Image Analysis. To ensure that all specimens were of the same length, they were resected 17 mm from the apex using a diamond disk. Two layers of nail polish were applied to the root surface, except for the apical 2 mm that remained exposed to the dye solution. The 2 teeth used as negative controls had the entire root surface sealed.

Specimens were then immersed in 1% methylene blue for 48 hours. After removal from the dye solution, the specimens were rinsed and dried. Then, roots were cut longitudinally following the principal axis of the root.

The roots were then photographed using a digital reflex camera (OLYMPUS EM 5). The distance to take pictures was standardized by a fixation device. The measurements were realized using ADOBE PS CS6 software. For more objectivity, many operators participated in the reading of the results. The Student's t-test was used to assess the results statistically and to compare differences in the depth of dye penetration between the three groups.

3. Results

In the negative control group, no sign of dye penetration was observed, which means there was no leakage.

In the positive control group, specimens showed maximum microleakage.

Group 1: Revealed a dye leakage variable between 0 and 2.7 mm with an average of 1.0220 (±0.8467)

Group 2: Revealed a dye leakage variable between 0 and 5 mm with an average of 1.3867 (±1.1344)

Group 3: Revealed a dye leakage variable between 0.6 and 9.4 mm with an average of 2.2907 (±2.2781)

$P > 0.05$ means that there are no significant differences in the apical leakage between the three different apical preparation sizes (20, 30, and 50).

The average, variance, and standard deviation for the three experimental groups are demonstrated in Table 1.

4. Discussion

There are two topics where no consensus was established.

4.1. The Limit of the Apical Preparation. The three dimensional preparation of the root canal with no instrumental excess is a well know principal, but many opinions were established about the choice of the appropriate apical limit [14].

4.1.1. The Apical Constriction. Apical constriction is a natural barrier which represents the smallest apical diameter and is located 0.5–1.5 mm inside the apical foramen [15]. This structure could coincide with the dentinocemental junction or very close to it. So, they are considered as a single anatomohistological entity elected as the apical limit of preparation [16, 17].

In fact, it would be appropriate to stop the shaping at the level where pulp tissue ends and leave the cement cone to permit a cemental reparation after the endodontic treatment. Therefore, the apical constriction (or CDJ) seems to be

Table 1: Calculation of the average, variance, and standard deviation of the dye penetration depths in the 3 experimental groups.

	Average (mm)	Variance	Standard deviation
Grp 1 (F1)	1.0220	0.7168	0.8467
Grp 2 (F3)	1.3867	1.2870	1.1344
Grp 3 (F5)	2.2907	5.1899	2.2781
		P value	0.08108

the ideal apical limit to be used as a matrix to support the closing material and avoid any overfilling [15–17].

4.1.2. The Apical Foramen. The working length is initially established as close as possible to the canal exit or slightly short of the apical foramen to clean the entire length of the canal [18]. With this choice, we avoid to leave a non-instrumented apical area with bacteria and dentin shavings stemming from the preparation [19].

However, since the root apex can be subject to several morphological variations especially in the presence of apical resorption, files placed to the apical extent of the root as viewed radiographically will likely be outside the confines of the canal and create potential damage such as a persistent inflammation at apical area [18].

Both of these two positions provide no evidence-based data to support them as the ideal working-length technique for instrumentation and obturation [18]. A meta-analysis evaluation of success/failure showed a better success rate when the obturation was confined to the canal space [8].

While the guideline of 1-2 mm from the radiographic apex remains rational, the point of apical end of the preparation and obturation remains empirical [20]. The need to compact the gutta-percha and sealer against the apical dentin matrix (apical constriction) is essential for success. Also, to prevent extrusion, the cleaning and shaping procedures must be confined to the radicular space. Canals filled to the radiographic apex are actually over-extended [20].

4.2. Degree of Apical Enlargement. Nowadays, two concepts oppose the modalities of apical enlargement.

4.2.1. An Important Enlargement. This concept is based on the presumption that the canal debridement would be improved by increasing the apical diameter [21]. It is justified by the fact that microorganismes colonize the dentinal tubules in a depth of 200 to 300 μm where they remain inaccessible [22]. Indeed, Falk and Sedgley have demonstrated that larger apical preparation ensures a higher efficiency of the irrigation solution and reduces the bacterial growth at the apical level [23]. Brunson et al. maintain that larger apical preparation increases the volume of the irrigation solution at the apical level and it eliminates the tissue debris [24]. Fornari et al. and De-Deus et al. report that the apical enlargement reduces the noninstrumented areas in the root canal [25, 26].

On the other hand, the study by coldero et al. did not show any significant difference in intracanal bacterial reduction with or without apical enlargement preparation and concluded that it was not necessary to remove dentine in the apical part of the root canal when a suitable coronal taper is achieved to allow efficient irrigation of the root canal system [27].

Thus, apical enlargement remains controversial until today: no study has ever shown a direct relationship between apical enlargement and clinical success or endodontic treatment failure.

In fact, the apical enlargement presents many inconveniences.

4.2.2. The Apical Debris Extrusion Risk. According to the results of the . study by Silva et al. that compared 4 systems of the canal preparation in a continuous rotation and reciprocating motions, apical debris extrusion occurred during large root apical preparations regardless of the file design and different kinematic motions (rotary or reciprocating) [28].

Extrusion of contaminated debris may be an important issue in the outcome of endodontic treatment. Besides bacterial extrusion due to mechanical and chemical aggression may cause flare-ups, and could also be responsible of post-operative pain and acute peri-apical lesions [29].

The root canal filling is technically more difficult to achieve. Few studies have been published comparing the apical diameter of preparation and apical sealing.

The study by Yared and Dagher evaluates the influence of apical enlargement on the sealing ability of vertical compaction and reports that the size 25 file group showed significantly less apical leakage than the size 40 file group [30]. Similarly, another study of Yared and Dagher showed that the canals instrumented to a size 40 file had significantly more overextensions than those instrumented to a size 25 file [31]. The study of Gomes-Filho et al. showed that greater dye leakage occurred after disruption and enlargement of the apical foramen [8]. Mente et al. evaluated the influence of the apical enlargement on sealing ability and observed a positive correlation between large apex diameter and greater leakage [32].

The results of our study are in accordance with all these studies since the most important values of the colorant infiltration have been observed in the group of larger apical diameter (F5) even if the comparison is statically not significant.

4.2.3. A Minimal Enlargement. This concept is the base of the crown-down technique and implies the maintenance of a narrow foramen. It has been shown that

(i) a canal with an initial small apical diameter and maintained during the shaping is not less cleaned, provided that a sufficient conicity is achieved [27]. In large canals, it is not a matter of increasing the diameter of the foramen, but rather increasing the conicity of the canal;

(ii) the necessary apical conicity to ensure the renewal of irrigation solution at the apical level, and thus disinfection, is at least 6% to 8% [33]. The advantage of the crown-down technique is to allow the cleaning of the canal as the instruments progress in the apical direction, which limits the extrusion in the periapex;

(iii) a continuously tapering preparation from the access cavity to apical foramen facilitates efficient delivery of irrigant and creates apical resistance, which maintains the gutta-percha in the canal space and reduces the possibility of overfilling [34];

(iv) in order to preserve apical foramen and to avoid the creation of apical zips or transport, it is important that instrumentation is performed according to all the principles of root canal therapy. Apical disruption violates one of these principles, which is to maintain the apical foramen in its original position [8].

5. Conclusion

Within the limitations of this study, there was no significant difference in the apical leakage between the three different apical preparation diameters. However, the most important infiltration was observed in the group prepared with the largest apical diameter.

There is still no real consensus to the exact size of the apical preparation. Moreover, it is necessary to construct a sufficient tapering along the root canal allowing the efficiency of the chemomechanical cleaning of the apical third and to guaranty a deep penetration of the irrigation, while preserving as much as possible the integrity of the noble anatomical structures of this apical area.

References

[1] L. M. Lin, P. A. Rosenberg, and J. Lin, "Do procedural errors cause endodontic treatment failure?," *Journal of the American Dental Association*, vol. 136, no. 2, pp. 187–193, 2005.

[2] G. Li, L. Niu, W. Zhang et al., "Ability of new obturation materials to improve the seal of the root canal system: a review," *Acta Biomaterialia*, vol. 10, no. 3, pp. 1050–1063, 2014.

[3] E. Olivier, "Leakage evaluation of root canal fillings: a literature review," *Revue d'Odonto-Stomatologie*, vol. 31, pp. 279–297, 2002.

[4] J. M. Laurichesse, F. Maestroni, and J. Breillat, *Endodontie Clinique*, Edition CDP, Paris, France, 1986.

[5] J. I. Ingle and L. K. Bakland, *Endodontics: Outcome of Endodontic Treatment and Retreatment*, chapter 13, vol. 153, p.668, BC Decker Inc., New York, NY, USA, 5th edition, 2002.

[6] A. Chaudhari, G. Asthana, G. Parmar, R. Vadher, and M. Kaur, "Significant of apical third: a review," *Scholars Journal of Applied Medical Sciences*, vol. 2, no. 5B, pp. 1613–1617, 2014.

[7] M. A. Schaeffer, R. R. White, and R. E. Walton, "Determining the optimal obturation length: a meta-analysis of literature," *Journal of Endodontics*, vol. 31, no. 4, pp. 271–274, 2005.

[8] J. E. Gomes-Filho, R. N. Hopp, P. F. Bernabé, M. J. Nery, J. A. Otoboni Filho, and E. Dezan Júnior, "Evaluation of the apical infiltration after root canal disruption and obturation," *Journal of Applied Oral Science*, vol. 16, no. 5, pp. 345–349, 2008.

[9] L. S. Buchanan, "The art of endodontics: files of greater taper," *Dentistry Today*, vol. 15, no. 2, pp. 42–51, 1996.

[10] L. S. Buchanan, "The standardised-taper root canal preparation. Part 1: concepts for variably tapered shaping instruments," *Dentistry Today*, vol. 17, no. 5, pp. 54–60, 1998.

[11] J. F. Siqueira Jr., K. C. Lima, F. A. C. Magalhaes, H. P. Lopes, and M. De Uzeda, "Mechanical reduction of the bacterial population in the root canal by three instrumentation techniques," *Journal of Endodontics*, vol. 25, no. 5, pp. 332–335, 1999.

[12] G. B. Shuping, D. Ørstavik, A. Sigurdsson, and M. Trope, "Reduction of intracanal bacteria using nickel-titanium rotary instrumentation and various medications," *Journal of Endodontics*, vol. 26, no. 12, pp. 751–755, 2000.

[13] A. ElAyouti, P. Kiefner, H. Hecker, A. Chu, C. Lost, and R. Weiger, "Homogeneity and adaptation of endodontic fillings in root canals with enlarged apical preparation," *Oral Surgery, Oral Medicine, Oral Pathology, Oral Radiology and Endodontics*, vol. 108, no. 3, pp. e141–e146, 2009.

[14] M. Fennich, M. Sakout, and F. Abdellaoui, "For a rational evaluation of working length in endodontics," *Revue d'Odonto-Stomatologie*, vol. 41, pp. 232–243, 2012.

[15] F. J. Vertucci, "Root canal morphology and its relationship to endodontic procedures," *Endodontic Topics*, vol. 10, no. 1, pp. 3–29, 2005.

[16] M. Hulsmann and E. Schaffer, *Problems in Endodontics*, Quintessence Publishing, New Malden, UK, 2009, Cat 3.

[17] D. Ricucci and K. Langeland, "Apical limit of root canal instrumentation and obturation, part 2. A histological study," *International Endodontic Journal*, vol. 31, no. 6, pp. 394–409, 1998.

[18] J. L. Gutmann, "Apical termination of root canal procedures-ambiguity or disambiguation?," *Evidence-Based Endodontics*, vol. 1, p. 4, 2016.

[19] S. Simon, P. Machtou, N. Adams, P. Tomson, and P. Lumley, "Apical limit and working length in endodontics," *Dental Update*, vol. 36, no. 3, pp. 146–153, 2009, Cat 3.

[20] W. T. Johnson and W. C. Noblett, "Cleaning and shaping," in *Endodontics: Principles and Practice*, M. Torabinejad and R. E. Walton, Eds., pp. 258–286, Saunders, St. Louis, MO, USA, 4th edition, 2009.

[21] A. Aminoshariae and J. C. Kulild, "Master apical file size-smaller or larger: a systematic review of healing outcomes," *International Endodontic Journal*, vol. 48, no. 7, pp. 639–647, 2015.

[22] N. Horiba, Y. Maekawa, T. Matsumoto, and H. Nakamura, "A study of the distribution of endotoxin in the dentinal wall of infected root canals," *Journal of Endodontics*, vol. 16, no. 7, pp. 331–334, 1990.

[23] K. W. Falk and C. M. Sedgley, "The influence of preparation size on the mechanical efficacy of root canal irrigation in vitro," *Journal of Endodontics*, vol. 31, no. 10, pp. 742–745, 2005.

[24] M. Brunson, C. Heilborn, D. J. Johnson, and N. Cohenca, "Effect of apical preparation size and preparation taper on irrigant volume delivered by using negative pressure irrigation system," *Journal of Endodontics*, vol. 36, no. 4, pp. 721–724, 2010.

[25] V. J. Fornari, Y. T. Silva-Sousa, J. R. Vanni, J. D. Pécora, M. A. Versiani, and M. D. Sousa-Neto, "Histological evaluation of the effectiveness of increased apical enlargement for cleaning the apical third of curved canals," *International Endodontic Journal*, vol. 43, no. 11, pp. 988–994, 2010.

[26] G. De-Deus, J. Marins, E. J. N. L. Silva et al., "Accumulated hard tissue debris produced during reciprocating and rotary nickel-titanium canal preparation," *Journal of Endodontics*, vol. 41, no. 5, pp. 676–681, 2015.

[27] L. G. Coldero, S. McHugh, D. MacKenzie, and W. P. Saunders, "Reduction in intracanal bacteria during root canal preparation with and without apical enlargement," *International Endodontic Journal*, vol. 35, no. 5, pp. 437–446, 2002.

[28] E. J. N. L. Silva, M. F. Carapia, R. M. Lopes et al., "Comparison of apically extruded debris after large apical preparations by full-sequence rotary and single-file reciprocating systems," *International Endodontic Journal*, vol. 49, no. 7, pp. 700–705, 2016.

[29] E. J. N. L. Silva, J. M. Teixeira, N. Kudsi, L. M. Sassone, R. L. Krebs, and T. S. Coutinho-Filho, "Influence of apical preparation size and working length on debris extrusion," *Brazilian Dental Journal*, vol. 27, no. 1, pp. 28–31, 2016.

[30] G. M. Yared and F. E. B. Dagher, "Apical enlargement: influence on the sealing ability of the vertical compaction technique," *Journal of Endodontics*, vol. 20, no. 7, pp. 313-314, 1994.

[31] G. M. Yared and F. E. B. Dagher, "Apical enlargement: influence on overextensions during in vitro vertical compaction," *Journal of Endodontics*, vol. 20, no. 6, pp. 269–271, 1994.

[32] J. Mente, S. Werner, M. J. Koch et al., "In vitro leakage associated with three root-filling techniques in large and extremely large root canals," *Journal of Endodontics*, vol. 33, no. 3, pp. 306–309, 2007.

[33] P. J. Lumley, "Cleaning efficacy of two apical preparation regimens following shaping with hand files of greater taper," *International Endodontic Journal*, vol. 33, no. 3, pp. 262–265, 2000.

[34] C. J. Ruddle, "Cleaning and shaping the root canal system," in *Pathways of the Pulp*, S. Cohen and R. C. Burns, Eds., pp. 231–291, Mosby, St. Louis, MO, USA, 8th edition, 2002.

Salivary Levels of Hemoglobin for Screening Periodontal Disease: A Systematic Review

Yoshiaki Nomura[1] **Ayako Okada,**[1] **Yoh Tamaki,**[2] **and Hiroko Miura**[3]

[1]*Department of Translational Research, School of Dental Medicine, Tsurumi University, 2-1-3 Tsurumi, Tsurumi-ku, Yokohama 230-8501, Japan*
[2]*Department of Health and Welfare Services, National Institute of Public Health, 2-3-6 Minami, Wako-shi, Saitama 351-0197, Japan*
[3]*Department of International Health and Collaboration, National Institute of Public Health, 2-3-6 Minami, Wako-shi, Saitama 351-0197, Japan*

Correspondence should be addressed to Yoshiaki Nomura; nomura-y@tsurumi-u.ac.jp

Academic Editor: Timo Sorsa

Periodontal disease is a common inflammatory disease. It affects about 20–50% of global population in both developed and developing countries. Early detection of slight changes of periodontal tissue plays an important role in prevention of onset and progression of periodontal disease. Hence, there is a need of a screening test to assess periodontal tissue for health check-ups. Salivary levels hemoglobin (Hb) has been proposed to assess the conditions of the inflammation of gingiva. The aim of this systematic review was to evaluate and summarize critically the current evidences for Hb as periodontal screening test. We performed a literature search of report published using PubMed databases. A total of 55 articles were retrieved and 16 were selected. Our review focuses on corelation coefficient with periodontal clinical parameters or sensitivity and specificity. As a result, fourteen studies calculated sensitivity and specificity of Hb. Six studies measured salivary levels hemoglobin at laboratory: three studies used polyclonal antibody reactions and other studies used colorimetric tests. Eight studies used paper strip method: 4 studies used monoclonal antibody reaction and 4 studies used colorimetric tests. Youden's indexes by antibody reaction were better than those of colorimetric methods. Evidences are described above and further studies are necessary to set the cut off values stratified by gender, age and number of remaining teeth.

1. Introduction

Periodontal diseases comprise a wide range of inflammatory conditions that affect the supporting structures of the teeth, which could lead to tooth loss and contribute to systemic inflammation. Periodontal disease is prevalent both in developed and developing countries and affect about 20–50% of global population. High prevalence of periodontal disease in adolescents, adults, and older individuals makes it a public health concern [1]. Early detection and treatment is important for periodontal disease to prevent the progression and to keep up systemic health.

In Japan, health check-up systems are established at each life stage, and the government regulates these check-up systems. In the health check-up system, oral examinations were included for pregnant women and infants at the age of 18 months and 36 months as maternal and child health, from elementary school children to high school student as school health. After that age, municipalities conduct dental check-ups for the resident at the age of 40, 50, and 60 years.

For laborers, company conducts annual medical check-ups for the prevention of noncommunicable disease. However, in this check-up system, oral examination is not included. Even though, periodontal disease symptoms appear at adults, and older individuals, the oral examinations at these ages are limited.

One of the obstacles for the popularization of periodontal check-ups is the cost. Dental professional is indispensable for the conventional oral examinations, and number of the subjects is limited for the oral examination. There is a pressing need for a reliable, low-cost method of assessing the gingival and periodontal status of large population groups.

Even the subjects with periodontal awareness did not visit dental clinics. Self-diagnosis of "Treatment not necessary" was found to be the common barrier for regular dental attendance [2]. Therefore, the results of screening tests may help for the regular dental attendance.

Salivary levels hemoglobin (Hb) is one of the candidates to assess the periodontal conditions without dental professionals and low-cost method alternative for oral examinations. Several advanced biomarkers had been proposed for assessing periodontal conditions; however, measuring these markers is not approved for extracorporeal diagnostic agents even for the blood tests. Especially, in Japan, only salivary levels hemoglobin i approved by the Pharmaceutical Affairs Law as extracorporeal diagnostic agents for assessing periodontal conditions.

In addition, saliva tests of Hb are an application of the fecal occult blood. It can detect subtle bleeding form gingival tissue. It may lead to early detection. If saliva tests can incorporate in medical check-up system, it may be the help of health promotion including oral health.

This study describes an evaluation of previously published article about salivary levels of hemoglobin as screening test for periodontal disease.

2. Materials and Methods

2.1. Search Strategy. Electronic database, PubMed was searched for eligible studies. Abstracts were reviewed, and full-text articles were inspected for inclusion criteria. The reference lists from reviewed studies were also examined to seek additional sources. The country of origin, study design, population, periodontal index used, method of measurement, sensitivity, and specificity were reviewed for each study.

Key word search terms using medical subject headings and text words included. Search details were as follows: ("hemoglobins" [MeSH Terms] OR "hemoglobins" [All Fields]) AND ("gingivitis" [MeSH Terms] OR "gingivitis" [All Fields]) OR ("periodontitis" [MeSH Terms] OR "periodontitis" [All Fields]) AND ("screening" [All Fields] OR "mass screening" [MeSH Terms] OR ("mass" [All Fields] AND "screening" [All Fields]) OR "mass screening" [All Fields] OR "screening" [All Fields]) AND ("saliva" [All Fields])

Studies were included if they tested human subjects for the screening of periodontal disease by salivary levels of Hb and were written in English.

2.2. Study Selection. An initial search for studies using saliva for the evaluation of periodontitis generated 55 articles. During the preliminary analysis, 39 studies were excluded because they reported HbA1c, not measuring salivary levels of Hb. Finally, 16 articles were reviewed. The investigators then independently evaluated 16 articles.

2.3. Outcome Measures. Two outcome measures were used. The effectiveness of saliva tests for the screening of periodontal disease was evaluated by mainly two methods: sensitivity and specificity or corelation coefficient with periodontal clinical parameters. From the sensitivity and specificity, positive likelihood ratio (sensitivity/(1 – specificity)) and negative likelihood ratio (specificity/(1 – sensitivity)) and Youden's index (sensitivity + specificity – 1) were calculated.

3. Results

3.1. Study Characteristics. One study was conducted to compare the performance of two commercially available products for measuring salivary levels of Hb [3]. One study calculated the corelation coefficient between salivary levels of Hb and periodontal index [4]. Other 14 studies calculated sensitivity and specificity for the screening of periodontal disease by salivary levels of Hb in Table 1 [5–18]. Table 2 showed the characteristics of the included the studies. Among these 14 studies, 6 studies measured Hb at laboratory by commercially available products like Hb in faeces or urine [9, 13–15, 17, 18]. Three used polyclonal antibody reaction and 3 other studies used colorimetric tests. Seven studies used paper strip method. Three studies used Perioscreen SUNSTAR (SUNSTAR, Osaka, Japan), which used monoclonal antibody against human Hb and 4 studies used colorimetric tests.

Periodontal indexes used as the gold standard varied between studies. One study used the criteria by the American Academy of Periodontology. Four studies used the Community Periodontal Index. One study used PD $\geq$ 4 mm. One study used progression of CAL > 3 mm. This study is the only one longitudinal study, and other studies were all cross-sectional studies.

Youden's indexes of Hb measured in laboratory by polyclonal antibody reaction ranged from 0.08 to 0.52. Those by colorimetric method ranged from 0 to 0.08. Youden's indexes of Perioscreen SUNSTAR were 0.24 to 0.50. Those of other paper strip methods were 0.17 to 0.57. Six studies used adjustment by statistical modeling.

4. Discussion

We reviewed studies for the screening periodontal disease by salivary levels of Hb. The measuring method of Hb, periodontal indexes used as a gold standard varied between studies. There are two methods for measuring Hb: colorimetric test and antibody reactions. The colorimetric tests are based on the reaction that the hemoglobin decomposes the hydrogen peroxide with the liberation of oxygen, oxidizing the orthotolidine to a blue colored derivative. For measuring Hb, the specificity of colorimetric tests is not superior to antibody reaction because it reacts with Hb of other animals contained in food. In general, the colorimetric method has been used for measuring Hb in urine. It is quite unlikely to contaminate blood form other animals in urine. Antibody reactions are used to detect Hb in fecal blood because, in feces, there may be remained various Hb from other animals

TABLE 1: Selected articles.

Author(s) and year published	Title of journal	Journal	Number of subjects	Results
Burt et al. 1978 [5]	Saliva-based colorimetric test as an index of gingival inflammation in epidemiologic studies	Community Dentistry and Oral Epidemiology	253	Colorimetric test may be a valid, reliable means of detecting major differences in the prevalence of gingival inflammation in most adult populations, although having little, if any, useful application among children at the mixed dentition stage.
Abbott and Caffesse 1978 [6]	The reliability of a colorimetric test in determining gingival inflammation	Journal of Periodontology	81	The G index chemical analysis may be a useful diagnostic aid for detecting the presence or absence of gingival inflammation in dental practice.
Kopczyk et al. 1995 [7]	The feasibility and reliability of using a home screening test to detect gingival inflammation	Journal of Periodontology	50	The test should be used as a home screening tool rather than a diagnostic aid. Patients who test positive for occult blood should seek advice from a dental professional.
Nomura et al. 2006 [8]	Screening of periodontitis with salivary enzyme tests	Journal of Oral Science	187	LDH level had the highest sensitivity and specificity (sensitivity, 0.66; specificity 0.67).
Kugahara et al. 2008 [9]	Screening for periodontitis in pregnant women with salivary enzymes	Journal of Obstetrics and Gynaecology Research	221	Combining LDH, ALP, and occult blood showed the highest diagnostic performance, with a sensitivity value of 0.90, specificity value of 0.62, positive predictive value of 0.18, and negative predictive value of 0.98.
Ohshima et al. 2009 [10]	Comparison of periodontal health status and oral health behavior between Japanese and Chinese dental students	Journal of Oral Science	92	Pain in gum, swollen gum, and bleeding gum had statistically significant corelation with the result of Perioscreen.
Shimazaki et al. 2011 [11]	Effectiveness of the salivary occult blood test as a screening method for periodontal status	Journal of Periodontology	1998	The sensitivity and specificity of the salivary occult blood test in screening for poor periodontal status were 0.72 and 0.52, respectively. In a multivariate logistic regression analysis, the results were significantly associated with the proportion of teeth with BOP and the proportion of teeth with PD ≥ 4 mm, independent of age, sex, use of antihypertensive medication, use of antidiabetic medication or insulin therapy, and the number of decayed or filled teeth.
Pham et al. 2011 [12]	Periodontal disease and related factors among Vietnamese dental patients	Oral Health & Preventive Dentistry	243	The perioscreen test showed moderate sensitivity (0.752) and specificity (0.746) to periodontal disease. The binary logistic regression analyses indicated that older subjects (OR = 2.5), or those who did not frequently visit a dentist (OR = 4.1), brushed their teeth only once a day (OR = 2.5), did not use dental floss (OR = 2.9), were past smokers (OR = 3.1), current smokers (OR = 4.1), or had positive BANA test results (OR = 12.0) were more likely to have periodontal disease.
Nomura et al. 2012 [13]	Screening for periodontal diseases using salivary lactate dehydrogenase, hemoglobin level, and statistical modeling	Journal of Dental Sciences	101	By the statistical modeling, sensitivity and specificity were improved for the screening of periodontal disease by the salivary levels of hemoglobin and LD.

Table 1: Continued.

Author(s) and year published	Title of journal	Journal	Number of subjects	Results
Nomura et al. 2012 [14]	Salivary biomarkers for predicting the progression of chronic periodontitis	Archives of Oral Biology	85	Salivary ALT level and the *P. gingivalis* ratio may be potential indicators for the progression of periodontitis. Such a salivary test could be a useful diagnostic tool for predicting periodontal disease progression.
Nam et al. 2015 [15]	Validity of screening methods for periodontitis using salivary hemoglobin level and self-report questionnaires in people with disabilities	Journal of Periodontology	195	The salivary hemoglobin level, self-report questionnaire, and the combined method demonstrated screening potential that could predict the population prevalence of CPI 3 or CPI 4.
Reed et al. 2015 [16]	Feasibility study of a salivary occult blood test to correlate with periodontal measures as indicators of periodontal inflammation in a population of pregnant women	Journal of Oral Science	23	Pearson correlation coefficient with the percent of sites with BOP was statistically significant (0.301, P value 0.0469), and with BOP as the sum of sites with bleeding on probing was 0.280, P value 0.0647.
Nomura et al. 2016 [17]	A new screening method for periodontitis: an alternative to the community periodontal index	BMC Oral Health	92	The sensitivity and specificity for hemoglobin levels were, respectively, 0.722 and 0.711, for lactate dehydrogenase levels. Combining these two tests, when samples tested positive for both hemoglobin and lactate dehydrogenase, the positive predictive value was 91.7%.
Maeng et al. 2016 [18]	Diagnostic accuracy of a combination of salivary hemoglobin levels, self-report questionnaires, and age in periodontitis screening	Journal of Periodontal & Implant Science	202	The combination of salivary hemoglobin levels and self-report questionnaires was shown to be a valuable screening method for detecting periodontitis.

by food. In this respect, antibody reactions are more suitable to detect Hb from oral cavity. In fact, Youden's indexes of antibody reaction measured in laboratory were better than that of the colorimetric method. The commercial products approved by Japanese Pharmaceutical Affairs Law to measure the Hb in saliva are all used antibody reactions including paper strip method (Perioscreen SUNSTAR).

The periodontal indexes used varied. It is likely that pure saliva from saliva ducts contains lilted or no Hb except for salivary gland inflammation. The Hb in saliva may be derived mainly from the bleeding of the periodontal tissue. Bleeding on probing (BOP) is the index that evaluates the bleeding from gum. When BOP was used as the gold standard of the screening, high sensitivity and specificity may be easily obtained when compared with other periodontal indexes. In fact, Youden's indexes by BOP ranged from 0.19 to 0.59. The index by PD 4 mm was 0.08 and that by American Academy of Periodontology was 0.52. The tooth that accompanied deep periodontal pockets does not always accompany bleeding from the periodontal pocket. Three studies used Community Periodontal Index (CPI) as a gold standard. Originally, CPI is a method for the survey proposed by the World Health Organization. It measured the sextant of representative 6 teeth. This method was sometimes used for the screening of periodontal disease. However, both saliva tests and CPI are a method for the screening of periodontal disease. Therefore, applying CPI as a gold standard for the saliva tests is not suitable. More precise definition of periodontal disease should be used for the standard.

For measuring Hb in laboratory (stimulated saliva) and Perioscreen SUNSTAR (resting saliva), method of saliva sampling is established because these reagents are approved by the Japanese Pharmaceutical Affairs Law. To obtain the approval, reporting the performance of the reagent, standardized measuring method, and established sampling method are indispensable.

Studies had shown that by the adjustment by statistical model, the sensitivity and specificity were improved. In the check-ups, to apply statistical model for every examination is insubstantial. These studies suggest that cut off values were in part dependent on the age, gender, number of remaining teeth, or subjective symptom of the subjects. Therefore, cut off values should be set separately by age, gender, or number of remaining teeth.

Table 2: Characteristics of the included the studies.

References	Subjects	Exclusion criteria	Definition of periodontitis	Measuring method		Saliva sample	Adjustment	Results				
				Reaction	Products			Sensitivity	Specificity	Positive likelihood ratio	Negative likelihood ratio	Youden's index
Laboratory examination												
Kugahara et al. [9]	221 pregnant women (mean age: 30 ± 4 years)	Current smokers and subjects with not sufficient saliva were excluded	Periodontitis (CPITN 3 and 4)	Colorimetric test	Salivastar-Bld	—		0.37	0.91	4.11	1.44	0.28
							Combination with LDH	0.68	0.74	2.62	2.31	0.42
Nomura et al. [13]	187 subjects (mean age: 37.2 ± 9.6 years)	—	PD ≥ 4 mm	Colorimetric test	—	Stimulated saliva	—	0.27	0.81	1.42	1.11	0.08
Nomura et al. [14]	85 patients with chronic periodontitis	Clinical attachment level (CAL) of 3 mm in at least three subsequent assessments	Progression of CAL ≥ 3 mm	Colorimetric test	—	Stimulated saliva	—	0.32	0.68	1.00	1.00	0.00
Nam et al. [15]	The participants were 195 patients with disabilities (aged >18 years)	—	CPI scores of 3-4	Polyclonal antibody reaction	OC-HEMODIA AUTO S	Stimulated saliva	—	0.41	0.77	1.78	1.31	0.18
			CPI scores of 4				—	0.53	0.75	2.12	1.60	0.28
			CPI scores of 3-4				With questionnaire	0.58	0.76	2.42	1.81	0.34
			CPI scores of 4				With questionnaire	0.73	0.74	2.81	2.74	0.47
			CPI scores of 3-4				With questionnaire and age	0.70	0.76	2.92	2.53	0.46
			CPI scores of 4				With questionnaire and age	0.71	0.80	3.55	2.76	0.51
Nomura et al. [17]	92 subjects (mean age: 50.03 years)	Patients older than 20 years who had more than 20 teeth remaining were included	Center for Disease Control and Prevention in partnership with the American Academy of Periodontology.	Polyclonal antibody reaction	OC-HEMODIA AUTO S	Stimulated saliva	—	0.76	0.76	3.20	3.17	0.52

Table 2: Continued.

References	Subjects	Exclusion criteria	Definition of periodontitis	Measuring method: Reaction	Measuring method: Products	Saliva sample	Adjustment	Results: Sensitivity	Results: Specificity	Results: Positive likelihood ratio	Results: Negative likelihood ratio	Results: Youden's index
Maeng et al. [18]	202 subjects (age: 20 to 79 years)	Pregnant, had undergone a periodontal operation within the past month, or had an injury accompanied by oral bleeding, such as a wound or ulcer	CPI scores of 3-4	Polyclonal antibody reaction	OC-HEMODIA AUTO S	Stimulated saliva	—	0.71	0.56	1.61	1.93	0.27
			CPI scores of 4				—	0.60	0.72	2.14	1.80	0.32
			CPI scores of 3-4				With questionnaire	0.71	0.68	2.25	2.38	0.40
			CPI scores of 4				With questionnaire	0.65	0.77	2.79	2.17	0.00
Paper strip												
Burt et al. [5]	136 school children, 52 adult dental hygene school students (age: 24 to 32) and 65 adults in correctional Institution (age: 18 to 66)	—	GI score (0–0.6, <1.2, <1.21, <0.2, <0.4, <0.41) GI > 0.6	Colorimetric test	G index	Resting saliva	School children	0.42	0.64	1.17	1.10	0.06
			GI > 1.2					0.50	0.63	1.35	1.26	0.13
			GI > 0.6				Innate correctional Institution	0.65	0.76	2.71	2.17	0.41
			GI > 1.2					0.67	0.53	1.43	1.61	0.20
			GI > 0.2				dental hygiene student	0.25	0.64	0.69	0.85	−0.11
			GI > 0.4					0.16	0.67	0.48	0.80	−0.17
Abbott and Caffesse [6]	81 subjects (age: 15 to 60 years)		GI > 0	Colorimetric test	G index	Before any clinical examination	—	0.83	0.63	2.24	3.71	0.46
			GI > 1					1.00	0.46	1.85	—	0.46
			GI > 2					1.00	0.29	1.41	—	0.29
Kopczyk et al. [7]	50 patients with less than 20 teeth 27 (age: 27 to 72 years)	Using aspirin or nonsteroidal anti-inflammatory drugs. Those with bleeding disorders, ulcerating oral lesions, or medical contraindications	BOP > 30%	Colorimetric test	Seracult	Resting saliva before and after tooth brush	Before tooth brush	0.19	1.00	—	1.23	0.19
			BOP > 50%					0.56	0.97	18.67	2.20	0.53
			BOP > 30%					0.75	0.82	4.17	3.28	0.57
			BOP > 50%				After tooth brush	0.85	0.66	2.50	4.40	0.51

Table 2: Continued.

References	Subjects	Exclusion criteria	Definition of periodontitis	Measuring method		Saliva sample	Adjustment	Results				
				Reaction	Products			Sensitivity	Specificity	Positive likelihood ratio	Negative likelihood ratio	Youden's index
Nomura et al. [8]	187 subjects (mean age 37.2 ± 9.6 years)	—	PD ≥ 4 mm	Colorimetric test	—	Stimulated saliva	—	0.27	0.81	1.42	1.11	0.08
Ohshima et al. [10]	92 dental school students (mean age: 22.1 years)	—	—	Monoclonal antibody reaction	Perioscreen SUNSTAR	—	—	—	—	—	—	—
Shimazaki et al. [11]	1998 subjects with less than 20 teeth (age: 40 to 79)	—	BOP ≥ 15% or at least one PD ≥ 4 mm	Monoclonal antibody reaction	Perioscreen SUNSTAR	Rinse 3 ml distilled water for 10 sec 8:00 am to 11:00 am before oral examination	—	0.69	0.55	1.53	1.77	0.24
Pham et al. [12]	243 subjects	—	—	Monoclonal antibody reaction	Perioscreen SUNSTAR	—	—	0.75	0.75	2.96	3.01	0.50
Reed et al. [16]	23 pregnant women (age: 18 to 45 years)	Preexisting parathyroid disease or uncontrolled thyroid disease, multiple fetuses (e.g., twins and triplets), preexisting sickle cell disease (not trait only), sarcoidosis, Crohn's disease, or ulcerative colitis	—	Monoclonal antibody reaction	Perioscreen SUNSTAR	—	—	—	—	—	—	—

5. Conclusions

Saliva tests can be applied by nonprofessional personnel. Further study is necessary to set the cut off values stratified by gender, age, and number of remaining teeth.

Acknowledgments

This work was supported by Health and Labour Sciences Research Grants, Research on Regional Medicine.

References

[1] M. A. Nazir, "Prevalence of periodontal disease, its association with systemic diseases and prevention," *International Journal of Health Sciences*, vol. 11, no. 2, pp. 72–80, 2017.

[2] D. Q. Taani, "Periodontal awareness and knowledge, and pattern of dental attendance among adults in Jordan," *International Dental Journal*, vol. 52, no. 2, pp. 94–98, 2002.

[3] A. Okada, Y. Nomura, K. Sogabe et al., "Comparison of salivary hemoglobin measurements for periodontitis screening," *Journal of Oral Science*, vol. 59, no. 1, pp. 63–69, 2017.

[4] Y. B. An, L. He, H. X. Meng et al., "Relationship between salivary occult blood and level of volatile sulphur compounds in oral cavity," *Zhonghua Kou Qiang Yi Xue Za Zhi*, vol. 45, no. 7, pp. 431–434, 2010.

[5] B. A. Burt, D. M. Roder, J. C. Cecil et al., "Saliva-based colorimetric test as an index of gingival inflammation in epidemiologic studies," *Community Dentistry and Oral Epidemiology*, vol. 6, no. 6, pp. 290–295, 1978.

[6] B. H. Abbott and R. G. Caffesse, "The reliability of a colorimetric test in determining gingival inflammation," *Journal of Periodontology*, vol. 49, no. 11, pp. 564–569, 1978.

[7] R. A. Kopczyk, R. Graham, H. Abrams et al., "The feasibility and reliability of using a home screening test to detect gingival inflammation," *Journal of Periodontology*, vol. 66, no. 1, pp. 52–54, 1995.

[8] Y. Nomura, Y. Tamaki, T. Tanaka et al., "Screening of periodontitis with salivary enzyme tests," *Journal of Oral Science*, vol. 48, no. 4, pp. 177–183, 2006.

[9] T. Kugahara, Y. Shosenji, and K. Ohashi, "Screening for periodontitis in pregnant women with salivary enzymes," *Journal of Obstetrics and Gynaecology Research*, vol. 34, no. 1, pp. 40–46, 2008.

[10] M. Ohshima, L. Zhu, Y. Yamaguchi et al., "Comparison of periodontal health status and oral health behavior between Japanese and Chinese dental students," *Journal of Oral Science*, vol. 51, no. 1, pp. 275–281, 2009.

[11] Y. Shimazaki, S. Akifusa, T. Takeshita et al., "Effectiveness of the salivary occult blood test as a screening method for periodontal status," *Journal of Periodontology*, vol. 82, no. 4, pp. 581–587, 2011.

[12] T. A. Pham, M. Ueno, K. Shinada et al., "Periodontal disease and related factors among Vietnamese dental patients," *Oral Health & Preventive Dentistry*, vol. 9, no. 2, pp. 185–194, 2011.

[13] Y. Nomura, Y. Tamaki, A. Eto et al., "Screening for periodontal diseases using salivary lactate dehydrogenase, hemoglobin level, and statistical modeling," *Journal of Dental Sciences*, vol. 7, no. 4, pp. 379–383, 2012.

[14] Y. Nomura, Y. Shimada, N. Hanada et al., "Salivary biomarkers for predicting the progression of chronic periodontitis," *Archives of Oral Biology*, vol. 57, no. 4, pp. 413–420, 2012.

[15] S. H. Nam, H. Jung, S. M. Kang et al., "Validity of screening methods for periodontitis using salivary hemoglobin level and self-report questionnaires in people with disabilities," *Journal of Periodontology*, vol. 86, no. 4, pp. 536–545, 2015.

[16] S. G. Reed, M. C. Manz, S. M. Snipe et al., "Feasibility study of a salivary occult blood test to correlate with periodontal measures as indicators of periodontal inflammation in a population of pregnant women," *Journal of Oral Science*, vol. 57, no. 1, pp. 55–58, 2015.

[17] Y. Nomura, A. Okada, E. Kakuta et al., "A new screening method for periodontitis: an alternative to the community periodontal index," *BMC Oral Health*, vol. 16, no. 1, p. 64, 2016.

[18] Y. J. Maeng, B. R. Kim, H. I. Jung et al., "Diagnostic accuracy of a combination of salivary hemoglobin levels, self-report questionnaires, and age in periodontitis screening," *Journal of Periodontal & Implant Science*, vol. 46, no. 1, pp. 10–21, 2016.

10

A Cone-Beam Computed Tomography Scanning of the Root Canal System of Permanent Teeth among the Moscow Population

Svetlana Razumova, Anzhela Brago, Lamara Khaskhanova, Ammar Howijieh, Haydar Barakat, and Ashot Manvelyan

Peoples' Friendship University of Russia (RUDN University), 6 Miklukho-Maklaya Street, Moscow 117198, Russia

Correspondence should be addressed to Haydar Barakat; dr.haydarbarakat@yahoo.com

Academic Editor: Gianrico Spagnuolo

Background. Successful endodontic treatment requires a significant knowledge of root canal anatomy. The aim of this study was to evaluate the root and root canal number of permanent teeth among the Moscow population using cone-beam computed tomography (CBCT) scanning. *Materials and methods.* 300 CBCT images of subjects were analyzed to study the anatomy of roots and root canal system of each tooth. The collected data were analyzed using IBM SPSS statistics software 22.0 version. *Results.* The maxillary incisors and canines had one root with one canal in 100%. Maxillary premolars had one root with one or two canals and two roots with two canals, while mandibular premolars were single-rooted with one or two canals. Maxillary first and second molar had three separated roots, and the prevalence of four canals was more often in first molars. Mandibular molars had two roots with different number of canals. *Conclusion.* The root canal system varies greatly among populations and even in different individuals within the same population; thus, using CBCT scanning is an effective technique in investigating the root canal system.

1. Background

The success of endodontic treatment depends on the precise knowledge of root and root canal anatomy, which is an important challenge due to the complexity of the root canal system and the anatomical variations [1, 2]. This knowledge helps the clinicians in endodontic treatment planning and decreases the percent of endodontic treatment failure. Many studies have been conducted to determine the anatomy and morphology of root canal system using different techniques [3–9]. Recently, with the development of cone-beam computed tomography (CBCT) technique, it became possible to study the anatomy of teeth, due to the high-quality three-dimensional (3D) images obtained from CBCT. This image allows studying the anatomy of the jaws, the morphology of teeth, and their root canal system [3]. Many studies have used this technique to find out the anatomy of root canal system especially in the molar regions [3, 6, 8].

Root canal morphology has been classified using different ways by several investigators in the literature [10–12]. Weine et al. [12] classified it into four types depending on the pattern of division of the main root canal of a tooth along its course from the floor of the pulp chamber to the root apex. Vertucci [10] also classified the root canal morphology in a more descriptive manner into eight types. This classification has been widely used by many researchers to classify the canal system of different teeth.

It is known that the number of teeth roots and the anatomy of root canal system vary among the world population, and to date, there are still no studies about the anatomy of roots and root canals in Russian Federation, where dental practitioners still use the data obtained from foreign authors on the anatomy of root canals in planning the endodontic treatment. The aim of this study was to investigate the anatomy of root and root canal system among the Moscow population using CBCT technique.

2. Materials and Methods

300 subjects aged 20–70 years were enrolled in this study, from those attending the diagnostic center (LLC Zolotoye Secheniye) for 3D radiological scanning in the period between January 2017 and November 2017. The study protocol was approved by the Ethics Committee in People's Friendship University of Russia (RUDN University), Moscow, Russia. A written consent was signed by all subjects, including who participated in this study. CBCT images were taken using a 3D eXam® dental tomography scanner (KaVo, Biberach, Germany) with standard exposure settings (23 ∗ 17 cm field of view; 0.3 mm voxel size; 110 kv; 1.6–20 s) and were viewed by three examiners in a semidark room using I-CAT viewer software (version 10, Hatfield, England). All teeth were evaluated in axial, coronal, and sagittal planes, and the number of roots and the number of canals in each tooth were recorded. The presence of additional canals especially in the molar regions was recorded.

2.1. Statistical Analysis. Data were processed using the software (SPSS v 22 for win, IBM, Chicago, IL), and descriptive data were processed to analyze the percentage of roots and root canals in each tooth.

3. Results

300 CBCT scans of 300 subjects with mean age of 49.91 ± 14.01 were analyzed. All the maxillary incisors had one root with 100% and one canal with 100%. First and second maxillary molars had three roots with 100%, and third molar recorded one root in 33.7% and three roots in 47.9%. Data for maxillary teeth including the number of roots and root canals are shown in (Table 1).

For mandibular teeth, data were the following: central and lateral incisors and canines showed one root and one canal in 99.4%, 99.2%, and 99.8%, respectively. First molars had two roots in 100%, and second molars had one root in 0.5% and two roots in 99.5%. Data for mandibular teeth are shown in (Table 2).

4. Discussion

The knowledge of the anatomy of the root canal system is the gold standard in successful endodontic treatment, and studying root and canal morphology has endodontic and anthropological significance. This study evaluated the roots and root canal system among the Moscow population using CBCT scanning. The advantages of CBCT scanning are its high accuracy, minimal distortion, and 3D visualization. Moreover, it is a nondestructive technique and can provide specific data [3].

When analyzing the anatomy of the maxillary anterior teeth, 510 central incisors, 500 lateral incisors, and 540 canines were recorded, and one root with one canal was identified in 100% of cases. These data are comparable with the results obtained from other studies on the anatomy of central incisors in USA [10], Mexico [11], Turkey [13], and Chennai urban [14]. The presence of two canals in lateral incisors was found in 13.7% of cases in a study by Calişkan et al. (Turkey) [13], in 9.5% of cases by Sert and BayirliIn (Turkey) [15], and in 2% in a study by Jain et al. (Chennai urban) [14]. The prevalence of two canals in canines was 3.9%, 2–4%, 4%, and 18.4% in studies by Calişkan et al. [13], Sert and Bayirli [15], Jain et al. [14], and Amardeep et al. [16] respectively. This difference in results could be attributed to the evaluation method, sample size, and racial differences.

According to the current study, the anatomy of root canals of maxillary first premolar was variable, two roots were identified in 91.3% of cases and 8.7% of cases were one rooted, and the first premolar recorded one root and two canals in 2.6% and one canal in 6.1% of cases. Similar data obtained in the studies of Bulut et al. (Turkey) [17], Pecora et. al. (Brazil) [18], Kerekes and Tronstad (Norway) [19], Green [20] (USA), Ok et al. (Turkey) [21], and Burklein et.al. (Germany) [22]. Pineda and Kuttler (Mexico) [11] have revealed in their studies a single-canal first premolar in 50.1% and two canals in 49.4% of cases.

The maxillary second premolar with one root was determined in 26.5% of observations and with two separated roots in 73.5% of cases according to the data of the current study, and two canals were recorded in 73.5% of cases. This coincides with the results of Awawdeh et al. (Jordan) [23], where one canal was found in 13.8% and 84.1% had two canals; the results of Elnour et al. (Saudi Arabia) [24], where two canals were recorded in 65% of cases; and the results of Bürklein et al. (Germany) [22], where 56.3% of cases had two canals. Bulut et al. (Turkey) [17] recorded one canal in 82.1% of the cases and two canals in 17.8%.

The maxillary first molar was analyzed by all researchers in detail by the number of canals in each root. Three separated roots were identified in 100% of cases. The number of canals varied from 3 to 5. The four-canal root system occurred in 59.8% of cases, and the localization of the two canals takes place more often in the mesiobuccal root (MB) and also occurred in the distobuccal root (DB). These results are comparable with the results of Pomeranz and Fishelberg (USA) [25], where 48% of cases had two canals in MB. Wasti et al. (Pakistan) [26] recorded a percent of two canals in MB in 43.4%, and Pineda and Kuttler (Mexico) [11] defined two canals in 48.5% of cases. This significantly varies from the results of Imura et al. (Japan) [27], where 88.2% of cases had two canals in the MB, and of Kim et al. (Korea) [8], where two canals in MB were found in 63.59% and 1.25% in DB. Ghoncheh et al. (Iran) [28], Martins et al. (Caucasian population) [29], Ratanajirasut et al. (Thai) [30], Silva et al. (Brazil) [31], and Guo et al. (North America) [32] recorded four-canal system in 46%, 71%, 63.6%, 42.63%, and 68.2% of cases, respectively. Ceperuelo et al. (Spain) [33] defined four-canal system in 92.3% of cases.

The maxillary second molar consisted of three separated roots in 100% of cases, and the prevalence of four canal systems was identified in 51.5% of cases (two canals in MB). This agreed with the published studies of Shalabi et al. (Ireland) 50% [34], Kulild and Peters (USA) 45.8% [35], Alavi et al. (Thailand) 44.6% [36], Kim et al. (Korea) 34.39% [8], Martins et al. (Caucasian population) 44% [29], and Ratanajirasut et al. (Thai) 29.4% [30] of the prevalence of two

Table 1: Anatomy of roots and root canals in maxillary teeth.

Tooth	Number of studied teeth	Roots	*N* (%)	Canals	*N* (%)
Central incisor	510	1	510 (100%)	1	510 (100%)
Lateral incisor	500	1	500 (100%)	1	500 (100%)
Canine	540	1	540 (100%)	1	540 (100%)
First premolar	460	1	40 (8.7%)	1	28 (6.1%)
				2	12 (2.6%)
		2	420 (91.3%)	2	420 (91.3%)
Second premolar	423	1	112 (26.5%)	1	75 (17.7%)
				2	37 (8.8%)
		2	311 (73.5%)	2	311 (73.5%)
First molar	410	3	410 (100%)	3	163 (39.7%)
				4	245 (59.8%)
				5	2 (0.5%)
Second molar	435	3	435 (100%)	3	210 (48.3%)
				4	224 (51.5%)
				5	1 (0.2%)
Third molar	238	1	114 (47.9%)	1	33 (13.8%)
				2	28 (11.8%)
				3	53 (22.3%)
		3	124 (52.1%)	3	119 (50%)
				4	5 (2.1%)

Table 2: Anatomy of roots and root canals in mandibular teeth.

Tooth	Number of studied teeth	Roots	*N* (%)	Canals	*N* (%)
Central incisor	512	1	512 (100%)	1	509 (99.4%)
				2	3 (0.6%)
Lateral incisor	500	1	500 (100%)	1	496 (99.2%)
				2	4 (0.8%)
Canine	521	1	521 (100%)	1	520 (99.8%)
					1 (0.2%)
First premolar	490	1	490 (100%)	1	437 (89.2%)
				2	53 (10.8%)
Second premolar	443	1	442 (99.8%)	1	399 (90.1%)
				2	43 (9.7%)
		2	1 (0.2%)	2	1(0.2%)
First molar	407	2	407 (100%)	2	2 (0.5%)
				3	320 (78.6%)
				4	85 (20.9%)
Second molar	398	1	2 (0.5%)	2	2 (0.5%)
		2	396 (99.5%)	2	47 (11.8%)
				3	327 (82.2%)
				4	22 (5.5%)
Third molar	210	1	42 (20%)	1	1 (0.5 %)
				2	41 (19.5%)
		2	168 (80%)	2	45 (21.4%)
				3	123 (58.6%)

canals in MB. Ghoncheh et al. (Iran) [28], Silva et al. (Brazil) [31], Ceperuelo et al. (Spain) [33], Betancourt et al. (Chili) [37], Al-Fouzan et al. (Saudi Arabia) [38], and Li et al. (China) [39] reported 14%, 32%, 75%, 48%, 19.7%, and 41.3%, respectively, of the prevalence of MB2 in maxillary second molar.

The maxillary third molar in our study was defined as single-rooted in 47.9% and three-rooted in 52.1%, and the system of root canals could consist of one, two, three, or more canals as shown in (Table 1). Similar results were found in a study of Sidow et al. (USA) [40], in which, it was found 15% of third molars had one root and 45% had three roots, and the number of canals ranged from 1 to 6 in teeth with one root and 2 to 5 in teeth with 3 roots. A study by Tomaszewska et al. (Poland) [41] reported the one-rooted maxillary third molar in 38.5% of cases and 61.5% were three-rooted. The prevalence of one, three, and four canals were 23.1%, 46.1%, and 15.4%, respectively. Singh and Pawar (India) [42] found three-canal system of maxillary third molar in 43% of cases and four-canal system in 5%.

In this study, for mandibular teeth, it was identified in central and lateral incisors and canines, one canal in 99.4%,

99.2%, and 99.8%, respectively, and two canals in 0.6%, 0.8%, and 0.2% of cases, respectively. These findings are consistent with other studies, where one canal was recorded in central incisors in 99.7% in Madeira and Hetem (Brazil) [43] and 99% in Walker (China) [44]. For lateral incisors, studies have reported the presence of 2 canals in 1.3% (Mexico) [11], 0.8% (Brazil) [43], and 1% (China) [44]. The presence of 2 canals in canines was 20.48% and 20.4% in studies by Rahimi et al. (Iran) [45] and Amardeep et al. (India) [16].

The mandibular first premolar was found as single-rooted in 100% of cases. One canal was found in 89.2%, and two canals in 10.8% of cases. This coincides with the results of Bulut (Turkey) [17], in which 1 canal was recorded in 94.2%, Llena et al. (Spain) [46], Alhadainy (Egypt) [47], and Sobhani et al. (Iran) [48], and one canal was found in 78.1%, 61.2%, and 90.8%, respectively. The presence of 2 canals was recorded by Zillich and Dowson (USA) [49] in 18.9%, Abraham and Gopinath (Emirate) [50] 35 %, Dou et al. (china) [51] with 34.27%, Bürklein et al. (Germany) [22] with 21.9%, and Singh and Pawar (India) [52] with 22%.

The mandibular second premolar had one root in 99.8%, and it had two roots in one clinical case (0.2%). When analyzing the root canal system, two canals were defined in 9.7% of cases. Similar data were found in studies by Bulut et al. (Turkey) [17] and Llena et al. (Spain) [46] with 98.9% and 90.6%, respectively, for the prevalence of one canal. Al-Qudah and Awawdeh (Jordan) [53], Bürklein et al. (Germany) [22], Bolhari et al. (Iran) [54], and Singh and Pawar (India) [52] recorded the prevalence of 2 canals in 22.8%, 3.6%, 8.7%, and 42% of cases, respectively.

The mandibular first molar had two roots in 100% of the cases. And, the anatomy of the root canal system could be two-canal, three-canal, and four-canal. Most often, there are three canals in 78.6% of observations. Similar data were found in Vertucci (USA) 59% [10], Pineda and Kuttler (Mexico) 57% [11], Celikten (Turkey) 84.6% [55], of cases of three-canal first molars. Skidmore and Bjorndal (USA) [56] have revealed 55.5% of cases. Zhang et al. (China) [57] recorded 56% and Caputo et al. (Brazil) [58] recorded 75.1% of cases of three-canals in mandibular first molars. The four-canal system of the first molar was defined in our study in 20.9% of cases; it was also described in the literature by Wasti et al. (Pakistan) [26] in 43.3% of cases, Caputo et al. (Brazil) [58] in 23.7%, Hung et al. (Taiwan) [59] in 40.5%, Celikten et al. (Turkey) [55] in 10.4%, Al-Qudah and Awawdeh (Jordan) [60] in 45.8%, and Pattanshetti et al. (Kuwait) [61] in 46.4%.

When analyzing the structure of the root canal system of the mandibular second molar, it was defined to be a two-, three-, and four-canal systems. 82.2% of cases had three canals. The most similar data were found in Celikten et al. (Turkey) [55], where 85.9% of three canals were recorded, and Neelakantan et al. (India) [62], in which most of second molars had two roots with three canals in 87.8%. Zhang et al. (China) [57] and Pawar et al. (India) [63] defined 3-canal system in 46% and 35.5% of cases.

The mandibular third molar was revealed as two-rooted in most cases (80%), and the canal system could have two- and three-canals, and these results agreed with other studies of the anatomy of third molar, as in Kuzekanani et al. (Iran) [64] where 73% of cases had 2 roots, and a study by Sidow et al. (USA) [40], where 77% of two roots were defined.

5. Conclusions

The root canal system varies greatly among populations and regions and even in different individuals within the same population, and using CBCT scanning is an effective technique in investigating the root canal system.

Abbreviations

CBCT: Cone-beam computed tomography
3D: Three-dimensional
MB: Mesiobuccal root
DB: Distobuccal root.

Acknowledgments

The publication has been prepared with the support of the "RUDN University Program 5-100."

References

[1] S. Rahimi and N. Ghasemi, "Maxillary first molar with two root canals," *Sultan Qaboos University Medical Journal*, vol. 13, no. 2, pp. 346–349, 2013.

[2] V. S. Blinov, M. V. Kartashov, S. E. Zholudev, and O. S. Zornikova, "Estimation of the cone-beam computed tomography in diagnostics of the molar root system anatomy of the mandible and maxilla," *Radiology—Practice*, vol. 59, no. 5, pp. 6–15, 2016.

[3] S. Patel, C. Durack, F. Abella, H. Shemesh, M. Roig, and K. Lemberg, "Cone beam computed tomography in Endodontics—a review," *International Endodontic Journal*, vol. 48, no. 1, pp. 3–15, 2015.

[4] V. V. Aliamovskii, O. A. Levenets, and A. A. Levenets, "Multiple anatomical variations of structure molars maxilla," *Endodontology Today*, no. 4, pp. 22–25, 2014.

[5] Y. A. Makedonova, I. V. Firsova, S. V. Poroyskyi, N. N. Trigolos, and E. B. Marymova, "Clinical-Radiological features of the structure of the tooth cavity and root canals of the upper," *Contemporary Problems of Science and Education*, no. 1, p. 1308, 2015.

[6] T. C. Blattner, N. George, C. C. Lee, V. Kumar, and C. D. Yelton, "Efficacy of cone-beam computed tomography as a modality to accurately identify the presence of second mesiobuccal canals in maxillary first and second molars: a pilot study," *Journal of Endodontics*, vol. 36, no. 5, pp. 867–870, 2010.

[7] J. Martos, C. Lubian, L. F. Silveria, L. A. Suita de Castro, and C. M. Ferrer Luque, "Morphologic analysis of the root apex in

human teeth," *Journal of Endodontics*, vol. 36, no. 4, pp. 664–667, 2010.

[8] Y. Kim, S. J. Lee, and J. Woo, "Morphology of maxillary first and second molars analyzed by cone-beam computed tomography in a Korean population: variations in the number of roots and canals and the incidence of fusion," *Journal of Endodontics*, vol. 38, no. 8, pp. 1063–1068, 2012.

[9] M. Iqbal and E. Fillmore, "Preoperative predictors of number of root canals clinically detected in maxillary molars: a pennendo database study," *Journal of Endodontics*, vol. 34, no. 4, pp. 413–416, 2008.

[10] F. J. Vertucci, "Root canal anatomy of the human permanent teeth," *Oral Surgery, Oral Medicine, Oral Pathology*, vol. 58, no. 5, pp. 589–599, 1984.

[11] F. Pineda and Y. Kuttler, "Mesiodistal and buccolingual roentgenographic investigation of 7,275 root canals," *Oral Surgery, Oral Medicine, Oral Pathology*, vol. 33, no. 1, pp. 101–110, 1972.

[12] F. S. Weine, H. J. Healey, H. Gerstein, and L. Evanson, "Canal configuration in the mesiobuccal root of the maxillary first molar and its endodontic significance," *Oral Surgery, Oral Medicine, Oral Pathology*, vol. 28, no. 3, pp. 419–425, 1969.

[13] M. K. Calişkan, Y. Pehlivan, F. Sepetcioğlu, M. Türkün, and S. Ş. Tuncer, "Root canal morphology of human permanent teeth in a Turkish population," *Journal of Endodontics*, vol. 21, no. 4, pp. 200–204, 1995.

[14] P. Jain, S. Balasubramanian, J. Sundaramurthy, and V. Natanasabapathy, "A cone beam computed tomography of the root canal morphology of maxillary anterior teeth in an institutional-based study in Chennai urban population: an in vitro study," *Journal of International Society of Preventive and Community Dentistry*, vol. 7, no. 8, pp. 68–74, 2017.

[15] S. Sert and G. S. Bayirli, "Evaluation of the root canal configurations of the mandibular and maxillary permanent teeth by gender in the Turkish population," *Journal of Endodontics*, vol. 30, no. 6, pp. 391–398, 2004.

[16] N. S. Amardeep, S. Raghu, and V. Natanasabapathy, "Root canal morphology of permanent maxillary and mandibular canines in Indian population using cone beam computed tomography," *Anatomy Research International*, vol. 2014, Article ID 731859, 7 pages, 2014.

[17] D. G. Bulut, E. Kose, G. Ozcan, A. E. Sekerci, E. M. Canger, and Y. Sisman, "Evaluation of root morphology and root canal configuration of premolars in the Turkish individuals using cone beam computed tomograpy," *European Journal of Dentistry*, vol. 9, no. 4, pp. 551–557, 2015.

[18] J. D. Pecora, P. C. Saquy, M. D. Sousa Neto, and J. B. Woelfel, "Root form and root canal anatomy of maxillary first premolars," *Brazilian Dental Journal*, vol. 2, no. 2, pp. 87–94, 1992.

[19] K. Kerekes and L. Tronstad, "Morphometric observations on root canals of human premolars," *Journal of Endodontics*, vol. 3, no. 2, pp. 74–79, 1977.

[20] D. Green, "Double canals in single roots," *Oral Surgery, Oral Medicine, Oral Pathology*, vol. 35, no. 5, pp. 689–696, 1973.

[21] E. Ok, M. Altunsoy, B. G. Nur, O. S. Aglarci, M. Çolak, and E. Güngör, "A cone-beam computed tomography study of root canal morphology of maxillary and mandibular premolars in a Turkish population," *Acta Odontologica Scandinavica*, vol. 72, no. 8, pp. 701–706, 2014.

[22] S. Bürklein, R. Heck, and E. Schäfer, "Evaluation of the root canal anatomy of maxillary and mandibular premolars in a selected German population using cone-beam computed tomographic data," *Journal of Endodontics*, vol. 43, no. 9, pp. 1448–1452, 2017.

[23] L. A. Awawdeh, H. Abdullah, and A. A. Al-Qudah, "Root form and canal morphology of Jordanian maxillary first premolars," *Journal of Endodontics*, vol. 34, no. 8, pp. 956–961, 2008.

[24] M. Elnour, A. Khabeer, and E. AlShwaimi, "Evaluation of root canal morphology of maxillary second premolars in a Saudi Arabian sub-population: an in vitro microcomputed tomography study," *Saudi Dental Journal*, vol. 28, no. 4, pp. 162–168, 2016.

[25] H. Pomeranz and G. Fishelberg, "The secondary mesiobuccal canal of maxillary molars," *Journal of the American Dental Association*, vol. 88, no. 1, pp. 119–124, 1974.

[26] F. Wasti, A. C. Shearer, and N. H. F. Wilson, "Root canal systems of the mandibular and maxillary first permanent molar teeth of south Asian Pakistanis," *International Endodontic Journal*, vol. 34, no. 4, pp. 263–266, 2001.

[27] N. Imura, G. I. Hata, and T. Toda, "Two canals in mesiobuccal roots of maxillary molars," *International Endodontic Journal*, vol. 31, no. 6, pp. 410–414, 1998.

[28] Z. Ghoncheh, B. M. Zade, and M. J. Kharazifard, "Root morphology of the maxillary first and second molars in an Iranian population using cone beam computed tomography," *Journal of Dentistry*, vol. 14, no. 3, pp. 115–122, 2017.

[29] J. N. R. Martins, D. Marques, A. Mata, and J. Caramês, "Root and root canal morphology of the permanent dentition in a Caucasian population: a cone-beam computed tomography study," *International Endodontic Journal*, vol. 50, no. 11, pp. 1013–1026, 2017.

[30] R. Ratanajirasut, A. Panichuttra, and S. Panmekiate, "A Cone-beam computed tomographic study of root and canal morphology of maxillary first and second permanent molars in a Thai population," *Journal of Endodontics*, vol. 44, no. 1, pp. 56–61, 2018.

[31] E. J. Silva, Y. Nejaim, A. I. Silva, F. Haiter-Neto, A. A. Zaia, and N. Cohenca, "Evaluation of root canal configuration of maxillary molars in a Brazilian population using cone-beam computed tomographic imaging: an in vivo study," *Journal of Endodontics*, vol. 40, no. 2, pp. 173–176, 2014.

[32] J. Guo, A. Vahidnia, P. Sedghizadeh, and R. Enciso, "Evaluation of root and canal morphology of maxillary permanent first molars in a north American population by cone-beam computed tomography," *Journal of Endodontics*, vol. 40, no. 5, pp. 635–639, 2014.

[33] D. Ceperuelo, M. Lozano, F. D. Sindreu, and M. Mercadé, "Root canal morphology of Chalcolithic and early bronze age human populations of El MiradorCave (Sierra de Atapuerca, Spain)," *Anatomical Record*, vol. 297, no. 12, pp. 2342–2348, 2014.

[34] R. M. A. Shalabi, O. E. Omer, J. Glennon, M. Jennings, and N. M. Claffey, "Root canal anatomy of maxillary first and second permanent molars," *International Endodontic Journal*, vol. 33, no. 5, pp. 405–414, 2000.

[35] J. C. Kulild and D. D. Peters, "Incidence and configuration of canal systems in the mesiobuccal root of maxillary first and second molars," *Journal of Endodontics*, vol. 16, no. 7, pp. 311–317, 1990.

[36] A. M. Alavi, A. Opasanon, Y. L. Ng, and K. Gulabivala, "Root and canal morphology of Thai maxillary molars," *International Endodontic Journal*, vol. 35, no. 5, pp. 478–485, 2002.

[37] P. Betancourt, P. Navarro, M. Cantin, and R. Fuentes, "Cone-beam computed tomography study of prevalence and location

of MB2canal in the mesiobuccal root of the maxillary second molar," *International Journal of Clinical and Experimental Medicine*, vol. 8, no. 6, pp. 9128–9134, 2015.

[38] K. S. Al-Fouzan, H. F. Ounis, K. Merdad, and K. Al-Hezaimi, "Incidence of canal systems in the mesio-buccal roots of maxillary first and second molarsin Saudi Arabian population," *Australian Endodontic Journal*, vol. 39, no. 3, pp. 98–101, 2013.

[39] L. Li, F. L. Zhan, and Y. W. Jin, "Preliminary study on root canal morphology of maxillary second molars," *Shanghai Kou Qiang Yi Xue*, vol. 23, no. 2, pp. 179–183, 2014.

[40] S. J. Sidow, L. A. West, F. R. Liewehr, and R. J. Loushine, "Root canal morphology of human maxillary and mandibular third molars," *Journal of Endodontics*, vol. 26, no. 11, pp. 675–678, 2000.

[41] I. M. Tomaszewska, B. Leszczyński, A. Wróbel, T. Gładysz, and H. F. Duncan, "A micro-computed tomographic (micro-CT) analysis of the root canal morphology of maxillary third molar teeth," *Annals of Anatomy—Anatomischer Anzeiger*, vol. 215, pp. 83–92, 2018.

[42] S. Singh and M. Pawar, "Root canal morphology of south Asian Indian maxillary molar teeth," *European Journal of Dentistry*, vol. 9, no. 1, pp. 133–144, 2015.

[43] M. C. Madeira and S. Hetem, "Incidence of bifurcations in mandibular incisors," *Oral Surgery, Oral Medicine, Oral Pathology*, vol. 36, no. 4, pp. 589–591, 1973.

[44] R. T. Walker, "The root canal anatomy of mandibular incisors in a southern Chinese population," *International Endodontic Journal*, vol. 21, no. 3, pp. 218–223, 1988.

[45] S. Rahimi, A. S. Milani, S. Shahi, Y. Sergiz, S. Nezafati, and M. Lotfi, "Prevalence of two root canals in human mandibular anterior teeth in an Iranian population," *Indian Journal of Dental Research*, vol. 24, no. 2, pp. 234–236, 2013.

[46] C. Llena, J. Fernandez, P. S. Ortolani, and L. Forner, "Cone-beam computed tomography analysis of root and canal morphology of mandibular premolars in a Spanish population," *Imaging Science in Dentistry*, vol. 44, no. 3, pp. 221–227, 2014.

[47] H. A. Alhadainy, "Canal configuration of mandibular first premolars in an Egyptian population," *Journal of Advanced Research*, vol. 4, no. 2, pp. 123–128, 2013.

[48] M. A. Sobhani, H. Razmi, and M. Sadegh, "Evaluation of anatomy and morphology of human mandibular premolar teeth by cone-beam computed tomography in Iranian population," *Journal of Dental Medicine*, vol. 26, no. 3, 2013.

[49] R. Zillich and J. Dowson, "Root canal morphology of mandibular first and second premolars," *Oral Surgery, Oral Medicine, Oral Pathology*, vol. 36, no. 5, pp. 738–744, 1973.

[50] S. B. Abraham and V. K. Gopinath, "Root canal anatomy of mandibular first premolars in an Emirati subpopulation: a laboratory study," *European Journal of Dentistry*, vol. 9, no. 4, pp. 476–482, 2015.

[51] L. Dou, D. Li, T. Xu, Y. Tang, and D. Yang, "Root anatomy and canal morphology of mandibular first premolars in a Chinese population," *Scientific Reports*, vol. 7, no. 1, p. 750, 2017.

[52] S. Singh and M. Pawar, "Root canal morphology of south Asian Indian mandibular premolar teeth," *Journal of Endodontics*, vol. 40, no. 9, pp. 1338–1341, 2014.

[53] A. A. Al-Qudah and L. A. Awawdeh, "Root form and canal morphology of mandibular premolars in a Jordanian population," *International Endodontic Journal*, vol. 41, no. 3, pp. 240–248, 2008.

[54] B. Bolhari, H. Assadian, and T. Fattah, "Evaluation of the root canal morphology of mandibular second premolars in an Iranian population," *Journal of Dentistry*, vol. 10, no. 6, pp. 516–521, 2013.

[55] B. Celikten, P. Tufenkci, U. Aksoy et al., "Cone beam CT evaluation of mandibular molar root canal morphology in a Turkish Cypriot population," *Clinical Oral Investigations*, vol. 20, no. 8, pp. 2221–2226, 2016.

[56] A. E. Skidmore and A. M. Bjorndal, "Root canal morphology of the human mandibular first molar," *Oral Surgery, Oral Medicine, Oral Pathology*, vol. 32, no. 5, pp. 778–784, 1971.

[57] R. Zhang, H. Wang, Y. Y. Tian, X. Yu, T. Hu, and P. M. Dummer, "Use of cone-beam computed tomography to evaluate root and canal morphology of mandibular molars in Chinese individuals," *International Endodontic Journal*, vol. 44, no. 11, pp. 990–999, 2011.

[58] B. V. Caputo, G. A. Noro Filho, D. M. de Andrade Salgado, C. Moura-Netto, E. M. Giovani, and C. Costa, "Evaluation of the root canal morphology of molars by using cone-beam computed tomography in a Brazilian population: part I," *Journal of Endodontics*, vol. 42, no. 11, pp. 1604–1607, 2016.

[59] C. C. Huang, Y. C. Chang, M. C. Chuang et al., "Evaluation of root and canal systems of mandibular first molars in Taiwanese individuals using cone-beam computed tomography," *Journal of the Formosan Medical Association*, vol. 109, no. 4, pp. 303–308, 2010.

[60] A. A. Al-Qudah and L. A. Awawdeh, "Root and canal morphology of mandibular first and second molar teeth in a Jordanian population," *International Endodontic Journal*, vol. 42, pp. 775–784, 2009.

[61] N. Pattanshetti, M. Gaidhane, and A. M. Al Kandari, "Root and canal morphology of the mesiobuccal and distal roots of permanent first molars in a Kuwait population: a clinical study," *International Endodontic Journal*, vol. 41, no. 9, pp. 755–762, 2008.

[62] P. Neelakantan, C. Subbarao, C. V. Subbarao, and M. Ravindranath, "Root and canal morphology of mandibular second molars in an Indian population," *Journal of Endodontics*, vol. 36, no. 8, pp. 1319–1322, 2010.

[63] A. M. Pawar, M. Pawar, A. Kfir et al., "Root canal morphology and variations in mandibular second molar teeth of an Indian population: an in vivo cone-beam computed tomography analysis," *Clinical Oral Investigations*, vol. 21, no. 9, pp. 2801–2809, 2017.

[64] M. Kuzekanani, J. Haghani, and H. Nosrati, "Root and canal morphology of mandibular third molars in an Iranian population," *Journal of Dental Research, Dental Clinics, Dental Prospects*, vol. 6, no. 3, pp. 85–88, 2012.

11

Specific Central Nervous System Medications Are Associated with Temporomandibular Joint Symptoms

John K. Drisdale III, Monica G. Thornhill, and Alexandre R. Vieira

Department of Oral Biology, University of Pittsburgh School of Dental Medicine, Pittsburgh, PA, USA

Correspondence should be addressed to Alexandre R. Vieira; arv11@pitt.edu

Academic Editor: Manal Awad

Aims. There is evidence of association between bruxism and the increasingly common central nervous system stimulants prescribed for attention deficit hyperactivity disorder (ADHD), as well as the selective serotonin reuptake inhibitors (SSRIs) often prescribed for depression or anxiety. However, the evidence is not clear on whether these medications inducing bruxism are directly associated with temporomandibular joint disorder (TMD). The aim of this work is to evaluate whether these medications are associated with TMD symptoms. *Methods.* Medical history and participant data were obtained for 469 patients from the University of Pittsburgh School of Dental Medicine, Dental Registry and DNA Repository, dating back to 2006. The chi-square test was used to determine any statistically significant associations. *Results.* There were no statistically significant associations between ADHD stimulant medications or SSRIs and reported TMD symptoms. However, there were significant differences seen between specific brands of medications and reported TMD symptoms. Individuals prescribed methylphenidate (Concerta) were less likely to report temporomandibular joint discomfort ($p = 0.01$). Conversely, individuals prescribed citalopram (Celexa) were more likely to report temporomandibular joint discomfort ($p = 0.04$). *Conclusion.* Signs and symptoms of temporomandibular joint dysfunction may be influenced by the use of certain medications prescribed for depression or attention deficit hyperactive disorder.

1. Introduction

As of 2012, more than 4.8 million Americans were prescribed stimulant medications to treat attention deficit hyperactivity disorder (ADHD) [1]. One out of ten Americans above the age of 12 are prescribed antidepressants, selective serotonin reuptake inhibitors (SSRIs) being the most common [2]. Central nervous system- (CNS-) stimulant ADHD medications have been associated with side effects such as bruxism [3] that can possibly cause TMD-like symptoms [4]. With the increasing use of stimulant ADHD medications, it is important to see if there is a relationship between these prescribed medications and TMD symptoms [5].

TMD can manifest in a variety of symptoms including pain or tenderness in the face muscles or jaw joint, a limited range of motion of the jaw, popping and clicking of the jaw, and headaches [6]. In addition to the adverse symptoms of TMD, treatment can often be extensive as well as expensive.

TMD symptoms are also more commonly seen in the female population. Of concern could be the recent increase in use of stimulant ADHD medications in women aged 26 to 34 [1]. The inherent predisposition to TMD symptoms in women combined with an increased use of ADHD medications could possibly put this patient population at an increased risk for developing TMD symptoms. Given this information, we hypothesize that there is an association between ADHD medications, as well as SSRIs, and the frequency of reported TMD symptoms.

2. Subjects and Methods

All subjects in this study were participants in the Dental Registry and DNA Repository of the University of Pittsburgh School of Dental Medicine [7–9]. All participants sought treatment at the University of Pittsburgh School of Dental Medicine dating back to September 2006. In April 2015, data from 4,959 individuals were queried from the registry and repository for this study and 469 individuals taking ADHD and SSRI medications were selected for this study. The records

Table 1: Comparison of the type of ADHD medication by the presence of TMD symptoms. The results show that Concerta is the ADHD medication that is significantly different compared to the rest.

	TMD diagnosis		Total
	No discomfort	Positive for discomfort	
Type of ADHD medication			
None			
Count	237	171	408
Expected count	243.6	164.4	408.0
% within type of medication	58.1%	41.9%	100.0%
Adjusted residual	−1.8	1.8	
Adderall			
Count	13	13	26
Expected count	15.5	10.5	26.0
% within type of medication	50.0%	50.0%	100.0%
Adjusted residual	−1.0	1.0	
Concerta			
Count	14	1	15
Expected count	9.0	6.0	15.0
% within type of medication	93.3%	6.7%	100.0%
Adjusted residual	**2.7**	**−2.7**	
Ritalin			
Count	11	4	15
Expected count	9.0	6.0	15.0
% within type of medication	73.3%	26.7%	100.0%
Adjusted residual	1.1	−1.1	
Vyvanse			
Count	3	0	3
Expected count	1.8	1.2	3.0
% within type of medication	100.0%	0.0%	100.0%
Adjusted residual	1.4	−1.4	
Adderall and Vyvanse			
Count	1	0	1
Expected count	.6	.4	1.0
% within type of medication	100.0%	0.0%	100.0%
Adjusted residual	.8	−.8	
Concerta and Ritalin			
Count	1	0	1
Expected count	.6	.4	1.0
% within type of medication	100.0%	0.0%	100.0%
Adjusted residual	.8	−.8	
Total			
Count	280	189	469
Expected count	280.0	189.0	469.0
% within type of medication	59.7%	40.3%	100.0%

Bold highlights the highest adjusted residual.

of these individuals were evaluated to determine if they had any TMD symptoms (pain or discomfort, cracking or clicking when opening the mouth).

Chi-square tests were used to determine associations between being prescribed any stimulant ADHD or SSRI medications and TMD symptoms. The same was performed for subjects prescribed any SSRI medication in search of a significant association between SSRIs and TMD symptoms. We used the likelihood ratio for comparisons when we violated the assumption of minimum expected cell count to be used for Pearson's chi-square. Alpha was established at 5%.

Standardized residuals were then compared to determine which medication in each category was responsible for a significantly different report rate of TMD symptoms.

TABLE 2: Comparison of the type of SSRI medication by the presence of TMD symptoms. The results show that Celexa is the SSRI that is significantly different compared to the rest.

	TMD diagnosis		Total
	No discomfort	Positive for discomfort	
Type of SSRI			
None			
Count	80	42	122
Expected count	72.8	49.2	122.0
% within type of SSRI	65.6%	34.4%	100.0%
Adjusted residual	1.5	−1.5	
Celexa			
Count	30	35	65
Expected count	38.8	26.2	65.0
% within type of SSRI	46.2%	53.8%	100.0%
Adjusted residual	**−2.4**	**2.4**	
Lexapro			
Count	40	30	70
Expected count	41.8	28.2	70.0
% within type of SSRI	57.1%	42.9%	100.0%
Adjusted residual	−.5	.5	
Prozac			
Count	58	27	85
Expected count	50.7	34.3	85.0
% within type of SSRI	68.2%	31.8%	100.0%
Adjusted residual	1.8	−1.8	
Luvox			
Count	8	4	12
Expected count	7.2	4.8	12.0
% within type of SSRI	66.7%	33.3%	100.0%
Adjusted residual	.5	−.5	
Paxil			
Count	17	12	29
Expected count	17.3	11.7	29.0
% within type of SSRI	58.6%	41.4%	100.0%
Adjusted residual	−.1	.1	
Zoloft			
Count	41	34	75
Expected count	44.8	30.2	75.0
% within type of SSRI	54.7%	45.3%	100.0%
Adjusted residual	−1.0	1.0	
Lexapro and Zoloft			
Count	2	3	5
Expected count	3.0	2.0	5.0
% within type of SSRI	40.0%	60.0%	100.0%
Adjusted residual	−.9	.9	
Lexapro and Prozac			
Count	2	0	2
Expected count	1.2	.8	2.0
% within type of SSRI	100.0%	0.0%	100.0%
Adjusted residual	1.2	−1.2	

Table 2: Continued.

	TMD diagnosis		Total
	No discomfort	Positive for discomfort	
Lexapro and Paxil			
Count	0	2	2
Expected count	1.2	.8	2.0
% within type of SSRI	0.0%	100.0%	100.0%
Adjusted residual	−1.7	1.7	
Celexa and Zoloft			
Count	2	0	2
Expected count	1.2	.8	2.0
% within type of SSRI	100.0%	0.0%	100.0%
Adjusted residual	1.2	−1.2	
Total			
Count	280	189	469
Expected count	280.0	189.0	469.0
% within type of SSRI	59.7%	40.3%	100.0%

Bold highlights the highest adjusted residual.

3. Results

The mean age of the 469 participants was 46 years, with 38% of participants identifying as male ($N = 179$) and 62% female ($N = 290$). Furthermore, the majority of participants were White ($N = 394$; 84%). The remaining 16% were comprised of Black individuals ($N = 52$), Hispanics ($N = 6$), and other groups ($N = 17$).

There was a trend, albeit not statistically significant, for being prescribed ADHD medication and reporting TMD symptoms ($p = 0.065$). Likewise, there was no significant association between taking SSRIs and reporting TMD symptoms ($p = 0.12$). We found differences in occurrence of reported TMD symptoms between the different ADHD stimulant medications ($p = 0.04$, six degrees of freedom). The likelihood ratio of .010 suggested that there is at least one medication that is statistically significant among the others in regard to reported TMD symptoms. Further testing by means of finding the expected counts and adjusted residuals for each ADHD medication determined that Concerta was the statistically significant medication when compared to the others (Table 1). Additionally, taking the observed counts versus the expected counts in Table 1 into consideration also depicts that subjects prescribed Concerta are less likely to report TMD symptoms than subjects prescribed any other ADHD stimulant. There were no differences based on sex or ethnic background (data not shown).

Similarly, the group of SSRIs also showed that there is a medication with a significant difference in regard to reported TMD symptoms ($p = 0.075$, 10 degrees of freedom); thus the likelihood ratio is of .040. Celexa showed a difference in expected reporting of TMD symptoms when compared to the other SSRIs (Table 2). Additionally, taking the observed counts versus the expected counts in Table 2 into consideration also depicts that subjects prescribed Celexa are more likely to report TMD symptoms than subjects prescribed any other SSRI. There were no differences based on sex or ethnic background (data not shown).

Being prescribed both an ADHD medication and SSRI showed a trend, albeit not statistically significant, for reporting TMD symptoms ($p = 0.074$).

4. Discussion

The results show that there is no formal significant difference in TMD symptoms between those that are prescribed ADHD medications and those that are not prescribed ADHD medications. This same statement also holds true for subjects prescribed SSRIs and those not prescribed SSRIs. However, there does seem to be a significant difference *between* the different medications prescribed. Our data shows that subjects prescribed Concerta for ADHD are less likely to report TMD symptoms when compared to subjects taking other ADHD medications. It is also important to consider that our data shows that subjects taking the SSRI Celexa are more likely to report experiencing TMD symptoms than those prescribed an SSRI other than Celexa.

This could be clinically important when treating patients who are already at an increased risk for TMD. According to numerous studies, including the National Institute of Dental and Craniofacial Research, women are at higher risk than are men for developing TMD symptoms [6]. Since TMD is a multifactorial disorder [10], it may be wise to limit the number of contributing factors targeted for intervention. For example, a patient that is already predisposed to TMD may benefit from being prescribed Concerta versus other ADHD stimulants due to Concerta's lower frequency of reported TMD symptoms. Similarly, the same patient population that requires a SSRI prescription may benefit from a SSRI other than Celexa. Understanding better the contributing factors to this multifactorial disorder could prove beneficial to the patient's health and ultimately their quality of life.

In summary, we report here for the first time that specific ADNH and SSRI drugs may impact risks for developing TMD.

Acknowledgments

The authors thank the individuals that enthusiastically participated in this study. The Dental Registry and DNA Repository project is supported by the University of Pittsburgh School of Dental Medicine.

References

[1] J. Austerman and D. J. Muzina, *Turning Attention to ADHD. U.S. Medication Trends for Attention Deficit Hyperactivity Disorder. An Express Scripts Report*, The Express Scripts Laboratory, 2014.

[2] National Institute of Mental Health, *Attention-Deficit/Hyperactivity Disorder (ADHD): The Basics*, vol. 8 of *NIH Publication no. QF-16-3572*, U.S. Department of Health and Human Services, 2016.

[3] F. Lobbezoo, R. J. van Denderen, J. G. Verheij, and M. Naeije, "Reports of SSRI-associated bruxism in the family physician's office," *Journal of Orofacial Pain*, vol. 15, no. 4, pp. 340–346, 2001.

[4] G. A. Malki, K. H. Zawawi, M. Melis, and C. V. Hughes, "Prevalence of bruxism in children receiving treatment for attention deficit hyperactivity disorder: A pilot study," *Journal of Clinical Pediatric Dentistry*, vol. 29, no. 1, pp. 63–67, 2004.

[5] D. M. Laskin, "Etiology of the pain-dysfunction syndrome.," *The Journal of the American Dental Association*, vol. 79, no. 1, pp. 147–153, 1969.

[6] B. Bagis, E. A. Ayaz, S. Turgut, R. Durkan, and M. Özcan, "Gender difference in prevalence of signs and symptoms of temporoman-dibular joint disorders: A retrospective study on 243 consecutive patients," *International Journal of Medical Sciences*, vol. 9, no. 7, pp. 539–544, 2012.

[7] I. Anjomshoaa, M. E. Cooper, and A. R. Vieira, "Caries is associated with asthma and epilepsy," *European Journal of Dentistry*, vol. 3, no. 4, pp. 297–303, 2009.

[8] L. Johnston and A. R. Vieira, "Caries experience and overall health status," *Oral Health & Preventive Dentistry*, vol. 12, no. 2, pp. 163–170, 2014.

[9] A. R. Vieira, K. M. Hilands, and T. W. Braun, "Saving more teeth—a case for personalized care," *Journal of Personalized Medicine*, vol. 5, no. 1, pp. 30–35, 2015.

[10] M. Oakley and A. R. Vieira, "The many faces of the genetics contribution to temporomandibular joint disorder," *Orthodontics and Craniofacial Research*, vol. 11, no. 3, pp. 125–135, 2008.

12

The Ball Welding Bar: A New Solution for the Immediate Loading of Screw-Retained, Mandibular Fixed Full Arch Prostheses

Danilo Bacchiocchi[1] and Andrea Guida[2]

[1] *Private Practice, Castelfidardo, 60022 Ancona, Italy*
[2] *Fundacao Universitaria Vida Crista (FUNVIC), 12400-010 Pindamonhangaba, SP, Brazil*

Correspondence should be addressed to Andrea Guida; prof.andreaguida@funvic.edu.br

Academic Editor: Eitan Mijiritsky

Purpose. To present a new intraoral welding technique, which can be used to manufacture screw-retained, mandibular fixed full-arch prostheses. *Methods.* Over a 4-year period, all patients with complete mandibular edentulism or irreparably compromised mandibular dentition, who will restore the masticatory function with a fixed mandibular prosthesis, were considered for inclusion in this study. The "Ball Welding Bar" (BWB) technique is characterised by smooth prosthetic cylinders, interconnected by means of titanium bars which are adjustable in terms of distance from ball terminals and are inserted in the rotating rings of the cylinders. All the components are welded and self-posing. *Results.* Forty-two patients (18 males; 24 females; mean age 64.2 ± 6.7 years) were enrolled and 210 fixtures were inserted to support 42 mandibular screw-retained, fixed full-arch prostheses. After two years of loading, 2 fixtures were lost, for an implant survival rate of 97.7%. Five implants suffered from peri-implant mucositis and 3 implants for peri-implantitis. Three of the prostheses (3/42) required repair for fracture (7.1%): the prosthetic success was 92.9%. *Conclusions.* The BWB technique seems to represent a reliable technique for the fabrication of screw-retained mandibular fixed full-arch prostheses. This study was registered in the ISRCTN register with number ISRCTN71229338.

1. Introduction

In 1982, P. L. Mondani and P. M. Mondani published an article in which they fully described the equipment and techniques necessary for intraoral welding, a welding procedure for intraoral implant abutments, developed to obtain an immediate fixed prosthesis without the need for complex and lengthy laboratory procedures [1]. The method was essentially based on the creation of an electric arc between two electrodes under an argon gas flux [1]. Current scientific literature has validated the use of intraoral welding techniques [2–6]. In 2002, Hruska et al. published a study reporting the results of 1301 immediately loaded implants, 436 of which were used to support fixed partial dentures and full arches built over intraorally welded frameworks [2]. In this paper, the authors reported a rather low incidence of implant failures, with three failed implants (0.7%), one due to fracturing and two due to peri-implantitis [2]. The authors showed how, in cases of extensive reconstruction, intraoral welding had the advantage of simplifying prosthetic procedures and in particular those involving highly disparallel abutments [2]. Intraorally welded frameworks acted as mesiostructures and reduced the incidence of fractures of the provisional prosthesis [2]. More than 20 years after the publication of Mondani's article [1], Degidi et al. published a study on the immediate loading of multiple implants using a preformed bar that was welded intraorally to the implant abutments and that supported a temporary, metal-reinforced bridge [3]. All 192 immediately loaded implants survived, and no prosthetic complications occurred at the level of the provisional prosthesis [3]. This structure proved to be capable of withstanding load better than a temporary restoration without reinforcement, as demonstrated by finite element analysis [3]. In a later work by the same authors [4], intraoral welding proved to be a reliable technique for the rehabilitation of completely edentulous mandibles. The process they described involved the delivery and immediate loading of a full arch prosthesis on the day of surgery, using fixtures with butt-joints and conical implant-abutment connections. Once again, in a further prospective clinical work, Degidi et al. showed the rehabilitation of the fully edentulous mandible by inserting 4 implants, splinted to each other through the intraoral welding of a bar to their titanium abutments [5]. The framework thus obtained was used to support an immediately loaded definitive prosthesis [5]. In brief, 22 patients treated with 88 implants were followed for a total period of one year. At the end of the period, only one implant was lost within a month of insertion, for an implant survival rate of 98.9% [5]. No fractures or alterations occurred to the intraorally welded framework, and no fractures of the prosthetic acrylic resin superstructure were recorded [5]. Finally, in 2013, Degidi et al. reported the 6-year follow-up results of the welding technique for the fabrication of immediately loaded maxillary and mandibular fixed full arches [6]. All the patients in this study were rehabilitated on the same day of surgery with a temporary, immediately loaded prosthesis built on a titanium framework obtained by the intraoral welding of a titanium bar to the implant abutments [6]. In total, there were 124 implants placed in the maxilla and 87 implants placed in the mandible; the fixtures were controlled for up to 6 years after loading [6]. Mean peri-implant bone resorption was measured as 1.39 mm (±0.67) and 1.29 mm (±0.71) for the maxilla and mandible, respectively [6]. The most frequent complication was the fracture of the resin superstructure. Overall, the intraoral welding technique proved to be effective and reliable in allowing the fabrication of immediately loaded prostheses in edentulous patients [6]. Some possible variations to the classic technique of intraoral welding have been presented in recent scientific literature [7–10]. In the most commonly used methods, the diameter of the bar (generally made of titanium grade 2) is chosen based on the distance between the implants, the extent of the arch, and the available prosthetic volumes. The bar is then shaped to be adherent to the titanium cylinders placed on the abutments and is then welded to them [2–6, 8, 10]. The purpose of our present work is therefore to present a new variant of the intraoral welding technique, which can be used to manufacture full arch screw-retained rehabilitations of the edentulous mandible, under an immediate loading protocol. This innovative type of prosthetic rehabilitation, which the authors refer to as the "Ball Welding Bar" (BWB) technique, is characterised by smooth prosthetic cylinders, interconnected by means of titanium bars (grade 4) which are adjustable in terms of distance from ball terminals and are inserted in the rotating rings of the cylinders. All the components are welded and self-posing and do not cause arcing or tension. This paper reports on a study tracking the results obtained two years after immediate loading of a full arch, screw-retained mandibular prosthesis (Toronto bridges) that was screwed onto the new intraorally welded Ball Welding Bars.

2. Materials and Methods

2.1. Patient Sample. In the period between January 2010 and December 2013, all patients who were referred to two different private dental centres (the private dental clinics of Professor Andrea Guida and Dr. Danilo Bacchiocchi) for rehabilitation using oral implants were considered for inclusion in this prospective clinical study. Patients considered for inclusion were those with

(1) complete mandibular edentulism, with functional and aesthetic problems related to the presence of a complete, removable conventional denture (i.e., lack of stability of the complete denture, discomfort during function, and aesthetic embarrassment),

(2) irreparably compromised mandibular dentition, due to advanced periodontal disease or destructive/massive tooth decay that made the residual dental elements unrestorable,

(3) sufficient bone volume (bone height × width) to allow for the placement of implants of at least 8 mm in length and 3.0 mm in diameter,

(4) will to restore the masticatory function with a fixed mandibular prosthesis supported by dental implants,

(5) the ability to understand and sign an informed consent form for implant treatment.

Patients excluded from the study were those

(1) with general medical conditions/systemic diseases that represented an absolute contraindication to surgical and implant treatment, such as severely immunocompromised patients or severely uncompensated diabetics, patients receiving radiotherapy to the head and neck area or chemotherapy, and patients receiving amino-bisphosphonates intravenously and/or orally,

(2) with psychiatric disorders,

(3) addicted to alcohol or drugs,

(4) who needed bone augmentation procedures with autogenous bone or other bone substitutes, to allow for proper implant insertion,

(5) who had previously undergone major regenerative bone surgery, preliminary to the placement of dental implants. Inclusion and exclusion criteria for the present study were also summarized in Table 1.

Cigarette smoking was not an exclusion criterion for enrollment in this study; nevertheless, patients that smoke were informed of the fact that cigarette smoking is a risk factor for the success of implant treatments [11]. All patients received detailed information about the planned therapy, the related risks, and possible alternatives. Patients were enrolled only after signing an informed consent form for implant treatment. Finally, the present clinical work was carried out in compliance with the principles set out in the Helsinki Declaration on Human Experimentation of 2000 (revised 2008). The present clinical study was registered in the ISRCTN, a publicly available register for clinical trials recognized by WHO and ICMJE, with number ISRCTN71229338.

Table 1: Inclusion and exclusion criteria for enrollment of patients in the study.

Inclusion criteria	Exclusion criteria
(1) Complete mandibular edentulism, with functional and aesthetic problems related to the presence of a complete, removable conventional denture.	(1) Severely immunocompromised status, severely uncompensated diabetes, radiotherapy of head and neck area, chemotherapy, and treatment with intravenous and/or intraoral amino-bisphosphonates.
(2) Irreparably compromised mandibular dentition, due to advanced periodontal disease or destructive/massive tooth decay that made the residual dental elements unrestorable.	(2) Psychiatric disorders.
(3) Sufficient bone volume to allow for the placement of implants of at least 8 mm in length and 3.0 mm in diameter.	(3) Alcohol and/or drugs addition.
(4) Will to restore the masticatory function with a fixed mandibular prosthesis supported by dental implants.	(4) Need for bone augmentation procedures with autogenous bone or other bone substitutes, to allow for proper implant insertion.
(5) Ability to understand and sign an informed consent form for implant treatment.	(5) Previous interventions of regenerative bone surgery.

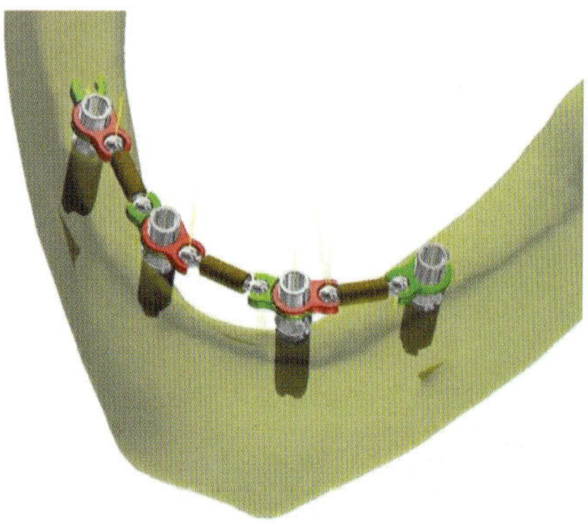

Figure 1: The BWB (Ball Welding Bar) consists of smooth prosthetic cylinders, interconnected by means of titanium bars (grade 4) adjustable in distance with ball terminals, which are inserted in the rotating rings of the cylinders. All the components are welded and self-posing, without arcing nor tensions. This BWB has been patented by the authors (patent number AN2014A000111 and variants).

2.2. The Ball Welding Bar (BWB) Concept. The BWB (Ball Welding Bar) consists of smooth prosthetic cylinders, interconnected by means of titanium bars (grade 4) which are adjustable in terms of distance from ball terminals and are inserted in the rotating rings of the cylinders. All the components are welded and self-posing and do not cause arcing or tension (Figure 1). This prosthetic device has been patented by the authors (patent number AN2014A000111 and variants).

2.3. The Implants Used in This Study. The fixtures used in the present work (BT Safe Bone Level®; Biotec BTK, Povolaro di Dueville, Vicenza, Italy) were made of titanium grade 4 (ASTM F67dISO 5832-2). These were tapered implants with double lead threads (Figure 2) and a hexagonal conical connection (11°) and integrated platform switching [12]. The dual acid etched (DAE) surface of these implants was the result of treatment with a mixture of strong inorganic acids (H2SO4, H3PO4, HCl, and HF) [13]. The implants were then rinsed and washed with distilled water, to neutralize acid residuals. Finally, implants were taken to a cleaning room (ISO 7 class) to be decontaminated through a plasma spray decontamination process, in an argon atmosphere.

The DAE implant surface (Figure 3) had the following roughness parameters:

(i) Ra (arithmetic mean of the absolute height of all points) = 1.12 (60.41) μm,

(ii) Rq (square root of the sum of the squared mean difference of all points) = 1.34 (60.69) μm,

(iii) Rt (difference between the highest and the lowest points) = 3.86 (61.40) μm [13].

2.4. Surgical and Prosthetic Phases. A preliminary clinical and radiographic evaluation with panoramic radiographs (Figure 4) preceded the surgery. Where needed, a cone beam computed tomography (CBCT) scan (I-Max Touch 3D®, Owandy Radiology, Oxford, CT, USA) was performed, in order to collect all anatomical information for optimal surgical and prosthetic planning. The digital imaging and communication in medicine (DICOM) files from CBCT were imported into three-dimensional (3D) reconstruction software, where the surgical and prosthetic planning was performed, and the feasibility of the protocol was investigated. The present protocol involved the fabrication of screw-retained, complete mandibular dentures (Toronto bridge) supported by 5 dental implants. Two implants had to be inserted in the molar areas (3.6 and 4.6, resp.), two in the first premolar areas (3.4 and 4.4, resp.), and the last one in midline or otherwise in the incisal areas (3.1 or 4.1). The prosthesis had to be immediately loaded, supported by multiunit abutments (MUA) splinted together with a Ball Welding Bar (BWB). Prior to surgery, a complete lower

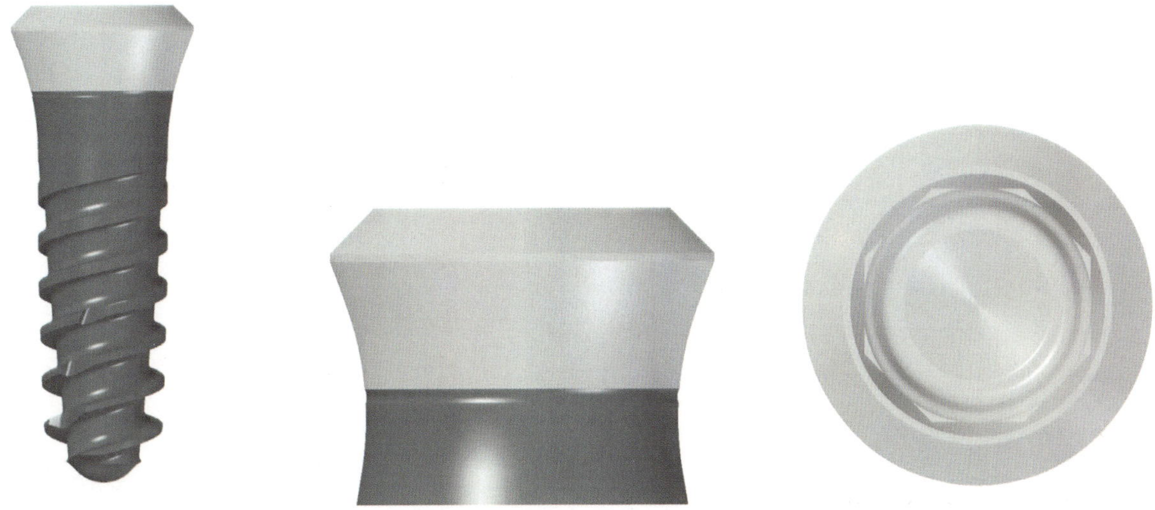

(a) (b) (c)

Figure 2: Drawing of the tapered, double lead threads implant used in this study. (a) Apical threads, deeper and cutting, favour insertion, and initial stability, whereas squared coronal thread enhances bone condensation. (b) Back-tapered collar provides excellent cortical bone management, improving soft tissue support. (c) Octagonal conical connection (2 mm in depth with 8° cone) that guarantees an excellent seal, reducing the risk of micromovements between the implant and the abutment.

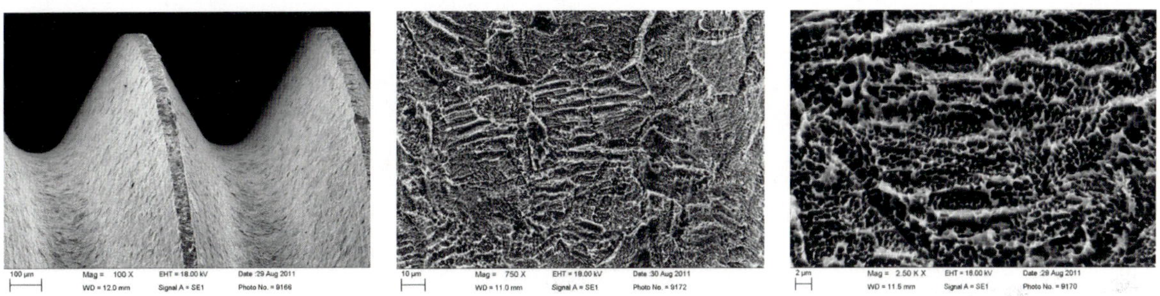

(a) (b) (c)

Figure 3: Scanning electron microscopy (SEM) evaluation of the dual acid etched (DAE) implant surface. The surface (a) presented micron-sized shallow cavities uniformly covered by submicroscopic pitting (b) limited by razor-sharp cusps and edges (c).

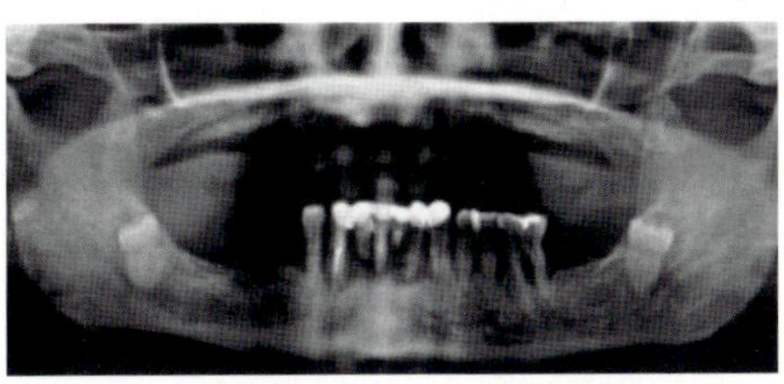

Figure 4: Preoperative situation. A 52-year female patient in good general health had a complete removable denture in the maxilla and a severe acute periodontitis in the mandible, with several teeth with reduced bone support and therefore high mobility. The patient asked for a full arch implant supported rehabilitation of the mandible, possibly involving an immediate loading protocol.

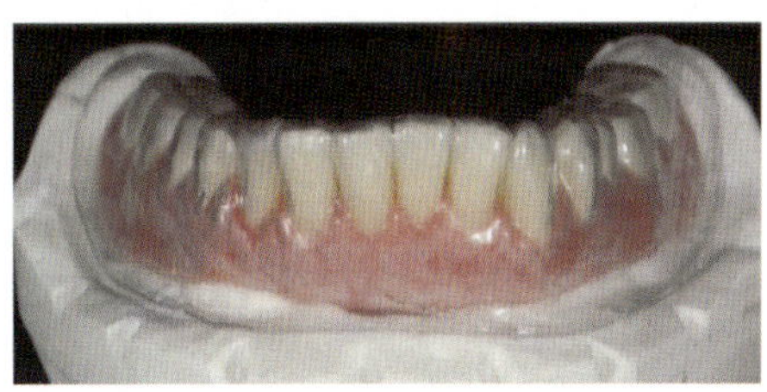

Figure 5: Prior to surgery, a complete lower denture was fabricated in the dental laboratory, made in composite resin with a transparent vacuum-formed template.

denture was fabricated in the dental laboratory, from composite resin with a transparent vacuum-formed template (Figure 5). In order to achieve this, impressions were taken and casts were developed and mounted in an articulator, with bite-in wax for definition of the proper occlusion and the selection of the colour and the shape of the teeth. This lower denture was then hollowed in order to be able to accommodate the intraorally welded titanium framework. Flanges

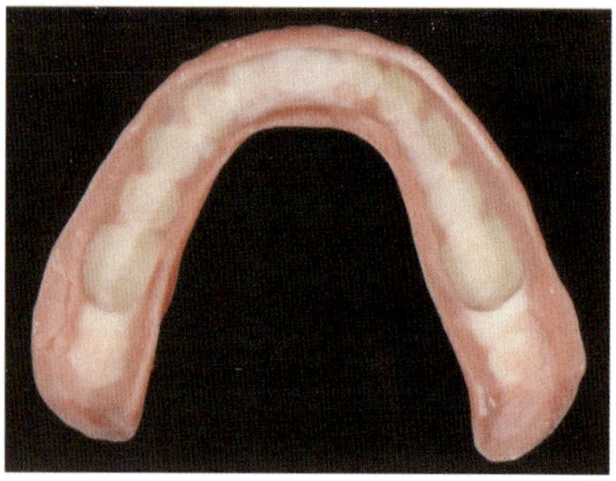

Figure 6: The lower denture was emptied internally, in order to subsequentially accommodate inside the future intraorally welded titanium framework. The flanges and the supports in the retromolar areas were preserved, in order to facilitate the positioning in the postwelding phase.

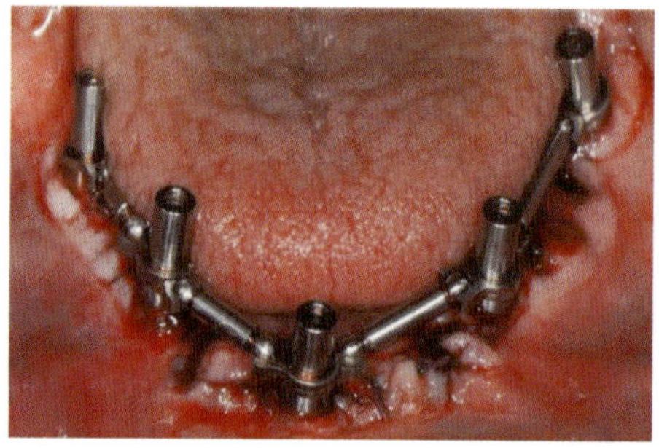

Figure 7: The prosthetic cylinders in titanium were screwed: over these cylinders, the adjustable rings and the rotating spheres were adapted both horizontally and vertically, paying attention to remain well above the bone crest.

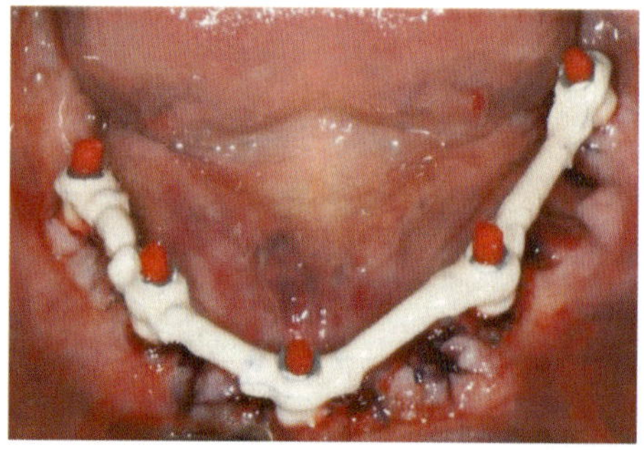

Figure 8: After the intraoral welding, the self-locating bar was removed from the mouth and finished, blasted, and then covered with a white opaque composite resin. The bar was subsequently repositioned onto the MUA abutments.

and supports were kept on the retromolar areas to facilitate positioning in the postwelding phase (Figure 6). Surgery commenced after infiltration of local anaesthesia. A full-thickness flap was raised after a crestal incision was performed, and two releasing vertical incisions were made. In the case of partially edentulous patients, the nonrestorable teeth affected by severe periodontal disease or decay were then removed, taking care not to damage the socket walls. This was followed by the preparation of the implant sites and the deepening of the apex of the socket (3-4 mm). In the case of fully edentulous patients with completely healed ridges, the preparation of the implant sites was performed in accordance with manufacturer recommendations, taking into account the clinical situation. The implants were then inserted in both extraction sockets and healed sites (the final insertion torque of the fixtures had to be ideally > 55 N/cm). The prosthetic phase started immediately with the placement of multiunit abutments (MUA) with a transmucosal height of 3 mm over the implants. The aforementioned MUA were screwed gently with a torque of 30 N/cm. In all immediate postextraction implants, the remaining gaps between the implant and the walls of the socket were filled and packed with a resorbable β-tricalcium phosphate [14] regenerative material (OXOFIX®, Biotec BTK, Povolaro di Dueville, Vicenza, Italy BTK, Italy). Finally, sutures were made. The prosthetic procedure went as follows. The prosthetic titanium cylinders provided by systematic BWB were first screwed in. Over these cylinders, the adjustable rings and rotating balls were adjusted both horizontally and vertically, taking care to remain well above the crest, and not to occupy extracrestal spaces (Figure 7). The self-locating bar was welded into the mouth, then removed, and finished; after blasting, it was covered with a white opaque light curing composite resin and repositioned onto the MUA abutments (Figure 8). The vacuum-formed template was placed over the bar to control the occlusal fairness and to verify the previously measured vertical dimensions (Figure 9(a)). Holes were made on the prosthesis using the vacuum-formed template which was already perforated in the direction of the cylinders (Figure 9(b)) in order to give access to the cylinders themselves after relining with composite resin flow (Figure 9(c)). Adhesive (Universal Futura B®, Voco, Cuxhaven, Germany) was positioned within the prosthesis and light cured, and the prosthesis was filled with a composite dual fluid (Rebilda, Voco, Cuxhave, Germany) and positioned above the bar. The prosthesis was self-centring, because it had all the support on the retromolar areas and the vestibules like a conventional full denture; therefore it found its natural position and occlusal vertical dimension without any error or unwanted movement (Figure 10(a)). When the dual composite resin was completely polymerized, the prosthesis was removed and sent to the laboratory, which after a few hours finished and returned it. The prosthesis was then delivered to the patient in less than 6 hours (Figures 10(b), 10(c), and 10(d)). The occlusion was carefully checked because it had to be perfectly balanced, and the holes were closed again with Teflon cylinders soaked in chlorhexidine 5% and a flowable light-cured composite. The patients received detailed instructions about oral hygiene and home care procedures and were enrolled in a series of scheduled follow-up controls, every 4 months, for professional oral hygiene sessions and clinical monitoring of their rehabilitation.

2.5. Outcome Variables and Statistical Evaluation. The main outcome variables for the present study were implant survival and the prosthetic success. With regard to implant survival, an implant was classified as "surviving" if it functioned

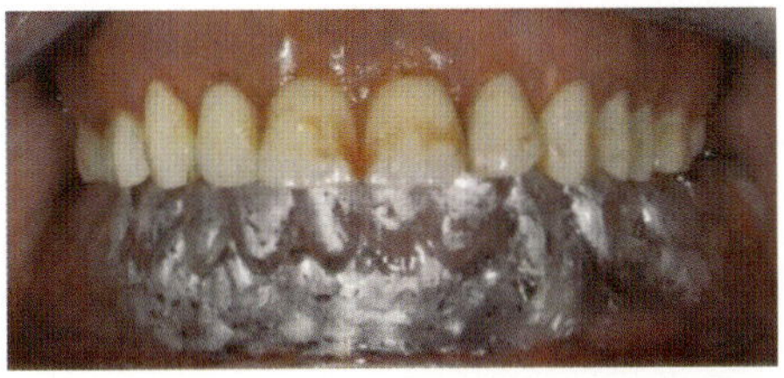

(a)

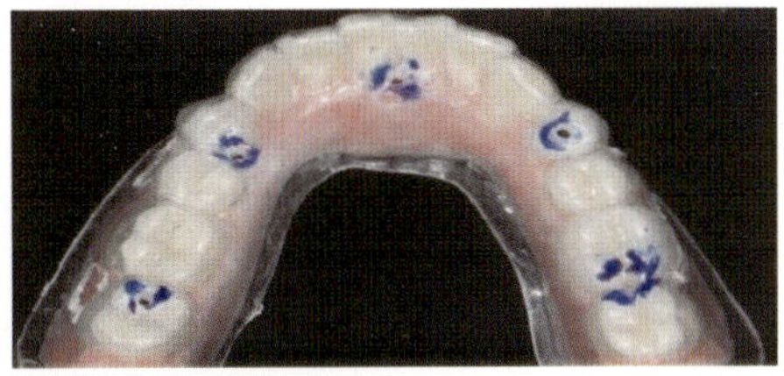

(b)

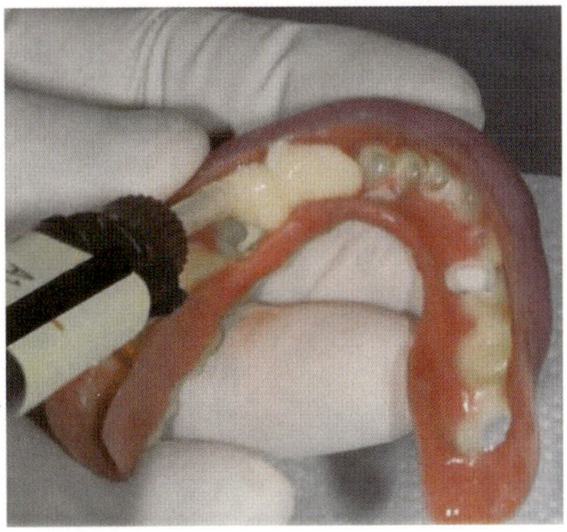

(c)

Figure 9: The vacuum-formed template was placed over the bar to control the occlusal fairness and to verify the previously measured vertical dimension (a). Holes were made on the prosthesis, using the vacuum-formed template already perforated in the direction of the cylinders, in order to access to the cylinders themselves (b). The prosthesis was relined with composite resin flow (c).

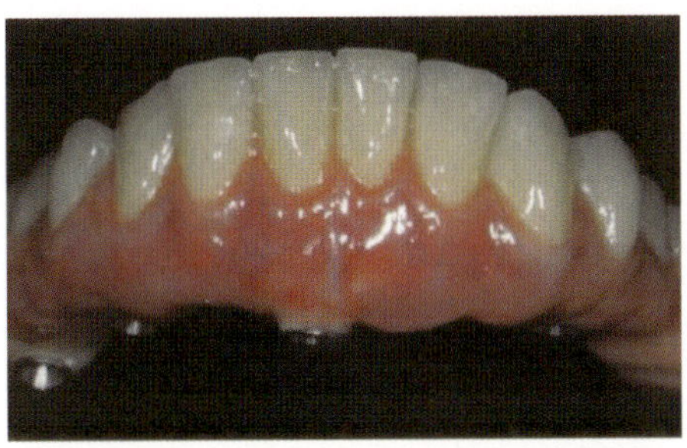

(a)

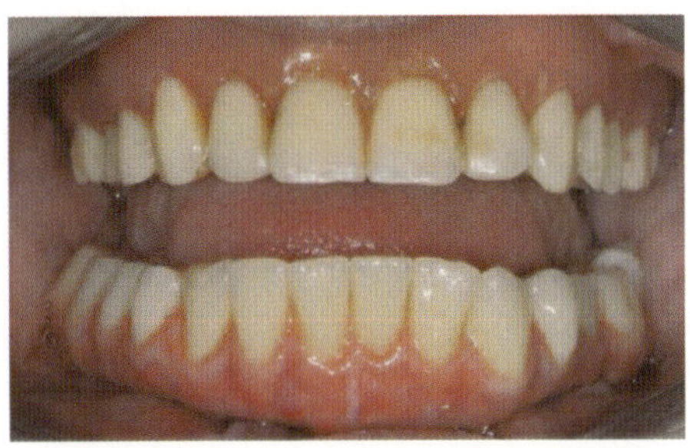

(b)

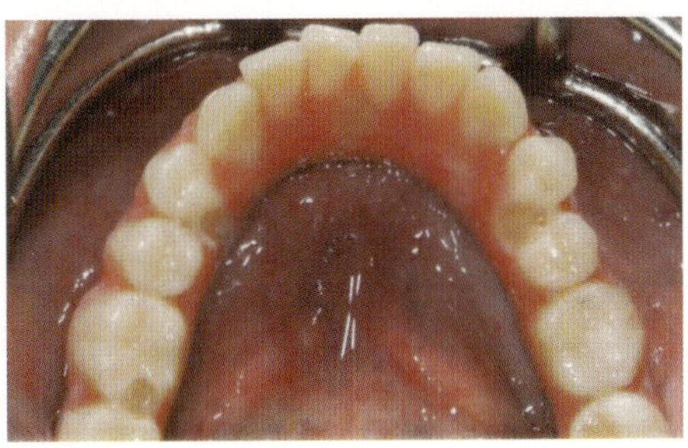

(c)

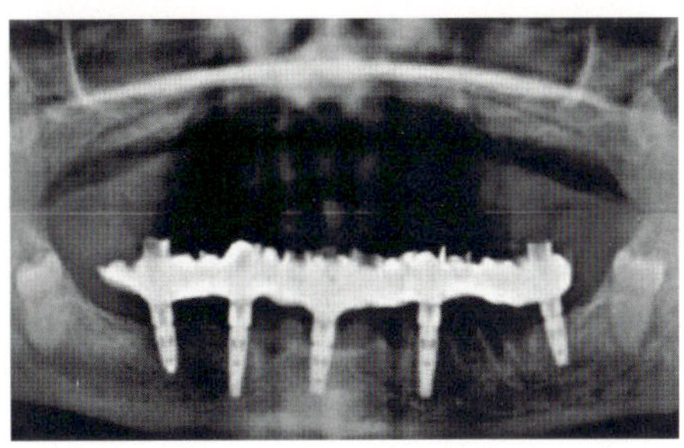

(d)

Figure 10: The fabrication of the prosthesis is completed in the laboratory (a), which after a few hours return the Toronto Bridge to the dentist for clinical application. The clinician delivers the prosthesis to the patient (b), after a careful check of the occlusion that must be perfectly balanced; then, the clinician closes the holes of the cylinders with Teflon soaked in chlorhexidine 5% and light curing flowable composite resin (c). The panoramic radiograph shows the titanium framework and the perfect adaptation of this structure on implant abutments (d).

regularly at the end of the study, two years after its placement and functional loading. In all cases in which the implant had to be removed, the fixture was defined as "failed." The causes for implant failure were as follows:

(1) mobility for lack of osseointegration, which occurred in the early healing period (not later than 4 months after insertion) but in the absence of symptoms/signs of infection,
(2) infection of the peri-implant tissue (peri-implantitis) that caused massive bone loss and subsequent loosening of the implant [15]. The threshold for diagnosis of peri-implantitis was a probing depth ≥4 mm, bleeding on probing, and/or pus secretion associated with evidence of radiographic bone loss (>2.5 mm) [15],
(3) progressive severe bone loss (>2.5 mm per year) in the absence of specific symptoms/signs of infection,
(4) fracture of the implant body.

With regard to prosthetic success, a prosthesis was considered successful when no adverse events (such as fractures/alterations of the resin superstructure and of the intraorally welded titanium framework) occurred [3–6, 16]. At the end of the study, after 2 years of functional loading, all relevant patient data (gender, age at surgery, and smoking habits), implant information (position, length, and diameter), and prosthesis information were collected in an Excel spreadsheet. Means (±SD) ranges, medians, and confidence intervals (95%) were calculated for quantitative variables and absolute and relative (%) frequency distributions were obtained for all qualitative variables. Implant survival and prosthesis success were finally calculated at the patient level, which meant that if even a single implant out of five failed, the procedure on that patient was classified as a failure, and in the presence of even a single prosthetic complication, the prosthesis could not be considered successful [17].

3. Results

In total, 42 patients (18 males and 24 females) were included in the present study. The mean age of patients was 64.2 (±6.7), range 54–79 years, median 63.5 years, and confidence interval (95%) 62.1–66.2. Among these patients, 12 (28.5%) were smokers. Overall, 210 fixtures were inserted to support 42 screw-retained, full arches restorations (Toronto bridges) in the edentulous mandible. The distribution of the implants was as follows: 18 fixtures (8.6%) were 3.7 mm in diameter × 12 mm in length, 40 fixtures (19%) were 3.7 × 14 mm, 46 fixtures (21.9%) were 3.7 × 16 mm, 18 fixtures (8.6%) were 4.1 × 12 mm, 48 fixtures (22.9%) were 4.1 × 14 mm, and 40 fixtures (19%) were 4.1 × 16 mm. The positions of the implants were the following: 84 molars (40%), 84 premolars (40%), and 42 incisors (20%). At the end of the study, only 2 fixtures were lost (2/210: 0.9%) during the first months after placement, in a single patient: the implant survival rate was 97.7% (patient-based). With regard to complications, during the follow-up, 5 implants suffered from peri-implant mucositis and 3 implants suffered for peri-implantitis: these fixtures were, however, successfully treated with dedicated professional oral hygiene sessions and no further biological problems were registered at the end of this work. With regard to prosthetic complication and therefore prosthetic success, 3/42 of the prostheses required repair for fracture (7.1%): this was considered a major complication. In addition, 4 multiunit abutments (1.9%) became loose during the entire follow-up: these were reinserted and screwed and no other abutment loosening was encountered in this study. The loosening of the multiunit abutments was considered as a minor complication.

4. Discussion

In recent years, several clinical studies have reported excellent results obtained using intraoral welding techniques for the rehabilitation of completely edentulous mandibles with screw-retained full arch immediately loaded prostheses and Toronto bridges [2–6]. Similar results have also been reported for procedures on the fully edentulous maxilla [6, 18, 19], giving the impression that intraoral welding can be successfully used for the rehabilitation of edentulous patients. In particular, Degidi et al. published a paper [18] in which 30 patients received 3 axial and 4 tilted implants in the edentulous maxilla and were rehabilitated with an immediately loaded definitive prosthesis achieved using intraoral welding. Patients were followed for a period of 3 years during which the 210 implants inserted were checked, and implant failures, marginal bone resorption around the fixtures, and prosthetic problems were carefully registered [18]. At the end of the study, three implants had biological problems, giving a success rate of 97.8% for axial implants and 99.2% for tilted implants, respectively. The mean marginal bone resorption was 0.92 mm (±0.75) for the axial and 1.03 mm (±0.69) for the tilted implants [18]. No fractures or alterations of the intraorally welded titanium framework occurred, for a prosthetic success of 100% [18]. One of the obvious advantages of the intraoral welding technique is the ability to rehabilitate in a very short timeframe and with limited costs fully edentulous patients, without going through lengthy and complex laboratory phases [2–6, 18]. Recently, some potential alternatives to the traditional technique originally proposed by P. L. Mondani and P. M. Mondani [1] and subsequently recovered by Degidi et al. [3, 5, 6, 18] have been proposed [7, 8]. Albiero and Benato [8] published a case report in which the technique of intraoral welding has been combined with modern guided surgical techniques. Using this "guided-welded approach," the authors were able to obtain a very precise passive fit of a maxillary complete denture supported by 4 implants, loaded immediately [8]. The passive fit contributed to the optimal healing of the implants and the use of guided surgery allowed for the reduction of surgery time and the adaptation of the bar to the implant abutments [8]. Fornaini et al. [7, 9, 10] have presented another possible variant of the intraoral welding technique, using a laser for the welding of a bar (previously prepared from a technician) to 4 implants placed in an edentulous maxilla. In particular, in their clinical report [7] preceded by an in vitro evaluation, the authors proved that the use of lasers can produce good results in terms of intraoral welding. The theoretical advantages of the use of lasers for the welding are different: lasers is effective on all metals and can be used without filler metal and shielding gas and thanks to the fact that the beam has extremely small dimensions and is well focused (0.6 mm), there is no adverse effect (overheating) on the surrounding tissue [7, 9, 10]. In addition, lasers can be used on all patients (even on patients with pacemakers) [7, 9, 10]. In our present clinical research, we have introduced a further possible variant of the classical intraoral welding technique procedure: the so-called "Ball Welding Bar" (BWB) technique. The BWB technique represents a new, simple treatment option for the fabrication of a screw-retained Toronto Bridge that has predictable results. The mechanical properties of this new bar (made of titanium grade 4) and the original assemblage designed and patented by the authors allow for the rapid fabrication of prostheses with no tension. This means that there will be good adaptation when using a variety of loading protocols (including immediate functional loading). Overall, 210 fixtures were inserted to support 42 screw-retained, full arches restorations (Toronto bridges) in the edentulous mandible. At the end of the study, only 2 fixtures were lost (2/210: 0.9%) during the first months after placement, in a single patient: the implant survival rate was 97.7% (patient-based). With regard to prosthetic complication and therefore prosthetic success, 3/42 of the prostheses required repair for fracture (7.1%): this was considered a major complication. The prosthetic success was therefore 92.9%. The main advantages of our method are that it makes it easy to centre the bars over the bone crest (for ease of orientation of the components in the vertical and horizontal dimensions), allows for fine regulation, and makes it easy to solder the framework without distortions. Finally, the procedure is very rapid and can be managed by a single operator, both of which allow for reduced rehabilitation costs. In the present study, we have used tapered implants with a hexagonal conical implant-abutment connection, because these fixtures had all the features necessary to meet the biological and mechanical requirements for immediate loading, both in fully healed edentulous ridges and in postextraction sockets [12]. The tapered design with double lead threads, in fact, allows the surgeon to obtain an excellent primary implant stability even in difficult clinical conditions [12], such as in the case of postextraction sockets [20]. At the same time, the dual acid etched surface of these implants has the potential to accelerate bone healing, as demonstrated by a recent histologic/histomorphometric human study [13]. In modern oral implantology, the presence of an adequate macrostructure (thread design) and microstructure (surface roughness) is considered critical for functional immediate loading [21–23]. Finally, new materials (such as composite resins) are now available for the fabrication of fixed full arch mandibular dentures [24, 25]. These composite resins can effectively replace more conventionally used materials (i.e., acrylic resins) because they offer greater hardness compared to conventional acrylic resins. In addition, they are better in terms of aesthetics, as they come in different shades of pink to mimic the colours of the gum [24, 25]. These features allow the technician to fabricate a prosthesis composed of a single material, in which the titanium framework/bar is incorporated and welded to the cylinders and the abutments. The resin composite, besides being stronger and more aesthetically pleasing than acrylic resin, has the potential to preserve the occlusion stability over time, and the maintenance and repair are similar to those of a common dental composite [25]. In our present study we have used these materials, and we have obtained excellent functional and aesthetic outcomes. Our present study has limitations, for example, the limited number of patients treated and prostheses fabricated; therefore further studies on a larger sample of patients are needed to confirm the positive clinical outcomes reported here. In addition, the present study has tracked outcomes for only two years and it is necessary to follow the progress of these patients in the long-term, before more specific conclusions can be drawn about the reliability of the new and innovative BWB technique.

5. Conclusions

Fulfilling patient demands for an immediate functional recovery is the main goal of modern dentistry. The novel "Ball Welding Bar" technique proposed in the present study is simple and makes it possible to immediately load a definitive screw-retained fixed full arch prosthesis, without the use of a provisional prosthesis. In our present study, 210 fixtures were inserted to support 42 mandibular screw-retained, fixed full arches restorations (Toronto bridges). After two years of loading, 2 fixtures were lost (2/210: 0.9%) during the first months after placement, in a single patient: the implant survival rate was 97.7% (patient-based). With regard to prosthetic complication and therefore prosthetic success, 3/42 of the prostheses required repair for fracture (7.1%): this was considered a major complication. The prosthetic success was therefore 92.9%. Further studies are needed to confirm these positive outcomes.

References

[1] P. L. Mondani and P. M. Mondani, "The Pierluigi Mondani intraoral electric solder. Principles of development and explanation of the solder using syncrystallization," *Rivista di odontostomatologia e implantoprotesi*, vol. 4, no. 4, pp. 28–32, 1982.

[2] A. Hruska, P. Borelli, A. C. Bordanaro, E. Marzaduri, and K.-L. Hruska, "Immediate loading implants: a clinical report of 1301 implants.," *The Journal of oral implantology*, vol. 28, no. 4, pp. 200–209, 2002.

[3] M. Degidi, P. Gehrke, A. Spanel, and A. Piattelli, "Syncrystallization: A technique for temporization of immediately loaded implants with metal-reinforced acrylic resin restorations," *Clinical Implant Dentistry and Related Research*, vol. 8, no. 3, pp. 123–134, 2006.

[4] M. Degidi, D. Nardi, and A. Piattelli, "Prospective study with a 2-year follow-up on immediate implant loading in the edentulous mandible with a definitive restoration using intra-oral

welding," *Clinical Oral Implants Research*, vol. 21, no. 4, pp. 379–385, 2010.

[5] M. Degidi, D. Nardi, G. Sighinolfi, and A. Piattelli, "Immediate rehabilitation of the edentulous mandible using AnkylosSynCone telescopic copings and a pilot study," in *Proceedings of the Immediate rehabilitation of the edentulous mandible using AnkylosSynCone telescopic copings and intraoral welding: a pilot study*, vol. 32, pp. 189–194, 2012.

[6] M. Degidi, D. Nardi, and A. Piattelli, "A six-year follow-up of full-arch immediate restorations fabricated with an intraoral welding technique," *Implant Dentistry*, vol. 22, no. 3, pp. 224–231, 2013.

[7] C. Fornaini, E. Merigo, I. Cernavin, G. Lòpez de Castro, and P. Vescovi, "Intraoral Laser Welding (ILW) in implant prosthetic dentistry: case report," *Case Reports in Dentistry*, vol. 2012, Article ID 839141, 4 pages, 2012.

[8] A. M. Albiero and R. Benato, "Computer-assisted surgery and intraoral welding technique for immediate implant-supported rehabilitation of the edentulous maxilla: case report and technical description," *International Journal of Medical Robotics and Computer Assisted Surgery*, vol. 12, no. 3, pp. 453–460, 2016.

[9] C. Fornaini, E. Merigo, P. Vescovi, M. Meleti, and S. Nammour, "Laser welding and syncristallization techniques comparison: *in vitro* study," *International Journal of Dentistry*, vol. 2012, Article ID 720538, 5 pages, 2012.

[10] C. Fornaini, P. Vescovi, E. Merigo et al., "Intraoral metal laser welding: a case report," *Lasers in Medical Science*, vol. 25, no. 2, pp. 303–307, 2010.

[11] B. R. Chrcanovic, T. Albrektsson, and A. Wennerberg, "Smoking and dental implants: a systematic review and meta-analysis," *Journal of Dentistry*, vol. 43, no. 5, pp. 487–498, 2015.

[12] G. A. Dolcini, M. Colombo, and C. Mangano, "From guided surgery to final prosthesis with a fully digital procedure: a prospective clinical study on 15 partially edentulous patients," *International Journal of Dentistry*, vol. 2016, Article ID 7358423, 7 pages, 2016.

[13] F. G. Mangano, J. T. Pires, J. A. Shibli et al., "Early bone response to dual acid-etched and machined dental implants placed in the posterior maxilla: a histologic and histomorphometric human study," *Implant Dentistry*, vol. 26, no. 1, pp. 24–29, 2017.

[14] A. Giuliani, A. Manescu, E. Larsson et al., "In vivo regenerative properties of coralline-derived (Biocoral) scaffold grafts in human maxillary defects: demonstrative and comparative study with beta-tricalcium phosphate and biphasic calcium phosphate bu synchrotron radiation x-ray microtopograph," *Clinical Implant Dentistry and Related Research*, vol. 16, no. 5, pp. 736–750, 2014.

[15] T. Albrektsson, L. Canullo, D. Cochran, and H. De Bruyn, "'Peri-implantitis': a complication of a foreign body or a man-made 'disease'. facts and fiction," *Clinical Implant Dentistry and Related Research*, vol. 18, no. 4, pp. 840–849, 2016.

[16] C. Mangano, F. Mangano, J. A. Shibli, M. Ricci, R. L. Sammons, and M. Figliuzzi, "Morse taper connection implants supporting "planned" maxillary and mandibular bar-retained overdentures: a 5-year prospective multicenter study," *Clinical Oral Implants Research*, vol. 22, no. 10, pp. 1117–1124, 2011.

[17] C. Mangano, F. Iaculli, A. Piattelli, and F. Mangano, "Fixed restorations supported by Morse-taper connection implants: a retrospective clinical study with 10–20 years of follow-up," *Clinical Oral Implants Research*, vol. 26, no. 10, pp. 1229–1236, 2015.

[18] M. Degidi, D. Nardi, and A. Piattelli, "Immediate loading of the edentulous maxilla with a definitive restoration supported by an intraorally welded titanium bar and tilted implants," *International Journal of Oral and Maxillofacial Implants*, vol. 25, no. 6, pp. 1175–1182, 2010.

[19] M. Marchesi, C. Ferrari, S. Superbi, R. Jimbo, and S. Galli, "Modified protocol of the intraoral welding technique for immediate implant-supported rehabilitation of the edentulous maxilla," *Implant Dentistry*, vol. 24, no. 1, pp. 110–116, 2015.

[20] F. G. Mangano, P. Mastrangelo, F. Luongo, A. Blay, S. Tunchel, and C. Mangano, "Aesthetic of immediately restored single implants placed in extraction sockets and healed sites of the anterior maxilla: a retrospective study on 103 patients with 3 of follow-up," *Clinical Oral Implants Research*, vol. 28, no. 3, pp. 272–282, 2017.

[21] H. De Bruyn, S. Raes, P.-O. Östman, and J. Cosyn, "Immediate loading in partially and completely edentulous jaws: a review of the literature with clinical guidelines," *Periodontology 2000*, vol. 66, no. 1, pp. 153–187, 2014.

[22] S. M. Meloni, M. Tallarico, M. Pisano, E. Xhanari, and L. Canullo, "Immediate loading of fixed complete denture prosthesis supported by 4–8 implants placed using guided surgery: a 5-year prospective study on 66 patients with 356 implants," *Clinical Implant Dentistry and Related Research*, vol. 19, no. 1, pp. 195–206, 2017.

[23] F. G. Mangano, A. Caprioglio, L. Levrini, D. Farronato, P. A. Zecca, and C. Mangano, "Immediate loading of mandibular overdentures supported by one-piece, direct metal laser sintering mini-implants: a short-term prospective clinical study," *Journal of Periodontology*, vol. 86, no. 2, pp. 192–200, 2015.

[24] F. Fieri, N. N. Aldini, M. Fini, and G. Corinaldesi, "Immediate occlusal loading of immediately placed implants supporting fixed restorations in completely edentulous arches: A 1-year prospective pilot study," *Journal of Periodontology*, vol. 80, no. 3, pp. 411–421, 2009.

[25] B.-W. Park, N.-J. Kim, J. Lee, and H.-H. Lee, "Technique for fabricating individualized dentures with a gingiva-shade composite resin," *Journal of Prosthetic Dentistry*, vol. 115, no. 5, pp. 547–550, 2016.

13

Shisha Smoking Habit among Dental School Students in the United Arab Emirates: Enabling Factors and Barriers

Natheer H. Al-Rawi,[1] Ahmed S. Alnuaimi,[2] and Asmaa T. Uthman[3]

[1]*College of Dental Medicine, University of Sharjah, Sharjah, UAE*
[2]*College of Medicine, University of Baghdad, Baghdad, Iraq*
[3]*College of Dental Medicine, Gulf Medical University, Ajman, UAE*

Correspondence should be addressed to Natheer H. Al-Rawi; nhabdulla@sharjah.ac.ae

Academic Editor: Louis M. Lin

Objectives. The objective of the present study was to assess shisha smoking among dental school students in Sharjah, United Arab Emirates (UAE). In addition, the role of suggested barriers and enabling factors in shisha smoking was also evaluated. *Methods.* A cross-sectional questionnaire-based survey was conducted at the College of Dental Medicine, University of Sharjah, between February and May 2016. The questions were adapted from previously published water pipe smoking studies. The collected data were analyzed to identify the relationship between shisha smoking and sociodemographic characteristics. Relevant questions were further categorized as enabling factors and barriers for shisha smoking. *Results.* Three enabling questionnaire items related to social environment were significantly associated with an increased risk of being a current smoker. The most powerful is peer pressure ("friends smoke shisha"), which increased the odds ratio of shisha smoking 11.3 times, followed by smoker sibling with increase in odd ratio by 4.52 times, then the belief of social acceptance with increase in odd ratio by 4.31 times. *Conclusion.* Shisha smoking is a serious problem among university students. Any intervention program in the university curricula should consider teaching students that shisha is no less risky than cigarettes and is addictive.

1. Introduction

Tobacco smoking is one of the ten leading health indicators proposed by the WHO Healthy People 2020 objectives [1]. According to the UN organization, by 2020, the current smoking pattern will cause about 10 million deaths every year [2]. It is estimated that death rate due to smoking will reach 8.3 million per year by the year 2030, where 70% of these deaths will occur in developing countries [3].

Tobacco consumption trend has been found constant over the past 3 decades in the Eastern Mediterranean region, especially in Iran; however, water pipe smoking was increasing in females and young people and decreasing in older people [4].

Shisha is another method of smoking that is attracting new younger customers, especially in the Middle East region. Worldwide, more than 100 million people are reported to smoke shisha [5]. The typical smoking session lasts between 45 and 50 minutes and may last for several hours [6]. Young people are attracted to shisha as the experience comes in a variety of flavors and is popular as a group activity. Many shisha users are under the misconception that shisha is less harmful than cigarettes. The reason for the drastic increase in shisha use is the false assumption that it is environmentally friendly and less harmful than cigarettes. Nevertheless, nicotine intake per shisha session has been reported as the equivalent of more than one pack of cigarettes [7]. Therefore, the type and magnitude of health adverse effects associated with shisha are prone to be different from those of cigarette smoking. Hadidi and Mohammed [7] stated that "smoking one head of flavored (Ma'assel) tobacco (204 mg/pack), containing an average of one-third of the nicotine present in 20 cigarettes, resulted in a 20% higher plasma nicotine level."

Table 1: Sociodemographic characteristics of the study participants ($n = 397$).

Variables	Categories	Number	Percentage (%)
Sex	Females	330	83.1
	Males	67	16.9
	Total	397	100.0
Grades	First and second	160	40.3
	Third and fourth	141	35.5
	Fifth and sixth	96	24.1
	Total	397	100.0
Being married	Single	368	92.7
	Married	29	7.3
	Total	397	100.0
Father education	Illiterate/read and write	18	4.6
	Elementary/intermediate school	19	4.8
	Secondary school	60	15.11
	University and higher education	296	75.55
	Not answered	4	0.01
	Total	397	100.0
Mother education	Illiterate/read and write	15	3.8
	Elementary/intermediate school	25	6.3
	Secondary school	86	21.66
	University and higher education	268	67.5
	Not answered	3	0.007
	Total	397	100.0
Nationality	UAE citizen	141	35.5
	Non-UAE citizen	256	64.5
	Total	397	100.0

Table 2: Knowledge and awareness about shisha smoking.

Variables	Number	Percentage (%)
Shisha contains nicotine	349	87.9
Shisha is addictive	304	76.6
Shisha is more addictive than cigarettes	150	37.6
Shisha is more harmful compared with cigarettes	331	83.4
Shisha smoking leads to lung cancer	367	92.4
Shisha smoking leads to cardiovascular diseases	369	92.9
Shisha smoking leads to dental problems	375	94.5
Shisha smoking reduces weight	183	46.1
Shisha contains carbon monoxide	363	91.4
Water in shisha filters toxins	139	35
Shisha is harmful to health	382	96.2
Shisha contains tar	284	71.5

Table 3: Social environment characteristics of the study participants.

Variables	Number	Percentage (%)
Father smokes shisha	48	12.1
Mother smokes shisha	23	5.8
Sibling smokes shisha	137	34.5
Friends can influence smoking	348	87.7
Parents influenced decision to start shisha smoking	192	48.4
Advertisement about shisha can influence smoking	276	69.5
Girls are more comfortable in smoking shisha compared to cigarette	283	71.3
People smoking shisha look cool	58	14.6
Shisha smoking is our cultural heritage	108	27.2
People smoking shisha have more friends	70	17.6

Table 4: Psychological factors involved in shisha smoking.

Variables	Number	Percentage (%)
University life burden leads to shisha smoking	186	46.9
Stress influences one to start shisha smoking	287	72.3
Problems with friends lead to shisha smoking	137	34.6
Husband-wife problems lead to shisha smoking	179	45.1
Family problems lead to shisha smoking	222	55.9
Financial problems lead to shisha smoking	143	36.0

Shisha smoking has been associated with a variety of diseases, like infertility [8], decreased respiratory function [9], infectious disease [10], and esophageal cancer [10]. The increased popularity of shisha could be attributed to its wide availability, low cost, and sociability. About 50% of university students report having used shisha, and about 25% of men currently smoke it [11]. Mohamed et al. in their study reported that around 9% of 5066 medical students in Cairo smoked both shisha and cigarettes. The prevalence of smoking was observed to be increasing from the first year through the final year despite an awareness of the hazards [12]. In Kuwait, more than 57% of men and 69% of women had used a water pipe at least once in their life [13]. In Lebanon, weekly use of water pipe was reported in 30.6% of male students and 23.4% of female students at Beirut Universities [14]. Medical student use is an example of the increased popularity of shisha smoking among educated peoples.

Among Iranian university students, 11.5% of females and 28.7% of males have been reported to smoke water pipe, compared to 2.5% of females and 18.3% of males who smoke cigarettes [15]. The sense of relaxing and energizing and a part of their culture are the main reasons behind water pipe smoking.

A systematic review of the prevalence of water pipe smoking from 38 studies found rates of current water pipe

Table 5: Prevalence rate of current shisha smoking stratified by grade and sex.

	Total N	Current shisha smoker N	%	95% confidence interval	P
Female					<0.001
First and second grade	131	10	7.6	(3.1 to 12.2)	
Third and fourth grade	121	3	2.5	(−0.3 to 5.2)	
Fifth and sixth grade	78	14	17.9	(9.4 to 26.5)	
Total female	330	27	8.2	(5.2 to 11.1)	
Male					0.04
First and second grade	29	16	55.2	(37.1 to 73.3)	
Third and fourth grade	20	4	20.0	(2.5 to 37.5)	
Fifth and sixth grade	18	9	50.0	(26.9 to 73.1)	
Total male	67	29	43.3	(31.4 to 55.1)	

P (chi-square) for male-female differences is <0.00.

Table 6: Prevalence rate of ever smoked shisha stratified by grade and sex.

	Total N	Ever smoked shisha N	%	95% confidence interval	P
Female					0.002
First and second grade	131	40	30.5	(22.6 to 38.4)	
Third and fourth grade	121	21	17.4	(10.6 to 24.1)	
Fifth and sixth grade	78	31	39.7	(28.9 to 50.6)	
Total female	330	92	27.9	(23 to 32.7)	
Male					0.12 (NS)
First and second grade	29	27	93.1	(83.9 to 102.3)	
Third and fourth grade	20	15	75.0	(56 to 94)	
Fifth and sixth grade	18	13	72.2	(51.5 to 92.9)	
Total male	67	55	82.1	(72.9 to 91.3)	

P (chi-square) for male-female differences is <0.00.

smoking in university students to be 15–28% in EMR countries, 33% in the South Asia region, 10% in the Americas, and 8% in Europe [16]. Most water pipe smokers in Ghafouri et al. study cited that social and fun aspects are the primary motivators for their continuing use of water pipe [17].

Table 7: The Modified Fagerström Nicotine Test for Dependence scale.

(1) How soon after you wake up do you smoke your first shisha:	
(i) Within 5 minutes	3
(ii) 6–30 minutes	2
(iii) 31–60 minutes	1
(iv) After 60 minutes	0
(2) Which shisha smoking would you hate most to give up?	
(i) The first one in the morning	1
(ii) Any other	0
(3) How many Hager/week?	
(i) 1 per week	0
(ii) 2–4 per week	1
(iii) More than 5 per week	2
(4) Do you smoke more frequently during the first hours after waking than during the rest of the day?	
(i) Yes	1
(ii) No	0
(5) Do you smoke if you are so ill that you are in bed most of the day?	
(i) Yes	1
(ii) No	0

Table 8: Nicotine dependence level among current shisha smokers by sex.

	Fagerström's Nicotine Tolerance score categories					
	Low level of dependence		Moderate level of dependence		Total	
	N	%	N	%	N	%
Sex						
Female	21	95.5	1	4.5	22	100
Male	22	84.6	4	15.4	26	100
P (Fisher's exact) = 0.35 (NS)						

A few articles have been published about shisha or water pipe smoking among university dental students [11, 18, 19]. Questionnaire-based study among Iranian dental students revealed that 23% are current cigarette, pipe, or water pipe users [20].

However, the authors are unaware of published studies assessing shisha smoking among students of dentistry in the UAE. The aims of the present study were to estimate the prevalence rate of shisha smoking (current and ever) among students categorized by grade and sex, the nicotine dependence among current shisha smokers, and the association between the suggested barriers and enabling factors, and the shisha smoking habit was also studied.

Table 9: The strength of association between selected barriers and enabling factors with current shisha smoking habits among females.

Sex = female	Current shisha smoking habit: Nonsmokers (*N* for total surveyed = 303)		Current smokers (*N* for total surveyed = 27)		OR	Inverse OR	95% confidence interval OR	*P*
	N	%	*N*	%				
Barriers								
(1) Shisha is more addictive than cigarettes	128	42.2	3	11.1	0.17	5.85	(0.05–0.58)	**0.005**
(2) Shisha is addictive	243	80.2	17	63	0.42	2.38	(0.18–0.96)	**0.041**
(3) Shisha smoking leads to lung cancer	286	94.4	24	88.9	0.48	2.10	(0.13–1.74)	0.261 (NS)
(4) Shisha smoking leads to dental problems	290	95.7	25	92.6	0.56	1.78	(0.12–2.62)	0.462 (NS)
(5) Shisha smoking reduces weight	150	49.5	10	37	0.60	1.67	(0.27–1.35)	0.218 (NS)
(6) Shisha is more harmful compared with cigarettes	254	83.8	21	77.8	0.68	1.48	(0.26–1.76)	0.421 (NS)
(7) Shisha contains carbon monoxide	277	91.4	24	88.9	0.75	1.33	(0.21–2.66)	0.657 (NS)
(8) Shisha is harmful to health	294	97	26	96.3	0.80	1.26	(0.1–6.53)	0.832 (NS)
(9) Shisha contains nicotine	273	90.1	24	88.9	0.88	1.14	(0.25–3.09)	0.841 (NS)
(10) Shisha smoking leads to cardiovascular diseases	282	93.1	25	92.6	0.93	1.07	(0.21–4.2)	0.926 (NS)
(11) Shisha contains tar	217	71.6	21	77.8	1.39	—	(0.54–3.55)	0.496 (NS)
Enabling factors								
(1) Friends smoke shisha	159	52.5	25	92.6	11.32	—	(2.63–48.65)	**0.001**
(2) Smoker sibling	93	30.7	18	66.7	4.52	—	(1.96–10.43)	**<0.001**
(3) Shisha smoking is more socially acceptable compared to cigarettes	153	50.5	22	81.5	4.31	—	(1.59–11.7)	**0.004**
(4) Friends can influence smoking	261	86.1	26	96.3	4.18	—	(0.55–31.7)	0.166 (NS)
(5) Father smokes shisha	33	10.9	9	33.3	4.09	—	(1.7–9.84)	**0.002**
(6) Mother smokes shisha	16	5.3	5	18.5	4.08	—	(1.37–12.17)	**0.012**
(7) Girls are more comfortable in smoking shisha compared to cigarettes	204	67.3	24	88.9	3.88	—	(1.14–13.22)	**0.03**
(8) People smoking shisha look cool	31	10.2	7	25.9	3.07	—	(1.2–7.84)	**0.019**
(9) Shisha smoking is our cultural heritage	71	23.4	9	33.3	1.63	—	(0.7–3.8)	0.254 (NS)
(10) People smoking shisha have more friends	47	15.5	6	22.2	1.56	—	(0.6–4.06)	0.366 (NS)
(11) University life burden leads to shisha smoking	143	47.2	12	44.4	0.90	1.12	(0.41–1.98)	0.784 (NS)
(12) Water in shisha filters toxins	105	34.7	7	25.9	0.66	1.52	(0.27–1.61)	0.362 (NS)
(13) Stress influences one to start shisha smoking	224	73.9	17	63	0.60	1.67	(0.26–1.36)	0.223 (NS)
(14) Problems with friends lead to shisha smoking	113	37.3	6	22.2	0.48	2.08	(0.19–1.23)	0.125 (NS)
(15) Shisha smoker parents influenced decision of children to start shisha smoking	181	59.7	11	40.7	0.46	2.16	(0.21–1.03)	0.06 (NS)

Table 9: Continued.

Sex = female	Current shisha smoking habit				OR	Inverse OR	95% confidence interval OR	*P*
	Nonsmokers (*N* for total surveyed = 303)		Current smokers (*N* for total surveyed = 27)					
	N	%	*N*	%				
(16) Parents influenced decision of children to start shisha smoking	160	52.8	9	33.3	0.45	2.24	(0.19–1.03)	0.058 (NS)
(17) Husband-wife or boyfriend-girlfriend problems lead to shisha smoking	149	49.2	8	29.6	0.44	2.30	(0.18–1.03)	0.057 (NS)
(18) Family problem leads to shisha smoking	183	60.4	9	33.3	0.33	3.05	(0.14–0.75)	**0.009**
(19) Financial problems lead to shisha smoking	122	40.3	4	14.8	0.26	3.88	(0.09–0.76)	**0.015**
(20) Advertisement about shisha can influence smoking	220	72.6	9	33.3	0.19	5.30	(0.08–0.44)	**<0.001**

2. Methods

A cross-sectional survey was conducted on students of the College of Dental Medicine at the University of Sharjah, UAE, between February and May 2016. All students from the dentistry baccalaureate program were included in the study. Students were informed about the aim of the study before the survey questionnaire was distributed.

The survey instrument was developed from a literature review and questions adapted from previously published water pipe smoking studies [19, 21].

Informed consent was obtained from each participant, and the study was approved by the research and ethics committee of the University of Sharjah. The survey questionnaire is categorized into five sections: The first section was about sociodemographic data (such as sex, age, marital status, family education, and nationality). The second section was information about the social environment like whether the student's parents, siblings, and friends smoked shisha. The third section of the questionnaire was about knowledge and awareness of shisha smoking. The fourth section consisted of questions about psychological factors involved in shisha smoking, such as stress, family and friends, and financial problems. The last section of the questionnaire addressed the personal smoking behavior of those who smoked shisha. The Modified Fagerström Test for Nicotine Dependence (MFTND) questionnaire with 5-item responses was used in this study to determine the level of dependence among the shisha smokers. The MFTND total score was calculated as the sum of the individual items, with a score of 5 or more indicating significant dependences and a score of 4 or less indicating low to moderate dependence.

The completed questionnaire was then collected and coded for data entry. Data were analyzed using IBM SPSS version 23 (IBM statistical package of social sciences program). The odds ratio was used to assess the strength of association between an independent categorical variable and an outcome dichotomous one.

3. Results

Out of 410 questionnaires distributed among all dental students (82 males and 328 females), only 397 students answered the questionnaire with a response rate of about 96.8%. Women constituted the highest proportion (83.1%) of the respondent students. Most of the students in the study sample were unmarried (92.7%), non-Emirati (64.6%), and had highly educated parents and high income (Table 1). The majority of participants (83.4%) mentioned that shisha was more harmful than cigarettes and that shisha smoking was addictive (76.7%), but only about one-third (37.6%) agreed that shisha was more addictive than cigarettes (Table 2). More than two-thirds of the participants acknowledged that women were more comfortable smoking shisha than cigarettes (71.3%). Most participants also acknowledged that friends could influence the shisha smoking habit (87.8%) (Table 3). Stress was found to be the most important factor influencing the start of shisha smoking (72.3%), followed by family problems (55.9%) (Table 4).

The prevalence rate of current shisha smoking among women was 8.2%, which is significantly lower than that of men (43.3%). In both sexes, the prevalence was lowest for third- and fourth-year students and varied significantly among the 3 grade categories. Among women, the prevalence was highest for the fifth and sixth years (17.9%), while among men, the prevalence was high for both the first and second and the fifth and sixth years (Table 5).

The prevalence of ever smoking shisha was much higher, being double in men compared with their current habit and triple in women. The prevalence rate of ever smoking shisha was significantly higher in men (82.1%) than in women (27.9%). Among men, the prevalence was slightly but not significantly higher among the lower grades (93.1% in the 1st to 2nd grade) and was lowest in the highest grades (72.2% in the 5th to 6th grades) (Table 6).

Of the 56 current shisha smokers, 48 completed the Modified Fagerström Nicotine Test for Dependence

Table 10: The strength of association between selected barriers and enabling factors with current shisha smoking habits among males.

Sex = male	Current shisha smoking habit				OR	Inverse OR	95% confidence interval OR	P
	Nonsmokers (N for total surveyed = 38)		Current smoker (N for total surveyed = 29)					
	N	%	N	%				
Barriers								
(1) Shisha is more addictive than cigarettes	36	94.7	26	89.7	0.48	2.08	(0.08–3.09)	0.441 (NS)
(2) Shisha is addictive	13	34.2	6	20.7	0.50	1.99	(0.16–1.54)	0.228 (NS)
(3) Shisha smoking leads to lung cancer	33	86.8	23	79.3	0.58	1.72	(0.16–2.13)	0.413 (NS)
(4) Shisha smoking leads to dental problems	26	68.4	18	62.1	0.76	1.32	(0.27–2.08)	0.588 (NS)
(5) Shisha smoking reduces weight	25	65.8	27	93.1	7.02	—	(1.44–34.29)	**0.016**
(6) Shisha is more harmful compared with cigarettes	34	89.5	28	96.6	3.29	—	(0.35–31.19)	0.299 (NS)
(7) Shisha contains carbon monoxide	32	84.2	25	86.2	1.17	—	(0.3–4.61)	0.82 (NS)
(8) Shisha is harmful to health	34	89.5	26	89.7	1.02	—	(0.21–4.96)	0.981 (NS)
(9) Shisha contains nicotine	13	34.2	10	34.5	1.01	—	(0.37–2.8)	0.981 (NS)
(10) Shisha smoking leads to cardiovascular diseases	34	89.5	28	96.6	3.29	—	(0.35–31.19)	0.299 (NS)
Enabling factors								
(1) Friends can influence shisha smoking	32	84.2	29	100	11.80	—	(1.37–101.5)	**0.025**
(2) Shisha smoking is more socially acceptable compared to cigarettes	21	55.3	25	86.2	5.06	—	(1.47–17.4)	**0.01**
(3) Girls are more comfortable in smoking shisha compared to cigarettes	28	73.7	27	93.1	4.82	—	(0.97–24.05)	0.055 (NS)
(4) People smoking shisha look cool	7	18.4	13	44.8	3.60	—	(1.2–10.81)	**0.022**
(5) Friends smoke shisha	31	81.6	27	93.1	3.05	—	(0.58–15.94)	0.187 (NS)
(6) Smoker sibling	12	31.6	14	48.3	2.02	—	(0.74–5.5)	0.167 (NS)
(7) Husband-wife or boyfriend-girlfriend problems lead to shisha smoking	10	26.3	12	41.4	1.98	—	(0.7–5.55)	0.196 (NS)
(8) Stress influences one to start shisha smoking	24	63.2	22	75.9	1.83	—	(0.63–5.38)	0.27 (NS)
(9) Water in shisha filters toxins	13	34.2	14	48.3	1.79	—	(0.67–4.83)	0.247 (NS)
(10) Financial problems lead to shisha smoking	8	21.1	9	31	1.69	—	(0.56–5.11)	0.355 (NS)
(11) Mother smokes shisha	1	2.6	1	3.4	1.32	—	(0.08–22.06)	0.846 (NS)
(12) Shisha smoker parents influenced decision of children to start shisha smoking	13	34.2	11	37.9	1.18	—	(0.43–3.21)	0.753 (NS)
(13) University life burden leads to shisha smoking	17	44.7	14	48.3	1.15	—	(0.44–3.04)	0.774 (NS)
(14) Problems with friends lead to shisha smoking	10	26.3	8	27.6	1.07	—	(0.36–3.17)	0.907 (NS)
(15) Family problem leads to shisha smoking	17	44.7	13	44.8	1.00	—	(0.38–2.65)	0.994 (NS)

TABLE 10: Continued.

Sex = male	Current shisha smoking habit				OR	Inverse OR	95% confidence interval OR	P
	Nonsmokers (N for total surveyed = 38)		Current smoker (N for total surveyed = 29)					
	N	%	N	%				
(16) People smoking shisha have more friends	10	26.3	7	24.1	0.89	1.12	(0.29–2.72)	0.839 (NS)
(17) Advertisement about shisha can influence smoking	28	73.7	19	65.5	0.68	1.47	(0.24–1.94)	0.47 (NS)
(18) Father smokes shisha	4	10.5	2	6.9	0.63	1.59	(0.11–3.7)	0.609 (NS)
(19) Parents influenced decision of children to start shisha smoking	15	39.5	8	27.6	0.58	1.71	(0.21–1.66)	0.312 (NS)
(20) Shisha smoking is our cultural heritage	18	47.4	10	34.5	0.58	1.71	(0.22–1.58)	0.291 (NS)

questionnaire (less than 20% nonresponse rate) (Table 7). A significant level of dependence was observed, which was significantly higher among men (15.4%) than among women (4.5%) (Table 8).

Some knowledge items were perceived as barriers, since they referred to the detrimental health consequences of shisha smoking and the toxic chemicals in the product. Other knowledge items were classified as enabling factors, since they encouraged shisha smoking behavior. The role of these barriers and enabling factors was tested for association with the current shisha smoking habit. This test was categorized by sex, since the perception of these knowledge items was different between the sexes.

All the 11 barrier knowledge items were more frequent among female nonsmokers than current smokers. However, only the first 2 items "shisha is more addictive than cigarettes" and "shisha is addictive" were positively identified and agreed upon by the interviewees as significantly reducing the risk of being a current shisha smoker by 5.85 and 2.38 times, respectively (Table 9). In men, 10 barriers were more frequent among nonsmokers than current shisha smokers. However, only 1 item "shisha contains nicotine" when positively identified significantly reduced the risk of being a current shisha smoker by 7.02 times. Only 3 enabling factors (items 1, 2, and 4) clearly increased the risk of being a current shisha smoker in men. These were "friends can influence shisha smoking," "shisha is more socially acceptable compared to cigarettes," and "people smoking shisha look cool" all of which significantly increased the risk of being current smokers by 11.08, 5.06, and 3.6, respectively (Table 10).

Among women, only 10 enabling factors clearly increased the risk of being current shisha smokers. The most powerful of these factors was item number (1) "friends smoke shisha," which significantly increased the risk of being a current smoker by 11.32 times.

The next 4 items (items 2, 3, 5, and 6) increased the risk of current shisha smoking by more than four times. These positive knowledge items included: "smoker sibling, father, and mother," believing that "friends can influence smoking," and feeling that "shisha smoking is more socially acceptable than cigarettes." In addition, agreeing that "girls are more comfortable smoking shisha compared to cigarettes" and feeling that "people smoking shisha look cool" significantly increased the risk of current shisha smoking as an outcome by more than three times. The remaining 2 knowledge items (9 and 10) "shisha smoking is our cultural heritage" and "people who smoke shisha have more friends" marginally increased the risk by between 56% and 63%. For women, the remaining 10 items originally classified as enabling factors not only did not increase the risk of current shisha smoking but also were inversely associated with this habit. These factors included stressful situations as a possible cause of smoking, including the life burden in university, the problems with friends, couple problems, and financial problems, "stress leads to shisha smoking." Advertising about shisha was not perceived by women as an enabling factor for shisha smoking (Table 9).

Tables 11 and 12 summarize the participants' smoking habits and personal smoking behavior.

4. Discussion

In the present study, men with a current shisha smoking habit comprised 43.3% of the male sample, which was nearly the same percentage reported among medical students in central Saudi Arabia (44.1%) [22]. The prevalence rate was the highest in senior year students. This high prevalence could be attributed to a common belief that shisha smoking is less harmful than cigarette smoking [23]. However, in the present study, most of the male participants (86.8% nonsmokers and 79.3% current smokers) acknowledged that shisha was more harmful than cigarettes. The increasing prevalence in shisha smoking among university dental students despite the high perception of its harmful effects and the increasing trend in shisha smoking is due to other factors, including peer pressure. Akers et al. [24] have stated that "the single most direct influence on smoking among young people is how many of their 5 best friends smoke." Initial cigarette workout occurs in the presence of other adolescents who are smoking [25, 26]. In the present study, 86.1% of surveyed nonsmokers and 96.3% of current shisha smokers supported this concept. The number of students

Table 11: Participant's smoking habits and dependence (current shisha smokers).

Variables	Number	Percentage (%)
Current shisha smoking	56	14.1
Share shisha	87	42.8
Smoke shisha at café	105	51.7
Smoke shisha with friends	96	42.2
Smoke cigarettes	41	20.1
Mixed smoker	43	21.1
How often do you smoke shisha?		
(i) 1/week	73	66.3
(ii) 2–4/week	21	19
(iii) More than 5/week	16	14.5
Number of Hager/day		
(i) One	28	77.7
(ii) More than 1	8	22.2
Number of Hager/week		
(i) One	23	53.5
(ii) 2–4	12	27.9
(iii) More than 5	8	18.6
Minutes to first shisha of the day		
(i) Less than hour	46	43.8
(ii) More than hour	59	56.2
How soon do you smoke after you wake up		
(i) Less than hour	46	43.8
(ii) More than hour	59	46.2
Which shisha smoking would you hate to give up		
(i) First one in the morning	18	18.9
(ii) Any other in the afternoon or evening	77	81.1
Do you find difficulty to refrain?		
(i) Yes	29	25.2
(ii) No	86	74.8
Do you smoke when ill		
(i) Yes	28	23.7
(ii) No	90	76.3
Do you inhale smoking		
(i) Yes	44	38.2
(ii) No	71	61.8
Do you want to quit?		
(i) Yes	51	44.7
(ii) No	63	55.3
Did you try to quit shisha smoking?		
(i) Yes	43	38
(ii) No	70	6262

who had ever smoked shisha was double among men and triple among women when compared with current shisha smokers (43.3% versus 82.1% for males and 8.2 versus 27.9% for females), as seen in Tables 5 and 6. More than 55.3% of nonsmokers and around 86.2% of male current smokers in the present study believed that shisha was more socially acceptable than cigarettes. Similar findings also showed that smokers do not see themselves as addicts and feel they can quit whenever they wish [27, 28]. Worldwide, more than 100 million people reported smoking shisha [4]. Young people are attracted to the water pipe as it comes in a variety of flavors and is popular as a group activity. For many years, the water pipe was considered less harmful than cigarettes; even worse many users did not consider it as a form of tobacco smoking. The use of the water pipe for smoking tobacco is a tradition in the Middle East region that goes back centuries. Since the early 1990s, however, its use has surged among new groups such as women, teenagers, and wealthy people. Shisha smoking is usually between 1 and 4 sessions/day, but with much more intense exposure per session when compared to cigarettes. Public health education and better informing health practitioners about the facts of water pipe tobacco exposure might correct the false concept of "safe smoking." In the present study, the overall prevalence of shisha smoking was 14.1% among dental students. A lower prevalence rate (5.6% and 7.3%) was reported among other nonmedical students at the University of Sharjah, UAE [1], and university students in Riyadh, Saudi Arabia [29].

A study conducted in the United Kingdom on 181 dental students showed that more than 90% of dental students had moderate or good knowledge and more than 80% had an appropriate attitude towards smoking [30]. However, appropriate knowledge and attitude alone cannot result in a proper behavior, and other confounding factors like socioeconomic and family issues [31, 32] should also be taken into account [3].

The Modified Fagerström Nicotine Test of Dependence (MFNTD) questionnaire with 5-item responses was used in the present study to determine the level of dependence (Table 7). The total score was calculated as the sum of the individual items; a significant level of dependence was observed in 15.4% of men with a current shisha habit (Table 8). Ghafouri et al. [17] found that 17.2% of their studied sample felt that shisha smoking was addictive.

Stress was found to be one of the enabling factors that leads to shisha smoking (22/29 men and 17/27 women) among current shisha smokers as shown in Tables 9 and 10. The high perception of the harmful effect of shisha smoking among participants does not prevent them from practicing this habit. This may be contributing to the widespread of this type and other types of tobacco use. Similarly, a study done at the American University of Beirut [32] reported that most students are aware about the effects of smoking on health but lacked detailed information about how these effects happened. These discrepancies reflect the failure of university curricula in this region to teach students about the harmful properties of tobacco effectively.

In addressing the concept of barriers, acknowledging the addictive nature of shisha and the fact that it is more addictive than cigarettes was found to reduce the risk of being a current shisha smoker among women. These barriers did not affect the male habit, in fact their knowledge about the nicotine content of shisha increased the risk of the habit.

Table 12: Personal smoking behavior.

		N	%
Current shisha smoking habit	Negative	341	85.9
	Current shisha smoker	56	14.1
	Total	397	100.0
Ever smoked shisha	Negative	250	63.0
	Positive	147	37.0
	Total	397	100.0
Shisha smoking habit	Negative	250	63.0
	Ex-shisha smoker	91	22.9
	Current shisha smoker	56	14.1
	Total	397	100.0
Shares shisha with others	Negative	14	25.0
	Positive	42	75.0
	Total	56	100.0
Smoke shisha usually at café	Negative	2	3.6
	Positive	54	96.4
	Total	56	100.0
Smoking shisha with friends/family	Negative	6	10.7
	Positive	50	89.3
	Total	56	100.0
Smokes shisha occasionally	Negative	10	17.9
	Positive	46	82.1
	Total	56	100.0
Smoke cigarettes	Negative	41	73.2
	Positive	15	26.8
	Total	56	100.0
Mixed smoker	Negative	38	67.9
	Positive	18	32.1
	Total	56	100.0
Frequency of smoking shisha	≤1/week	38	67.9
	2–4 sessions/week	11	19.6
	5 ± week	7	12.5
	Total	56	100.0
Dose of smoking per week (Hager/week)-categories	Only one	34	66.7
	2–4	10	19.6
	5–9	6	11.8
	10+	1	2.0
	Total	51	100.0
Duration of first shisha of the day	0	32	61.5
	1	20	38.5
	Total	52	100.0
Do you smoke more during the first 2 hours of the day than during the rest of the day	Negative	50	92.6
	Positive	4	7.4
	Total	54	100.0
How soon after you wake up do you smoke your first shisha	In the afternoon or evening	49	94.2
	>30 min but before noon	2	3.8
	<30 min	1	1.9
	Total	52	100.0
Which shisha smoking would you hate to give up	Any other in the afternoon or in the evening	4	8.0
	First one in the morning	46	92.0
	Total	50	100.0
Difficult to refrain from shisha smoking in places where it is forbidden	Negative	44	81.5
	Positive	10	18.5
	Total	54	100.0

Table 12: Continued.

		N	%
Smoking when ill	Negative	43	78.2
	Positive	12	21.8
	Total	55	100.0
Inhalation of smoking	Negative	35	64.8
	Positive	19	35.2
	Total	54	100.0
Want to quit shisha smoking	Negative	30	54.5
	Positive	25	45.5
	Total	55	100.0
Attempt to quit shisha smoking	Negative	36	65.5
	Positive	19	34.5
	Total	55	100.0
Modified Fagerström Test for Nicotine Dependence score categories	Low level of dependence	43	89.6
	Moderate level of dependence	5	10.4
	Total	48	100.0

Among the factors that promote the habit of smoking shisha, both sexes agreed on the positive peer effect. However, current female shisha smokers were more likely to have a friend with the shisha smoking habit. In addition, both sexes were significantly affected by the positive social image of shisha. They used the word "cool" to describe the habit. In addition, they thought that shisha smoking was more acceptable than cigarettes. Socially, women are more comfortable with shisha smoking than cigarette smoking. Finally, the role of family members (father, mother, and siblings) was an important promoter for women.

If dental students are to become advocates for reducing smoking, the dental schools' curricula should stress more about the awareness of tobacco-related diseases. The positive social image of shisha for both sexes and the role model of family members in fostering this habit among women should be addressed to prevent its spread. The increasing number of women smoking water pipes may become an epidemic unless robust health education programs are designed to combat water pipe smoking, especially in these age groups.

5. Conclusion

Water pipe smoking among university students is of growing concern. Acknowledging the addictive nature of shisha and the fact that it is more addictive than cigarettes is an important barrier for the habit among women users. Among the factors that promote the habit in both sexes were the positive peer effect and the positive social image of shisha. The influential role model of other family members smoking shisha was an important promoter only for women. An intervention program to prevent this health problem must teach the public that water pipes are no less risky than cigarettes. Water pipe smoking should be bound by the same regulations and laws as cigarette smoking, including banning it in public places.

Furthermore, teachers and faculty at schools and universities should be engaged to include tobacco and water pipe prevention programs in their curriculum.

References

[1] World Health Organization, *TobReg Advisory Note: Waterpipe Tobacco Smoking: Health Effects, Research Needs and Recommended Actions by Regulators*, World Health Organization, Geneva, Switzerland, 2005.

[2] World Health Organization, *Waterpipe Tobacco Smoking: Health Effects, Research Needs and Recommended Actions for Regulators*, World Health Organization, Geneva, Switzerland, 2nd edition, 2015.

[3] M. Garcia, A. Jemal, E. M. Ward et al., *Global Cancer Facts and Figures 2007*, vol. 1, American Cancer Society, Atlanta, GA, USA, 2007.

[4] G. Heydari, M. Yousefifard, M. Hosseini, A. Ramezankhani, and M. R. Masjedi, "Cigarette smoking, knowledge, attitude and prediction of smoking between male students, teachers and Clergymen in Tehran, Iran, 2009," *International Journal of Preventive Medicine*, vol. 4, no. 5, pp. 557–564, 2013.

[5] A. Chattopadhyay, "Emperor Akbar as a healer and his eminent physicians," *Bulletin of the Indian Institute of History of Medicine*, vol. 30, no. 2, pp. 151–157, 2000.

[6] W. Maziak, K. D. Ward, F. Mzayek, S. Rastam, and M. E. Bachir, "Mapping the health and environmental situation in informal zones of Aleppo, Syria: report from the Aleppo household survey," *International Archives of Occupational and Environmental Health*, vol. 78, no. 7, pp. 547–558, 2005.

[7] K. A. Hadidi and F. I. Mohammed, "Nicotine content in tobacco used in hubble-bubble smoking," *Saudi Medical Journal*, vol. 25, no. 7, pp. 912–917, 2004.

[8] M. C. Inhorn and K. A. Buss, "Ethnography, epidemiology and infertility in Egypt," *Social Science & Medicine*, vol. 39, no. 5, pp. 671–686, 1994.

[9] G. Kiter, E. S. Ucan, E. Ceylan, and O. Kilinc, "Water-pipe smoking and pulmonary functions," *Respiratory Medicine*, vol. 94, no. 9, pp. 891–894, 2000.

[10] W. J. Munckhof, A. Konstantinos, M. Wamsley, M. Mortlock, and C. Gilpin, "A cluster of tuberculosis associated with use of marijuana water pipe," *International Journal of Tuberculosis and Lung Disease*, vol. 7, no. 9, pp. 860–865, 2003.

[11] W. Maziak, F. M. Fouad, T. Asfar et al., "Prevalence and characteristics of narghile smoking among university students in Syria," *International Journal of Tuberculosis and Lung Disease*, vol. 8, no. 7, pp. 882–889, 2004.

[12] F. M. Mohamed, A. Khatab, T. El-Naggar, and M. Farrag, *Smoking Habits in Medical Students of Ain Shams Faculty of Medicine*, MSc Thesis, Faculty of Medicine, Ain Shams University 2001.

[13] A. Memon, P. M. Moody, T. N. Sugathan et al., "Epidemiology of smoking among Kuwaiti adults: prevalence, characterstics, and attitudes," *Bulletin of the World Health Organization*, vol. 78, pp. 1306–1315, 2000.

[14] H. Tamim, A. Terro, H. Kassem et al., "Tobacco use by university students, Lebanon, 2001," *Addiction*, vol. 98, no. 7, pp. 933–939, 2003.

[15] H. Roohafza, M. Sadeghi, M. Shahnam, A. Bahonar, and N. Sarafzadegan, "Perceived factors related to cigarette and waterpipe (ghelyan) initiation and maintenance in university students of Iran," *International Journal of Public Health*, vol. 56, no. 2, pp. 175–180, 2011.

[16] E. A. Akl, S. K. Gunukula, S. Aleem et al., "The prevalence of waterpipe tobacco smoking among the general and specific populations: a systematic review," *BMC Public Health*, vol. 11, no. 1, p. 244, 2011.

[17] N. Ghafouri, J. D. Hirsch, G. Heydari, C. M. Morello, G. M. Kuo, and R. F. Singh, "Waterpipe smoking among health sciences university students in Iran: perceptions, practices and patterns of use," *BMC Research Notes*, vol. 4, no. 1, p. 496, 2011.

[18] A. A. Gunaid, A. A. Sumairi, R. G. Shidrawi et al., "Oesophageal and gastric carcinoma in the Republic of Yemen," *British Journal of Cancer*, vol. 71, no. 2, pp. 409-410, 1995.

[19] R. A. AL-Naggar and F. S. A. Saghir, "Water pipe (shisha) smoking and associated factors among Malaysian University students," *Asian Pacific Journal of Cancer Prevention*, vol. 12, no. 11, pp. 3041–3047, 2011.

[20] M. R. Khami, H. Murtomaa, S. Razeghi, and J. I. Virtanen, "Smoking and its determinants among Iranian dental students," *Medical Principles and Practice*, vol. 19, no. 5, pp. 390–394, 2010.

[21] A. Z. Taha, A. A. Sabra, Z. Z. Al-Mustafa, H. R. Al-Awami, M. A. Al-Khalaf, and M. M. Al-Momen, "Water pipe (shisha) smoking among male students of medical colleges in the eastern region of Saudi Arabia," *Annals of Saudi Medicine*, vol. 30, no. 3, pp. 222–226, 2010.

[22] Y. A. Al-Turki, "Smoking habit among medical students in Central Saudi Arabia," *Saudi Medical Journal*, vol. 27, no. 5, pp. 700–703, 2006.

[23] L. S. Friedman, E. Lichtenstein, and A. Biglan, "Smoking onset among teens: an empirical analysis of initial situations," *Addictive Behaviors*, vol. 10, no. 1, pp. 1–13, 1985.

[24] R. L. Akers, M. D. Krohn, L. Lanza-Kaduce, and M. Radosevich, "Social learning and deviant behavior: a specific test of a general theory," *American Sociological Review*, vol. 44, no. 4, pp. 636–655, 1979.

[25] H. R. Mohammed, Y. Zhang, M. Newman, and D. F. Shell, "Water pipe smoking in Kuwait," *Eastern Mediterranean Health Journal*, vol. 16, pp. 1115–1120, 2010.

[26] S. Smith-Simone, W. Maziak, K. Ward, and T. Eissenberg, "Water pipe tobacco smoking: knowledge, attitude, beliefs, and behavior in two U.S. samples," *Nicotine & Tobacco Research*, vol. 10, pp. 393–398, 2008.

[27] B. A. Primack, J. Sidani, A. A. Agarwal, W. G. Shadel, E. C. Donny, and T. E. Eisenberg, "Prevalence of and associations with waterpipe tobacco smoking among U.S. University students," *Annals of Behavioral Medicine*, vol. 36, no. 1, pp. 81–86, 2008.

[28] A. Mandil, A. Hussein, H. Omer, G. Turki, and I. Gaber, "Characteristics and risk factors of tobacco consumption among University of Sharjah students, 2005," *Eastern Mediterranean Health Journal*, vol. 13, no. 6, pp. 1449–1458, 2007.

[29] S. Clareboets, V. Sivarajasingam, and I. G. Chestnutt, "Smoking cessation advice: knowledge, attitude and practice among clinical dental students," *British Dental Journal*, vol. 208, no. 4, pp. 173–177, 2010.

[30] R. Kelishadi, "Tobacco use prevention for Iranian adolescents: time for family-centered counseling programs," *International Journal of Preventive Medicine*, vol. 2, no. 4, pp. 201-202, 2011.

[31] F. Rezaei, S. Nedjat, B. Golestan, and R. Majdzadeh, "Reasons for smoking among male teenagers in Tehran, Iran: two case-control studies using snowball sampling," *International Journal of Preventive Medicine*, vol. 2, no. 4, pp. 216–223, 2011.

14

Relationship between the Necessary Support Level for Oral Hygiene and Performance of Physical, Daily Activity, and Cognitive Functions

Yoh Tamaki, [1] **Yoshimune Hiratsuka**, [1,2] **Toshiro Kumakawa**, [1,3] **and Hiroko Miura** [4]

[1] *Department of Health and Welfare Services, National Institute of Public Health, 2-3-6 Minami, Wako, Saitama 351-0197, Japan*
[2] *Department of Ophthalmology, Juntendo University School of Medicine, 3-1-3, Hongo, Bunkyo-ku, Tokyo 113-8431, Japan*
[3] *The University of Fukuchiyama, 3370, Aza Hori, Fukuchiyama-shi, Kyoto 620-0886, Japan*
[4] *Department of International Health and Collaboration, National Institute of Public Health, 2-3-6 Minami, Wako-shi, Saitama 351-0197, Japan*

Correspondence should be addressed to Yoh Tamaki; pxz11337@nifty.com

Academic Editor: Manal Awad

To maintain good oral hygiene on their own, elderly adults need comprehensive abilities, such as physical, daily activity, and cognitive functions. In the long-term care certification, care support specialists conduct surveys that include a total of 74 items about physical function, daily activity function, living functions, cognitive function, mental/behavioral disorders, and adaption to social life. The data of the long-term care certification survey contain three items related to oral health: the necessary support level for oral hygiene, ability to swallow, and assistance with food intake. The aims of this study were to identify which functions are absent in elderly individuals who cannot maintain proper oral hygiene and to clarify at which stage it is necessary to assist elderly individuals with their oral hygiene and provide professional oral care. In this study, an analysis was conducted to identify the relationship between the necessary support level for oral hygiene and the performance of physical, daily activity, and cognitive functions. The results of the long-term care certification surveys were analyzed for 23,423 cases that involved 9,571 individuals who submitted a claim using long-term care statements between January 2009 and March 2018. The results of a multivariable logistic regression analysis showed that the following items had high odds ratios: "walk" and "stand up" in the physical and daily activity functions and the ability to "understand the everyday routine" and "make daily decisions" in the cognitive functions. The results of a decision tree analysis revealed that in order for elderly individuals to maintain good oral hygiene on their own, they must have adequate physical functioning as well as adequate performance of cognitive functions. Our study's findings suggest that comprehensive ability in both physical and cognitive functions is required for elderly adults to maintain their oral hygiene.

1. Introduction

The population of elderly individuals in Japan has been dramatically increasing over the past three decades. According to a report by the Ministry of Internal Affairs and Communications of Japan, the percentage of older individuals aged 65 years or more increased from 7.1% in 1970 to 25.2% in 2013 [1]. One in every three individuals will be aged 65 years or older, and one in every five will be aged 75 years or older by 2035 [1]. By 2060, elderly adults will account for no less than 39.9% of the Japanese population, or 1 in 2.5 individuals, according to the medium-fertility projection [1].

Oral health is a significant factor affecting the quality of life and overall health and well-being of elderly individuals [2, 3]. In elderly adults, poor oral health affects the ability to chew and eat a variety of foods, causing poor dietary intake and weight loss [4, 5]. In addition, aspiration pneumonia is linked to poor oral health [6, 7]. Thus, maintaining good oral hygiene is important for elderly individuals [8, 9]. However, frail elderly individuals often have poor oral hygiene due to a decline in physical performance and cognitive function [10]. To maintain good oral hygiene on their own, elderly adults need comprehensive abilities, such as in their physical function, daily activity function, and cognitive function [11]. However, there is currently no research that has examined which functions are missing in elderly individuals who cannot maintain proper oral hygiene.

In Japan, long-term care insurance is a mandatory social insurance system, in which individuals who are aged 40 years or older are required to participate. Various long-term care services are provided for those who need care if they pay part of the cost [12]. Under the long-term care insurance, individuals aged 65 years or over (Category 1) and those aged 40–64 years (Category 2) are covered by the health insurance program. Long-term care insurance services are provided when individuals aged 65 years or over require care or support for any reason or when individuals aged 40–64 years develop age-related diseases, such as terminal cancer or rheumatoid arthritis, and thereby require care or support. The number of beneficiaries in Japan who required care under this system and eligible individuals (including those in need of support) was 2.18 million in 2000, which increased to 6.19 million in December 2015. Approximately 18% of Japanese people aged 65 years and older are eligible for long-term care certification [13].

To receive long-term care services in Japan, it is necessary to apply for the long-term care certification that is required in the municipality where each individual lives and has to be certified for the level of long-term care that they need. The survey for the need for long-term care certification assesses the mental and physical conditions of the certificate applicant and determines what level of care the applicant needs. This system is used to determine the necessary care level for several millions of individuals. The assessment data collected during this process are developed at the national level, are entered into a database, and are expected to be used for the analysis of regional and clinical issues, including quality of care. In the long-term care certification process, care support specialists conduct surveys that contain a total of 74 items about physical function, daily activity function, living functions, cognitive function, mental/behavioral disorders, and adaption to social life. The necessary care level is then evaluated using a total of seven levels (support need levels 1–2 and care need levels 1–5). The data of the long-term care certification survey contain three items related to oral health: the necessary support level for oral hygiene, ability to swallow, and assistance with food intake.

In this study, an analysis was conducted to identify the relationship between the necessary support level for oral hygiene and the performance of physical, daily activity, and cognitive functions. The aims of this study were to identify which functions are absent in elderly individuals who cannot maintain proper oral hygiene and to clarify at which stage it is necessary to assist elderly individuals with their oral hygiene and provide professional oral care.

2. Methods

The results of the long-term care certification surveys were analyzed for 23,423 cases that involved 9,571 individuals (3,640 males and 5,931 females; average age 85.8 ± 9 years, range 44–111 years) who submitted a claim using long-term care statements between January 2009 and March 2018. The study population was selected from 68,000 insured individuals in Mishima City, Shizuoka Prefecture (which has a total population of about 110,000). The results of the surveys conducted by the long-term care support specialists for the long-term care certification regarding physical function, daily activity function, living functions (10 items), cognitive function (eight items), mental/behavioral disorders, and adaption to social life were used. The data were analyzed to identify the relationship between the necessary support level for oral hygiene and the performance of other physical and daily activity functions (10 items: roll-over, get up, maintain a seated posture, maintain a standing position on both feet, walk, stand up, stand on one foot, vision, hearing, and swallowing) and cognitive function (eight items: communicate one's will, understand the everyday routine, state one's birthday and age, recall from short-term memory, state one's name, know what the current season is, know the environment, and make daily decisions).

First, cross-tabulation was performed of each item, including the necessary support level for oral hygiene and the evaluation items for the physical, daily activity, and cognitive functions. In addition, a multivariable logistic regression analysis was conducted with the necessary support level for oral hygiene as the dependent variable (total assistance—partial assistance/can do by their self) and the other performance evaluation items (a total of 20 items related to sex, age, physical function, daily activity function, and cognitive function) as the independent variables.

A more detailed analysis was conducted for similar items using a decision tree analysis; specifically, the Classification and Regression Trees method. The analyses were conducted using IBM SPSS version 24 and SPSS Modeler 17.1 (IBM Japan Ltd., Tokyo, Japan).

This survey was approved by the ethics committee of the National Institute of Public Health (NIPH-IBRA #12137) and the city council of Mishima City. All methods were performed in accordance with the International Ethical Guidelines for Epidemiological Studies [14], Guideline for the Provision of the Database for National Health Insurance Claim/Specific Medical Checkup/Specific Health Guidance [15], and Security Guidelines for Health Information Systems [16]. In compliance with the above guidelines, the researchers conducted the analyses once any information that could be identified as personal data was made anonymous by the local government.

3. Results

Table 1 shows the results of the cross-tabulation of the evaluation items of physical function and daily activity function, and the necessary support level for oral hygiene. Table 2 shows the results of the cross-tabulation for the

Table 1: Results of cross-tabulation for evaluation items of physical and daily activity functions and level of assistance needed for oral hygiene.

Ability items			Oral hygiene: Can do on one's own	Oral hygiene: Partial assistance	Oral hygiene: Total assistance	Total	p value*
Roll-over	Can do without holding on to something	N	6963	1696	170	8829	<0.001
		%	78.9%	19.2%	1.9%	100.0%	
	Can do with holding on to something	N	5234	3131	397	8762	
		%	59.7%	35.7%	4.5%	100.0%	
	Cannot do on one's own	N	650	902	1531	3083	
		%	21.1%	29.3%	49.7%	100.0%	
Get up	Can do without holding on to something	N	1821	421	35	2277	<0.001
		%	80.0%	18.5%	1.5%	100.0%	
	Can do with holding on to something	N	10582	3556	249	14387	
		%	73.6%	24.7%	1.7%	100.0%	
	Cannot do on one's own	N	444	1752	1814	4010	
		%	11.1%	43.7%	45.2%	100.0%	
Maintain a seated posture	1: Can do on their own	N	7466	1823	130	9419	<0.001
		%	79.3%	19.4%	1.4%	100.0%	
	2: Can do if supported using one's own arms	N	3729	1673	130	5532	
		%	67.4%	30.2%	2.3%	100.0%	
	3: Can do with support	N	1631	2171	1617	5419	
		%	30.1%	40.1%	29.8%	100.0%	
	4: Cannot do	N	21	62	221	304	
		%	6.9%	20.4%	72.7%	100.0%	
Maintain a standing position on both feet	Can do without support	N	8447	1766	100	10313	<0.001
		%	81.9%	17.1%	1.0%	100.0%	
	Can do with support of something	N	4202	2627	297	7126	
		%	59.0%	36.9%	4.2%	100.0%	
	Cannot do on one's own	N	198	1336	1701	3235	
		%	6.1%	41.3%	52.6%	100.0%	
Walk	1: Can do without holding on to something	N	4622	850	63	5535	<0.001
		%	83.5%	15.4%	1.1%	100.0%	
	2: Can do with holding on to something	N	6975	2041	196	9212	
		%	75.7%	22.2%	2.1%	100.0%	
	3: Cannot do	N	1250	2838	1839	5927	
		%	21.1%	47.9%	31.0%	100.0%	
Stand up	Can do without holding on to something	N	1247	248	24	1519	<0.001
		%	82.1%	16.3%	1.6%	100.0%	
	Can do with holding on to something	N	11369	3694	241	15304	
		%	74.3%	24.1%	1.6%	100.0%	
	Cannot do	N	231	1787	1833	3851	
		%	6.0%	46.4%	47.6%	100.0%	
Stand on one foot	Can do without support	N	2435	400	14	2849	<0.001
		%	85.5%	14.0%	0.5%	100.0%	
	Can do with support of something	N	9445	2905	166	12516	
		%	75.5%	23.2%	1.3%	100.0%	
	Cannot do on one's own	N	967	2424	1918	5309	
		%	18.2%	45.7%	36.1%	100.0%	
Vision	Normal	N	11729	4862	880	17471	<0.001
		%	67.1%	27.8%	5.0%	100.0%	
	Cannot see the letters in newspapers or magazines but can see a picture one meter away	N	715	500	218	1433	
		%	49.9%	34.9%	15.2%	100.0%	
	Cannot see a picture one meter away but can see a picture directly in front of them	N	275	222	129	626	
		%	43.9%	35.5%	20.6%	100.0%	
	Cannot hardly see	N	119	88	50	257	
		%	46.3%	34.2%	19.5%	100.0%	

TABLE 1: Continued.

Ability items			Oral hygiene: Can do on one's own	Oral hygiene: Partial assistance	Oral hygiene: Total assistance	Total	p value*
Hearing	Normal	N	9325	4006	1190	14521	<0.001
		%	64.2%	27.6%	8.2%	100.0%	
	Cannot hear a normal voice easily	N	2826	1169	361	4356	
		%	64.9%	26.8%	8.3%	100.0%	
	Can hear a loud voice	N	655	511	239	1405	
		%	46.6%	36.4%	17.0%	100.0%	
	Can hardly hear	N	40	42	19	101	
		%	39.6%	41.6%	18.8%	100.0%	
Swallowing	1: Can do on their own	N	12284	5188	1019	18491	<0.001
		%	66.4%	28.1%	5.5%	100.0%	
	2: Monitoring needed	N	547	513	593	1653	
		%	33.1%	31.0%	35.9%	100.0%	
	3: Cannot do	N	16	28	486	530	
		%	3.0%	5.3%	91.7%	100.0%	
Total		N	12847	5729	2098	20674	
		% of the total	62.1%	27.7%	10.1%	100.0%	

*Chi-square test.

TABLE 2: Results of cross-tabulation for evaluation items of cognitive functions and level of assistance needed oral hygiene.

Item			Oral hygiene: Can do on one's own	Oral hygiene: Partial assistance	Oral hygiene: Total assistance	Total	p value*
Communicate one's will	Can do	N	12272	4570	500	17342	<0.001
		%	70.8%	26.4%	2.9%	100.0%	
	Can sometimes do	N	526	926	457	1909	
		%	27.6%	48.5%	23.9%	100.0%	
	Can hardly do	N	47	224	696	967	
		%	4.9%	23.2%	72.0%	100.0%	
	Cannot do	N	2	9	445	456	
		%	0.4%	2.0%	97.6%	100.0%	
Understand the everyday routine	Can do	N	12042	3356	261	15659	<0.001
		%	76.9%	21.4%	1.7%	100.0%	
	Cannot do	N	805	2373	1837	5015	
		%	16.1%	47.3%	36.6%	100.0%	
State one's birthday and age	Can do	N	12588	4720	680	17988	<0.001
		%	70.0%	26.2%	3.8%	100.0%	
	Cannot do	N	259	1009	1418	2686	
		%	9.6%	37.6%	52.8%	100.0%	
Recall from short-term memory	Can do	N	10005	2618	255	12878	<0.001
		%	77.7%	20.3%	2.0%	100.0%	
	Cannot do	N	2842	3111	1843	7796	
		%	36.5%	39.9%	23.6%	100.0%	
State one's own name	Can do	N	12827	5605	1191	19623	<0.001
		%	65.4%	28.6%	6.1%	100.0%	
	Cannot do	N	20	124	907	1051	
		%	1.9%	11.8%	86.3%	100.0%	
Know what the current season is	Can do	N	11660	3436	389	15485	
		%	75.3%	22.2%	2.5%	100.0%	
	Cannot do	N	1187	2293	1709	5189	
		%	22.9%	44.2%	32.9%	100.0%	
Know the environment	Can do	N	12719	4966	751	18436	<0.001
		%	69.0%	26.9%	4.1%	100.0%	
	Cannot do	N	128	763	1347	2238	
		%	5.7%	34.1%	60.2%	100.0%	

TABLE 2: Continued.

Item			Oral hygiene: Can do on one's own	Partial assistance	Total assistance	Total	p value*
Make daily decisions	Can do	N	7102	1099	79	8280	<0.001
		%	85.8%	13.3%	1.0%	100.0%	
	Can do except for special cases	N	5529	3409	361	9299	
		%	59.5%	36.7%	3.9%	100.0%	
	Daily difficulties	N	211	1159	953	2323	
		%	9.1%	49.9%	41.0%	100.0%	
	Cannot do	N	5	62	705	772	
		%	0.6%	8.0%	91.3%	100.0%	
Total		N	12847	5729	2098	20674	
		% of total	62.1%	27.7%	10.1%	100.0%	

*Chi-square test.

TABLE 3: Results of multivariate logistic regression analysis.

	Item	Multivariate adjusted odds ratio	95% CI Lower limit	95% CI Upper limit	p value
Physical and daily activity functions	Age	1.00	0.99	1.00	0.473
	Sex (female/male)	0.64	0.58	0.70	<0.001
	Roll-over	1.16	1.08	1.26	<0.001
	Get up	1.77	1.57	1.99	<0.001
	Maintain a seated posture	1.08	1.01	1.15	0.015
	Maintain a standing position on both feet	1.53	1.39	1.69	<0.001
	Walk	2.35	2.15	2.56	<0.001
	Stand up	2.10	1.81	2.43	<0.001
	Stand on one foot	1.31	1.18	1.46	<0.001
	Vision	1.19	1.10	1.29	<0.001
	Hearing	0.90	0.84	0.97	0.005
	Swallowing	1.15	0.99	1.34	0.077
Cognitive functions	Communicate one's will	1.12	0.97	1.28	0.113
	Understand the everyday routine	3.08	2.68	3.55	<0.001
	State one's birthday and age	2.00	1.63	2.44	<0.001
	Recall from short-term memory	1.88	1.67	2.10	<0.001
	State one's own name	1.03	0.50	2.11	0.934
	Know what the current season is	1.96	1.73	2.22	<0.001
	Know the environment	2.25	1.73	2.92	<0.001
	Make daily decisions	2.55	2.33	2.79	<0.001

A total of 20 items were entered simultaneously as the explanatory variables.

evaluation items of cognitive function and necessary support level for oral hygiene. The results of the multivariable logistic regression analysis showed that there was a significant odds ratio (OR) with regards to the necessary support level for oral hygiene for 16 items, including sex, and the evaluation items of the other physical, daily activity, and cognitive functions. Women had a lower risk in the necessary support level for oral hygiene than the men (OR 0.64). The following items had high ORs: walk (OR 2.3) and stand up (OR 2.10) in the physical and daily activity functions, and the ability to understand the everyday routine (OR 3.1) and make daily decisions (OR 2.55) in the cognitive function (Table 3). No significant OR was obtained for the ability to swallow, which is one of the ability indexes of oral health. For cognitive function, no significant OR was obtained in the ability to communicate one's will or state one's name.

Furthermore, the results of the decision tree analysis revealed that 92.1% of respondents needed complete assistance with their oral hygiene if they could not stand on one's own and if they could not communicate their will (Figure 1). On the contrary, 83.1% of respondents did not require assistance with oral hygiene if they could stand or could stand if holding on to something, and could understand the everyday routine. In addition, more than 80% did not need assistance or partially needed assistance if they could or sometimes could communicate their will and if

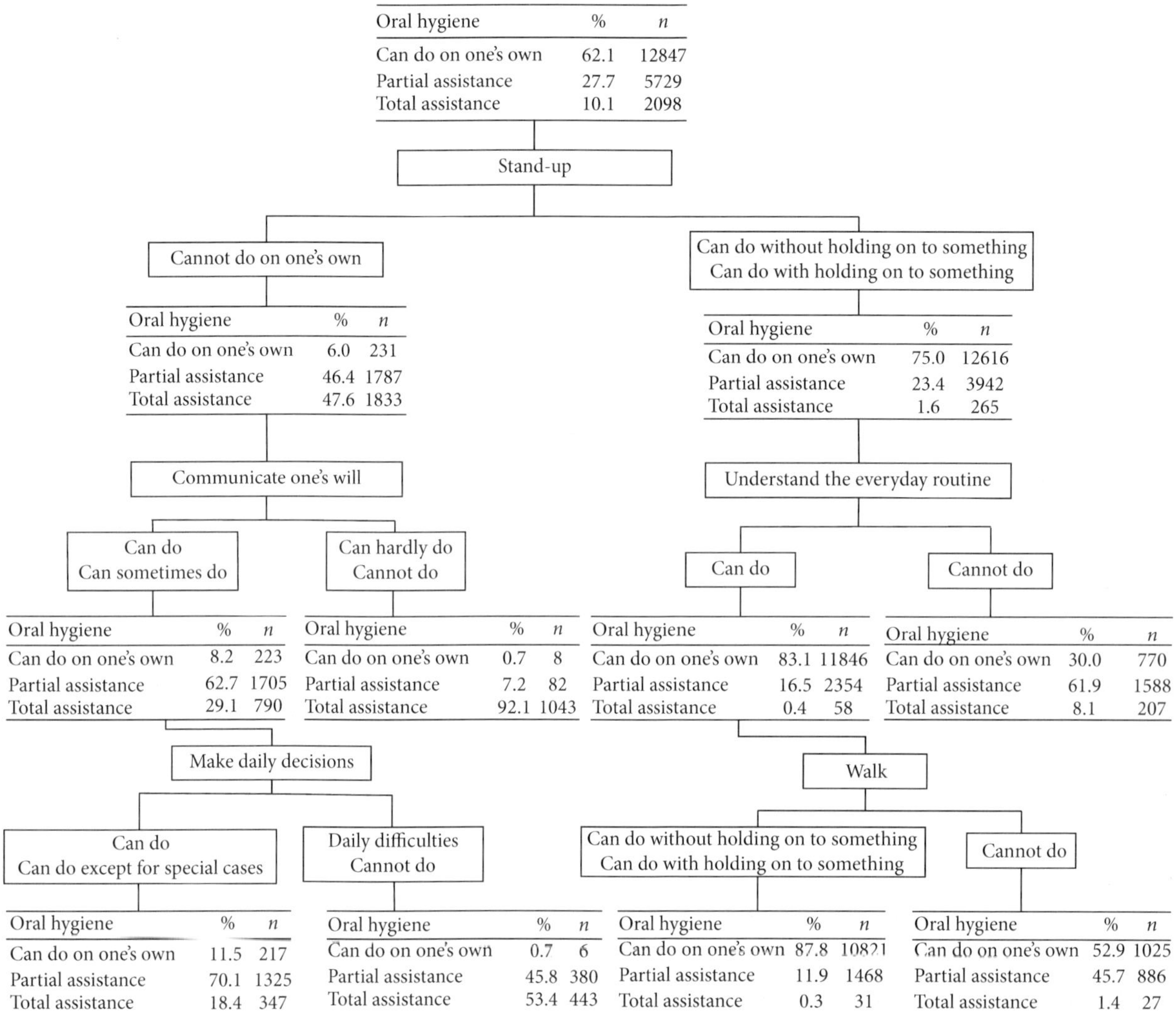

FIGURE 1: Results of decision tree analysis.

they could make daily decisions or could make daily decisions except in special cases, even if they could not stand up.

4. Discussion

This study found significant ORs for many of the survey items for physical function, daily activity function, and cognitive function regarding oral hygiene, which suggests that a comprehensive ability is required in terms of both physical function and cognitive function in order to maintain oral hygiene. Regarding the indexes of physical and daily activity functions, at least 80% of respondents were capable of maintaining oral hygiene with no assistance or partial assistance if they could or sometimes could not communicate their will, and if they could make daily decisions or could make daily decisions except for in special cases, even if they could not stand up. Therefore, for elderly individuals to maintain good oral hygiene on their own, they must have adequate physical functioning as well as adequate cognitive functioning.

Previous studies have confirmed that dementia can reduce the efficiency and stability of people to clean themselves; thus, the patients' oral hygiene condition worsens, and they develop more caries [17–19] and periodontal disease [20, 21] than people without dementia. Accordingly, it is presumed that patients with a moderate or higher level of dementia, who have many remaining teeth and who care for themselves without oral care assistance, have a high risk of oral diseases. For patients with mild dementia who can converse and understand well, there is a risk of multiple developments, such as periodontal diseases and caries, because oral self-care becomes poor owing to decreased self-motivation and finger dexterity, as well as visuospatial cognitive disorders. In this study, we found that respondents with a lower ability to understand everyday routines and to make daily decisions need assistance with oral hygiene because they are expected to have a higher risk of periodontal diseases and caries.

Physical functions deteriorate rapidly during dementia compared with during normal aging. It has also been reported that physiological vulnerability and vulnerability to stress increase the decline in general muscle mass and flexibility, as well as lowering the speed of a reaction to a fall, because physiological preparatory ability declines, and nutrition intake may decrease according to the level of severity [22, 23]. Moreover, the swallowing function deteriorates during Alzheimer's disease (AD), and there is a high risk of physical complications, such as aspiration pneumonia and acute disease episodes [24]. In the case of dementia with Lewy bodies, it is reported that decline in physical functions, such as swallowing functions, occur earlier than in AD [25]. Therefore, assistance with oral hygiene can be said to lead to a reduced risk of physical complications, such as aspiration pneumonia and the occurrence of acute diseases in elderly individuals with decreased cognitive function.

According to the report presented by the World Health Organization (WHO) entitled "Dementia: A Public Health Priority" (2012) [26], there are about 35.6 million individuals with dementia worldwide. The WHO estimates that this number will nearly double every 20 years, reaching an estimated 65.7 million in 2030 and 115.4 million in 2050 [27]. In 2013, a research group at the Ministry of Health, Labour, and Welfare reported that there are 4.62 million individuals with dementia in Japan [28].

If dementia is recognized in the early stages and early countermeasures are taken, patients will have more opportunities to receive support and become more independent. When plaque control suddenly deteriorates or when increased cavities and periodontal are noticed during a dental examination, it is important to treat elderly patients with the understanding that dementia is possible instead of assuming the condition is only the result of aging. In these patients, it is necessary to start a dental intervention, such as providing regular professional oral care, from the mild stage as much as possible, taking into consideration that dental treatment and special oral care become more difficult as dementia advances. In the dental treatment of patients with dementia, the proposed treatment plan should include a projection of the progress of the disease conditions as well as flexible measures that take into account the subsequent changes in condition. To achieve this, it is important to understand the dementia diseases and make appropriate plans for treatment and continuous care. Currently, patients with dementia who cannot visit dental clinics miss opportunities to receive dental treatment (including special oral care). These patients often do not request dental treatment until they develop bad breath, toothache, loosening teeth, difficulty with dentures, and difficulty eating. In many cases, by the time the family members or caregivers notice the change, the patient has already reached the stage where they cannot accurately describe the condition due to the severity of the dementia. In such cases, proactive dental treatment becomes difficult and, most of the time, only urgent care can be provided, which results in worse oral conditions. It is therefore important to understand the conditions of dementia and to continuously provide preventive dental treatment and oral health management for patients with dementia.

In this study, 23.2% of the elderly adults who required total assistance with oral hygiene had a swallowing disorder. On the contrary, 3% of those who had a swallowing disorder did not receive assistance with oral hygiene (data not shown). In the case of the care recipients who need total assistance, assistance with daily life is prioritized, and care often cannot be extended to oral hygiene. To better prevent aspiration pneumonia and other complications, providing assistance with oral hygiene at an early stage is crucial for elderly adults whose physical and cognitive functions have declined.

5. Conclusion

Our study's findings suggest that comprehensive ability in both physical and cognitive functions is required for elderly adults to maintain their oral hygiene. In the future, it will be necessary to assist elderly individuals with their oral hygiene and to provide professional oral care at an earlier stage for those who have reduced physical and cognitive functions.

Authors' Contributions

Yoh Tamaki, Hiroko Miura, Yoshimune Hiratsuka, and Toshiro Kumakawa made substantial contributions to the study's conception, data acquisition, study design, statistical analysis, interpretation of the results, and drafting of the manuscript.

Acknowledgments

This work was supported by the Japan Agency for Medical Research and Development (grant 15dk0107014h0002).

References

[1] Institute of Population and Social Security Research, *Population Projections for Japan (January 2012): 2011 to 2060*, Institute of Population and Social Security Research, Tokyo, Japan, 2012, http://www.ipss.go.jp/index-e.asp.

[2] N. Kshetrimayum, C. V. Reddy, S. Siddhana et al., "Oral health-related quality of life and nutritional status of institutionalized elderly population aged 60 years and above in Mysore City, India," *Gerodontology*, vol. 30, no. 2, pp. 119–125, 2013.

[3] T. A. Saliba, M. M. Ortega, K. K. Goya, S. A. S. Moimaz, and C. A. S. Garbin, "Influence of oral health on the quality of life of institutionalized and noninstitutionalized elderly people," *Dental Research Journal (Isfahan)*, vol. 15, no. 4, pp. 256–263, 2018.

[4] M. Furuta, M. Komiya-Nonaka, S. Akifusa et al., "Interrelationship of oral health status, swallowing function, nutritional status, and cognitive ability with activities of daily living in Japanese elderly people receiving home care services

due to physical disabilities," *Community Dentistry and Oral Epidemiology*, vol. 41, no. 2, pp. 173–181, 2013.

[5] F. B. de Andrade, M. L. Lebrão, Y. A. de Oliveira Duarte, and J. L. Santos, "Oral health and changes in weight and waist circumference among community-dwelling older adults in Brazil," *Journal of the American Dental Association*, vol. 145, no. 7, pp. 731–736, 2014.

[6] F. A. Scannapieco and K. Shay, "Oral health disparities in older adults: oral bacteria, inflammation, and aspiration pneumonia," *Dental Clinics of North America*, vol. 58, no. 4, pp. 771–782, 2014.

[7] J. Sarin, R. Balasubramaniam, A. M. Corcoran, J. M. Laudenbach, and E. T. Stoopler, "Reducing the risk of aspiration pneumonia among elderly patients in long-term care facilities through oral health interventions," *Journal of the American Medical Directors Association*, vol. 9, no. 2, pp. 128–135, 2008.

[8] F. B. 1 de Andrade, M. L. Lebrão, J. L. Santos, and Y. A. Duarte, "Relationship between oral health and frailty in community-dwelling elderly individuals in Brazil," *Journal of the American Geriatrics Society*, vol. 61, no. 5, pp. 809–814, 2013.

[9] Á. Ástvaldsdóttir, A. M. Boström, T. Davidson et al., "Oral health and dental care of older persons-A systematic map of systematic reviews," *Gerontology*, 2018.

[10] K. H. Lee, B. L. Plassman, W. Pan, and B. Wu, "Mediation effect of oral hygiene on the relationship between cognitive function and oral health in older adults," *Journal of Gerontological Nursing*, vol. 42, no. 5, pp. 30–37, 2016.

[11] P. A. Steinmassl, O. Steinmassl, G. Kraus, H. Dumfahrt, and I. Grunert, "Is cognitive status related to oral hygiene level and appropriate for determining need for oral hygiene assistance?," *Journal of Periodontology*, vol. 87, no. 1, pp. 41–47, 2016.

[12] Long-Term Care, *Health and Welfare Services for the Elderly*, Japanese Ministry of Health, Labour and Welfare, Tokyo, Japan, http://www.mhlw.go.jp/english/policy/care-welfare/care-welfare-elderly/.

[13] Japanese Ministry of Health, Labour and Welfare, Long-Term Care Insurance Business Situation, Japanese Ministry of Health, Labour and Welfare, Tokyo, Japan, https://www.e-stat.go.jp/stat-search/files?page=1&toukei=00450351&tstat=000001031648.

[14] Ethical Guidelines for Epidemiological Research, *Ministry of Education, Culture, Sports, Science and Technology*, Ministry of Health, Labour and Welfare Japan, Japan, 2013, http://www.lifescience.mext.go.jp/files/pdf/n796_01.pdf.

[15] Ministry of Health, Labour and Welfare Japan, *Guideline for Provision of Database for National Health Insurance Claim and the Specific Medical Checkup and Specific Health Guidance*, Ministry of Health, Labour and Welfare Japan, Japan, 2015, http://www.mhlw.go.jp/file/05-Shingikai-12401000-Hokenkyoku-Soumuka/0000064238_3.pdf.

[16] Ministry of Health, Labour and Welfare Japan, *Security Guidelines for Health Information Systems*, Ministry of Health, Labour and Welfare Japan, Japan, 2017, http://www.mhlw.go.jp/file/05-Shingikai-12601000-Seisakutoukatsukan-Sanjikanshitsu_Shakaihoshoutantou/0000166260.pdf.

[17] B. 1 Wu, B. L. Plassman, R. J. Crout, and J. Liang, "Cognitive function and oral health among community-dwelling older adults," *Journals of Gerontology Series A: Biological Sciences and Medical Sciences*, vol. 63, no. 5, pp. 495–500, 2008.

[18] A. M. Syrjälä, P. Ylöstalo, P. Ruoppi et al., "Dementia and oral health among subjects aged 75 years or older," *Gerodontology*, vol. 29, no. 1, pp. 36–42, 2012.

[19] W. Sabbah, R. G. Watt, A. Sheiham, and G. Tsakos, "The role of cognitive ability in socio-economic inequalities in oral health," *Journal of Dental Research*, vol. 88, no. 4, pp. 351–355, 2009.

[20] J. M. 1 Noble, L. N. Borrell, P. N. Papapanou, M. S. Elkind, N. Scarmeas, and C. B. Wright, "Periodontitis is associated with cognitive impairment among older adults: analysis of NHANES-III," *Journal of Neurology, Neurosurgery and Psychiatry*, vol. 80, no. 11, pp. 1206–1211, 2009.

[21] H. l Agüero-Torres, L. Fratiglioni, Z. Guo, M. Viitanen, E. von Strauss, and B. Winblad, "Dementia is the major cause of functional dependence in the elderly: 3-year follow-up data from a population-based study," *American Journal of Public Health*, vol. 88, no. 10, pp. 1452–1456, 1998.

[22] T. W. Auyeung, T. Kwok, J. Lee, P. C. Leung, J. Leung, and J. Woo, "Functional decline in cognitive impairment--the relationship between physical and cognitive function," *Neuroepidemiology*, vol. 31, no. 3, pp. 167–173, 2008.

[23] D. Putcha and G. Tremont, "Predictors of independence in instrumental activities of daily living: amnestic versus non-amnestic MCI," *Journal of Clinical and Experimental Neuropsychology*, vol. 38, no. 9, pp. 991–1004, 2016.

[24] E. Sato, H. Hirano, Y. Watanabe et al., "Detecting signs of dysphagia in patients with Alzheimer's disease with oral feeding in daily life," *Geriatrics and Gerontology International*, vol. 14, no. 3, pp. 549–555, 2014.

[25] S. Shinagawa, H. Adachi, Y. Toyota et al., "Characteristics of eating and swallowing problems in patients who have dementia with Lewy bodies," *International Psychogeriatrics*, vol. 21, no. 3, pp. 520–525, 2009.

[26] Dementia, *A Public Health Priority*, World Health Organization, Geneva, Switzerland, 2012, http://apps.who.int/iris/bitstream/10665/75263/1/9789241564458_eng.pdf?ua=1.

[27] UK to host G8 dementia summit, https://www.gov.uk/government/news/uk-to-host-g8-dementia-summit.

[28] The Ministry of Health, Labour and Welfare Scientific Research Fund, *Measures of the Dementia Prevalence and Life Function Disorders of Dementia in the City Areas, Dementia Countermeasure Total Research Project*, The Ministry of Health, Labour and Welfare Scientific Research Fund, Japan, 2013, http://www.tsukuba-psychiatry.com/wp-content/uploads/2013/06/H24Report_Part1.pdf.

15

A Competition between Care Teams Improved Recording of Diagnoses in Primary Dental Care: A Longitudinal Follow-Up Study

Jouko Kallio,[1] Timo Kauppila,[2] Lasse Suominen,[1] and Anna Maria Heikkinen[3,4]

[1]*Social and Health Services of Espoo, City of Espoo, Finland*
[2]*Department of General Practice and Primary Healthcare, Institute of Clinical Medicine, University of Helsinki, Helsinki, Finland*
[3]*Department of Oral and Maxillofacial Diseases and Surgery, Head and Neck Center, Helsinki University Hospital, HUS, Helsinki, Finland*
[4]*Department of Oral and Maxillofacial Diseases, University of Helsinki and Helsinki University Hospital, Helsinki, Finland*

Correspondence should be addressed to Timo Kauppila; timo.kauppila@fimnet.fi

Academic Editor: Louis M. Lin

Introduction. A playful competition was launched in a primary dental health care system to improve the recording of diagnoses into an electronic patient chart system and to study what diagnoses were used in primary dental care. *Methods.* This was a longitudinal follow-up study with public sector primary dental care practices in a Finnish city. A one-year-lasting playful competition between the dental care teams was launched and the monthly percentage of dentists' visits with recorded diagnosis before, during, and after the intervention was recorded. The assessed diagnoses were recorded with the International Classification of Diseases (ICD-10). *Results.* Before the competition, the level of diagnosis recordings was practically zero. At the end of this intervention, about 25% of the visits had a recorded diagnosis. Two years after the competition, this percentage was 35% without any additional measures. The most frequent diagnoses were dental caries (K02, 38.6%), other diseases of hard tissues of teeth (K03, 14.8%), and diseases of pulp and periapical tissues (K04, 11.4%). *Conclusions.* Commitment to the idea that recording of diagnoses was beneficial improved the recording of dental diagnoses. However, the diagnoses obtained did not accurately reflect the reputed prevalence of oral diseases in the Finnish population.

1. Introduction

In primary care, the recording of diagnoses is important for ensuring sufficient treatment actions and for planning activities and for managing the resources of primary care [1–4]. Recording of diagnoses makes it possible to document the types and frequency of conditions the dentists encounter, enhance communication with patients and clinicians, enable outcomes-tracking, and facilitate data sharing and different kinds of research [5]. It also supports educational aims by enhancing learning of diagnostic skills and emphasizing link between diagnosis, treatment, and patient care [5]. Electronic patient information systems allow the recording of diagnoses and allow dentists time for clinical work instead of administrative tasks [6]. Yet, despite their availability, use of those systems has been infrequent for recording diagnoses and it has not been possible to gain a clear idea about the diagnostic distribution of treated oral diseases in primary dental care.

In the primary dental care of Espoo, the basic level of the frequency of recording oral disease diagnoses was practically 0% [4]. A higher frequency of recorded diagnoses was deemed necessary for planning activities and for managing the resources of primary care. In primary care of Espoo, it was possible to increase the frequency of recording diagnoses from 55% of all visits to general practitioners to a level of 90% by using financial group bonuses for care teams [4]. The primary dental care had no resources for financial incentives. As a solution to this problem, the administration of Espoo primary dental care started a playful competition for the dental health care teams to improve recording oral diseases diagnoses.

The aim of this study was to discover whether the competition between the dental care teams increased the rate of recording oral disease diagnoses. We also wanted to explore what diagnoses were recorded in primary dental care.

2. Methods

2.1. Design and Setting. The present work is a retrospective longitudinal quasi-experimental study with a before-and-after design in the primary dental care of the second largest city of Finland. This study was performed in Espoo city, where, in 2009, there were 230,000 inhabitants (254,000 in 2012) and 21 communal dental care teams, for example, cells. The number of dentists varied from 2 to 12 per team. There was the same number of dental nurses (including dental hygienists) supporting work of dentists in these teams, too.

2.2. Primary Outcomes and Data Extraction. The proportion of monthly visits having a recorded diagnosis (out of all communal primary care dentists' visits in Espoo) was our main measure to study the effect of implementing group bonuses. Diagnoses were recorded by ICD-10 system (the International Classification of Diseases (ICD), http://www.who.int/classifications/icd/en/HistoryOfICD.pdf) by the dentists. To commit the staff to the change in function, a competition was announced in December 2008 by the head of primary dental care. The nature of the reward was not revealed and it was promised solely to the team where the percentage of the dentists' visit with recorded diagnosis was the highest during the year 2009. Thus, the intervention itself took place between 1 January and 31 December 2009 (12 months). The data was obtained from the electronic Effica patient chart system (Tieto LTD, Helsinki, Finland) from which the data were reliably obtainable from 1.5.2003. No ethical approval was required because this study was performed directly by computer from the patient register without identifying the patients. According to the Finnish law about register studies, no ethical approval was required (https://rekisteritutkimusen.wordpress.com/data-protection-and-permissions/). The registry keeper (the health authorities of Espoo) granted permission to carry out the study. The report generator automatically allowed following the monthly number of recorded diagnoses for each individual doctor and therefore also by each individual communal dental care cell.

The obtained data were analyzed in a quasi-experimental design, where the recording of diagnoses was compared between similar periods of time before and after the initiation of group bonuses to all persons belonging to the cells (intervention) in primary care of Espoo city. Both the absolute and proportional amounts of visits with recorded diagnoses were available from Espoo.

The competition was closed and the reward was revealed in January 2010: the winning staff of the team got tickets to one show in the Finnish National Theatre in Helsinki with refreshments in February 2010. We continued to collect the data during 2010–2012 after the cessation of the intervention. To study what diagnoses primary care dentists used, all diagnoses were recorded during the last year of the follow-up (2012).

2.3. Statistical Methods. The rate of change in diagnosis marking in Espoo primary care was analyzed with a regression analysis followed by t-test (GLM procedure of SigmaPlot 10.0 Statistical Software, Systat Software Inc., Richmond, CA, USA) and these rates were compared with t-test [4]. The monthly frequencies of marking the diagnoses were analyzed by calculating monthly percentages of visits with recorded diagnoses during each of the follow-up years and comparing them with each other. The statistical significance was tested with One-Way Repeated-Measures Analysis of Variance followed by Bonferroni correction for multiple comparisons. $p < 0.05$ was considered to be statistically significant [4].

3. Results

The rate of change in the recording of diagnoses was 0.040 ± 0.003%/month (mean ± SEM) in 2003–2008, for example, before the intervention. During the intervention (2009), this rate increased to 0.60 ± 0.30%/month ($p < 0.001$, t-test). After cessation of the intervention, for example, in 2010–2012, the increased rate of recording diagnoses (0.58 ± 0.18%/month) did not differ from the rate during intervention. However, this rate was statistically significantly higher than during the preintervention level ($p < 0.001$, Figure 1(a)). Practically, this led to a situation where the monthly percentage of dentist visits having a recorded diagnosis increased every year after intervention. Once started, this increase continued every year even without any specific intervention (One-Way Repeated-Measures ANOVA, $p < 0.001$, Figure 1(b)).

According to the reported distribution of diagnoses (Table 1), the most common diagnosis assessed by the dentists was dental caries (K02). The next frequent diagnoses were other diseases of hard tissues of teeth (K03), diseases of pulp and periapical tissues (K04), and periodontal diseases (K05).

4. Discussion

A playful competition enhanced the marking of diagnoses significantly. Financial incentives are useful in altering the behavior of primary care dentists [7]. However, in this case, practically no financial incentives were required because the financial value of a theatre evening to one team was really a minimal investment. Furthermore, the rate of recording diagnosis in primary dental care increased after intervention, although no extra attempt to enhance this activity was performed. Thus, commitment to the idea that the recording of diagnoses was beneficial had the effect of improving the recording of diagnoses, not the competition itself. In this case, the competition just guided the attention of the primary care dentists to a significant problem which was shortage of knowledge about the quality of local clinical activities. The dentists just decided that recording diagnoses was worth doing disregarding whether they were rewarded for it or not. This led to observed improvements even after

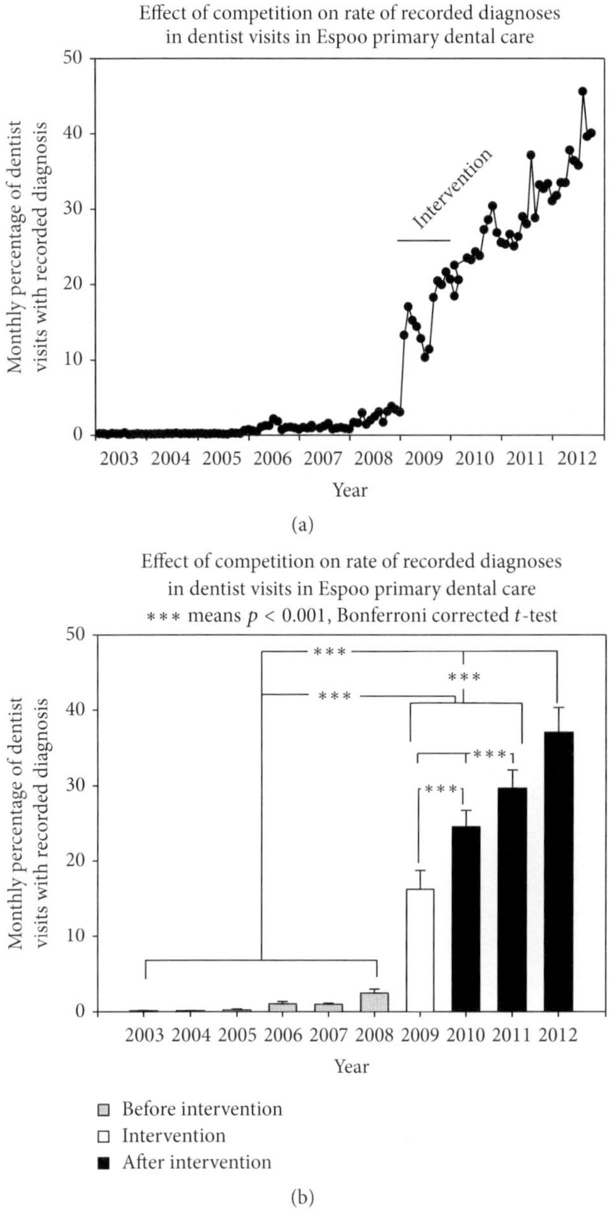

FIGURE 1: (a) Monthly percentage of dentists' visits with recorded diagnoses before, during, and after the playful competition in 2009. (b) Year-based percentage of monthly dentists' visits with recorded diagnoses during the same observation periods. Means (bars) and SDs (brackets) are presented.

TABLE 1: Diagnoses made by primary care dentists.

%	Diagnosis (ICD-10 group)
2.1	Disorders of tooth development and eruption (K00-K01)
38.6	Dental caries (K02)
14.8	Other diseases of hard tissues of teeth (K03)
11.4	Diseases of pulp and periapical tissues (K04)
9.6	Gingivitis and periodontal diseases (K05)
0.2	Other disorders of gingiva and edentulous alveolar ridge (K06)
2.4	Dentofacial anomalies [including malocclusion] (K07)
1.0	Other disorders of teeth and supporting structures (K08)
0.3	Other diseases of jaws (K10)
0.1	Diseases of salivary glands (K11)
0.1	Stomatitis and related lesions (K12)
0.1	Other diseases of lip and oral mucosa (K13)
7.9	Fracture of tooth (S02)
0.3	Dislocation of tooth (S03)
10.8	Others *Includes:* *5.7%, dental examination (Z01.2)* *3.3%, a patient with former gastrointestinal disease (Z87.1)* *0.8%, bruxism (F45.8)*

cessation of the intervention, although ICD-10 standardized oral disease diagnostic terms have not obtained a widespread extent [8, 9]. The present result is in line with former studies demonstrating that commitment of the staff is equally or even more important than financial demands when improving the quality of clinical work [10].

To the best of our knowledge, there are no former reports about the diagnoses recorded by primary care dentists. About half of the diagnostic terms entered to electronic patient chart considered dental caries, other diseases of hard tissues of teeth, or diseases of pulp and periapical tissue. The observed diagnostic terms did not accurately reflect the reputed prevalence of oral diseases in the Finnish population. According to epidemiologic surveys, periodontitis is a major common oral disease among adults in Finland and over 60% of Finnish population suffers from it [11]. However, only less than 10% of ICD-10 terms included codes related to gingivitis or periodontitis in the present study. Either communal dentists fail to diagnose these diseases, they do not record these diagnoses despite the fact that they observe their presence, or they do not record them under correct terms. Reason for this discrepancy requires further studies.

There are former studies suggesting that factors related to use of the applied diagnostic terminology itself, use of the electronic patient chart interface, or use of the terminology as part of clinic workflow may modify the frequency to record diagnoses and the quality of these recordings in dental care [12, 13]. There may also be aspects such as cultural traditions (instead of recording diagnoses, dentists are used to record treatments and procedures), extra work required to learn to use novel, possibly changing terminology, financial incentives, and fear of loss of autonomy which may decrease enthusiasm to record diagnoses [9, 14]. There is variance in how diagnostic terms are set up for use in electronic patent chart systems, and if the terms are not easy to be navigated in the category/subcategory, they may end up in the wrong place in the ICD-10 system [14]. This might be a reason why ICD-10 terms are not used in dental practice so frequently. In line with other previous findings, just ICD-10 system has been shown to be prone to misclassification bias in dental practice [15]. Yet, systems using other dental diagnostic terms are not totally protected against this type of bias either [16]. Improving electronic patient charts in accordance with existing systems of dental diagnostic terms could also enhance better recording of diagnosis in primary dental care.

The frequent use of diagnostic terms of oral disease by dentists should provide valuable data for management and for targeting proper treatments given to oral diseases and help primary dental health care to be more effective [17]. Recording diagnosis might promote diagnostic thinking and thereby enhance rational judgement of treatment options which then may lead to better treatment outcomes and increased patient safety [18]. It might also facilitate use of computer-based clinical decision support systems [18]. Habitual recording of a structured dental diagnosis would allow for the aggregation and secondary analyses of clinical data to support downstream analyses for quality improvement and epidemiological assessments and give basis for reasonable incentive systems [16]. It could also support formation of group practices, which is a current trend in dentistry [13]. As already stated in Introduction, frequent recording of diagnosis supports also educational functions in various ways [5].

5. Conclusion

The present data suggest that even a playful competition may be an effective primer in interventions of primary dental care. Commitment to the idea that the recording of diagnoses was beneficial had the effect of improving the recording of diagnoses. However, the quality of obtained diagnoses did not reflect well the prospected distribution of oral diseases in Finnish primary dental care.

Abbreviations

ICD: The International Classification of Diseases.

Acknowledgments

The authors thank Michael Horwood, Ph.D., for reviewing the language of this manuscript.

References

[1] D. Fleming, F. Schellevis, and W. Paget, "Health monitoring in sentinel practice networks: the contribution of primary care," *European Journal of Public Health*, vol. 13, supplement 3, pp. 80–84, 2003.

[2] P. Hjerpe, J. Merlo, H. Ohlsson, K. Bengtsson Boström, and U. Lindblad, "Validity of registration of ICD codes and prescriptions in a research database in Swedish primary care: a cross-sectional study in Skaraborg primary care database," *BMC Medical Informatics and Decision Making*, vol. 10, no. 1, article 23, 2010.

[3] E. B. Dosumu, O. O. Dosumu, and F. B. Lawal, "Quality of records keeping by undergraduate dental students in Ibadan, Nigeria," *Annals of Ibadan Postgraduate Medicine*, vol. 10, no. 1, pp. 13–17, 2012.

[4] T. Lehtovuori, T. Kauppila, J. Kallio, M. Raina, L. Suominen, and A. M. Heikkinen, "Financial team incentives improved recording of diagnoses in primary care: a quasi-experimental longitudinal follow-up study with controls," *BMC Research Notes*, vol. 8, no. 1, article 668, 2015.

[5] E. Kalenderian, R. L. Ramoni, J. M. White et al., "The development of a dental diagnostic terminology," *Journal of Dental Education*, vol. 75, no. 1, pp. 68–76, 2011.

[6] F. Masic, "Information systems in dentistry," *Acta Informatica Medica*, vol. 20, no. 1, pp. 47–55, 2012.

[7] P. Brocklehurst, J. Price, A. M. Glenny et al., "The effect of different methods of remuneration on the behaviour of primary care dentists," *Cochrane Database of Systematic Reviews*, 2013.

[8] J. M. White, E. Kalenderian, P. C. Stark, R. L. Ramoni, R. Vaderhobli, and M. F. Walji, "Evaluating a dental diagnostic terminology in an electronic health record," *Journal of Dental Education*, vol. 75, no. 5, pp. 605–615, 2011.

[9] R. B. Ramoni, J. Etolue, O. Tokede et al., "Adoption of dental innovations: the case of a standardized dental diagnostic terminology," *The Journal of the American Dental Association*, vol. 148, no. 5, pp. 319–327, 2017.

[10] S. Mc Hugh, P. Marsden, C. Brennan et al., "Counting on commitment; the quality of primary care-led diabetes management in a system with minimal incentives," *BMC Health Services Research*, vol. 11, article 348, 2011.

[11] L. Suominen-Taipale, A. Nordblad, M. Vehkalahti, and A. Aromaa, "Oral health in the finnish adult population: health 2000 survey," KTL B 25/2008, Kansanterveyslaitos, Terveyden ja toimintakyvyn osasto, KTL-National Public Health Institute, Health and Functional Capacity, Helsinki, Finland, 2008.

[12] M. F. Walji, E. Kalenderian, D. Tran et al., "Detection and characterization of usability problems in structured data entry interfaces in dentistry," *International Journal of Medical Informatics*, vol. 82, no. 2, pp. 128–138, 2013.

[13] E. Obadan-Udoh, L. Simon, J. Etolue et al., "Dental providers' perspectives on diagnosis-driven dentistry: strategies to enhance adoption of dental diagnostic terminology," *International Journal of Environmental Research and Public Health*, vol. 14, no. 7, article 767, 2017.

[14] O. Tokede, J. White, P. C. Stark et al., "Assessing use of a standardized dental diagnostic terminology in an electronic health record," *Journal of Dental Education*, vol. 77, no. 1, pp. 24–36, 2013.

[15] R. L. F. Figueiredo, S. Singhal, L. Dempster, S. W. Hwang, and C. Quinonez, "The accuracy of International Classification of Diseases coding for dental problems not associated with trauma in a hospital emergency department," *Journal of Public Health Dentistry*, vol. 75, no. 4, pp. 343–347, 2015.

[16] E. Kalenderian, B. Tokede, R. Ramoni et al., "Dental clinical research: an illustration of the value of standardized diagnostic terms," *Journal of Public Health Dentistry*, vol. 76, no. 2, pp. 152–156, 2016.

16

Oral Health Status of Syrian Children in the Refugee Center of Melilla, Spain

Sabrina Gonçalves Riatto,[1,2] Javier Montero,[3] David Ribas Pérez,[2] Antonio Castaño-Séiquer,[2] and Abraham Dib[3]

[1]*Faculty of Dentistry, IESP, Joao Pessoa, PB, Brazil*
[2]*Department of Stomatology, University of Seville, Seville, Spain*
[3]*Department of Surgery, University of Salamanca, Salamanca, Spain*

Correspondence should be addressed to Javier Montero; javimont@usal.es

Academic Editor: Manal Awad

Introduction. Little is known about the state of oral health among immigrants from conflict zones, such as the refugee children from the Syrian Civil War. *Aim.* To determine the oral health status of Syrian immigrant children refugee at the Center for Temporary Stay of Immigrants in Melilla to plan prevention and care programs. *Design.* Using the criteria set by the World Health Organization, an exploration of the oral cavity of all Syrian children aged 5–13 living at that center was conducted in May 2015. All subjects were clinically evaluated by a calibrated and standardized examiner, accompanied by a dentist who registered the clinical variables, and translators. The sociodemographic and clinical variables were analyzed through a descriptive and analytical study, respectively. *Results.* The prevalence of caries in both the permanent and deciduous dentition was 75% and 50% in 6- and 12-year-olds, respectively. The dft was 3.2 ± 2.9 in 6-year-old children. At 12 years old, the DMFT was 1.6 ± 2.6 teeth, the DMFM was 1.1 ± 1.7 teeth, the SiC was 3.2, and the IR was 5%. Eighty-six percent of the examined sextants were periodontally healthy. *Conclusions.* The prevalence of caries was high in the sample population studied, confirming the need for a comprehensive primary oral health care program.

1. Introduction

According to the World Health Organization (WHO), oral disease is one of the most prevalent health care problems [1]. Dental caries are the most frequent form of oral disease and are considered a public health problem affecting both children and adults worldwide and often lead to a significant reduction in the quality of life of individuals and communities [2, 3]. Periodontal disease also significantly contributes to global oral disease, affecting all age groups [4]. The WHO regularly monitors the health status of the main age groups, with the intention of promoting better oral health. Recent studies have shown that immigrant populations are more affected by dental caries than native populations [5–8]. However, very little is known about the state of oral health among immigrants originating from conflict zones.

In 2011, a civil war began in Syria, which has caused one of the largest refugee exoduses of recent history [9]. According to the United Nations High Commissioner for Refugees (UNHCR available at http://data.unhcr.org/syrianrefugees/regional.php), as of May 2016, almost 5 million Syrian refugees have been registered since the beginning of the armed struggle. The vast majority of refugees are located in Turkey, Lebanon, Jordan, Iraq, Egypt, and North Africa, and 53% of them are aged younger than 18 years. Although this number of people is low (10%) compared to the number of refugees originating from other neighboring countries in conflict, the amount of Syrians seeking asylum in Europe is still rising. Nevertheless, according to the abovementioned website, applications for international protection have been registered in 37 European countries: 62% in Serbia and Germany; 27% in Sweden, Hungary, Austria, Netherlands, and Denmark; and 11% in all of the other countries, including Spain, with almost 9000 applications. The Syrian immigrants arrive to Spain by the so-called "southern route" where they hope to find in the Spanish city of

Melilla, located in the north of the African continent, a gateway to Europe.

The extreme situation in which people live along the border between Melilla and the Moroccan city of Nador has resulted in the concentration of approximately 2000 refugees in the Center for Temporary Stay of Immigrants (CETI), which has a maximum capacity of accommodating 480 individuals. Among this population are around 300 children living in overcrowded conditions and exposed to general health risks, as affirmed by the Spanish Government. This community faces economic, cultural, and linguistic barriers that hinder their access to oral health services deployed in the city. To address this problem, proper planning of oral health services is needed to be able to evaluate the current status of oral health and to identify the main type of treatments needed in order to set priorities and plan the different preventive and curative strategies.

This study sought to explore the state of oral health in the population of Syrian immigrant refugee children living at the CETI in Melilla, Spain, which have otherwise not received help to control oral disease.

2. Materials and Methods

In May 2015, refugee Syrian children living at the Center for Temporary Stay of Immigrants (CETI) in Melilla (Spain) were evaluated, following the guidelines recommended by the WHO [10]. Of the 300 children at the CETI, only those aged 5 to 13 years were included within the study.

This work was approved by the Ethics Committee of Andalusia (approval protocol number: 057575944–0905N14) and authorized by the CETI of Melilla, and signed consent was obtained from the individuals responsible for each child participating in the study.

The oral examination of each participant was carried out by a dentist (first author) who had been previously trained in the basic methods and standardized diagnostic criteria outlined by the WHO [10] for the evaluation of different oral conditions. Previous to the start of the study, the examiner was tested using calibration tests of intraexaminer concordance and showed excellent results that supported their suitability to carry out the work. The results obtained were in accordance with test kappa = 0.90, which represents a level of agreement of "almost complete agreement," according to the scale of Landis and Koch [11].

During clinical examinations, the examiner was next to the patient accommodated in a reclining chair. Natural and artificial lighting was supplemented using a portable front focus white light lamp of 100 W (Kopfleuchte Heine SL 350 Optotechnik, Germany). The clinical variables were measured using a basic disposable plane oral mirror and a WHO periodontal probe.

The exploration was attended by a dentist who registered the clinical variables and a bilingual organizer assistant (Arabic and Spanish speaker) who completed the general descriptive information about each child. Arabic translators were present to facilitate communication between the review team with children and/or parents who did not speak Spanish. One of the translators observed while the questionnaire/form was being filled in to ensure that no mistakes were made in recording the information. The average scan time for each child was around 4-5 minutes.

Table 1: Sociodemographic description.

Sociodemographic variables		All ages		5–7 years old		8–10 years old		11–13 years old	
		%	n	%	n	%	n	%	n
		100	156	33	51	42	66	25	39
Gender	Male	57	89	57	29	44	37	59	23
	Female	43	67	43	22	56	29	41	16
Ethnicity	Caucasian	36	56	37	19	35	23	36	14
	Arab	64	100	63	32	65	43	64	25

(Age groups: 5–7, 8–10, 11–13 years old.)

The oral health assessment questionnaire/form was developed based on the model proposed by the WHO [10] in which sociodemographic variables (age, gender, religious beliefs, and ethnicity) and clinical variables (healthy teeth, decayed teeth, missing or filled teeth, healthy sextants, bleeding sextants, or sextants with calculus) were registered.

The following indexes of caries history were calculated: DMFT (mean of decayed, missing, and filled permanent teeth) [12], dft (mean of decayed and filled primary teeth) [13], and DMFM (mean of decayed, missing, and filled first permanent molars); significant caries index (SiC), which reflects the mean of decayed teeth in the third of the population with the highest decayed teeth component in the DMFT [14], and the index of restoration (IR) for the filled teeth.

The global DMFT was calculated by computing the decayed, missing, or filled teeth independent of the type of dentition, since the dentition in this age group (5–13 years) was mostly mixed.

The SiC was calculated using the program developed by the WHO available at http://www.whocollab.od.mah.se/expl/siccalculation.xls.

Periodontal status was registered using the community periodontal index (CPI) recommended by the WHO for children under 15 years [10]. The mean number of sextants with healthy periodontal tissues, bleeding teeth, and teeth with calculus was calculated to describe the periodontal health.

The statistical analysis of the data was carried out using the program SPSS Statistics 20. The statistics carried out on the descriptive data used means, standard deviations (SD), number of subjects (n), and percentages. In addition, comparisons of the quantitative variables between two or more groups were performed using Student's t-test and ANOVA with Bonferroni correction, respectively. The influence of age on the state of the oral health of the children examined was analyzed by the Pearson correlation.

3. Results

According to Table 1, which shows the sociodemographic description, most children were between the ages of 8 and 10 years (42%), followed by one group of 5- to 7-year-olds (33%) and one group of 11- to 13-year-olds (25%). Of the

TABLE 2: Oral health status within the distinct age groups.

Variables	Age groups					
	5–7 yrs (n = 51)	8–10 yrs (n = 66)	11–13 yrs (n = 39)	6 yrs (n = 28)	12 yrs (n = 10)	5–13 yrs (n = 156)
Global caries prevalence (DMFT or dft > 1) (% of subjects)	74.5	74.2	59.0	75.0	50.0	70.5
Caries prevalence in permanent dentition (% of subjects)	7.8	34.8	41.0	7.1	50.0	27.6
Caries prevalence in deciduous dentition (% of subjects)	72.5	60.6	25.6	75.0	0.0	55.8
DMFT (mean ± SD)^{††a,b,c}	0.1 ± 0.4	0.7 ± 1.1	1.8 ± 3.1	0.1 ± 0.5	1.6 ± 2.6	0.8 ± 1.8
Decayed permanent teeth (mean ± SD)^{††a,b,c}	0.1 ± 0.4	0.7 ± 1.0	1.5 ± 2.8	0.1 ± 0.5	1.4 ± 2.5	0.7 ± 1.7
Missing permanent teeth (mean ± SD)	0.0 ± 0.0	0.0 ± 0.1	0.1 ± 0.2	0.0 ± 0.0	0.0 ± 0.0	0.0 ± 0.1
Filled permanent teeth (mean ± SD)$^{†(a/b),c}$	0.0 ± 0.0	0.0 ± 0.0	0.2 ± 0.8	0.0 ± 0.0	0.2 ± 0.6	0.1 ± 0.4
IR (mean ± SD)	0.6 ± 4.7	2.8 ± 13.6	4.2 ± 14.2	0.0 ± 0.0	5.0 ± 15.8	2.5 ± 11.6
DMFM (mean ± SD)$^{††a,(b/c)}$	0.1 ± 0.4	0.6 ± 0.9	0.9 ± 1.4	0.1 ± 0.5	1.1 ± 1.7	0.5 ± 1.0
dft (mean ± SD)^{††a,c}	3.2 ± 3.6	2.2 ± 2.5	0.9 ± 2.2	3.2 ± 2.9	0.0 ± 0.0	2.2 ± 2.9
CPI 0 = healthy sextants (mean ± SD)$^{††a,(b/c)}$	4.0 ± 2.5	5.8 ± 0.6	5.5 ± 1.0	2.8 ± 2.7	5.4 ± 1.4	5.1 ± 1.8
CPI 1 = bleeding sextants (mean ± SD)	0.0 ± 0.0	0.0 ± 0.4	0.1 ± 0.4	0.0 ± 0.0	0.0 ± 0.0	0.1 ± 0.3
CPI 2 = sextants with calculus (mean ± SD)$^{††(a/b,c)}$	0.0 ± 0.0	0.0 ± 0.3	0.4 ± 0.9	0.0 ± 0.0	0.6 ± 1.4	0.1 ± 0.5

DMFT: mean of decayed, missing, and filled permanent teeth; IR: index of restoration for the filled teeth (permanent and deciduous); DMFM: mean of decayed, missing, and filled first permanent molars; dft: mean of decayed and filled primary teeth; CPI: community periodontal index. †Statistically significant intergroup comparisons according to ANOVA test ($p < 0.05$). ††Statistically significant intergroup comparisons according to ANOVA test ($p < 0.01$). a,b,cThe letters beside the symbol "†" indicate the subgroups (a = 5–7 yrs; b = 8–10 yrs; and c = 11–13 yrs) that are statistically different after post hoc Bonferroni correction.

TABLE 3: Influence of ethnicity and gender in the oral health status of Syrian children in the CETI of Melilla (n = 156).

Sociodemographic variables			Oral health variables					
			Healthy teeth	Decayed teeth	Global DMFT	Global IR	Healthy sextants	Bleeding sextants
Ethnicity (mean ± SD)	Caucasian		21.3 ± 3.9*	2.3 ± 2.9*	2.7 ± 3.6	1.8 ± 8.2	5.2 ± 1.6	0.0 ± 0.3
	Arab		20.0 ± 4.3*	3.2 ± 3.3*	3.5 ± 3.6	2.8 ± 13.3	5.1 ± 1.9	0.0 ± 0.3
Gender (mean ± SD)	All the sample	Male	20.5 ± 3.7	2.9 ± 3.0	3.1 ± 3.1	2.2 ± 12.6	5.0 ± 1.9	0.1 ± 0.4
		Female	20.4 ± 4.8	2.8 ± 3.5	3.3 ± 4.1	2.7 ± 10.3	5.4 ± 1.5	0.0 ± 0.0
	5–7 years old	Male	19.2 ± 3.6	2.5 ± 2.9*	2.6 ± 3.0*	0.0 ± 0.0	3.6 ± 2.7	0.0 ± 0.0
		Female	17.9 ± 5.0	4.4 ± 4.4*	4.9 ± 5.1*	1.5 ± 7.1	4.5 ± 2.3	0.0 ± 0.0
	8–10 years old	Male	20.4 ± 2.8	2.9 ± 2.3	3.2 ± 2.5	3.6 ± 17.2	5.8 ± 0.7	0.0 ± 0.5
		Female	20.1 ± 4.1	2.7 ± 3.1	3.2 ± 3.8	1.7 ± 6.8	5.9 ± 0.4	0.0 ± 0.0
	11–13 years old	Male	22.1 ± 4.6*	3.3 ± 3.9*	3.7 ± 4.1*	2.8 ± 11.9	5.4 ± 1.2	0.2 ± 0.5*
		Female	24.5 ± 2.5*	0.9 ± 1.6*	1.3 ± 1.9*	6.3 ± 17.1	5.7 ± 0.7	0.0 ± 0.0

*Significant difference with $p < 0.05$ between both groups after Student's t-test.

total sample, 57% were males and mainly of Arab origin (64%), where 36% were of Caucasians. The sample had a mean age of 9.0 ± 2.2 years.

Table 2 depicts the oral health status of the sample and the comparisons regarding several indexes among the three age groups after the analysis of variance (ANOVA). When the focus was directed towards the estimation of the global caries (in both deciduous and permanent dentition), it was found that prevalence of caries (59%) was lower in the older children (11–13 years) than in the children of the younger age groups (over 74%). However, caries in the permanent dentition increase with age, and the prevalence in the deciduous dentition decreases with aging. Furthermore, it was observed that, in the oldest children, there were fewer active caries (decayed teeth + teeth filled with caries) and therefore a greater number of decay-free teeth (healthy teeth + filled teeth + with crown + fractured). Regarding the indicators indexes of caries history, an increase was observed in the DMFT, DMFM, and IR, according to the age, whereas the dft decreased in the oldest group of children. After analyzing the sextants using the different CPI codes, the majority of the sextants were found to be healthy in all of the age groups studied. A SiC of 3.2 ± 3.0 decayed teeth was obtained for the 12-year-old children. The index of restoration was zero in the majority of the children of every subgroup (≥90%), reflecting that dental caries were mostly untreated.

Table 3 shows the influence of ethnicity and gender in the oral health of Syrian children after comparison with Student's t-test. Significant differences were observed in the number of healthy and decayed teeth, with the best oral health status within the non-Arab group. Additionally, it was established that gender had no significant influence on the oral health status of the whole sample after analyzing the corresponding data. However, when analyzing the various age groups separately, significant differences in the number of decayed teeth, global DMFT, and sextants with bleeding were found. The 5- to 7-year-old girls had higher values than the boys of the same age and, therefore, had a worse state of general oral health. In contrast, the group of 11- to 13-year-old boys had significant worse oral health than the girls.

The analysis of the influence of age on the oral health status by the Pearson linear correlation is displayed in Figure 1. Age was found to be positively correlated with the presence of healthy nonrestored teeth (r: 0.44; $p < 0.01$) and consequently with the number of first molars needing sealants (r: 0.33; $p < 0.01$) but also with the number of filled teeth without caries (r: 0.18; $p < 0.05$). Similarly, age was inversely correlated with the number of decayed teeth needing fillings. In periodontal terms, age was directly related with both the presence of healthy periodontal sextants (r: 0.36; $p < 0.01$), but also with the presence of sextants with calculus (r: 0.31; $p < 0.01$).

These data demonstrate that within this short age range (5–13 years) which comprises the eruption period of the permanent teeth, the older children in the sample population have more healthy standing teeth with optimal health (crown and periodontium). However, paradoxically, an increase in the presence of calculus is also observed around the gingival margin of the targeted teeth for the CPI.

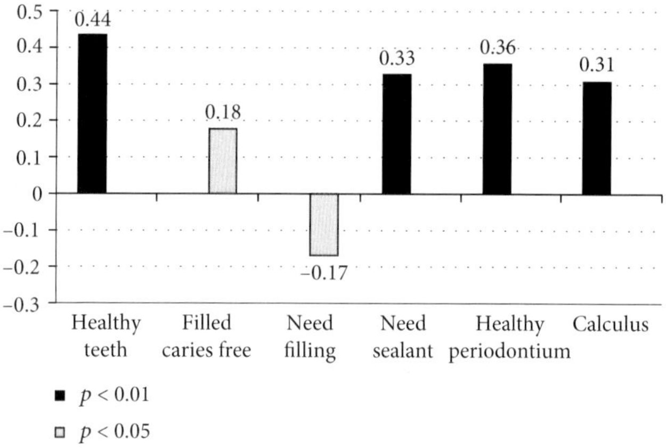

FIGURE 1: Influence of age on the oral health of Syrian children in the CETI of Melilla. Pearson correlation coefficients between age and oral health variables.

4. Discussion

The aim of this study was to register the oral health status of Syrian refugee children living in the CETI in Melilla, Spain, during 2015, using the methodological dossier established by the WHO [10]. All 5- to 13-year-old Syrians were examined and, for logistical reasons, were divided into three age cohorts according to the activities that were taking place within the center. In addition, a microanalysis of the 6- and 12-year-old children was conducted with the intention of comparing the oral health status of this group with other paediatric populations. In order to compare the results, reference studies involving immigrants in Spain [5], North Africans [2, 15–21], Syrians [22–24], and Middle East children [18, 25–27] were used.

It can be expected that the immigrants from war zones have very poor oral health. However, paradoxically, the results obtained were not so negative and may be attributed to the average socioeconomic level of the population studied, where the parents of the children had jobs and incomes, before they were affected by conflict, therefore coming from wealthier families. Also, a low global index of restoration (5.0 ± 15.8% teeth at 12 years old), in accordance with the goals of oral health (IR ≥ 60%) proposed by Spain for children of this age by 2015 [28], was observed. The IR is considered to be an indicator of the level of dental care received by the target population and may be linked to its economic power, as well as the degree of information and access to health services. This fact may be attributed to the young age of the children at the start of the armed struggle, an event which drastically changed the routine of these families, where reparative oral health treatments become a total nonpriority [29]. In any case, immigrant children are expected to climb down the levels of oral health of the host countries [30].

The high prevalence of dental caries in children is linked to the habits and cultural factors of each population [31], which include eating habits (unhealthy or high sugar), poor dental hygiene, lack of dental care services and prevention programs [32], as well as the widespread use of fluorides from different sources [33].

In many Middle Eastern countries, the prevalence and severity of dental caries is one of the main problems of oral health due to the deficiency of prevention programs [34]. In regard to African countries, the incidence of caries is less prevalent or severe than in developed countries. However, this situation is changing, and the incidence of caries is expected to increase as a result of a higher consumption of sugars, the popularity of western food, and also to the difficulties to access dental care [18].

Figure 2 shows a higher prevalence of caries in 5- to 6-year-olds in the Middle Eastern countries than in African countries. Also, other studies involving children of these ages showed that the countries with the highest prevalence of caries were Saudi Arabia [25], Arab Emirates [26], and Jordan [27]; countries with an intermediate prevalence of caries were Syria [24], Tunisia [17], and Niger [16]; and countries with the lowest prevalence of caries were Algeria [15] and Burkina Faso [20, 21].

According to the WHO [10], DMFT values are considered: very low up to 1.1 teeth; low between 1.2 and 2.6 teeth; moderate between 2.7 and 4.4 teeth; high between 4.5 and 6.5 teeth; and very high up to 6.5 teeth. Figure 3 exhibits the results of studies involving 12-year-old children from different countries, where it can be observed that very low DMFT values were found in Burkina Faso [21], Nigeria [19], United Republic of Tanzania [18], Ghana [18], Nigeria 2 [18], Senegal [18], Kenya [18], Eritrea [18], Burkina Faso 2 [20], Zimbabwe [18], Uganda [18], Spain [5], South Africa [18], Qatar [18], and Jordan [18]. Low DMFT values were found in Oman [18], Tunisia [17], Niger [16], Pakistan [18], Ethiopia [18], Iraq [18], Algeria [15], Seychelles [18], Islamic Republic of

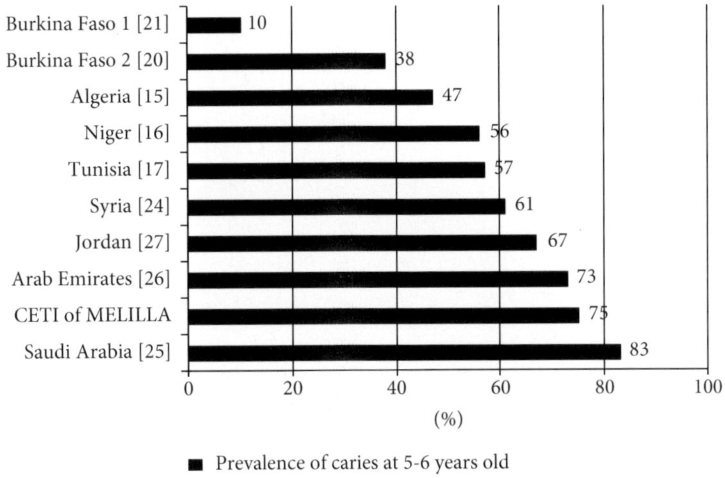

Figure 2: Prevalence of caries in 5- to 6-year-old children in some countries within Africa and in the Middle East, as well as in the CETI of Melilla.

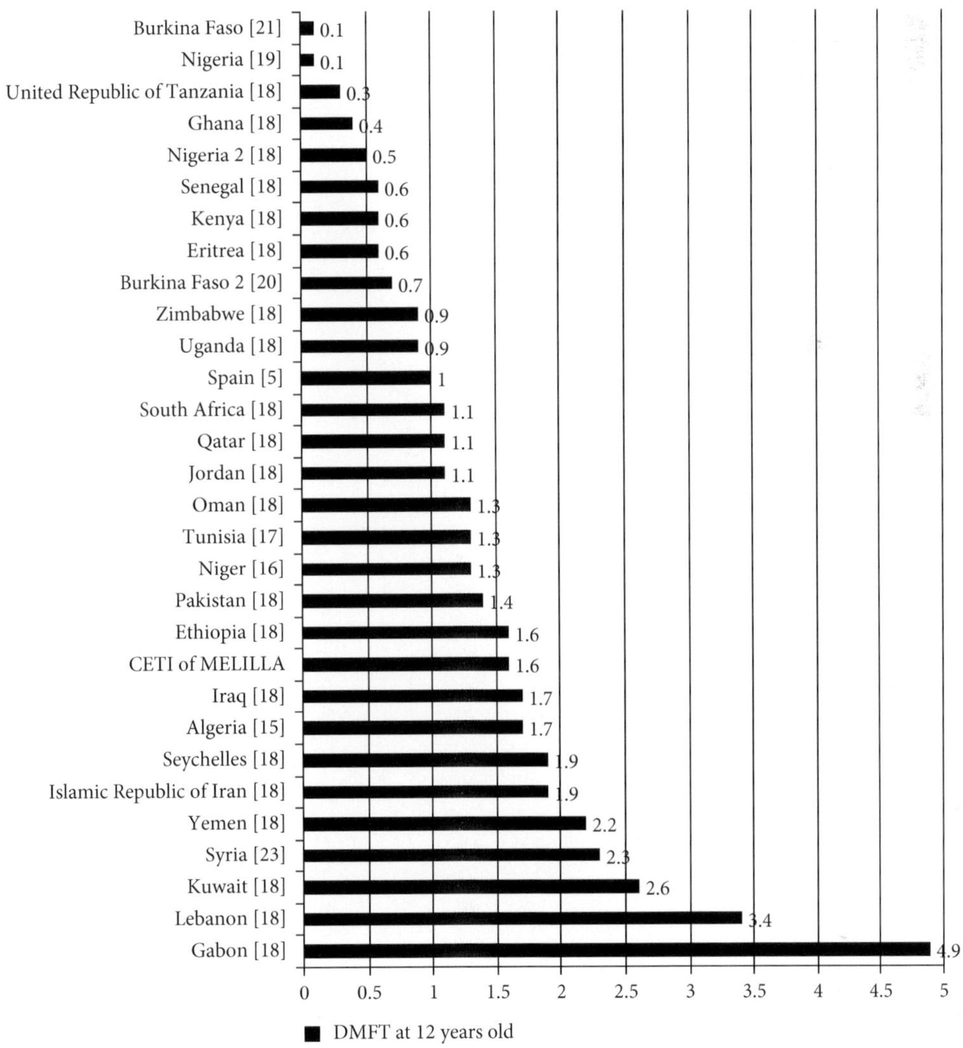

Figure 3: DMFT of 12-year-olds in some countries within the Middle East and Africa, as well as in Spain and in the CETI of Melilla.

Iran [18], Yemen [18], Syria [23], and Kuwait [18]. A moderate DMFT value was found in Lebanon [18], and a high DMFT value was found in Gabon [18].

Also, the result of the low level of dental caries registered by Almerich-Silla et al. [15] in children studied in the southern region of Algeria (Sahara) was attributed to the exposure of the population to high concentrations of fluoride in the drinking water.

The 12-year-old Syrian children studied by Beiruti et al. [23] presented a DMFT of 2.3 teeth, which is higher than the findings of this study for children of the same age (1.6 ± 2.6 teeth). However, we need to be cautious in interpreting this data because our sample only included ten 12-year-olds. Furthermore, we found a greater DMFT in the children living at the CETI in Melilla than in Spain—although lower than in Syria.

Among African populations, conditions of oral hygiene are generally deficient, and the methods used for oral cleaning can be unconventional (such as using sticks or sponges gum, banana stems with carbon powder, plants leaves with ash used with cotton, cloth, or fingers), and lead to plaque formation and consequently calculus formation, even at early ages [35]. Furthermore, in Syria the use of conventional oral hygiene methods was reported, and Dashash et al. [24] also found a strong association between the oral hygiene habits of the parents and the children, where 53% of the children with poor oral hygiene came from families who did not report having good oral hygiene habits. Beiruti et al. [22] reported that 26% of Syrian adolescents have healthy periodontium. Some years later, the same authors in another study reported that 94% of the adolescents examined had an accumulation of dental plaque due to poor oral hygiene [23]. These various studies help to confirm that the population examined in the CETI of Melilla had a better level of periodontal health for all age groups (86% of the sextants were healthy, 12% were not evaluable, and only 3% had bleeding and/or calculus and 8% of the 12-year-old children had bleeding and/or calculus).

The main limitation of this study was that no information regarding the frequency and techniques of oral hygiene, the use of fluoride toothpaste or mouth rinses, or the diet of the Syrian children before entering into the CETI was collected. In any case, each child in the CETI had access to an oral hygiene kit consisting of a toothbrush and toothpaste and was instructed to brush their teeth after each meal and before to continue educational activities aimed at them. Future studies need to be conducted that accurately assess these behavioral factors that are jointly responsible for the inherent risk of oral diseases, considered desirable to know what the oral health circumstances and maintenance before being housed as immigrants.

5. Conclusion

The oral health status of Syrian children refugee in the CETI of Melilla showed a high prevalence of caries, especially, in primary teeth as well as in permanent teeth (affecting 75% in children under 10 years). The index of restoration observed was very low (5%); however, the periodontal health was satisfactory where most of the sextants were healthy (86%).

Disclosure

This work was presented in part in the poster session of the 26th International Association of Paediatric Dentistry Congress held in Chile, October 4–7, 2017 (poster number: P10.36// "Oral health status of Syrian children in the refugee center of Melilla, Spain"; the special issue is available at Poster Sessions, *International Journal of Paediatric Dentistry*, vol. 27, pp. 36–140, 2017, doi: 10.1111/ipd.12332).

References

[1] WHO (World Health Organization), *Global Oral Health Data Bank*, WHO, Geneva, Switzerland, 2000.

[2] D. M. Bourgeois and J. C. Llodra, "Global burden of dental condition among children in nine countries participating in an international oral health promotion programme, 2012-2013," *International Dental Journal*, vol. 64, pp. 27–34, 2014.

[3] A. Sheiham, "Oral health, general health and quality of life," *Bulletin of the World Health Organization*, vol. 83, no. 9, pp. 644-645, 2005.

[4] P. E. Petersen, D. Bourgeois, H. Ogawa, S. Estupinan-day, and C. Ndiaye, "The global burden of oral diseases and risks to oral health," *Bulletin of the World Health Organization*, vol. 83, no. 9, pp. 661–669, 2005.

[5] J. M. Almerich-Silla and J. M. Montiel-Company, "Influence of immigration and other factors on caries in 12- and 15-yr-old children," *European Journal of Oral Sciences*, vol. 115, no. 5, pp. 378–383, 2007.

[6] B. Cvikl, G. Haubenberger-Praml, P. Drabo et al., "Migration background is associated with caries in Viennese school children, even if parents have received a higher education," *BMC Oral Health*, vol. 14, no. 1, pp. 51–56, 2014.

[7] E. Riggs, M. Gussy, L. Gibbs et al., "Assessing the cultural competence of oral health research conducted with migrant children," *Community Dentistry and Oral Epidemiology*, vol. 42, no. 1, pp. 43–52, 2014.

[8] C. C. Chen, S. J. Chiou, C. C. Ting et al., "Immigrant-native differences in caries-related knowledge, attitude, and oral health behaviors: a cross-sectional study in Taiwan," *BMC Oral Health*, vol. 14, no. 1, pp. 3–11, 2014.

[9] R. Bahelah, F. M. Fouad, A. Coutts, M. Wilcox, and W. Maziak, "Syria: health in a country undergoing tragic transition," *International Journal of Public Health*, vol. 60, no. S1, pp. 63–72, 2014.

[10] WHO, *Oral Health Surveys: Basic Methods*, World Health Organization, Geneva, Switzerland, 4th edition, 1997.

[11] J. R. Landis and G. G. Koch, "The measurement of observer agreement for categorical data," *Biometrics*, vol. 33, no. 1, pp. 159–174, 1977.

[12] H. Klein and C. E. Palmer, *Dental Caries in the American Indian Children*, U.S. Government Printing Office, Washington, DC, USA, 1938.

[13] A. O. Gruebbel, "A measurement of dental caries prevalence and treatment service for deciduous teeth," *Journal of Dental Research*, vol. 23, no. 3, pp. 163–168, 1944.

[14] D. Bratthall, "Introducing the Significant Caries Index together with a proposal for a new global oral health goal for 12-year-olds," *International Dental Journal*, vol. 50, no. 6, pp. 378–384, 2000.

[15] J. M. Almerich-Silla, J. M. Montiel-Company, and A. Ruiz-Miravet, "Caries and dental fluorosis in a western Saharan population of refugee children," *European Journal of Oral Sciences*, vol. 116, no. 6, pp. 512–517, 2008.

[16] P. E. Petersen and M. Kaka, "Oral health status of children and adults in the Republic of Niger, Africa," *International Dental Journal*, vol. 49, no. 3, pp. 159–164, 1999.

[17] A. Abid, "Oral health in Tunisia," *International Dental Journal*, vol. 54, no. S6, pp. 389–394, 2004.

[18] A. Abid, F. Maatouk, L. Berrezouga et al., "Prevalence and severity of oral diseases in the Africa and Middle East Region," *Advances in Dental Research*, vol. 27, no. 1, pp. 10–17, 2015.

[19] C. A. Adekoya-Sofowora, W. O. Nasir, A. O. Oginni, and M. Taiwo, "Dental caries in 12 year old suburban Nigerian school children," *African Health Sciences*, vol. 6, no. 3, pp. 145–150, 2006.

[20] B. Varenne, P. E. Petersen, and S. Ouattara, "Oral health status of children and adults in urban and rural areas of Burkina Faso, Africa," *International Dental Journal*, vol. 54, no. 2, pp. 83–89, 2004.

[21] C. Mazza, L. Strohmenger, G. Campus, G. Cagetti, F. Caruso, and P. E. Petersen, "Oral health status of children living in Gorom-Gorom, Oudalan District, Burkina Faso," *International Journal of Dentistry*, vol. 2010, pp. 1–6, 2010.

[22] N. Beiruti, D. Taifour, W. H. van Palenstein-Helderman, and J. E. Frencken, "A review of the oral health status in Syria," *International Dental Journal*, vol. 51, no. 1, pp. 7–10, 2001.

[23] N. Beiruti and W. H. van Palenstein-Helderman, "Oral health in Syria," *International Dental Journal*, vol. 54, no. 1, pp. 383–388, 2004.

[24] M. Dashash and A. Blinkhorn, "The dental health of 5 year-old children living in Damascus, Syria," *Community Dental Health*, vol. 29, no. 3, pp. 209–213, 2012.

[25] T. R. Paul, "Dental health status and caries pattern of preschool children in Al-Kharj, Saudi Arabia," *Saudi Medical Journal*, vol. 24, no. 12, pp. 1347–1351, 2003.

[26] R. Hashim, S. M. Williams, W. M. Thomson, and M. A. Awad, "Caries prevalence and intra-oral pattern among young children in Ajman," *Community Dental Health*, vol. 27, no. 2, pp. 109–113, 2010.

[27] A. Sayegh, E. L. Dini, R. D. Holt, and R. Bedi, "Oral health, sociodemographic factors, dietary and oral hygiene practices in Jordanian children," *Journal of Dentistry*, vol. 33, no. 5, pp. 379–388, 2005.

[28] M. Bravo, F. J. Cortés, E. Casals, C. Llena, J. M. Almerich-Silla, and E. Cuenca, "Basic oral health goals for Spain 2015/2020," *International Dental Journal*, vol. 59, no. 2, pp. 78–82, 2009.

[29] H. Saltaji and H. Alfakir, "Oral health consequences of the crisis in Syria," *British Dental Journal*, vol. 219, no. 2, p. 49, 2015.

[30] UNHCR, *2005 Global Refugee Trends. Statistical Overview of Populations of Refugees, Asylum-Seekers, Internally Displaced Persons, Stateless Persons, and Other Persons of Concern to UNHCR*, pp. 1–10, UNHCR, Geneva, Switzerland, 2006.

[31] P. E. Petersen, "Challenges to improvement of oral health in the 21st century–the approach of the WHO Global Oral Health Programme," *International Dental Journal*, vol. 54, no. S6, pp. 329–343, 2004.

[32] P. E. Petersen, "Sociobehavioural risk factors in dental caries–international perspectives," *Community Dentistry and Oral Epidemiology*, vol. 33, no. 4, pp. 274–279, 2005.

[33] O. Fejerskov, M. J. Larsen, A. Richards, and V. Baelum, "Dental tissue effects of fluoride," *Advances in Dental Research*, vol. 8, no. 1, pp. 15–31, 1994.

[34] T. T. Amin and B. M. Al-Abad, "Oral hygiene practices, dental knowledge, dietary habits and their relation to caries among male primary school children in Al Hassa, Saudi Arabia," *International Journal of Dental Hygiene*, vol. 6, no. 4, pp. 361–370, 2008.

[35] V. Baelum and F. Scheutz, "Periodontal diseases in Europe," *Periodontol 2000*, vol. 29, no. 1, pp. 79–103, 2002.

17

Endodontic and Restorative Treatment Patterns of Pulpally Involved Immature Permanent Posterior Teeth

Ebtissam M. Al-Madi,[1,2] Samar A. Al Saleh,[3] Sundus M. Bukhary,[3] and Maha M. Al-Ghofaily[3]

[1]*Department of Restorative Dentistry, College of Dentistry, King Saud University, P.O. Box 60169, Riyadh 11545, Saudi Arabia*
[2]*Department of Clinical Dental Sciences, College of Dentistry, Princess Nourah bint AbdulRahman University, P.O. Box 84428, Riyadh 11671, Saudi Arabia*
[3]*Department of Prosthetic Dental Sciences, College of Dentistry, King Saud University, P.O. Box 60169, Riyadh 11545, Saudi Arabia*

Correspondence should be addressed to Ebtissam M. Al-Madi; ealmadi@gmail.com

Academic Editor: Carlos A. Munoz-Viveros

Objective. The study aims at investigating the treatment patterns for young permanent posterior teeth with pulp involvement. *Materials and Methods.* A random sample of 1793 dental records of patients aged 6–18 years old who had received dental treatment was investigated. 663 permanent posterior treated teeth had pulp involvement. Demographic and treatment data were gathered from patients' records. *Results.* Prevalence of young permanent teeth with pulp involvement was 36.9%. Treatments received significantly increased as patients' age increased ($P = 0.001$). The first mandibular molar had the most pulp involvement among all teeth (43.89%). Temporary restoration was the most received restoration (59%). The most common pulpal diagnosis, leading to treatment, was irreversible pulpitis (43.04%). Only 19.8% of treated teeth received completed root canal treatment. *Conclusion.* There is a high percentage of children and adolescents with immature permanent posterior teeth with pulp involvement. Similarly, a variety of treatment patterns is present, with a small percentage of completed root canal treatment. *Clinical Relevance.* The study has identified the need to provide guidelines to provide high-quality root canal treatments for young permanent posterior teeth that have pulpal involvement. Only 21.8% of root canal treatments were completed, while 24% of teeth were extracted, and 59% of patients received temporary restorative treatments. This suggests that there might be several factors that might prevent completion of the dental treatment, such as patient preference, insurance coverage, or dentist capability. These factors and guidelines for patient care should be investigated and resolved.

1. Introduction

Dental caries is the most common infectious disease of childhood and adolescence and is rated the highest among dental problems [1, 2]. Caries prevalence has increased in the last three decades in Saudi Arabia [3]. If the cariogenic environment persists in the oral cavity, the newly erupted permanent teeth, specifically the first molar, may get decayed [4]. Young permanent teeth have wide dentinal tubules, a large pulp chamber, and high pulp horns [5], shortening the distance for decay to reach the pulp. If not treated early, infection of the dental pulp will eventually occur [6]. A high prevalence (35.8%) of young permanent teeth with pulp involvement was found in Saudi schoolchildren aged 6–18 years [7].

Treatment of pulpal infection in young permanent teeth in children and adolescence presents a unique challenge to dental clinicians [8]. Although there are many treatment options, evidence-based treatments are limited. Vital pulp techniques are associated with poor clinical outcomes, in the case of symptoms referring to irreversible pulpitis, such as unprovoked pain [9]. In addition, when the infectious process cannot be arrested by treatment methods to preserve vitality, such as protective liner, apexogenesis, indirect pulp treatment, direct pulp cap, and partial pulpotomy [10], then nonvital treatment options should be attempted, such as pulpectomy or

Table 1: Distribution of posterior permanent teeth with pulpal involvement treated teeth according to patients' age.

Age group	Max1PM	Max2PM	Mand1PM	Mand2PM	Max1M	Max2M	Mand1M	Mand2M	Total
6–9	0	0	0	0	5	0	5	0	10
10–12	1	4	0	1	15	2	40	1	64
13–15	13	6	2	3	61	8	99	12	204
16–18	26	27	4	23	97	34	147	27	385
Total	40	37	6	27	178	44	291	40	663
Total (%)	6.0%	5.6%	0.9%	4.1%	26.8%	6.6%	43.9%	6.0%	100%

Max1PM : maxillary first premolar; Max2PM : maxillary second premolar; Mand1PM : mandibular first premolar; Mand2PM : mandibular second premolar; Max1M : maxillary first molar; Max2M : maxillary second molar; Mand1M : mandibular first molar; Mand2M : mandibular second molar.

apexification [11]. Extraction should only be considered if bony support cannot be regained, inadequate tooth structure remains for a restoration, or excessive pathologic root resorption exists [10, 12, 13]. If the tooth is preserved, it is imperative that the overlying intermediate and/or final restoration must be tight-sealed to decrease bacterial leakage from the restoration-dentin interface [14–18]. Root canal systems are morphologically complex, which makes them difficult to clean and fill. Therefore, root canal filling does not always prevent coronal bacterial contamination. This type of restoration poses a dilemma, especially in severely decayed permanent teeth, as the instability of occlusion at an early age presents a changing environment for a permanent restoration [19]. Therefore, in many instances, the decision is deferred, and consequences of delayed treatment increase the likelihood of failure.

This study aims to analyze the current treatment patterns for young permanent teeth with pulpal involvement (deep carious lesions and/or root canal treatment) in patients aged 6–18 years old in multiple centers in Riyadh, Saudi Arabia.

2. Methods and Materials

The Institutional Review Board (IRB) of the College of Dentistry, King Saud University, has deemed this study as exempt from IRB approval, due to the minimum risk to participants. In addition, written consents were embedded in the medical records of both institutes, and these have been approved by the IRB.

A retrospective evaluation of a random sample of 1793 dental records of male and female patients aged 6–18 years old who had received dental treatment at two different institutes (dental college clinics and military hospital) was performed. Dental records that indicated deep carious lesions and/or root canal treatment in young permanent posterior teeth were further analyzed.

Demographic data (patient file number, gender, and date of birth), treatment data (tooth number, pulpal diagnosis, and treatment provided), date of pulp extirpation and complete root canal treatment (if performed), and type of restoration placed were recorded. The periapical radiograph was examined to evaluate presence of any periapical lesions.

Prior to the analysis, data were anonymized and de-identified, and data were analyzed by using the Statistical Package for the Social Sciences (SPSS; Version #16). Frequency distribution was used for the descriptive analysis, and the chi-square test was used for statistical association between the variables. The significance level was set at 0.05.

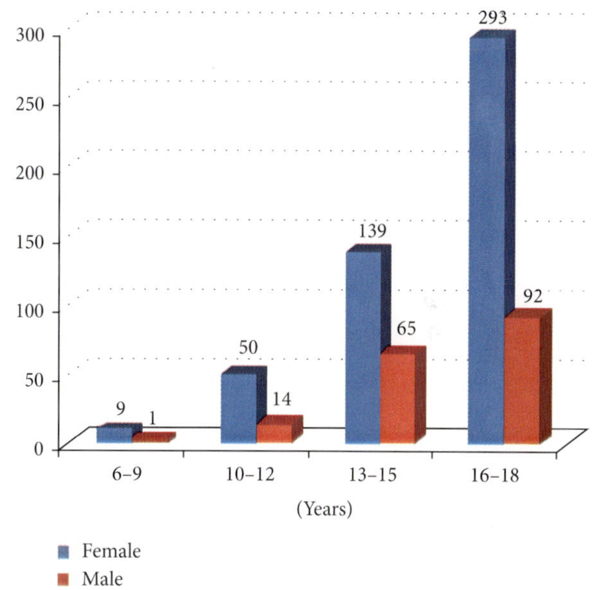

Figure 1: Distribution of young permanent teeth with pulpal involvement according to patients' age and gender.

3. Results

Six hundred sixty-three young permanent posterior teeth with pulpal involvement (deep carious lesions and/or root canal treatment) were identified and analyzed. The prevalence of immature permanent posterior teeth with pulpal involvement was 36.9%.

The number of teeth with pulpal involvement significantly increased as patients' age increased ($P = 0.001$). Significantly more molars had pulpal involvement than premolars ($P < 0.05$). The mandibular first molar was the most affected tooth (43.9%). The distribution of posterior teeth with pulpal involvement with regards to patient age is shown in Table 1. More than twice the number of female patients (73.3%) presented with pulpal involvement than males (26.7%). The distribution of young permanent teeth with pulpal involvement per patient age and gender is shown in Figure 1.

The most common pulpal diagnosis leading to treatment was irreversible pulpitis (43%) followed by pulp necrosis (33.27%) and reversible pulpitis (12.84%), while only 10.85% were diagnosed as vital pulp. The most common treatment was pulp extirpation (35.6%), while the least was apexification (0.2%). All teeth with vital diagnosis and 97% of teeth with reversible pulpitis were treated by vital pulp

Table 2: Distribution of pulpal diagnosis according to treatment rendered.

	Extraction	Pulp extirpation	Vital pulp therapy	Root canal treatment	Apexification	Total
Vital	0	0	60	0	0	60 (10.8%)
Reversible	0	1	69	1	0	71 (12.8%)
Irreversible	4	167	6	61	0	238 (43%)
Necrosis	58	64	1	60	1	184 (33.3%)
Total	62 (11.2%)	232 (42%)	136 (24.6%)	122 (22%)	1 (0%)	553 (100%)

Vital : vital pulp; reversible : reversible pulpitis; irreversible : irreversible pulpitis: necrosis : necrotic.

Table 3: Distribution of treatment according to patients' age.

Age group	Extraction	Pulp extirpation	Vital pulp therapy	Root canal treatment	Apexification	Total (%)
6–9	3	1	5	0	1	10 (1.5%)
10–12	23	18	14	9	0	64 (9.7%)
13–15	36	78	46	44	0	204 (30.8%)
16–18	97	139	71	78	0	385 (58.1%)
Total	159	236	136	131	1	663
Total (%)	24%	35.6%	20.5%	19.8%	0.2%	100%

therapy. On the other hand, within teeth diagnosed with irreversible pulpitis, 70% had pulp extirpation performed, 25.6% had completed root canal treatment, and 0.1% were extracted. Among teeth with necrotic pulps, 34.7% had cleaning and shaping only, 32.6% had completed root canal treatment, while 31.5% were extracted. Distribution of pulpal diagnosis per treatment rendered is displayed in Table 2. All types of rendered treatments increased significantly as patients' age increased ($P = 0.001$). The distribution of the treatment for teeth with pulpal involvement per patient age is shown in Table 3.

Although no radiographs were taken for 41.9% of the cases, in those which radiographs were taken, there was a periapical lesion associated with 32.7% of the teeth.

Overall, most of the teeth with pulpal involvement (59%) received temporary restorations (37.1% IRM and 21.9% Cavit), and only 17% received permanent restorations (9.4% GIC, 4% amalgam, 2.1% crowns, and 1.5% composite), while 24% of the involved teeth were extracted.

4. Discussion

Prevalence of young permanent posterior teeth with pulp involvement was found to be very high (36.9%) in the sample group. This is in agreement with a previous investigation that showed comparable results of 35.8% prevalence [7]. On the contrary, it contrasts with reports from American and European countries, where prevalence is much lower [20–23].

A significantly higher number of females had pulpal involvement in young permanent posterior teeth (74%) compared to males (26%). Tooth eruption occurs earlier in girls than boys; therefore, caries exposure and subsequently pulpal involvement could occur earlier [24]. Females have also been reported to visit the dentist more frequently than males [25]. Females might also be more able to vocalize their complaints about their teeth to their parents [7].

The number of young permanent posterior teeth with pulpal involvement and their treatment significantly increased as age increased. The largest age group with posterior teeth with pulpal involvement was the 16–18-year-old group. This is likely due to the cumulative nature of caries and pulpal involvement [26]. The most treatment provided was pulp extirpation (35.6%), followed by extraction (24%), despite the negative consequences to extraction. Although extraction might be a viable solution for teeth with irreversible pulpitis or necrosis in younger children, this is not a suitable solution for older adolescents [27]. Optimal treatment would involve complete endodontic therapy, followed by core buildup and a cusp protecting indirect restoration [28]. In this instance, only 1.5% of the involved cases in 6–9-year-olds were extracted, while an alarming 58.1% of the involved cases were extracted in the 16–18-year-old group. This warrants a review of the knowledge of guidelines for pediatric dental therapy among dentists in the area, as well as awareness among patients.

There were significantly more molars involved than premolars. The first mandibular molar was more prevalent within all age groups. The first molar has been quoted as the most caries-prone tooth in permanent dentition, probably due to its early exposure to the oral environment and its morphological features being pitted and fissured, inducing plaque and caries formation [29]. The most restoration used was temporary restoration, regardless of treatment rendered (59%). Most likely, as most treatment consisted of incomplete root canal therapy, the restoration of choice would be a temporary one. Another explanation would be that many clinicians would be unable to decide on a final treatment plan for the patient, as the final prognosis and outcome was unclear to them. It is difficult to attempt to perform final and permanent restorations in a young age group, since the lack of occlusal stability might provide a restorative dilemma. On the other hand, glass ionomer cements (GIC) with or without an IRM base have been suggested as a favorable long-term seal. IRM and GIC over a Cavit base over a one-month period have been suggested to provide a significantly superior seal against penetration of *S. mutans* when compared to Cavit alone [30].

Although most cases of irreversible pulpitis and necrosis (76.3%) had root canal treatment initiated, only a small number (21.8%) of these were completed. This could be explained by lack of ability of clinicians to commit to the completion of RCT, as the restorative choices are unclear.

Teeth with vital pulps or reversible pulpitis were treated by vital pulp therapy, while teeth with irreversible pulpitis were treated by pulp extirpation in most cases. Only a quarter of cases had a full root canal treatment completed. Within the group of teeth with necrotic pulps, an equal distribution of initiated RCT, complete RCT, and extractions were performed. Further investigations into the reasons behind the differences in treatment of cases of necrosis versus irreversible pulpitis need to be investigated.

Although many of the teeth proved to have periapical involvement, many had no documentation of X-rays to prove periapical involvement. There might be more periapical involvement in these teeth. This would warrant further treatment to eliminate disease progress by RCT completion and adequate restoration [31].

Overall, within the limitations of this study, results show a disturbingly high percentage of children and adolescence with pulpal involvement of young permanent teeth. Most of these teeth have partial pulpal treatment, with temporary restorations. Further investigations into clinicians' opinions regarding treatment options are currently being investigated to recognize the reasons behind this large variation in treatment patterns. Further prognostic studies are needed to establish the clear guidelines to the most advantageous restorative treatment options after endodontic therapy for this population.

5. Conclusion

Prevalence of young permanent posterior teeth with pulp involvement was found to be very high (36.9%) in Saudi Arabia. More females had young permanent posterior teeth with pulpal involvement (74%) compared to males (26%). The largest age group with immature permanent posterior teeth with pulp involvement was the 16–18-year-old group. The first mandibular molar was the most commonly affected tooth. The most treatment provided was pulp extirpation (35.6%), followed by extraction (24%). The most common restoration used was temporary restoration (59%), and although cases of irreversible pulpitis and necrosis (76.3%) had root canal treatment initiated, only a small number (21.8%) of these were completed. Further investigations and prognostic studies are needed to evaluate the reasons and prognosis of these treatment patterns.

References

[1] R. A. Bagramian, F. Garcia-Godoy, and A. R. Volpe, "The global increase in dental caries–A pending public health crisis," *American Journal of Dentistry*, vol. 22, no. 1, pp. 3–8, 2009.

[2] M. Mortazavi, M. Mesbahi, M. R. Azar, and G. Ansari, "MTA pulpotomy in primary molars–A prospective study," *Research Journal of Biological Sciences*, vol. 4, pp. 599–603, 2009.

[3] D. E. AlAgili, "A systematic review of population-based dental caries studies among children in Saudi Arabia," *Saudi Dental Journal*, vol. 25, no. 1, pp. 3–11, 2013.

[4] P. Carrotte, "Endodontic treatment for children," *British Dental Journal*, vol. 198, no. 1, pp. 9–15, 2005.

[5] D. H. Pashley, R. E. Walton, and H. C. Slavkin, *Histology and Physiology of the Dental Pulp. Endodontics*, BC Decker Inc., Hamilton, ON, Canada, 5th edition, 2002.

[6] F. E. Martin, "Carious pulpitis: microbiological and histopathological considerations," *Australian Endodontic Journal*, vol. 29, no. 3, pp. 134–137, 2003.

[7] E. M. Al-Madi, "Prevalence of pulpally involved permanent teeth in Saudi schoolchildren," *International Dental Journal*, vol. 54, no. 4, pp. 206–210, 2004.

[8] J. Ingle, *Pediatric Endodontics*, BC Decker, Hamilton, New Zealand, 5th edition, 2005.

[9] R. Gruythuysen, G. van Strijp, and M. K. Wu, "Long-term survival of indirect pulp treatment performed in primary and permanent teeth with clinically diagnosed deep carious lesions," *Journal of Endodontics*, vol. 36, no. 9, pp. 1490–1493, 2010.

[10] American Academy of Pediatric Dentistry–Clinical Practice Guidelines, *Guidelines of Pulp therapy for Primary and Immature Permanent Teeth*, Council on Clinical Affairs, Chicago, IL, USA, 2014.

[11] American Association Endodontists, *American Association of Endodontists Glossary of Endodontic Terms*, American Association Endodontists, Chicago, IL, USA, 7th edition, 2003.

[12] A. B. Fuks, "Pulp therapy for the primary dentition," in *Pediatric Dentistry: Infancy through Adolescence*, J. R. Pinkham, P. S. Casamassimo, H. W. Fields Jr., D. J. McTigue, and A. Nowak, Eds., pp. 331–351, Elsevier Saunders Co., St. Louis, MO, USA, 5th edition, 2013.

[13] P. J. Waterhouse, J. Whitworth, J. Camp, and A. Fuks, "Pediatric endodontics: endodontic treatment for the primary and young permanent dentition," in *Pathways of the Pulp*, pp. 808–857, Mosby Elsevier, St Louis, MO, USA, 10th edition, 2011.

[14] P. Aguilar and P. Linsuwanont, "Vital pulp therapy in vital permanent teeth with cariously exposed pulp: a systematic review," *Journal of Endodontics*, vol. 37, no. 5, pp. 581–587, 2011.

[15] G. Bergenholtz and L. Spångberg, "Controversies in endodontics," *Critical Reviews in Oral Biology and Medicine*, vol. 15, no. 2, pp. 99–114, 2004.

[16] N. Cohenca, A. Paranjpe, and J. Berg, "Vital pulp therapy," *Dental Clinics of North America*, vol. 57, no. 1, pp. 59–73, 2013.

[17] J. Ward, "Vital pulp therapy in cariously exposed permanent teeth and its limitations," *Australian Endodontic Journal*, vol. 28, no. 1, pp. 29–37, 2002.

[18] P. E. Murray, A. A. Hafez, A. J. Smith, and C. F. Cox, "Bacterial microleakage and pulp inflammation associated with various restorative materials," *Dental Materials*, vol. 18, no. 6, pp. 470–478, 2002.

[19] J. Penchas, B. Peretz, and A. Becker, "The dilemma of treating severely decayed first permanent molars in children: to restore or to extract," *ASDC Journal of Dentistry for Children*, vol. 61, no. 3, p. 199, 1994.

[20] M. Buckley and L. S. Spangberg, "The prevalence and technical quality of endodontic treatment in an American subpopulation," *Oral Surgery, Oral Medicine, Oral Pathology, Oral Radiology, and Endodontology*, vol. 79, no. 1, pp. 92–100, 1995.

[21] L. L. Kirkevang, D. Ørstavik, P. Hörsted-Bindslev, and A. Wenzel, "Periapical status and quality of root fillings and coronal restorations in a Danish population," *International Endodontic Journal*, vol. 33, no. 6, pp. 509–515, 2000.

[22] Y. Boucher, L. Matossian, F. Rilliard, and P. Machtou, "Radiographic evaluation of the prevalence and technical quality of root canal treatment in a French subpopulation," *International Endodontic Journal*, vol. 35, no. 3, pp. 229–238, 2002.
[23] A. Hugoson, G. Koch, A. N. Helkimo, and S. Å. Lundin, "Caries prevalence and distribution in individuals aged 3–20 years in Jönköping, Sweden, over a 30-year period 1973–2003," *International Journal of Paediatric Dentistry*, vol. 1, no. 18, pp. 18–26, 2008.
[24] J. R. Lukacs and L. L. Largaespada, "Explaining sex differences in dental caries prevalence: saliva, hormones, and "life-history" etiologies," *American Journal of Human Biology*, vol. 18, no. 4, pp. 540–555, 2006.
[25] G. Horst and C. A. De Wit, "Review of behavioural research in dentistry 1987-1992: dental anxiety, dentist-patient relationship, compliance and dental attendance," *International Dental Journal*, vol. 43, no. 3, p. 265, 1993.
[26] A. Thysltrup and O. Fejerskov, *Textbook of Cariology*, Munksgaard, Copenhagen, Denmark, 1986.
[27] P. J. Sandler, R. Atkinson, and A. M. Murray, "For four sixes," *American Journal of Orthodontics and Dentofacial Orthopedics*, vol. 117, no. 4, pp. 418–435, 2000.
[28] T. A. DeRosa, "A retrospective evaluation of pulpotomy as an alternative to extraction," *General Dentistry*, vol. 54, no. 1, pp. 37–40, 2006.
[29] S. J. Nelson, *Wheeler's Dental Anatomy, Physiology and Occlusion*, Elsevier Health Sciences, Berlin, Germany, 2014.
[30] H. J. Naoum and N. P. Chandler, "Temporization for endodontics," *International Endodontic Journal*, vol. 35, no. 12, pp. 964–978, 2002.
[31] K. Ridell, A. Petersson, L. Matsson, and I. Mejàre, "Periapical status and technical quality of root-filled teeth in Swedish adolescents and young adults. A retrospective study," *Acta Odontologica Scandinavica*, vol. 64, no. 2, pp. 104–110, 2006.

18

TheraCal LC: From Biochemical and Bioactive Properties to Clinical Applications

Naji Ziad Arandi[1] **and Tarek Rabi**[2]

[1]Department of Conservative Dentistry and Prosthodontics, Faculty of Dentistry, Arab American University, Jenin, State of Palestine
[2]Department of Conservative Dentistry, Al-Quds University, Jerusalem, State of Palestine

Correspondence should be addressed to Naji Ziad Arandi; naji.arandi@aauj.edu

Academic Editor: Louis M. Lin

Background. Direct pulp capping is a popular treatment modality among dentists. TheraCal LC is a calcium silicate-based material that is designed as a direct/indirect pulp capping material. The material might be very attractive for clinicians because of its ease of handling. Unlike other calcium silicate-based materials, TheraCal LC is resin-based and does not require any conditioning of the dentine surface. The material can be bonded with different types of adhesives directly after application. There has been considerable research performed on this material since its launching; however, there are no review articles that collates information and data obtained from these studies. This review discusses the various characteristics of the material with the aim of establishing a better understanding for its clinical use. *Methods.* A search was conducted using search engines (PubMed and Cochrane databases) in addition to reference mining of the articles that was used to locate other papers. The process of searching for the relevant studies was performed using the keywords pulp protection, pulp capping, TheraCal, and calcium silicates. Only articles in English published in peer-reviewed journals were included in the review. *Conclusion.* This review underlines the fact that further *in vitro* and *in vivo* studies are required before TheraCal LC can be used as a direct pulp capping material.

1. Introduction

The primary objective of restorative dentistry is to preserve pulpal health of vital teeth. Currently, there is no single pulp protection protocol for clinicians to follow [1, 2]. A direct pulp cap is a procedure in which the exposed vital pulp is treated with a therapeutic material, followed by a base and restoration, to promote healing, to maintain pulp vitality, and to protect the pulp from thermal, chemical, and noxious stimuli [1]. Calcium hydroxide has traditionally been used as the pulp capping material of choice for pulpal exposures in permanent teeth [3]. The effect of calcium hydroxide is the result of the chemical injury caused by the hydroxyl ions released during the hydration reaction into the surrounding environment [2]. Calcium hydroxide stimulates the pulp to defend and repair to form a reparative dentin bridge. It has been reported that 89% of 192 dentin bridges formed by calcium hydroxide cement in monkeys contained tunnel defects that might fail to provide a permanent barrier and a long-term biological seal against bacterial infection [4]. However, the major disadvantage of calcium hydroxide is its high solubility which leads to the disappearance of the material and the formation of defects in reparative dentin underneath the capping material, thereby failing to provide a permanent seal against bacterial invasion [5].

Calcium silicate-based materials are bioactive materials capable of forming apatite by using calcium silicates or calcium aluminates. These materials are also biointeractive [6]; they release ions needed to stimulate dentin bridging. Mineral trioxide aggregate (MTA) is a calcium silicate-based material that is used in direct and indirect pulp capping in primary and permanent teeth. MTA has been reported superior to calcium hydroxide for pulp capping of mechanically exposed human teeth [7–9]. However, MTA exhibits many drawbacks as a capping material such as difficult handling, long setting time, induction of tooth discoloration, and incompatibility with other dental materials when layered [10].

New calcium silicate materials have appeared recently, and among them, Biodentine (Septodont, Saint Maur-des-Fosses, France) is a modified MTA-like material that was introduced to overcome the drawbacks presented by MTA as a pulp capping material. Biodentine is a calcium silicate-based dentin substitute presented as a powder in a capsule composed of tricalcium silicate cement, zirconium oxide, and calcium carbonate. The liquid in the ampule is composed of water, calcium chloride, and a water-based polymer [11]. Biodentine can be applied directly into the prepared cavity as a bioactive bulk dentin substitute that induces dentin bridge formation. Biodentine has been reported to form a mineral-rich interfacial layer and a tag-like structure extending from the interfacial layer to the dentinal tubules that anchors the material micromechanically to the underlying dentine [12]. It has good mechanical properties as well as excellent biocompatibility and bioactive behavior. In addition, it sets in approximately 12 minutes and does not cause tooth discoloration [11]. Brizuela et al. [13] conducted a randomized clinical trial to investigate the outcome of direct pulp capping of permanent young teeth with Biodentine and compare the results with MTA (ProRoot MTA, Dentsply, Maillefer) and calcium hydroxide. The study showed that Biodentine had no failures after 12 months while each of calcium hydroxide and MTA had a 13.6% failure rate after the same time period. However, the study reported that there were no statistically significant differences among the materials studied at different time intervals, that is, 3, 6, and 12 months. Similar results were reported in a split-mouth study by Katge and Patil [14]. The study reported 100% success rate at 6 and 12 months with both MTA and Biodentine when used as direct pulp capping agent in first permanent molars in 7- to 9-year-old children. Nowicka et al. [15] also reported similar clinical results for both MTA and Biodentine in premolars extracted for orthodontic reasons after 6 weeks of follow-up. However, the main drawback with using Biodentine is its water-based chemistry and thus poor bonding as the bond is mainly micromechanical to the overlying resin restoration. To overcome this limitation, a light-curable resin-modified tricalcium silicate (TheraCal LC) was introduced as a pulp capping material.

TheraCal LC is a single paste calcium silicate-based material promoted by the manufacturer for use as a pulp capping agent and as a protective liner for use with restorative materials, cement, or other base materials. This material has been classified as a 4th generation calcium silicate material [16]. According to ISO 9917-2017 part 2 clause 4.1, TheraCal LC is a class 2 cement material "in which the setting reaction of the polymerizable component is light-activated."

2. Search Methodology

An electronic search was conducted in the PubMed and Cochrane databases with appropriate MeSH headings and keywords related to the physical, chemical, sealing ability, biocompatibility, antibacterial properties, clinical applications, drawbacks, and mechanism of action of TheraCal LC. Combinations of the following keywords were used for the identification of the studies to be considered in this review: "TheraCal LC," "pulp capping," "vital pulp therapy," "calcium silicate cements," "pulp protection," and "bioactive liners." To enrich the results, a hand-search was conducted of the last 2 years' worth of issues of the following major endodontic and dental material journals: *International Endodontic Journal; Journal of Endodontics; Dental Materials;* Reference mining of the articles that were identified was used to locate other papers. The process of cross-referencing continued until no new articles were identified. Only articles in English published in peer-reviewed journals were included in the review.

3. Review

TheraCal LC is a hybrid material [16]. The original patent sheet stated that TheraCal LC consists of Portland type III cement (45%), fumed silica as a thickening agent (7%), resin (43%), bismuth oxide (3%), and barium sulfate (3%) as radiopaquers [17]. The safety data sheet provided from the manufacturer (dated August 2011) shows that TheraCal LC is mainly composed of Portland cement type III (20–60%), poly(ethylene glycol) dimethacrylate (10–50%), bis-GMA (5–20%), and barium zirconate (1–10%) [18]. However, safety data sheets dated March 2012 show that the material is HEMA-free and composed of Portland cement (30–50%), polyethelyene glycol dimethacrylate (10–30%), and barium zirconate (1–10%) [19]. This was confirmed by the study of Nilsen and Einar [18] which reported that Bis-GMA was not detected in the UPLC-MS analysis of TheraCal LC, despite being listed in the safety data sheet provided by the supplier (dated 2011).

TheraCal LC is claimed to be a hydraulic silicate material that sets by hydration. Hydration is the chemical reaction that leads to the setting of a hydrophilic cement. The setting starts with the contact of the material and water. TheraCal LC does not include water for material hydration. It depends on the water taken up from the environment and its diffusion within the material. Hence, the manufacturer instructions implement placing the material on moist dentin. A study by Camilleri et al. [20] reported that TheraCal LC hydration is incomplete because of the limitation of moisture diffusion from the pulp-dentine complex into the set TheraCal LC.

TheraCal LC has displayed calcium release properties [6, 20–23]. The bioavailability of calcium ions plays a key role in the material-induced proliferation and differentiation of human dental pulp cells and the new formation of mineralized hard tissues. The amount of calcium ions released from TheraCal LC was in the concentration range with potential stimulatory activity for dental pulp and odontoblasts [22, 24]. In a study by Gandolfi et al. [22], TheraCal LC was found to release significantly more calcium than Dycal throughout the tested period (28 days). However, the amount of leached calcium decreased with the time for all the materials (28 days). Another study by Gandolfi et al. stated that the calcium release of ProRoot MTA and TheraCal LC was not marked but constant (no statistically significant changes over time) [21]. This is in contrast to a study by Camilleri et al. which investigated the hydration of TheraCal LC and compared it with Biodentine. The study reported that both materials leached calcium ions in solution. However, TheraCal LC displayed lower calcium ion release and a slower reaction rate than Biodentine [6]. Similarly, the calcium-releasing ability of TheraCal LC was reported to be significantly less than Biodentine [20]. Camilleri et al. [6] attributed the differences in the results due to the different methodologies used in each study. Moreover, Yamamoto et al. [23] and that ProRoot MTA released significantly greater amounts of calcium ions than the TheraCal LC. The study also showed that TheraCal LC does not form calcium hydroxide after setting, although it releases calcium ions and produces calcium apatite on its surface. The absence of calcium hydroxide in set TheraCal LC suggests that calcium ions leached from this material are not in the hydroxide form [6].

On the other hand, the release of hydroxyl ions raises the pH of the surrounding environment and causes irritation of the pulp tissue. This develops superficial necrosis on exposed pulp, provoking mineralization directly against the necrotic zone [25]. An alkaline pH also creates a hostile environment for bacterial survival and proliferation. TheraCal LC has provided a very alkaline (10.66) pH after 3 hours and displayed a nonsignificant reduction in pH (9.85) after 24 hours [25]. Gandolfi et al. [21] reported that TheraCal LC induced lower pH alkalization than the conventional self-setting Dycal did. However, the moderate alkalizing activity of TheraCal LC was constant (9.53 after 3 hours and 8.12 at 28 days) while Dycal maintained the pH 9.81 at 28 days. Yamamoto et al. [23] reported a pH of 9.30 at 5 hours which gradually decreased to 8.4 at 6 hours and 8 at 25 and 144 hours which was significantly lower the pH values recorded for ProRoot MTA at all time periods.

TheraCal LC secures a protective physical lining despite contact with dentinal or pulpal fluids. Its solubility is lower than that of Dycal, ProRoot MTA, Angelus MTA, and Biodentine [21, 22], and its water sorption and porosity is similar to ProRoot MTA and Biodentine, and lower than Angelus MTA [21]. Hence, TheraCal LC may act as a scaffold for reparative dentine formation. Dentinal fluids are absorbed within it, resulting in the release of calcium and hydroxide ions, and the tooth responds to form apatite and a bond, supporting the natural sealing ability of the apatite, plays a crucial role in pulpal protection. TheraCal LC is reported to have an apatite-forming ability [23]. The resultant "apatite coating" plays a key role is dentine repair and mineralization [23]. Its ability to induce the formation of hydroxyapatite-like crystals could contribute to the chemical bond to dentine and provides a biological seal [20, 21]. The sealing ability of MTA, Biodentine, and TheraCal LC was investigated using a confocal laser scanning microscope. The study reported no significant difference in the interfacial microleakage between MTA and Biodentine. However, TheraCal LC exhibited better sealing ability and less interfacial microleakage than the other tested materials [26].

Hydraulic calcium silicate cements are also materials of interest to serve as remineralization agents [27]. TheraCal LC has been developed for indirect (and direct) pulp capping as well. Li et al. [27] compared the remineralization potential of TheraCal LC, Biodentine, and ProRoot MTA. They reported that the hydraulic calcium silicate cements (Biodentine and ProRoot MTA) clearly induced remineralization of artificially demineralized dentine at a higher speed and intensity than the resin-based and resin-free hydraulic calcium silicate cement was attributed to the difference in Ca-ion release kinetics displayed by each material [6, 20, 27]. However, the study reported that the remineralization induced by all the investigated hydraulic calcium silicate cements was incomplete in terms of relative remineralization depth and intensity.

TheraCal LC is a light-cured resin-based material that facilitates the placement of the final restoration as no delay is necessary as shown for water-based pulp capping materials such as Biodentine. The bond strength between restorative and pulp capping materials is important for the success of restorations. TheraCal LC, which is a resin-based material, facilitates layering with composite resin. The effectiveness of layering TheraCal LC with resin composite (Evetric, Ivoclar) bonded with either total-etch adhesives (ExciTe F) or self-etch adhesives (AdheSe One F), and glass ionomer (Fuji IX) was investigated by Meraji and Camilleri [28]. They found that the bond strength between TheraCal LC and composite using the total-etch technique displayed better bond strength values when compared with the self-etch primer. TheraCal LC had higher bond strength values than Biodentine when layered with either composite or glass ionomer cement [28]. However, the study concluded that glass ionomer cements are not indicated for the restoration of teeth in which TheraCal LC is used as a dentine replacement material. Karadas et al. [29] investigated the bond strength of different adhesive agents to TheraCal LC. They reported that etch and rinse adhesives provided the overlying composite restoration with better shear bond strength when compared with self-etch adhesives [29]. The study also showed that two-step self-etch adhesives had higher bond strength values when compared with one-step self-etch adhesives with the exception of the one-step Clearfil S^3 bond which was attributed to the fact that it contains 10-metacryloxydecyl dihydrogen phosphate (MDP), which has been reported to chemically bond to calcium within the tooth [29, 30]. No correlation was found between the pH of the self-etch adhesives and their bond strength to TheraCal LC [29]. Deepa et al. [31] compared and evaluated the bonding ability of resin composite to three different liners: TheraCal LC, Biodentine, and Fuji II LC using a universal silane-containing adhesive (Single Bond Universal). They found that the bond strength of composite resin to TheraCal LC and Fuji II LC was similar and significantly higher than that of Biodentine following the application of universal adhesive. The bond strength of TheraCal to methacrylate-based composite was significantly higher than that with silorane-based composites and GI cement [32].

TheraCal LC has been referred to as a light-curable MTA-cement [22]. This description has caused some confusion in the literature since there is no light-initiated setting of the Portland cement. The setting reaction depends upon polymerization of the resin component, thus excluding this material from the classification of hygroscopic dental cements that encompasses MTA as well as cements based on bioceramics, calcium silicate, or calcium sulfate [33]. The polymerization of TheraCal LC is associated with low heat generation, and this could reduce adverse pulpal effects when used in pulp capping procedures [34]. TheraCal LC is opaque and "whitish" in color. It should be kept in thin layers so as not to show through composite materials that are very translucent affecting final restoration shade. The manufacturer recommends placing it in 1 mm layers and curing it for 20 seconds. However, Gandolfi et al. [21], reported that the material can be placed in 1.7 mm layers after irradiation for 20 seconds. Nilsen et al. [18] found that TheraCal LC leeched the most camphorquinone of all the investigated materials (Calcimol LC and Ultra-Blend plus), and it was also the only material to leech a co-initiator (DMABEE) which may suggest that the composition of TheraCal LC is not properly suited for light curing.

A pulp capping material should be able to exert antimicrobial activity. Calcium silicate-based materials have better antibacterial activity than calcium hydroxide-based materials [35, 36]. Poggio et al. studied the antimicrobial activity of different pulp capping materials using agar diffusion tests. They found that TheraCal LC had a significantly lower effect on *S. salivarius* and *S. sanguis* when compared with a calcium hydroxide liner (Dycal). However TheraCal LC had similar activity to Dycal when tested against *S. mutans* [35]. The study also demonstrated that the antimicrobial activity of TheraCal LC was similar to the light-cured calcium hydroxide liner Calcimol LC (Voco). Arias-Moliz et al. [36] investigated the antimicrobial activity of leachates from TheraCal LC by means of the minimal inhibitory concentration against *S. mutans*, *S. sobrinus*, and *S. gordonii*. The study reported the absence of antimicrobial activity of the eluents and suggested that the antimicrobial activity might be influenced by the pH.

The cytotoxicity and biocompatibility of a pulp capping material is of particular importance in order to avoid pulp irritation and maintain pulp vitality. Lee et al. [37] conducted a study to evaluate and compare pulpal responses to ProRoot MTA (Dentsply Tulsa Dental, Tulsa, OK), Retro-MTA (Meta Biomed Co., Ltd., Seoul, Korea), and TheraCal (BiscoInc, Schamburg, IL) in dog partial pulpotomy cases, whereas a complete dentinal bridge was formed only in 33% of the teeth. They found that TheraCal LC produced the least favorable pulpal responses among the materials used in the study. TheraCal induced an extensive pulp inflammatory reaction in 75% of the lower biocompatibility of the material, which caused a higher degree of inflammation. The study attributed this to the acrylic monomer Bis-GMA present in the material. Poggio et al. [38] studied the cytocompatibility of pulp capping *in vitro* using the Transwell method and reported that TheraCal LC showed very low cytocompatibility. Hebling et al. [39] evaluated the cytotoxic effects of resin-based light-cured liners (TheraCal LC, Vitrabond, Ultra-Blend plus) on pulp cells and reported that all the resin-based liners tested were toxic to the cultured odontoblast-like cells. However, among the tested materials, the light-cured resin-based MTA cement presented the lowest cytopathic effects. Jeanneau et al. [40] studied the consequences of adding resins to tricalcium silicates by investigating TheraCal LC and Biodentine interactions with the dental pulp. Their work showed that TheraCal is toxic to pulp fibroblasts and has a higher inflammatory effect and a lower bioactive potential than Biodentine. Jeanneau and her colleagues stated that upon their preclinical results, TheraCal cannot be recommended for direct pulp capping. Bakhtiar et al. [41] compared the use of TheraCal LC, ProRoot MTA, and Biodentine for partial pulpotomy of sound human third molars. Biodentine performed better than TheraCal LC when used as partial pulpotomy agent and presented the best clinical outcomes. TheraCal LC treatment resulted in pulp disorganization in 66.7% ($n = 9$) of the cases beneath the material and in the entire pulp in 22.2% of the cases. Discontinued dentinal bridge was noted in most cases treated with TheraCal. Bakhtiar et al. [41] stated that they do not support the use of TheraCal LC in partial pulpotomy and considered Biodentine and ProRoot MTA more reliable for long-term protection of dental pulp.

In the previous studies [37, 38, 40, 41], the cytotoxicity of TheraCal LC was attributed to its resin components which may remain unpolymerized after contact with pulp tissue. The studies owed the low biocompatibility to the presence of monomers like BisGMA, HEMA, TEGDMA, and UDMA. Nevertheless, it should be noted that the safety data sheet for TheraCal LC does not list BisGMA as a component of TheraCal LC [19]; a fact that was confirmed by the study of Nilsen and Einar [18] which reported that Bis-GMA was not detected in the UPLC-MS analysis of TheraCal LC, despite being listed in the safety data sheet provided by the supplier (dated 2011). This implies that changes in the composition of TheraCal LC might have occurred without the supplier and/or clinicians being notified. Studies on TheraCal LC could, in that case, have been performed with a material of dissimilar composition to the material tested in other studies. Nilsen and Einar [18] investigated the organic composition and eluates of TheraCal LC in relation to its indications and safety data sheets and reported that TheraCal LC contains and elutes several reactive, organic substances that are not declared in the safety data sheets of the material and stated that the use of these materials should be questioned by further *in vitro* and *in vivo* studies.

Nevertheless, TheraCal LC has been reported successful in short term studies. A 2-year *in vivo* study demonstrated that TheraCal LC had a higher success rate (93.3%) for direct pulp capping compared with an antibacterial adhesive system (Protect Bond, Kurary) (83.3%) and glass ionomer cement (Fuji IX, GC) (66.6%) [42]. TheraCal LC had the highest success rates when compared with other test groups treated with self-etch adhesives and Glass Ionomer restorative materials in a 6-month *in vivo* study [43]. Cannon et al. [44] compared the effectiveness of TheraCal LC, pure Portland cement, resin-based calcium hydroxide, or glass ionomer in the healing of bacterially contaminated primate pulps. They found no statistical difference between the groups in regard to pulpal inflammation. However, they reported that the light-cured TheraCal LC groups had significantly more frequent hard tissue bridge formation, a greater thickness of the dentinal bridge and better dentinal bridge qualities than the Glass ionomer and VLC Dycal groups. Gopika et al. [45] compared and evaluated the response of the human pulp following direct pulp capping with TheraCal LC, Septocal LC, and Dycal. Their study found that TheraCal LC and Septocal LC (Calcium hydroxide with hydroxyapatite) cements were as effective as Dycal in inducing the formation of reparative dentin and evoking an inflammatory response. There are a scarcity of studies reporting the outcome of using TheraCal LC in indirect pulp capping procedures. Only one randomized clinical trial reported successful clinical (no pain and absence of sinus tract) and radiographic (no sign of external and internal resorption and presence of bridge) outcomes following the use of MTA and TheraCal LC when used for indirect pulp capping in primary teeth [46].

4. Conclusion

Materials with new compositions should be evaluated comprehensively before their clinical application. Future studies should examine whether the lower calcium ion releasing ability , together with the cy totoxic effect due to unpoly merized resin monomers of TheraCal LC has an influence on its biological and clinical performance. Further *in vitro* and *in vivo* studies are required before TheraCal LC can be used as a direct pulp capping material.

References

[1] T. J. Hilton, "Keys to clinical success with pulp capping: a review of the literature," *Operative Dentistry*, vol. 34, no. 5, pp. 615–625, 2009.

[2] N. Arandi, "Calcium hydroxide liners: a literature review," *Clinical, Cosmetic and Investigational Dentistry*, vol. 9, pp. 67–72, 2017.

[3] L. Stangvaltaite, F. Schwendicke, C. Holmgren et al., "Management of pulps exposed during carious tissue removal in adults: a multi-national questionnaire-based survey," *Clinical Oral Investigations*, vol. 21, no. 7, pp. 2303–2309, 2016.

[4] C. F. Cox, R. K. Sübay, E. Ostro, S. Suzuki, and S. H. Suzuki, "Tunnel defects in dentin bridges: their formation following direct pulp capping," *Operative Dentistry*, vol. 21, no. 1, pp. 4–11, 1996.

[5] M. J. Tyas, "Pulp protection under restorations-do you need a liner?," *Australian Endodontic Journal*, vol. 24, no. 3, pp. 104–108, 1998.

[6] J. Camilleri, "Hydration characteristics of biodentine and theracal used as pulp capping materials," *Dental Materials*, vol. 30, no. 7, pp. 709–715, 2014.

[7] P. N. R. Nair, H. F. Duncan, T. R. Pitt Ford, and H. U. Luder, "Histological, ultrastructural and quantitative investigations on the response of healthy human pulps to experimental capping with mineral trioxide aggregate: a randomized controlled trial," *International Endodontic Journal*, vol. 41, no. 2, pp. 128–150, 2008.

[8] I. M. Faraco and R. Holland, "Response of the pulp of dogs to capping with mineral trioxide aggregate or a calcium hydroxide cement," *Dental Traumatology*, vol. 17, no. 4, pp. 163–166, 2001.

[9] M. Aeinehchi, B. Eslami, M. Ghanbariha, and A. S. Saffar, "Mineral trioxide aggregate (MTA) and calcium hydroxide as pulp-capping agents in human teeth: a preliminary report," *International Endodontic Journal*, vol. 36, no. 3, pp. 225–231, 2002.

[10] T. Komabayashi, Q. Zhu, R. Eberhart, and Y. Imai, "Current status of direct pulp-capping materials for permanent teeth," *Dental Material Journal*, vol. 35, no. 1, pp. 1–12, 2016.

[11] I. About, "Biodentine: from biochemical and bioactive properties to clinical applications," *Giornale Italiano di Endodonzia*, vol. 30, no. 2, pp. 81–88, 2016.

[12] A. R. Atmeh, E. Z. Chong, G. Richard, F. Festy, and T. F. Watson, "Dentin-cement interfacial interaction: calcium silicates and polyalkenoates," *Journal of Dental Research*, vol. 91, no. 5, pp. 454–459, 2012.

[13] C. Brizuela, A. Ormeño, C. Cabrera et al., "Direct pulp capping with calcium hydroxide, mineral trioxide aggregate, and biodentine in permanent young teeth with caries: a randomized clinical trial," *Journal of Endodontics*, vol. 43, no. 11, pp. 10–14, 2017.

[14] F. A. Katge and D. P. Patil, "Comparative analysis of 2 calcium silicate-based cements (biodentine and mineral trioxide aggregate) as direct pulp-capping agent in young permanent molars: a split mouth study," *Journal of Endodontics*, vol. 43, no. 4, pp. 507–513, 2017.

[15] A. Nowicka, M. Lipski, M. Parafiniuk et al., "Response of human dental pulp capped with biodentine and mineral trioxide aggregate," *Journal of Endodontics*, vol. 39, no. 6, pp. 743–747, 2013.

[16] A. Dutta and W. Saunders, "Calcium silicate materials in endodontics," *Dental Updates*, vol. 41, no. 8, pp. 708–722, 2014.

[17] B. I. Suh, R. Yin, M. Cannon, and D. Martin, "Polymerizable dental pulp healing, capping, and lining material and method for use," International Patent A61k33/42;A61K33/42, vol. 1, 2008.

[18] B. Nilsen and J. Einar, "Analysis of organic components in resin-modified pulp capping materials: critical considerations," *European Journal of Oral Sciences*, vol. 125, no. 3, pp. 183–194, 2017.

[19] Federal Register (USA), "TheraCal LC safety data sheet," vol. 77, pp. 1–7, 2016.

[20] J. Camilleri, P. Laurent, and I. About, "Hydration of biodentine, theracal LC, and a prototype tricalcium silicate-based dentin replacement material after pulp capping in entire tooth cultures," *Journal of Endodontics*, vol. 40, no. 11, pp. 1846–1854, 2014.

[21] M. G. Gandolfi, F. Siboni, T. Botero, M. Bossù, F. Riccitiello, and C. Prati, "Calcium silicate and calcium hydroxide materials for pulp capping: biointeractivity, porosity, solubility and bioactivity of current formulations," *Journal of Applied Biomaterials and Fundamental Materials*, vol. 13, no. 1, pp. 43–60, 2014.

[22] M. G. Gandolfi, F. Siboni, and C. Prati, "Chemical-physical properties of TheraCal, a novel light-curable MTA-like material for pulp capping," *International Endodontic Journal*, vol. 45, no. 6, pp. 571–579, 2012.

[23] S. Yamamoto, L. Han, Y. Noiri, and T. Okiji, "Evaluation of the Ca ion release, pH and surface apatite formation of

a prototype tricalcium silicate cement," *International Endodontic Journal*, vol. 50, pp. 1–10, 2017.

[24] A. E. Dawood, P. Parashos, R. H. K. Wong, E. C. Reynolds, and D. J. Manton, "Calcium silicate-based cements: composition, properties, and clinical applications," *Journal of Investigative and Clinical Dentistry*, vol. 8, no. 2, pp. 1–15, 2017.

[25] C. Poggio, M. Lombardini, M. Colombo, R. Beltrami, and S. Rindi, "Solubility and pH of direct pulp capping materials: a comparative study," *Journal of Applied Biomaterials & Functional Materials*, vol. 13, no. 2, pp. e73–e193, 2015.

[26] S. Makkar, H. Kaur, A. Anurag, and R. Vashisht, "A confocal laser scanning microscopic study evaluating the sealing ability of mineral trioxide aggregate, biodentine and a new pulp capping agent-theracal," *Dental Journal of Advance Studies*, vol. 3, no. 1, pp. 19–25, 2016.

[27] X. Li, J. De Munck, K. Van Landuyt, M. Pedano, Z. Chen, and B. Van Meerbeek, "How effectively do hydraulic calcium-silicate cements re-mineralize demineralized dentin," *Dental Materials*, vol. 33, no. 4, pp. 434–445, 2017.

[28] N. Meraji and J. Camilleri, "Bonding over dentin replacement materials," *Journal of Endodontics*, vol. 43, no. 8, pp. 1343–1349, 2017.

[29] M. Karadas, K. Cantekin, H. Gumus, S. M. Ateş, and Z. Y. Duymuş, "Evaluation of the bond strength of different adhesive agents to a resin-modified calcium silicate material (TheraCal LC)," *Scanning*, vol. 38, no. 5, pp. 403–411, 2016.

[30] Y. Yoshida, K. Nagakane, R. Fukuda et al., "Comparative study on adhesive performance of functional monomers," *Journal of Dental Research*, vol. 83, no. 6, pp. 454–458, 2004.

[31] L. Deepa, B. Dhamaraju, I. P. Bollu, and T. S. Balaji, "Shear bond strength evaluation of resin composite bonded to three different liners: TheraCal LC, biodentine, and resin-modified glass ionomer cement using universal adhesive: an in vitro study," *Journal of Conservative Dentistry*, vol. 19, no. 2, pp. 166–170, 2016.

[32] K. Cantekin, "Bond strength of different restorative materials to light-curable mineral trioxide aggregate," *Journal of Clinical Pediatric Dentistry*, vol. 39, no. 2, pp. 143–148, 2015.

[33] W. Ha, B. Kahler, and L. J. Walsh, "Classification and nomanclature of commercial hygroscopic dental cements," *European Endodontic Journal*, vol. 2, no. 1, p. 27, 2017.

[34] S. Savas, M. S. Botsali, E. Kucukyilmaz, and T. Sari, "Evaluation of temperature changes in the pulp chamber during polymerization of light-cured pulp-capping materials by using a VALO LED light curing unit at different curing distances," *Dental Materials Journal*, vol. 33, no. 6, pp. 764–769, 2014.

[35] C. Poggio, C. R. Arciola, R. Beltrami et al., "Cytocompatibility and antibacterial properties of capping materials," *Scientific World Journal*, vol. 2014, Article ID 181945, 10 pages, 2014.

[36] M. T. Arias-Moliz, C. Farrugia, C. Y. K. Lung, P. S. Wismayer, and J. Camilleri, "Antimicrobial and biological activity of leachate from light curable pulp capping materials," *Journal of Dentistry*, vol. 64, pp. 45–51, 2017.

[37] H. Lee, Y. Shin, S.-O. Kim, H.-S. Lee, H.-J. Choi, and J. S. Song, "Comparative study of pulpal responses to pulpotomy with ProRoot MTA, RetroMTA, and TheraCal in Dogs" teeth," *Journal of Endodontics*, vol. 41, no. 8, pp. 1317–1324, 2015.

[38] C. Poggio, R. Beltrami, M. Colombo, M. Ceci, A. Dagna, and M. Chiesa, "In vitro antibacterial activity of different pulp capping materials," *Journal of Clinical Experimental Dentistry*, vol. 7, pp. e584–e588, 2015.

[39] J. Hebling, F. C. R. Lessa, I. Nogueira, R. M. de Carvalho, and C. A. S. de Costa, "Cytotoxicity of resin-based light-cured liners," *American Journal of Dentistry*, vol. 22, no. 3, pp. 137–142, 2009.

[40] C. Jeanneau, P. Laurent, C. Rombouts, T. Giraud, and I. About, "Light-cured tricalcium silicate toxicity to the dental pulp," *Journal of Endodontics*, vol. 43, no. 12, pp. 2074–2080, 2017.

[41] H. Bakhtiar, M. H. Nekoofar, P. Aminishakib et al., "Human pulp responses to partial pulpotomy treatment with TheraCal as compared with biodentine and ProRoot MTA: a clinical trial," *Journal of Endodontics*, vol. 43, no. 11, pp. 1786–1791, 2017.

[42] F. Petrolo, A. Comba, M. Scansetti et al., "Effects of light-cured MTA like material on direct pulp capping," *Dental Materials*, vol. 30, p. e15, 2014.

[43] A. Comba, F. Petrolo, M. Scansetti et al., "Effect of a novel light-cured MTA-like material on direct pulp capping outcome," *Dental Materials*, vol. 29, p. e38, 2013.

[44] M. Cannon, N. Gerodias, A. Viera, C. Percinoto, and R. Jurado, "Primate pulpal healing after exposure and TheraCal application," *Journal of Clinical Pediatric Dentistry*, vol. 38, no. 4, pp. 333–337, 2014.

[45] G. J. Gopika, S. Ramarao, C. Usha et al., "Histological evaluation of human pulp capped with light-cured calcium based cements: a randomized controlled clinical trial," *International Journal of Scientific Reports*, vol. 3, no. 5, pp. 120–127, 2017.

[46] N. P. Menon, B. R. Varma, S. Janardhanan, P. Kumaran, A. M. Xavier, and B. S. Govinda, "Clinical and radiographic comparison of indirect pulp treatment using light-cured calcium silicate and mineral trioxide aggregate in primary molars: a randomized clinical trial," *Contemporary Clinical Dentistry*, vol. 7, no. 4, pp. 475–480, 2016.

19

Effect of Surgical Installation of Dental Implants on Surface Topography and Its Influence on Osteoblast Proliferation

Helder H. M. Menezes,[1] **Marina M. Naves**,[2] **Henara L. Costa**,[3,4] **Tarsis P. Barbosa**,[3,5] **Jéssica A. Ferreira**,[2] **Denildo Magalhães**,[2] **and Elizabeth F. Martinez**[6]

[1]*Department of Periodontology and Implant Dentistry, HD Post Graduation Dental School, Uberlândia 38408-394, Brazil*
[2]*School of Dentistry, Federal University of Uberlandia, Uberlândia 38405-320, Brazil*
[3]*School of Mechanical Engineering, Federal University of Uberlandia, Uberlandia 38400-901, Brazil*
[4]*School of Engineering, Federal University of Rio Grande, Rio Grande 96203-900, Brazil*
[5]*Department of Telecommunications and Mechatronics, Federal University of Sao Joao Del-Rei, Ouro Branco 36420-000, Brazil*
[6]*Department of Cellular and Mollecular Biology, São Leopoldo Mandic Research, Campinas 13045-755, Brazil*

Correspondence should be addressed to Elizabeth F. Martinez; dr.efmartinez@gmail.com

Academic Editor: Andreas Stavropoulos

Surface treatment alone does not determine the final microtopography of a dental implant, which can be influenced by implant design and the surgical procedure. This study investigated the effect of surgical placement of dental implants with same surface treatments on surface roughness. Three implants (SIN) of each group with different macrogeometries (Strong, Stylus, and Tryon) were analyzed using laser interferometry and scanning electron microscopy to evaluate surface topography. All threaded regions of the implants, namely, top, flank, and valley, were analyzed individually. Relevant surface parameters (S_a, S_{sk}, S_{ku}, S_{tr}, and S_{dq}) were calculated for the different regions on each implant before (B) ($n = 9$) and after (A) ($n = 9$) placement into porcine rib bones. The behavior and proliferation of a preosteoblastic cell line MC3T3-E1 on titanium surface, cell viability, and osteopontin secretion were evaluated after 24 h, 48 h, and 96 h, also before ($n = 18$) and after ($n = 18$) implant placement into porcine ribs bone. As results, the valleys of all implants had an increase in S_a values after implant placement. By contrast, the tops of the Stylus A implant and the flanks of the Tryon A implant showed a significant decrease in mean height of the irregularities (S_a), 0.16 μm and 1.25 μm, respectively. The Stylus implant presented significantly ($p < 0.05$) higher asymmetry values on the distribution curve for irregularity heights (S_{ku}) in all regions after insertion into bone (6.99 for tops, 9.54 for flanks, and 17.64 for valleys), indicating a greater preponderance of peaks over valleys. An increase in roughness gradients (S_{dq}) was observed for all macrogeometries after insertion into bone. The cell culture results showed no significant difference ($p > 0.05$) for all macrogeometries after bone placement. In conclusion, a subtle change in implant surface roughness was detected after insertion into bone for all the macrogeometries, without significantly affecting the cellular parameters studied.

1. Introduction

Long-term success of dental implants is based on several factors [1–3] including osseointegration [4–6]. In addition, the chemical biocompatibility of the material and the microgeometry of the implant surface are important for implant success and long-term osseointegration, affecting the cellular response, resulting in greater/better quality bone formation and, therefore, improving secondary implant stability [7–12].

In order to increase long-term implant success/survival rates, research has focused on implant modifications, including surface topography and macrogeometry [13]. The design of most recent implants seeks to minimize potential osseointegration issues, such as low-density bone or patients with systemic diseases that compromise bone repair, and also to reduce bone trauma and prosthetic fractures, especially when immediate loading is applied [13]. With modification of any of the mechanical or chemical properties of an implant, host tissue response is expected to improve, thus optimizing the bond with the bone tissue [5, 14].

Furthermore, implant morphology can also influence bone metabolism: rougher surfaces stimulate differentiation, growth, and attachment of bone cells and increase mineralization. Implants may have "smooth" (machined) or rough surfaces. The main methods that are reported in the literature to create implant roughness are titanium plasma spraying, hydroxyapatite (HA) coating, sandblasting, and acid etching. A current tendency is the manufacturing of implants with submicro (nano) topography and microtopography. Furthermore, the biofunctionalization of implant surfaces, by adding different substances to improve its biological characteristics, has also been recently investigated [15–17].

The development of bone-implant interfaces depends on the direct interactions of bone matrix and osteoblasts with the biomaterial [18]. Osteoblast adhesion is essential for bone-biomaterial interactions [19]. Consequently, maximization of bone integration has become a goal of the treatment, which apparently can be improved by varying surface roughness of the implant [20]. Therefore, cell adhesion is a fundamental process directly involved in cell growth, cell migration, and cell differentiation. It is concerned in embryogenesis, maintenance of tissue integrity, wound healing, immune response, and biomaterial tissue integration. Several proteins are involved in cell adhesion, such as extracellular matrix proteins (collagen, fibronectin, and vitronectin) and membrane receptors (integrins). Interactions between these proteins and their specific receptors induce signal transduction and consequently influence cell growth and differentiation.

Studies have shown that implants with roughened surfaces have better bone apposition and higher BIC when compared with smooth surfaces [2, 21]. In 2004, Albrektsson and Wennerberg [2] described the topographical properties by a literature review, and the findings showed that moderate roughened surfaces (S_a between 1.0 and 2.0 μm) present better osseous response than rougher or smoother surfaces.

Changes in implant macrogeometry also contribute to implant success by directly affecting primary stability [22–25]. First, for tapered implants, the macrogeometry of the implant body and the thread design are directly related to the surface contact area of the implant. The area of surface contact with the host tissue will determine contact pressures, affecting implant stability [26–28]. Second, the insertion torque of tapered implants is normally greater than that of cylindrical implants [26]. Among tapered implants, the insertion torque is affected by the thread design (shape, width, depth, pitch, face, and helix angle) and thread pitch (angle and width). The insertion torque will affect the amount of deformation in the bone, changing the amount of bone around the implant and the degree of bone apposition, which will influence bone remodeling, affecting implant success [29–32]. Third, the thread design will affect micromovements of the implant in relation to the bone since it will affect mechanical interlocking.

In screw-type implants, it is necessary to measure topography in three regions of the threads: flank, top, and valley [32–35]. Although this characterization is well defined, it is unclear whether increasingly complex surface features found in modern dental implants are maintained after bone placement.

During implant placement, the insertion torque may result in varying levels of compression stress transmitted to the adjacent bone, since the diameter of the osteotomy is somewhat narrower than that of the diameter of the implant to optimize primary stability [35, 36]. Clinical studies have demonstrated a close relationship between initial stability and implant success [37–40], where the former can be measured by insertion torque during implant placement [38]. Insertion torque, in most cases, should be higher than 30 N cm for predictable outcomes [38], thus preventing implant micromovement and, consequently, connective tissue formation [39]. An excessively high insertion torque above 50 N cm [36] may occur during implant installation in dense bones [37, 40], resulting in compression stress to the adjacent bone and compromising osseointegration [41]. In addition, some studies have shown that shear force during placement may alter implant surface features [42–44].

Considering the lack of studies investigating the stability of surface characteristics after implant placement as well as a lack of clarity in the methods reported to analyze implant design in such context, the present study investigated *ex vivo* the influence of different implant macrogeometry and insertion torque to cortical and cancellous bone in the surface microtopography and cellular parameters *in vitro*, considering cellular proliferation and viability assays, as well as, osteopontin expression.

2. Materials and Methods

2.1. Sample Description. This study analyzed commercially pure titanium implants (grade 4) of the types Strong, Stylus, and Tryon, marketed by SIN (Implant System, São Paulo, Brazil). All implants presented an external hexagon connection with a 4.1 mm platform. The Strong and Tryon implants had a diameter of 3.75 mm, and the Stylus implants had a diameter of 4.0 mm, all of which were 13 mm long with different macrogeometries, as shown in Figure 1. For the topographic characterization of the surfaces, three samples from each type of implant were analyzed before (B) and three after (A) installation into 3 porcine rib bones. For the *in vitro* cellular analysis, six samples from each type of implant were analyzed before and after installation into 3 porcine bones.

All samples with the same type of surface treatment were purchased directly from the manufacturer. The treatment consisted of nitric acid followed by sulfuric acid (DAA, double acid etching) baths, according to the description by the manufacturer.

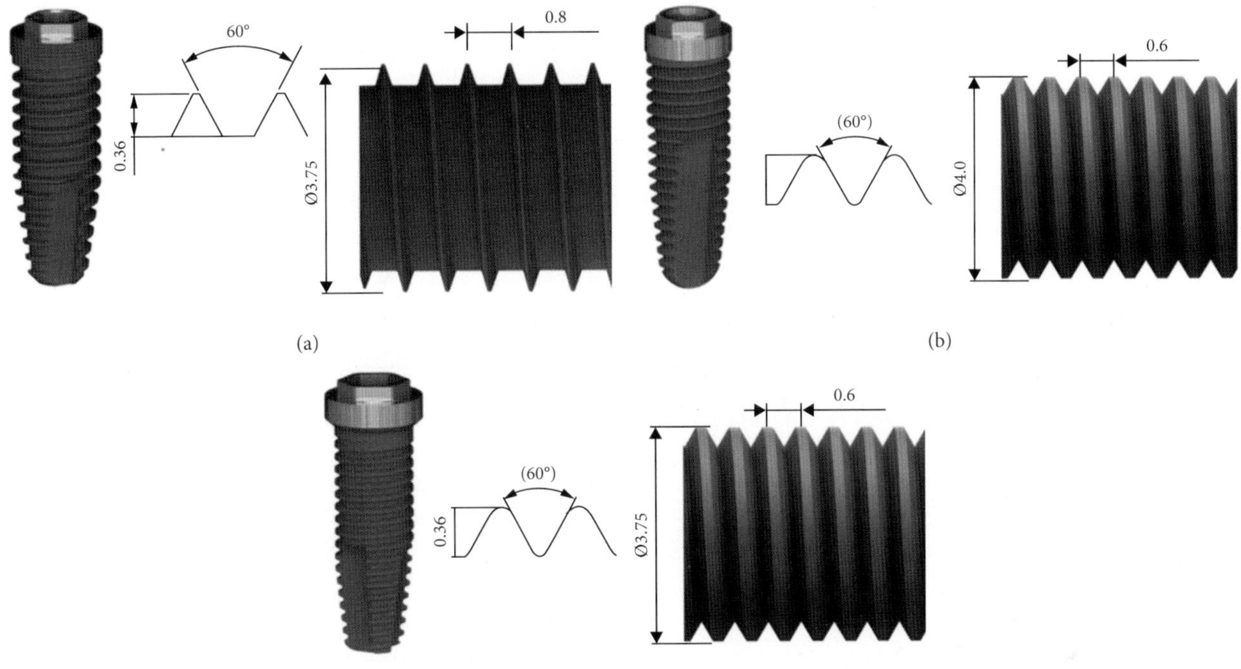

Figure 1: Macrogeometry of the implants and detail of their diameter and threads. (a) Sample of group Strong—implant with smaller thread heights/triangular V shaped (size: 3.75 mm × 13 mm). (b) Sample of Stylus—implant with lower internal thread angles/square and buttress thread-l (size: 4.0 mm × 13 mm). (c) Sample of Tryon—implant with lower internal thread angles/square and buttress thread-(size: 3.75 mm × 13 mm); all implants are hybrid (cervical part of the implant body in cylindrical shape and apical part of the implant body in tapered shape).

2.2. Implant Placement into Porcine Ribs. Nine fresh porcine ribs (bone quality D3) [45] with 15 mm high and 15 cm long were used as an experimental model. Three implants of each macrogeometry were placed into 3 porcine ribs for the implant surfaces analysis ($n = 9$), and six implants of each macrogeometry ($n = 18$) were placed into three ribs for cellular assays analysis. Considering that the animals were not sacrificed for research purposes, this study was exempt from approval by the Animal Ethics Committee [46, 47].

Dental implants were placed into 13 mm deep perforations, following the manufacturer's instructions (Figures 2(a) and 2(b)), by one expert surgeon, and final drill with dimension of 3.0 mm. The distance between the implants was 20 mm. Implant fixation was measured by the same manufacturer using a manual torque wrench, with a maximum torque of 60 N cm, as recommended by the manufacturer. Computed tomography (CT) was performed to ascertain the exact position of each implant (Figures 2(c) and 2(d)). After installation, the implants were removed using a piezoelectric ultrasonic tip (PiezoSurgery® White, Mectron, Italy) cutting the bone laterally to the implant, taking care not to damage the implant surface and allow passive release of the implants from the bone.

Implants were cleaned to remove bone debris from the surface by immersion in filtered water (30 minutes) and then in acetone (10 minutes) as suggested by Senna et al. [44].

2.3. Characterization of Implant Surfaces. Laser interferometry and scanning electron microscopy (SEM) were used to characterize the surface of the implants. A 3D laser interferometer (UBM MESSTECHNIK MicroFocus, Ettlingen, Germany) was used to analyze surface topography at densities of 1000 × 1000 points and measurement rate of 300 points/s, using the continuous method. The measurement area was 0.8 × 0.4 mm to allow the inclusion of at least one thread for all regions without losing focus [48].

Due to the complex macrogeometry of the implants, different areas were measured for each implant, as shown in Figure 3. From all the samples evaluated ($n = 18$), 9 were measured before installation and 9 after, from which 6 were model Strong, 6 Stylus, and 6 Tryon. Each implant was divided into three macroregions for analysis: 4 mm within the cervical region [1], 5 mm within the implant body [2], and 4 mm at the apical end [3] (Figure 3(a)). Thus, for each region, three tops, three valleys, and three consecutively threaded flanks (Figure 3(a)) measuring 0.8 × 0.4 mm were analyzed and measured, totaling 27 measurements for each implant in each macroregion. All the implants were randomized to minimize the effects of subjective bias.

The characterization of surface topography consisted of three components: shape, waviness, and roughness, where filters were necessary to isolate each of these components for analysis. The software Mountains Map (Digital Surf, Besançon, France) was used for this purpose, which also permitted collation of the 2D and 3D images based on

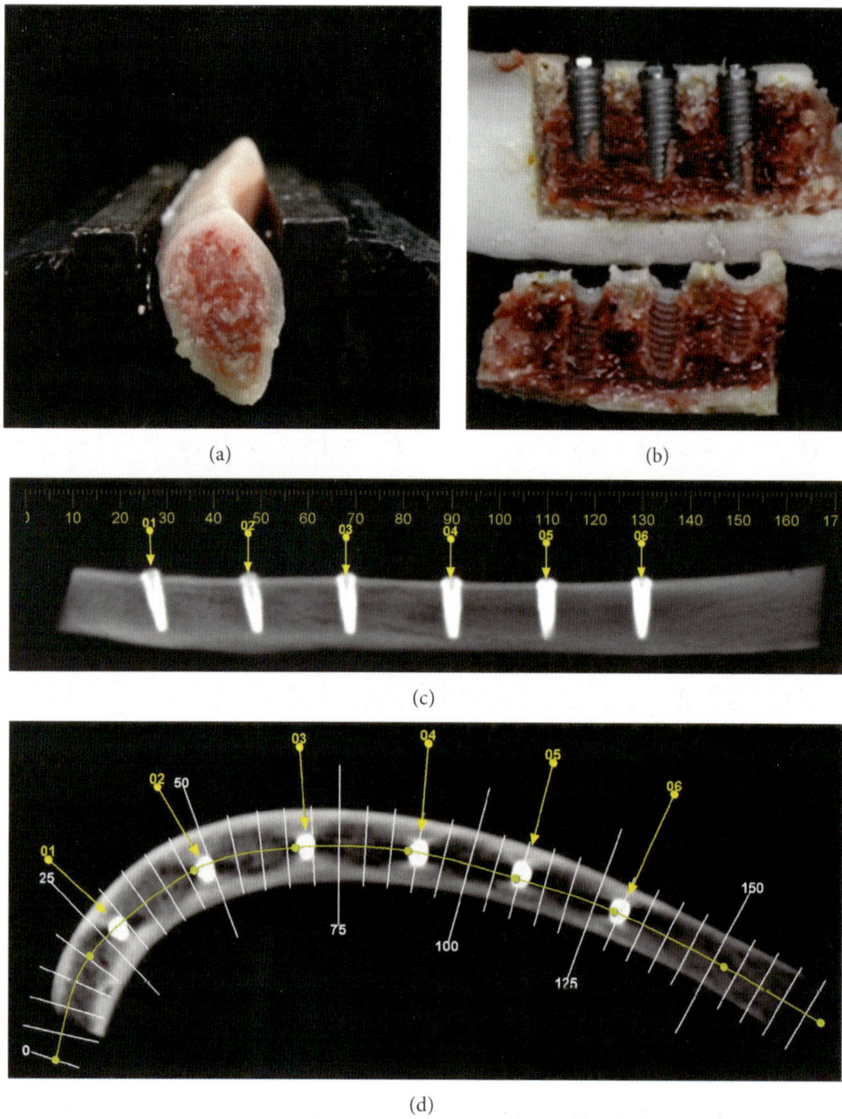

FIGURE 2: (a) Porcine rib positioned on the vise for implant installation. (b) Vertically sectioned porcine rib with Strong implants after osteotomy with piezoelectric ultrasound. (c, d) Transverse CT of implants into porcine rib.

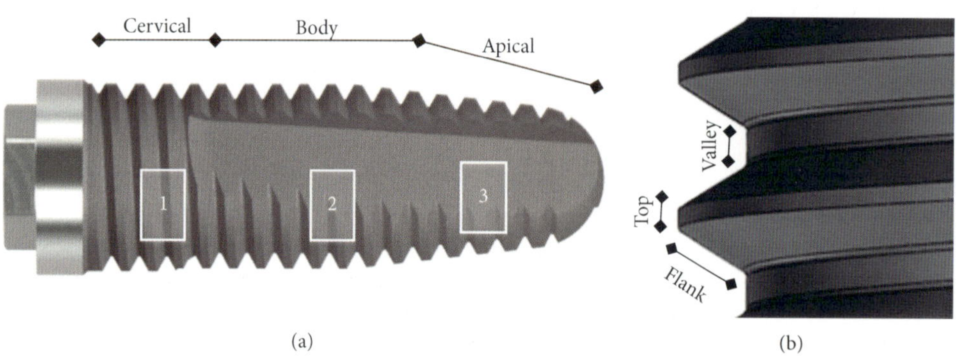

FIGURE 3: (a) Implant macroregions for analysis: 1-cervical, 2-body, and 3-apical. (b) Analyzed areas of each thread (top, flank, and valley) of regions 1, 2, and 3.

numerical description of the parameters for surface roughness. To characterize the shape of the implants (macrogeometry), profiles of the threads were selected. Vertical heights and thread angles were measured in the profiles. The MB Ruler software (MarkusBader MB-Software solutions, Iffezheim, Germany) was used to calculate the angles of the implant threads, the total length of the implant thread profile, and the specific lengths of every flanks, tops, and valleys [47]. Dividing the total length by the specific lengths of each region, the percentage of the area of each region in relation to the whole surface of the implant was estimated. For the calculation of the roughness parameters, the first step was to use a filter to remove the shape of the implant. Then, a 50 × 50 μm Gaussian filter was used to separate waviness from roughness.

The numerical description of surface roughness at the different regions used three height parameters (S_a, S_{sk}, and S_{ku}), one spatial parameter (S_{tr}), and one hybrid parameter (S_{dq}). S_a, also referred to as mean roughness, is the arithmetic mean height of the asperities. S_{sk} and S_{ku} are related to the height distribution curve, where S_{sk} is a measure of asymmetry of surface deviations about the mean plane, and S_{ku} is a measure of the peakedness or sharpness of the surface height distribution. S_{tr} is the texture aspect ratio of the surface, used to identify uniformity of texture aspect. S_{dq} is the root mean square slope of the asperities. The mathematical description of these parameters can be found in the study by Stout et al. [49]. Other studies in the literature [31, 48] have used the same parameters to characterize the surface topography of dental implants.

Ultrastructural SEM images of the tops, flanks, and valleys were performed before and after implant installation to provide a qualitative analysis of the surfaces (EVO MA 10, Carl Zeiss, Germany) at different magnifications and 15 kV voltage acceleration. This surface characterization was performed in three implants of each macrogeometry before installation in the porcine rib (B implants) and in three implants after installation in the porcine rib (A implants).

Osteoblast cell proliferation and viability assays, as well as osteopontin quantification were performed on the different surfaces, before and after implants installation. All the assays were performed in triplicates at a density of 1.9×10^4/well on 24-well tissue culture plates. In order to stabilize the implants inside the 24-well tissue culture plate, orthodontic wire segments were used (nickel-titanium (NiTi) (Morelli Ortodontia™--Sorocaba, SP, Brazil).

The preosteoblastic cell line MC3T3-E1 was obtained from the ATCC (American Type Culture Collection, ATCC, VC, USA) and cultured at 4th to 6th passage in DMEM/F-12 medium (LGC Biotechnology, São Paulo, SP, Brazil), supplemented with 10% bovine fetal serum (LGC Biotechnology) and 100 U/ml penicillin and 100 μg/ml streptomycin (Sigma, St. Louis, Missouri, USA). During the culture period, cells were incubated at 37°C in a humidified atmosphere of 5% CO_2 and 95% air, and the medium was changed every 2-3 days [48].

For the evaluation of cell proliferation, the trypan blue vital exclusion method was used at 24 h, 48 h, and 96 h from cell seeding onto the surfaces. The cells were enzymatically detached from the surfaces with 1 mM EDTA (Gibco) and 0.25% trypsin solution (Gibco). The cells were then counted using a hemocytometer (Hausser Scientific, Horsham, PA). Cell proliferation was expressed as number of cells × 10^4.

Cell viability was evaluated by 3-[4,5-dimethylthiazol-2-yl]-2,5-diphenyl tetrazolium bromide (MTT; Sigma) assay after 24, 48, and 72 h. Briefly, the cells were incubated with 10% of MTT (5 mg/mL) in culture medium at 37°C for 4 h. The MTT solution was then aspirated from the well, and 200 μL of dimethyl sulfoxide (Sigma) was added to each well. Then, the plates were agitated on a plate shaker for 5 min, and 150 μL of this solution was transferred to a new 96-well plate. The optical density was read at 570–650 nm on the plate reader (Epoch; Bio-Tek, Winooski, VT), and data were expressed as absorbance.

Quantification of secreted osteopontin by the osteoblastic cells cultured on the different surfaces was evaluated by enzyme immunoassay (ELISA). The supernatant was collected and centrifuged at 336 g for 10 min, and the resulting supernatant was collected, aliquoted, and stored at −80°C. The osteopontin quantification was carried out using Mouse Osteopontin kit (R&D Systems, Minneapolis, USA) according to the manufacturer's instructions. The values were expressed as ng/ml.

2.4. Statistical Analysis. For each parameter, mean and standard deviation values were calculated for the implants before and after installation. In order to evaluate statistical significance, the topographical parameters (B and A) were analyzed using the paired t-test ($\alpha = 0.05$) (SPSS Statistics Base 17.0-IBM, Chicago, USA).

The Shapiro–Wilk test was used to test normality on the data collected, which did not conform to the assumptions of normality. The Wilcoxon test was paired and used to better compare the mesurements between two samples statistically similar, on dependent samples. The morphological aspects before (B) and after (A) implant installation into bone were compared for the Strong, Stylus, and Tryon macrogeometries. The entire study was performed considering a confidence level of 95%. The comparison among implants from different macrogeometries was not performed because the cell sedimentation region within the flanks and valleys were different across the groups.

3. Results and Discussion

3.1. Surface Characterization. The implant insertion torque did not exceed the maximum values recommended by the manufacturer, and there was considerable variation in insertion torque among the three implants, possibly due to the influence of the macrogeometry on the porcine rib bone, which is D3. The mean insertion torque (N.cm) was 48.3 3 (±10.98) for Strong, 33.88 (±15.58) for Stylus, and 33.05 (±13.84) for Tryon. The porcine rib was chosen due to its cortical thickness (2 mm thick) and microscopic bone structure that resembles the human jaw bone.

Table 1 shows the values of the parameters used to characterize the threads in the different regions for each

Table 1: Macrogeometric measurements of the implants, where α_1 and α_2 are the internal angles between flanks, and h is the thread height.

Implant	Insertion torque (mean ± SD)	Region	α_1 (degrees)	α_2 (degrees)	Height, h (μm)	Percentage of area in relation to total implant length
Strong	48.33 N cm ± 10.98	Region 1-cervical	59.3	59.9	331.6	Top: 10.25%
		Region 2-body	59.7	61.7	349.5	Flank: 63.03%
		Region 3-apical	59.7	59.2	250.1	Valley: 26.70%
		Mean	**59.9**		**310.4**	
Stylus	33.88 N cm ±15.58	Region 1-cervical	58.7	62.1	389.4	Top: 15.14%
		Region 2-body	59.6	57.1	380.0	Flank: 75.35%
		Region 3-apical	50.7	59.2	283.6	Valley: 9.49%
		Mean	**57.9**		**351.0**	
Tryon	33.05 N cm ±13.84	Region 1-cervical	55.8	55.6	350.1	Top: 17.11%
		Region 2-body	55.9	59.7	362.1	Flank: 73.72%
		Region 3-apical	63.2	58.1	312.5	Valley: 9.79%
		Mean	**58.0**		**341.6**	

implant. Some variation in angles and heights between regions for the same implant were observed. The Strong implant presented threads with smaller thread heights, while the Stylus implant had lower internal thread angles. It was possible to observe that the flanks corresponded to the larger area for all implants. The tops were the second largest areas in the Stylus and Tryon implants, while the valleys were the second largest areas in the Strong implant.

The mean values ±standard deviation of the surface roughness parameters (S_a, S_{sk}, S_{ku}, S_{tr}, and S_{dq}) were the means of all regions 1, 2, and 3 for each type of dental implant (B and A) and are shown in Table 2. The values of total Δ are the difference between the mean of all areas (top, flank, and valley) before and after the implant placement for each implant type, shown in Table 2. Considering the evaluation methods, other studies that evaluated surface alterations also used scanning electron microscopy and interferometry [41–43]. As laser interferometry is suggested as an excellent quantification method for screw-type implant topography [31, 51, 52], the same surface roughness (3D) parameters were evaluated before and after installation in the porcine rib.

For the tops, flanks, and valleys, implant macrogeometry had a significant influence in S_a values, mainly for Strong and Tryon implants. Regarding the effects of bone insertion, it was observed that the parameter S_a, which represents the mean height of the surface irregularities, showed significant reduction in the top regions after insertion in the bone for the Stylus (Stylus top $p = 0.000$). It must be pointed out that for this implant, the top regions did not present regular topography, i.e., the surface treatment did not seem to have been effective to change the whole area (Figure 4(b)).This seemed to occur as a result of the flattening of the asperities observed from the SEM images, which was much less significant for the top of the implant Tryon. On the contrary, for the Strong implant, S_a showed a tendency to increase with bone insertion, although the standard deviation was very high. The area of the tops of those implants were smaller compared with the other implants (Table 1), which probably resulted in higher contact pressures during the insertion process. This could lead to more intense generation of bone debris, which may justify their higher values of S_a and also the larger scattering of the results. Some evidence of bone debris is indicated by the arrow in Figure 4(d) relative to the top of the Strong implant after insertion. Significant reduction in S_a values on the flanks of the implants was observed for the Tryon implants (Tryon flank $p = 0.000$). Regarding the thread valleys, all values of S_a increased after placement into bone, which was statistically significant in the Strong implants ($p = 0.001$) and Tryon ($p = 0.000$). This is probably related to the accommodation of bone debris resulting from bone insertion in the valleys of the threads and/or to damage to the valleys of the threads.

According to Albrektsson and Wennerberg [2], implants can be divided into four categories depending on surface roughness: smooth ($S_a < 0.5\,\mu$m), minimally rough (S_a between 0.5 and 1.0 μm), moderately rough (S_a between 1.0 and 2.0 μm), and rough ($S_a > 2.0\,\mu$m). Some studies have suggested that an ideal implant surface should have S_a values between 1.0 and 2.0 μm [29, 50, 51]. In this study, most implants showed S_a values below 1.0 μm (minimally rough) prior to insertion into bone (B). One exception was the Tryon implant (B), which presented values of S_a in the flank of 1.98 ± 0.68 (Table 2). Before insertion into porcine ribs, macrogeometries had little effect on S_a values, but the insertion process into bone may have led to the formation of bone debris that accommodated in the valleys of the threads and/or simply damaged the thread valleys for the Tryon (A) and Strong (A) implants, increasing S_a values in these regions. At the tops of the Stylus (A) implant and flanks of the Tryon (A) implant, the S_a values decreased, apparently due to flattening of the surface irregularities. The fact that roughness parameters were calculated in the different regions (tops, flanks, and valleys) enabled identifying different phenomena occurring during insertion, i.e., flattening of asperities at the flanks and tops of some implants and debris accumulation at the valleys of some implants. Another possible reason for changes in S_a after the insertion process is the accommodation of smaller bone debris in the valleys of the surface topography, but this should be accompanied by an increase in the values of S_{sk}, which did not occur, as described below.

The parameters associated with height distribution of surface irregularities are S_{sk} and S_{ku}. The parameter S_{sk} is associated with asymmetry of the height distribution curve, where curves with approximately normal distribution

TABLE 2: Surface roughness parameters (S_a, S_{sk}, S_{ku}, S_{tr} and S_{dq}) measured in three different areas (top, flank, and valley) in threaded implants before (B) and after (A) insertion into bone using laser interferometry. Mean values ±standard deviation (SD) (* $p < 0.05$ between implants before and after insertion).

Implant	Before (B) after (A)	Top	Flank	Valley	Δ total (B-A)
S_a μm					
Strong	B	0.21 ± 0.02	0.69 ± 0.11	0.57 ± 0.24	0.02
	A	0.55 ± 1.21	0.75 ± 0.31	1.35 ± 1.55*	
Stylus	B	0.23 ± 0.03	0.70 ± 0.10	0.26 ± 0.13	0.42
	A	0.16 ± 0.11*	0.99 ± 1.04	2.38 ± 3.85	
Tryon	B	0.48 ± 0.26	1.98 ± 0.68	0.10 ± 0.07	0.17
	A	0.47 ± 0.64	1.25 ± 0.46*	3.68 ± 2.46*	
S_{sk}					
Strong	B	−0.34 ± 0.31	0.06 ± 0.37	−0.12 ± 0.27	−0.01
	A	−0.20 ± 0.39	0.01 ± 0.31	−0.14 ± 0.38	
Stylus	B	−0.17 ± 0.19	0.07 ± 0.51	−0.13 ± 0.52	0.01
	A	−0.17 ± 0.20	0.06 ± 0.61	−0.63 ± 1.48	
Tryon	B	−0.12 ± 0.45	0.06 ± 0.57	−0.02 ± 0.32	−0.02
	A	−0.11 ± 0.61	0.19 ± 0.63	0.17 ± 0.82	
S_{ku}					
Strong	B	4.21 ± 1.45	3.23 ± 0.81	3.58 ± 0.49	−0.04
	A	13.54 ± 4.88	3.50 ± 0.73	3.40 ± 0.99	
Stylus	B	3.63 ± 0.50	3.36 ± 4.60	3.52 ± 1.06	−0.02
	A	6.99 ± 4.36*	9.54 ± 6.68*	17.64 ± 33.52*	
Tryon	B	4.60 ± 1.75	3.69 ± 1.78	3.01 ± 0.56	−0.05
	A	8.48 ± 7.18*	4.72 ± 3.21	4.92 ± 5.89	
S_{tr} μm					
Strong	B	0.21 ± 0.05	0.10 ± 0,13	0.17 ± 0.07	0.01
	A	0.22 ± 0.14	0.05 ± 0,06	0.19 ± 0.18	
Stylus	B	0.21 ± 0.05	0.08 ± 0.01	0.09 ± 0.03	0.01
	A	0.21 ± 0.11	0.03 ± 0.02*	0.03 ± 0.02*	
Tryon	B	0.15 ± 0.10	0.11 ± 0.11	0.08 ± 0.02	−0.01
	A	0.15 ± 0.10	0.04 ± 0.01*	0.04 ± 0.02*	
S_{dq} μm					
Strong	B	0.03 ± 0.03	1.12 ± 0.19	0.40 ± 0.08	−0.05
	A	0.53 ± 0.34*	1.20 ± 0.58	2.07 ± 2.30*	
Stylus	B	0.42 ± 0.05	1.14 ± 1.11	5.02 ± 2.27	0.53
	A	0.36 ± 0.11*	1.80 ± 1.66*	4.67 ± 7.14	
Tryon	B	0.85 ± 0.46	3.15 ± 1.11	1.15 ± 0.40	−0.01
	A	0.88 ± 0.99	1.95 ± 0.73*	5.77 ± 4.40*	

present S_{sk} values close to 0. S_{ku} is associated with the flatness of the height distribution curve, where curves with approximately normal distribution have S_{ku} values close to 3. All implant regions of B and A showed S_{sk} values close to 0 and S_{ku} values close to 3 (Table 2). The S_{sk} values for all implants B and A showed no significant changes (Table 2).

Since all regions of all implants showed values close to 0, no top or valley predominance was observed in any region of the implants before or after placement. The deviations of S_{sk} from 0 (corresponding to a normal distribution), whether slightly positive or negative, may be considered too small to represent any relevant asymmetry [54]. Although S_{ku} values for top and flank increased across all implants after insertion into bone, such findings do not represent physical significance overall, indicating only discrete deformation at the top surfaces. The mean S_{ku} values were close to 3 in all regions for all (B) implants. There was a mild increase in these values for the top, flank, and valley of the Stylus (A) implant and to the top of the Tryon (A) implant. Such an increase in S_{ku} values may be due to surface roughness modifications during the insertion process [42–44], creating a small number of very sharp peaks. S_{ku} values close to 3, presented together with S_{sk} values close to 0, confirm that the distribution of irregularity heights is close to a normal distribution, regardless of macrogeometry or implant region.

As these parameters may vary greatly with discrete changes in topography, such as residues, it is prudent to evaluate a plot of morphological space $S_{ku} \times S_{sk}$ before and after bone insertion rather than numbers alone [55]. Figure 5 shows the $S_{ku} \times S_{sk}$ morphological space for all the different regions of each implant analyzed before (B) and after (A) insertion. For all the tops, shown in the plot with the symbols "∗," S_{ku} values increased. The flattening effect due to possible plastic deformation observed for the tops of the implants results that the vast majority of the asperities have similar heights, with the presence of very few sharp peaks, which increases S_{ku}. For the flanks of the Stylus implant, S_{ku} also increased after bone insertion, but no evident flattening mechanism was detected from the SEM images. This increase might be simply due the presence of

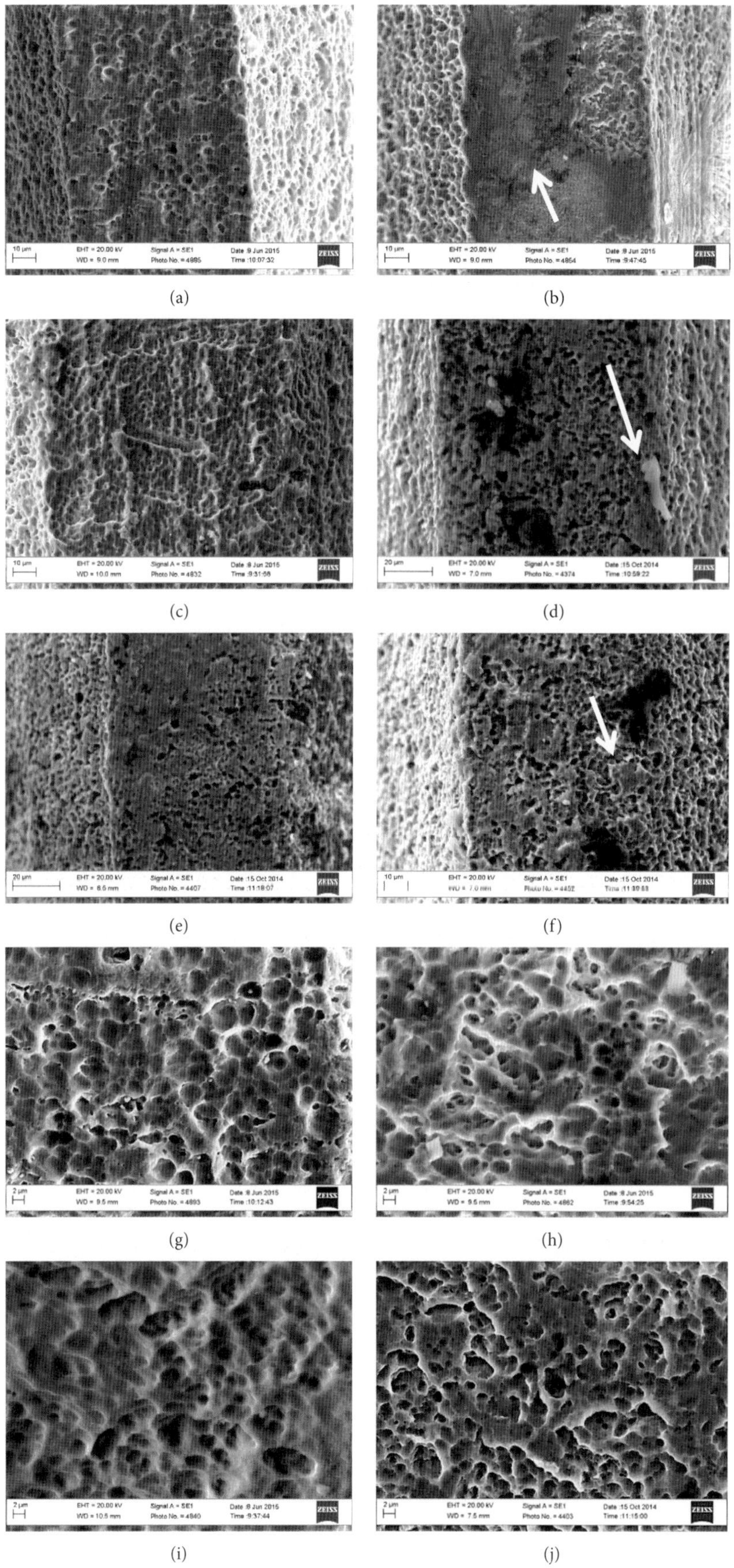

Figure 4: Continued.

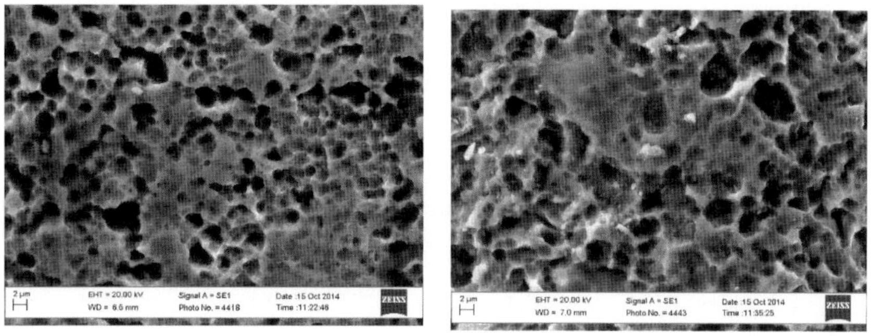

(k) (l)

FIGURE 4: Representative images of the implants prior to placement (a–c) and after removal from the bone (d–f). Although the images are very similar qualitatively in both conditions, it is possible to observe discrete deformation (arrow, (f)) and residue (arrow, (d)) on the implant surface after insertion/removal (A). Surface treatment in some implants appears not effective in covering all regions, such as those indicated by the arrow in Figure 4(b), which has a different surface topography. When the thread tops were seen at higher magnification, their surface morphology was very similar across all implants (g–i). After insertion (A), minimal changes may be noticed, suggesting small plastic deformation in surface irregularities for the three different implants (j–l).

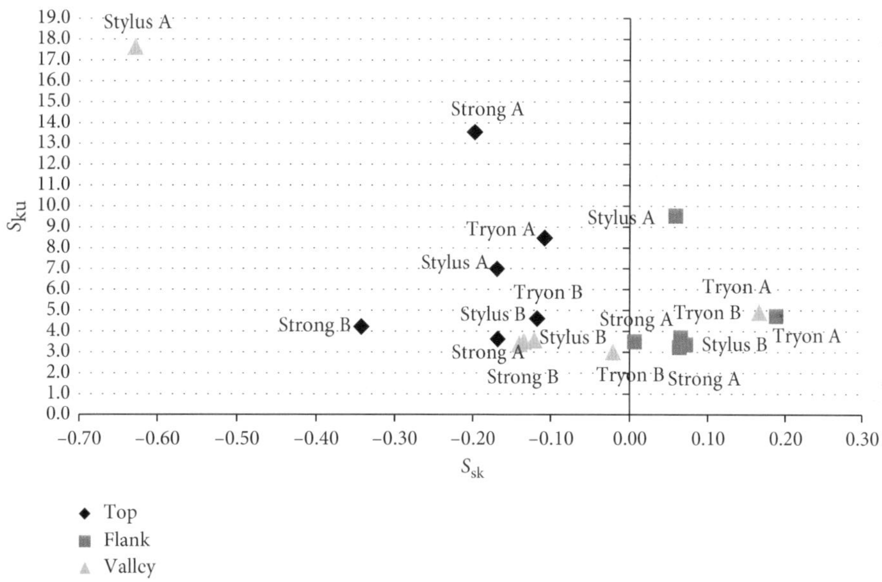

FIGURE 5: Morphological space of the parameters $S_{sk}(x) \times S_{ku}(y)$ for implants B and A.

a few residues such as bone debris, so that, in comparison with the large debris, the heights of the other asperities seem “flattened.”

To quantify the texture strength, i.e., the uniformity of surface texture, the parameter S_{tr} was used, which evaluates the texture aspect ratio of the surfaces. Values of $S_{tr} > 0.5$ indicate a uniform texture in all directions, i.e., the surface is topographically isotropic; whereas $S_{tr} < 0.3$ indicates strong directionality of the texture (anisotropy) [49]. The results for implants B and A are shown in Table 2. Initially, it was observed that all implants presented $S_{tr} < 0.3$, i.e., strong anisotropy. All implants B and A presented lower S_{tr} values for the flanks and valleys compared with the tops, suggesting a more evident directionality in these regions. After insertion into bone, all implants maintained their anisotropic surface characteristics in all regions. The flanks and valleys of the Stylus and Tryon implants increased their directionality after insertion into bone, presenting a significant reduction in S_{tr} values (Stylus flank, $p = 0.000$ and $p = 0.000$; Tryon flank, $p = 0.008$ and $p = 0.000$). It was verified that the same surface treatment in different implants resulted in differences in roughness parameters, due probably to variables relating to the double-etching process itself, particularly depending on the macrogeometry of the implant and the thread region within each implant. In general, implants B and A maintained their anisotropic characteristics. Moreover, as this study did not apply reverse torque for implant removal, as suggested by Mint [42] and Senna [44], the results presented herein are more reliable when compared with the Salerno study [43], where values of topography deformation did not show any significant change, due probably to the process of removal, which was based on reverse torque.

The S_{dq} values, which represent the mean square values of the roughness slopes, are also shown in Table 2. In general, the flanks and the valleys showed roughness with steeper inclination. After bone insertion, (A) implants showed increased S_{dq} values at the tops for all macrogeometries, but only the Strong and Stylus implants were statistically different after placement into bone ($p = 0.035$ and $p = 0.004$, respectively). Particular attention should be given to the tops of the Strong implant, which showed large increase in the slope of the asperities after bone insertion. It was previously postulated that the contact pressures acting on the tops are higher during bone insertion for this implant due to the reduced top area, and therefore, it is plausible the presence of steeper asperities after bone implantation (Figure 4(b)) and it can be noted that surface finish treatment did not produce a regular topography on the top of those implants. The highest and most dispersed values for S_{dq} were observed in the flanks and valleys of the Stylus A and Tryon A implants, and after insertion into the bone, the top of the Stylus and the flank of the Tryon implants were the only regions that showed a significant reduction ($p = .004$ and $p = .000$, respectively).

The present study characterized the surface topography of implants using laser interferometry and scanning electron microscopy before and after insertion into the porcine rib bone. Differences in topography were observed, depending on the area and macrogeometry of the implant. After insertion into bone, surface topography subtly changed in different regions of the screws for all evaluated implants. Within the limitations of this *in vitro* evaluation, it could be observed that the methodology applied herein seemed appropriate for quantitative surface evaluation of different screw-type implants.

3.2. Cell Assays. Representative results of the cell proliferation assay are expressed in Table 3, and all showed $p > 0.05$ by the Wilcoxon test.

At 24 h, 48 h, and 96 h, no significant difference was observed between the groups before and after placement of the implants into the porcine bone ($p > 0.05$) for the three types of implants evaluated.

For the cell viability assay, the mean absorbance values (±standard deviation) generated by the test (at 24 h, 48 h, and 96 h) showed no significant difference between groups (B) and (A) for the three types of implants evaluated ($p > 0.05$). Values are presented in Table 4, and all presented $p > 0.05$ on the Wilcoxon test.

Surface treatments, such as double acid etching, may influence cell adhesion, morphology, and proliferation, with a significant increase in osteoblastic cell activity and biocompatibility on porous coatings, favoring the osseointegration process [53, 55]. The surface evaluated in

Table 3: Mean (±standard deviation) of cell proliferation on implants B and A by the trypan blue vital exclusion method in osteoblasts.

Time	Cell × 10^4 mean ± SD	Cell × 10^4 mean ± SD
	Strong B	*Strong A*
24 h	1.25 ± 0.46	1.77 ± 0.45
48 h	5.25 ± 0.34	4.07 ± 0.26
96 h	8.22 ± 0.22	8.14 ± 0.56
	Stylus B	*Stylus A*
24 h	2.14 ± 0.46	1.48 ± 0.25
48 h	5.62 ± 0.25	4.22 ± 0.22
96 h	8.81 ± 0.46	9.03 ± 0.26
	Tryon B	*Tryon A*
24 h	2.07 ± 0.13	1.63 ± 0.34
48 h	6.00 ± 0.23	3.55 ± 0.22
96 h	8.88 ± 0.67	9.40 ± 0.34

this study had roughness with different characteristics for top, flank, and valley. Nevertheless, cell proliferation and cell viability results showed no significant differences among any of the implant types before and after placement into bone at the time points evaluated.

Osteopontin is a phosphorylated and sulfated glycoprotein, secreted by several cell types including osteoblasts, allowing adhesion of such cells to the extracellular matrix [56, 57]. It is described as an early marker of bone development and osteoblastic differentiation, expressing strongly in the immature matrix, mineralization fronts, having greater expression in osteoblasts [57]. Based on the ELISA assay, the results for osteopontin secretion by the preosteoblastic cells on the different surfaces are shown in Table 5, and all of them presented $p > 0.05$ by the Wilcoxon test.

The results revealed no change in osteopontin expression on any of the surfaces tested ($p > 0.05$). A slight increase in osteopontin at 96 hours could be observed for the three types of implants after installation into the porcine rib, although this did not reach statistical significance. Despite a slight increase in osteopontin at 96 h for all macrogeometries in the implants (B), no difference was significant for the implants (A) at any evaluated time.

As the cell culture method kept the implants in a horizontal position, sedimentation of cells occurred into the valleys and flanks of the threads. Within this study, this factor is regarded as a limitation because it was not possible to accurately assess the behavior of cells at the top, flank, and valley separately, as per the physical surface analysis. In order to assess whether the surface modification caused by insertion into bone alters cell behavior, such methodology was, however, efficient.

Therefore, within the limitations of this study, the results showed herein revealed no significant difference in cell behavior for implant surface before and after the placement of the implant into bone. For future studies, the cell culture method should be optimized to prevent cell sedimentation within the implant threads.

Table 4: Mean (±standard deviation) of cell viability using the MTT assay in osteoblasts.

Time	Optical density = 590 nm mean ± SD	Optical density = 590 nm mean ± SD
	Strong A	*Strong D*
24 h	0.16 ± 0.00	0.11 ± 0.01
48 h	0.40 ± 0.03	0.30 ± 0.03
96 h	0.82 ± 0.02	0.73 ± 0.06
	Stylus A	*Stylus D*
24 h	0.15 ± 0.01	0.12 ± 0.02
48 h	0.39 ± 0.03	0.29 ± 0.04
96 h	1.00 ± 0.00	0.58 ± 0.09
	Tryon A	*Tryon D*
24 h	0.16 ± 0.02	0.11 ± 0.00
48 h	0.39 ± 0.01	0.30 ± 0.03
96 h	0.87 ± 0.01	0.73 ± 0.13

Table 5: Mean (±standard deviation) in pg/mL of osteopontin synthesis on implants B and A as quantified via the ELISA assay.

Time	Mean ± SD	Mean ± SD
	Strong B	*Strong A*
24 h	986.28 ± 81.42	1103.2 ± 34.21
48 h	156.75 ± 27.99	1321.12 ± 117.46
96 h	1224.72 ± 161.74	1941.33 ± 107.66
	Stylus B	*Stylus A*
24 h	1120.01 ± 54.63	1222.85 ± 15.38
48 h	1891.62 ± 54.72	1266.86 ± 104.97
96 h	1292.05 ± 59.8	1935.2 ± 116.28
	Tryon B	*Tryon A*
24 h	964.15 ± 220.98	1171.05 ± 96.22
48 h	1769.25 ± 146.94	1390.77 ± 159.43
96 h	1360.34 ± 58.66	2078.06 ± 131.64

4. Conclusions

A subtle change in surface roughness was detected on implants after insertion into bone for all the macrogeometries tested, without significantly affecting the cellular parameters studied.

Acknowledgments

The authors wish to thank Pollyanna Tombini Montaldi for her excellent technical expertise.

References

[1] A. Schroeder, E. Van der Zypen, H. Stich et al., "The reactions of bone, connective tissue, and epithelium to endosteal implants with titanium-sprayed surfaces," *Journal of Maxillofacial Surgery*, vol. 22, no. 2, pp. 135–142, 2011.

[2] T. Albrektsson and A. Wennerberg, "Oral implant surfaces: part 1—review focusing on topographic and chemical properties of different surfaces and in vivo responses to them," *International Journal of Prosthodontic*, vol. 17, no. 5, pp. 536–543, 2004.

[3] P. Papaspyridakos, C. J. Chen, M. Singh et al., "Success criteria in implant dentistry: a systematic review," *Journal of Dental Research*, vol. 91, no. 3, pp. 242–248, 2012.

[4] L. Carlsson, T. Röstlund, B. Albrektsson et al., "Osseointegration of titanium implants," *Acta Orthopaedica Scandinavica*, vol. 57, no. 4, pp. 285–289, 1986.

[5] M. Esposito, J. M. Hirsch, U. Lekholm et al., "Biological factors contributing to failures of osseointegrated oral implants (II): Etiopathogenesis," *European Journal of Oral Sciences*, vol. 106, no. 3, pp. 721–764, 1998.

[6] L. Le Guéhennec, A. Soueidan, P. Layrolle et al., "Surface treatments of titanium dental implants for rapid osseointegration," *Dental Materials*, vol. 23, no. 7, pp. 844–854, 2007.

[7] T. Albrektsson, P. I. Branemark, H. A. Hansson, and J. Lindstrom, "Osseointegrated titanium implants. Requirements for ensuring a long-lasting, direct bone-to-implant anchorage in man," *Acta Orthopaedica Scandinavica*, vol. 52, no. 2, pp. 155–170, 1981.

[8] V. Bucci-Sabattini, C. Cassinelli, P. G. Coelho et al., "Effect of titanium implant surface nanoroughness and calcium phosphate low impregnation on bone cell activity in vitro," *Oral Surgery, Oral Medicine, Oral Pathology, Oral Radiology, and Endodontology*, vol. 109, no. 2, pp. 217–224, 2010.

[9] L. Meirelles, *On Nano Size Structures for Enhanced Early Bone Formation*, Department of Prosthodontics/Dental Material

Science, Department of Biomaterials, Göteborg University, Göteborg, Sweden, 2007.

[10] A. Wennerberg and T. Albrektsson, "A review of current knowledge, opinions and suggestions for possible common mechanisms behind the increased bone response reported to different types of modern oral implant surfaces," *International Journal of Oral & Maxillofacial Implants*, vol. 25, pp. 63–74, 2010.

[11] N. Deyneka-Dupriez, B. Kocdemir, U. Herr et al., "Interfacial shear strength of titanium implants in bone is significantly improved by surface topographies with high pit density and microroughness," *Journal of Biomedical Materials Research Part B: Applied Biomaterials*, vol. 82, no. 2, pp. 305–312, 2007.

[12] T. J. Webster and J. U. Ejiofor, "Increased osteoblast adhesion on nanophase metals: Ti, Ti_6Al_4V, and CoCrMo," *Biomaterials*, vol. 25, no. 19, pp. 4731–4739, 2004.

[13] P. Trisi, R. Lazzara, A. Rebaudi, W. Rao, T. Testori, and S. S. Porter, "Bone implant contact on machined and dual acid-etched surfaces after 2 months of healing in the human maxilla," *Journal of Periodontology*, vol. 74, no. 7, pp. 945–956, 2003.

[14] A. Rebaudi, "The ray setting procedure: a new method for implant planning and immediate prosthesis delivery," *International Journal of Periodontics & Restorative Dentistry*, vol. 27, no. 3, pp. 267–275, 2007.

[15] R. Beutner, J. Michael, B. Schwenzer, and D. Scharnweber, "Biological nano-functionalization of titanium-based biomaterial surfaces: a flexible toolbox," *Journal of The Royal Society Interface*, vol. 7, no. 1, pp. S93–S105, 2010.

[16] R. R. Barros, A. B. Novaes, V. Papalexiou et al., "Effect of biofunctionalized implant surface on osseointegration: a histomorphometric study in dogs," *Brazilian Dental Journal*, vol. 20, no. 2, pp. 91–98, 2009.

[17] R. Lutz, S. Srour, J. Nonhoff, T. Weisel, C. J. Damien, and K. A. Schlegel, "Biofunctionalization of titanium implants with a biomimetic active peptide (P-15) promotes early osseointegration," *Clinical Oral Implants Research*, vol. 21, no. 7, pp. 726–734, 2010.

[18] P. I. Brånemark, "Osseointegration and its experimental background," *Journal of Prosthetic Dentistry*, vol. 50, no. 3, pp. 399–410, 1983.

[19] K. Anselme, M. Bigerelle, B. Noel et al., "Qualitative and quantitative study of human osteoblast adhesion on materials with various surface roughnesses," *Journal of Biomedical Materials Research*, vol. 49, no. 2, pp. 155–166, 2000.

[20] A. Wennerberg and T. Albrektsson, "Effects of titanium surface topography on bone integration: a systematic review," *Clinical Oral Implants Research*, vol. 20, no. 4, pp. 172–184, 2009.

[21] P. G. Coelho, R. Granato, C. Marin, and H. S. Teixeira, "The effect of different implant macrogeometries and surface treatment in early biomechanical fixation: an experimental study in dogs," *Journal of the Mechanical Behavior of Biomedical Materials*, vol. 4, no. 8, pp. 1974–1981, 2011.

[22] D. Deporter, "Dental implant design and optimal treatment outcomes," *International Journal of Periodontics and Restorative Dentistry*, vol. 29, no. 6, pp. 625–633, 2009.

[23] M. Degidi and A. Piattelli, "7-year follow-up of 93 immediately loaded titanium dental implants," *Journal of Oral Implantology*, vol. 31, no. 1, pp. 25–31, 2005.

[24] F. Javed and G. E. Romanos, "The role of primary stability for successful immediate loading of dental implants: a literature review," *Journal of Dentistry*, vol. 38, no. 8, pp. 612–620, 2010.

[25] C. E. Misch, "Density of bone: effect on treatment plans, surgical approach, healing, and progressive bone loading," *International Journal of Oral Implantology*, vol. 6, no. 2, pp. 23–31, 1990.

[26] C. E. Misch, M. L. Perel, H. L. Wang et al., "Implant success, survival, and failure: the international congress of oral implantologists (ICOI) pisa consensus conference," *Implant Dentistry*, vol. 17, no. 1, pp. 5–15, 2008.

[27] C. N. Elias, F. A. Rocha, A. L. Nascimento, and P. G. Coelho, "Influence of implant shape, surface morphology, surgical technique and bone quality on the primary stability of dental implants," *Journal of the Mechanical Behavior of Biomedical Materials*, vol. 16, pp. 169–180, 2012.

[28] J. E. Lemons, R. M. Meffert, J. A. Hahn, J. T. Krauser, and R. A. James, "HA-coated root-form implants-is there cause for concern?," *Dental Implantology Update*, vol. 4, no. 5, pp. 37–42, 1993.

[29] J. Steigenga, K. Al-Shammari, C. Misch, F. H. Nociti, and H. L. Wang, "Effects of implant thread geometry on percentage of osseointegration and resistance to reverse torque in the tibia of rabbits," *Journal of Periodontology*, vol. 75, no. 9, pp. 1233–1241, 2004.

[30] M. V. Cardoso, K. Vandamme, A. Chaudhari et al., "Dental implant macro-design features can impact the dynamics of osseointegration," *Clinical Implant Dentistry and Related Research*, vol. 17, no. 4, pp. 639–645, 2015.

[31] A. Wennerberg and T. Albrektsson, "Suggested guidelines for the topographic evaluation of implant surfaces," *International Journal of Oral & Maxillofacial Implants*, vol. 15, no. 3, pp. 331–344, 2000.

[32] M. B. Rosa, T. Albrektsson, C. E. Francischone, H. O. Filho, and A. Wennerberg, "Micrometric characterization of the implant surfaces from the five largest companies in Brazil, the second largest worldwide implant market," *International Journal of Oral & Maxillofacial Implants*, vol. 28, no. 2, pp. 358–365, 2013.

[33] T. P. Barbosa, M. M. Naves, H. H. M. Menezes, P. H. C. Pinto, D. B. de Mello, and H. L. Costa, "Topography and surface energy of dental implants: a methodological approach," *Journal of the Brazilian Society of Mechanical Sciences and Engineering*, vol. 39, no. 6, pp. 1895–1907, 2017.

[34] A. N. Natali, E. L. Carniel, and P. G. Pavan, "Investigation of viscoelastoplastic response of bone tissue in oral implants press fit process," *Journal of Biomedical Materials Research Part B: Applied Biomaterials*, vol. 91, no. 2, pp. 868–875, 2009.

[35] A. N. Natali, E. L. Carniel, and P. G. Pavan, "Dental implants press fit phenomenon: biomechanical analysis considering bone inelastic response," *Dental Materials*, vol. 25, no. 5, pp. 573–581, 2009.

[36] K. Akca, T. L. Chang, I. Tekdemir, and M. I. Fanuscu, "Biomechanical aspects of initial intraosseous stability and implant design: a quantitative micro-morphometric analysis," *Clinical Oral Implants Research*, vol. 17, no. 4, pp. 465–472, 2006.

[37] T. Irinakis and C. Wiebe, "Initial torque stability of a new bone condensing dental implant. A cohort study of 140 consecutively placed implants," *Journal of Oral Implantology*, vol. 35, no. 6, pp. 277–282, 2009.

[38] D. Rodrigo, L. Aracil, C. Martin, and M. Sanz, "Diagnosis of implant stability and its impact on implant survival: a prospective case series study," *Clinical Oral Implants Research*, vol. 21, no. 3, pp. 255–261, 2010.

[39] J. Duyck, L. Corpas, S. Vermeiren et al., "Histological, histomorphometrical, and radiological evaluation of an

experimental implant design with a high insertion torque," *Clinical Oral Implants Research*, vol. 21, no. 8, pp. 877–884, 2010.

[40] A. Tabassum, G. J. Meijer, J. G. C. Wolke, and J. A. Jansen, "Influence of surgical technique and surface roughness on the primary stability of an implant in artificial bone with different cortical thickness: a laboratory study," *Clinical Oral Implants Research*, vol. 21, no. 2, pp. 213–220, 2010.

[41] A. P. R. Filho, F. S. F. Fernandes, F. G. Straioto, W. J. Silva, and A. A. Del Bel Cury, "Preload loss and bacterial penetration on different implant-abutment connection systems," *Brazilian Dental Journal*, vol. 21, no. 2, pp. 123–129, 2010.

[42] D. Mints, C. Elias, P. Funkenbusch et al., "Integrity of implant surface modifications after insertion," *International Journal of Oral & Maxillofacial Implants*, vol. 29, no. 1, pp. 97–104, 2014.

[43] M. Salerno, A. Itri, M. Frezzato, and A. Rebaudi, "Surface microstructure of dental implants before and after insertion: an in vitro study by means of scanning probe microscopy," *Implant Dentistry*, vol. 24, no. 3, pp. 248–255, 2015.

[44] P. Senna, A. A. Del Bel Cury, S. Kates et al., "Surface damage on dental implants with release of loose particles after insertion into bone," *Clinical Implant Dentistry and Related Research*, vol. 17, no. 4, pp. 681–692, 2015.

[45] C. E. Misch, "Implant design considerations for the posterior regions of the mouth," *Implant Dentistry*, vol. 8, no. 4, pp. 376–386, 1999.

[46] C. Ercoli, P. D. Funkenbusch, H. J. Lee, M. E. Moss, and G. N. Graser, "The influence of drill wear on cutting efficiency and heat production during osteotomy preparation for dental implants: a study of drill durability," *International Journal of Oral & Maxillofacial Implants*, vol. 19, no. 3, pp. 335–349, 2004.

[47] B. H. Harris and S. S. Kohles, "Effects of mechanical and thermal fatigue on dental drill performance," *International Journal of Oral & Maxillofacial Implants*, vol. 16, no. 6, pp. 819–826, 2001.

[48] M. M. Naves, H. H. M. Menezes, D. Magalhães et al., "Effect of macrogeometry on the surface topography of dental implants," *International Journal of Oral & Maxillofacial Implants*, vol. 30, no. 4, pp. 789–799, 2015.

[49] K. J. Stout, P. J. Sullivan, W. P. Dong et al., *The Development of Methods for the Characterization of Roughness in Three Dimensions*, University of Birmingham and L'Ecole Centrale de Lyon, Pub no. EUR 15178EN, Penton press, Cleveland, OH, USA, 1993.

[50] E. F. Martinez, G. J. Ishikawa, A. B. de Lemos, F. J. Barbosa Bezerra, M. Sperandio, and M. H. Napimoga, "Evaluation of a titanium surface treated with hydroxyapatite nanocrystals on osteoblastic cell behavior: an in vitro study," *International Journal of Oral & Maxillofacial Implants*, vol. 33, no. 3, pp. 597–602, 2018.

[51] D. Kilpadi and J. Lemons, "Surface energy characterization of unalloyed titanium implants," *Journal of Biomedical Materials Research*, vol. 28, no. 12, pp. 1419–1425, 1994.

[52] S. Vercaigne, J. G. C. Wolke, I. Naert, and J. A. Jansen, "The effect of titanium plasma-sprayed implants on trabecular bone healing in the goat," *Biomaterials*, vol. 19, no. 11-12, pp. 1093–1099, 1998.

[53] C. N. Elias and L. Meirelles, "Improving osseointegration of dental implants," *Expert Review of Medical Devices*, vol. 7, no. 2, pp. 241–256, 2010.

[54] W. P. Dong, P. J. Sullivan, and K. J. Stout, "Comprehensive study of parameters for characterizing 3-dimensional surface-topography. 3. Parameters for characterizing amplitude and some functional-properties," *Wear*, vol. 178, no. 1-2, pp. 29–43, 1994.

[55] J. D. B. De Mello, M. Durand-Charre, and T. Mathia, "Abrasion mechanisms of white cast iron II: influence of the metallurgical structure of V-Cr white cast irons," *Materials Science and Engineering*, vol. 78, no. 2, pp. 127–134, 1986.

[56] J. E. Aubin, "Advances in the osteoblast lineage," *Biochemistry and Cell Biology*, vol. 76, no. 6, pp. 899–910, 1998.

[57] Y. Sasano, H. C. Li, J. X. Zhu, K. Imanaka-Yoshida, I. Mizoguchi, and M. Kagayama, "Immunohistochemical localization of type I collagen, fibronectin and tenascin C during embryonic osteogenesis in the dentary of mandibles and tibias in rats," *Histochemical Journal*, vol. 32, no. 10, pp. 591–598, 2000.

Impact of Orthognathic Surgery on Quality of Life in Patients with Dentofacial Deformities

Faezeh Eslamipour,[1] Arash Najimi,[2] Azade Tadayonfard,[3] and Zeinab Azamian[4]

[1] *Torabinejad Dental Research Center, Department of Oral Public Health, School of Dentistry, Isfahan University of Medical Sciences, Isfahan, Iran*
[2] *Department of Medical Education, Medical Education Research Center, Isfahan University of Medical Sciences, Isfahan, Iran*
[3] *Department of Prosthodontics, School of Dentistry, Shahid Beheshti University of Medical Sciences, Tehran, Iran*
[4] *Department of Orthodontics, School of Dentistry, Isfahan University of Medical Sciences, Isfahan, Iran*

Correspondence should be addressed to Azade Tadayonfard; azdtadayon@gmail.com

Academic Editor: Vincent Everts

The aim of this investigation was to determine the impact of orthognathic surgery on quality of life in patients with dentofacial deformities at immediate presurgery and at 3-week, 3-month, and 6-month intervals following the surgery. Subjects included forty-three 18–40-year-old Iranian orthognathic patients who were referred to private offices in Isfahan. Data collection was performed using the 22-item Orthognathic Quality of Life Questionnaire (OQLQ). Participants completed the questionnaire prior to surgery and 3 weeks, 3 months, and 6 months after it. Differences and correlations were calculated by the two-tailed t-test, ANOVA with Repeated Measure test, and the Pearson correlation coefficient. The results showed significant reduction returned to baseline in OQLQ mean scores and aesthetic, awareness, and social subdomains in all 3 intervals after surgery. However oral function domain showed an increase at T_2 and then a decrease at next intervals. Maximum and minimum effect size were observed in aesthetic (ES = 0.7) and oral function (ES = 0.3) domain, respectively. Based on the finding of this study, in 6-month interval after surgery, orthognathic surgery causes significant improvements in quality of life in patients with dentofacial deformities as assessed in emotional, psychological, oral function, and social domains and maximum changes occurred in emotional domain.

1. Introduction

Dentofacial deformities have been described as changes that primarily affect the jaws and teeth, although the multiple craniofacial structures may also be affected [1]. In most cases, they are the result of moderate or severe genetic distortions of the normal development process (such as mandibular prognathism, bimaxillary prognathism or retrognathism, maxillary vertical excess) and should be corrected using an integrated treatment of orthodontics and orthognathic surgery in adult orthodontic [2]. Some study reported these deformities affect 20% of the population with various degrees of functional and esthetic compromise [3]. In a study, Proffit and White revealed that a large part of the population in the USA suffer from significant malocclusion. In many of these cases, the facial proportions were abnormal and approximately 5% were so severe that the patients could be regarded as handicapped [4]. Borzabadi-Farahani et al. reported that 36% of Iranian young population need orthodontic treatment and nearly 12% of them had severe malocclusion which needs compound orthodontics and orthognathic surgery treatments [5, 6].

One of the important risk factors in low appearance self-esteem is determined to be severe dentofacial deformity [7]. Over the years, the patients with dentofacial deformities have lower mean quality of life values in comparison with those who have not [8]. At present, the combination of the two treatment modalities, maxillofacial surgery and orthodontics, is one of the most important parts in the corrective treatment of malocclusion and facial deformities [9]. Current advances in diagnostic and planning methods and surgical techniques have made orthognathic surgery safe and common for treating these deformities [10]. Modern fixation techniques (i.e., internal rigid fixation) and improvements in facial esthetics have increased patients' trust in this type of surgery, resulting in an increased demand for orthognathic procedures [11].

Patients' motivation for the surgical option is the hope for improvement of their quality of life [12]. The information about the effect of orthognathic surgery on patients during the recovery phase enables surgeons to better inform patients on their expectations from surgery [13].

Al-Bitar et al. in a study revealed that Jordanian patients with dentofacial deformities as an Arab population had generally lower score and therefore a poorer QOL than reported in British, Japanese, and Chinese populations. They concluded that these differences may be cultural or may be due to differences in healthcare system's criteria for funding. The differences may refer to socially and culturally unique definitions and concepts of health and quality of life and awareness of higher level needs [13]. Due to paucity of published studies investigating QOL in Iranian orthognathic patients, the aim of this study was to determine changes in QOL among Iranian patients with dentofacial deformities who had undergone orthognathic surgery after completion of presurgical orthodontic treatment for dental decompensation.

2. Methods

2.1. Participants. This prospective study was carried out on sixty 18–40-year-old orthognathic patients who had completed presurgical orthodontic phase in the orthodontists private offices in Isfahan, Iran, and were scheduled to undergo orthognathic surgery. A convenient sampling was used. All the subjects mainly had sagittal and/or vertical discrepancy or asymmetric jaw relation and underwent bimaxillary osteotomies. Exclusion criteria were patients with cleft lip and palate or craniofacial syndromes, patients who were scheduled to undergo orthognathic surgery without orthodontic treatment or with additional features, e.g., genioplasty or distraction device, and patients reluctant to participate in the study. The study trend was approved by the research committee, Faculty of dentistry, Isfahan University of Medical Sciences, Iran (no. 388488). The research protocol was described to patients and a written consent was obtained before participating in the study. This study has been conducted in full accordance with the World Medical Association Declaration of Helsinki.

2.2. Instruments and Data Collection. Data were collected using self-administered 22-item Orthognathic Quality of Life Questionnaire (OQLQ a condition-specific QOL assessment). The Orthognathic Quality of Life Questionnaire (OQLQ) was developed as an instrument to estimate quality of life in patients treated with orthognathic surgery in 2000 and validated in 2002 by Cunningham et al. [14, 15].

The questionnaire was translated into Persian using a standardized forward-backward linguistic translation method. The content validity of the questionnaire was approved by orthodontic and psychiatric specialists. In a pilot study the face validity was checked and the internal consistency reliability was assessed by measuring Cronbach's alpha ($\alpha = 0.93$).

The OQLQ questionnaire consists of 22 questions which is rated on a 5-point Likert scale ranging from "does not bother me at all" (score 0) to "bothers me a lot" (score 4). The total score is 0 to 88. A lower score indicates a better QOL and vice versa. This questionnaire consists of 4 subscales: aesthetic impact (items 1, 7, 10, 11, and 14, range 0 to 20), oral function (2 to 6, range 0 to 20), awareness impact (8, 9, 12, and 13, range 0 to 16), and social impact (items 15 to 22, range 0 to 32).

The questionnaire was distributed to the patients and asked them to complete it during their routine visits in orthodontist offices at 4 times (T_1–T_4), first, the last visit before surgery (about 10–20 days before surgery), second, in 3 weeks after surgery, third, in 3 months after surgery, and the last, 6 months after surgery. Before completing the questionnaire by patients, instructions were given regarding the study.

In the copy of the last questionnaire, which the patients filled 6 months after surgery, global measures were included to rate patient satisfaction with two questions as follows: "How would you rate your satisfaction with the outcome? Rate your satisfaction with a score from 0 to 5 where 0 means completely dissatisfied and 5 means completely satisfied." The other question was "would you recommend this surgery to other people?" with a "yes" or "no" answer. The average time for a patient to fill the questionnaire ranged from 5 to 7 minutes.

2.3. Data Analysis. Data were analyzed using the statistical software SPSS version 18 (Inc., Chicago, IL) The Kolmogorov Smirnov normality test was performed to determine if the samples conformed to a normal distribution. Differences between subgroups and correlations between QOL as dependent variables and age, sex, skeletal problem, and level of their education as independent variables were calculated by the two-tailed t-test. Regarding nonnormal distribution of OQLQ and its subdomains scores, Friedman and Wilcoxon analysis were performed. The magnitude of the statistical difference in scores was determined by calculating effect sizes (ES); ES (effect size) was calculated with division of mean changes by standard deviation for evaluating the efficacy of orthognathic surgery in terms of clinical importance on patient's quality of life. An ES of less than 0.2 is considered as minimal; 0.2 to 0.49 as small; 0.5 to 0.8 as moderate; and greater than 0.8 as large. The larger the ES, the greater the magnitude of change as a result of the intervention. A $P < 0.05$ was considered significant. Reliability analyses were conducted to assess the consistency by calculating Cronbach's alpha. To be evaluated as a reliable scale, an α of at least 0.70 was required.

3. Results

From sixty patients who agreed to participate in the study only 43 patients had completed the questionnaires at all-time points, which were used in the final analyses so the response rate was 71.6%. Demographic characteristics of patients are presented in Table 1.

Table 1: Demographic characteristics of patients.

Variables	N	(%)
Sex		
Male	13	30.2
Female	30	69.8
Age group		
≤25	31	72.1
>25	12	27.9
Problem		
Class II	13	30.2
Class III	30	69.8
Education		
≤Diploma	13	31.7
>Diploma	28	69.3

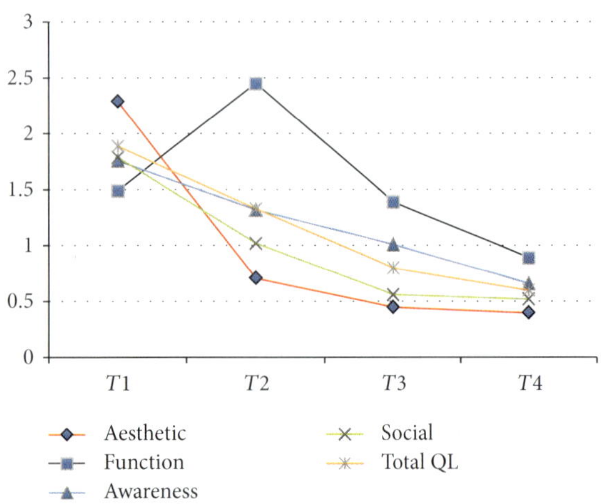

Figure 1: Mean of total OQLQ and subdomains (range 0–4) in different stage of treatment.

Mean change values of OQLQ and its subdomains scores in different stage of treatment are showed in Table 2. A significant reduction in OQLQ and all subdomains mean scores was observed over the trajectory of treatment (Figure 1).

There was not any statistically significant relation between OQLQ mean scores and demographic characteristics of samples except gender at presurgical stage T_1 and type of dentofacial problem at 6-month postsurgical stage T_4 (Table 3).

Based on our results effect size value of change in OQLQ was 0.63. Throughout the treatment period, variation in subdomain scores differed significantly compared with the baseline. Maximum and minimum ES were observed in aesthetic (ES = 0.7, $P < 0.001$) and oral function (ES = 0.3, $P = 0.001$) domain, respectively. An exception was seen in oral function domain over the time of assessment. It showed an increase at T_2 and then a decrease at T_3 and T_4 (Table 4).

At 6 months, 81.4% of patients reported their global satisfaction above 3 (score 0–5) and the mean score of it was 4.07 ± 1.18 and 79.1% claimed they would recommend the surgery to others.

4. Discussion

Patients with dentofacial deformities, who visit a clinic for the first time, frequently behave in a shy, defensive, and passive manner because of a lack of confidence in their appearance [12, 16]. Their appearance leads to impacts and influences on many aspects of life such as social interactions, chances when seeking employment, being chosen as a partner, and their personality characteristics; therefore it affects their QOL. In these patients orthognathic surgery has become more important because it has been widely performed to improve dentofacial deformities [17, 18].

This study showed that there were significant improvements in patients' quality of life both at 3 and 6 months after orthognathic surgery compared with baseline levels. This finding is consistent with similar studies conducted in China and USA using the same questionnaire [9, 19]. Moreover, this finding is supported by many other studies that show remarkable improvements in patients' wellbeing in different aspects including psychological, functional, social, emotional, and physical wellbeing [4, 7, 10, 15, 20–23]. These findings illustrate the effectiveness of orthognathic surgery beyond its complications like swelling, pain, and so forth.

In this study, at 6 months there was a significant improvement in QOL compared with 3 months' interval. This gradual postsurgical improvement is supported by Choi et al.'s study which reported moderate to large improvement in this interval [9].

In terms of different aspects of patients' QOL, maximum changes occurred in emotional domain and then social, psychological, and functional aspects, respectively. These results are similar to previous studies [3, 4, 9]. Based on our results minimum changes occurred in the functional domain and no significant change occurred as early as 3 months. This is also similar to the results of Choi et al. which revealed no significant or even some reduction in patient's short-term wellbeing after the surgery [9]. Desforges et al. showed that improvement in this domain occurred later than other domains [22]. This finding is expected, because surgical intervention is not without complication in itself. Pain, swelling, neurosensory disturbances, limitation in mouth opening, and reduced muscular efficiency are common morbidities [19, 20, 24, 25].

Previous studies comparing the total score of patients in pre- and postsurgical periods suggested that changes in self-esteem and self-confidence had occurred [4, 26, 27]. Some investigations reported that patients had received more psychological benefits such as improvement of body image, facial image [28], and higher interpersonal relationship [27].

The results indicate short-term effects of orthognathic surgery are more remarkable and rapid on emotional and social wellbeing rather than physical status. This can be a reflection of orthodontic treatment phase and also the patient's dental and neuromuscular adaptation. In terms of improvement period, minimum period was seen in emotional domain in the same early stages after the surgery [9, 29].

According to this study, women's overall QOL score in all four domains (specially, in emotional and social subscales) showed a poorer status compared with men before surgery.

TABLE 2: Mean values of OQLQ and its subdomains scores in different stage of treatment.

Variables	T_1 Mean (SD)	T_2 Mean (SD)	T_3 Mean (SD)	T_4 Mean (SD)
OQLQ (0–88)	40.5 (21.0)	29.2 (18.5)	17.6 (13.0)	13.1 (11.0)
Aesthetic (0–20)	11.4 (6.0)	3.6 (4.3)	2.3 (3.2)	2.0(2.9)
Function (0–20)	7.4 (5.1)	12.2 (5.5)	6.7 (4.8)	4.4(4.1)
Awareness (0–16)	7.0 (4.5)	5.1 (4.7)	4.0 (4.1)	2.5 (2.9)
Social (0–32)	14.5 (9.6)	8.1 (8.5)	4.5 (4.5)	4.1 (4.0)

TABLE 3: Mean OQLQ scores of the sample based on demographic characteristics and phase of treatment.

OQLQ	T_1 Mean ± SD	T_2 Mean ± SD	T_3 Mean ± SD	T_4 Mean ± SD
Sex				
Male	30.1 ± 20.9	24.0 ± 11.8	20.1 ± 16.0	10.0 ± 9.1
Female	45.0 ± 19.7	31.7 ± 20.7	16.5 ± 11.7	14.5 ± 11.6
P value	<0.03*	0.2	0.42	0.23
Age group				
≤25	37.7 ± 19.7	28.8 ± 18.6	19.0 ± 14.4	13.9 ± 12.2
>25	47.8 ± 23.3	30.1 ± 19.2	13.7 ± 17.6	11.2 ± 7.0
P value	0.16	0.86	0.25	0.48
Problem				
Class II	43.7 ± 19.8	31.9 ± 23.9	21.3 ± 11.1	19.1 ± 12.1
Class III	39.1 ± 21.7	28.0 ± 16.1	16.0 ± 13.6	10.5 ± 9.6
P value	0.51	0.57	0.24	0.018*
Education				
≤Diploma	38.8 ± 23.0	25.9 ± 19.0	16.7 ± 12.8	14.1 ± 14.4
>Diploma	40.5 ± 20.0	30.6 ± 18.5	18.1 ± 13.6	13.4 ± 9.4
P value	0.75	0.48	0.76	0.84

*$P < 0.05$ is significant.

TABLE 4: Comparison of OQLQ and its subdomains from baseline ($T1$) to postoperative 6+ months ($T4$).

Variables	T_1-T_2 Mean (SD)	P^*	ES**	T_1-T_3 Mean (SD)	P^*	ES**	T_1-T_4 Mean (SD)	P^*	ES**	T_2-T_3 Mean (SD)	P^*	ES**	T_2-T_4 Mean (SD)	P^*	ES**	T_3-T_4 Mean (SD)	P^*	ES**
OQLQ	9.27 (23.2)	0.02	.22	21.95 (23.9)	<0.001	.54	27.37 (22.0)	<0.001	.63	10.85 (17.2)	0.001	.32	16.35 (14.2)	<0.001	.47	5.02 (8.3)	<0.001	.20
Aesthetic	7.64 (7.3)	<0.001	.59	8.95 (7.0)	<0.001	.67	9.48 (6.3)	<0.001	.70	1 (4.7)	0.219	.12	1.83 (2.9)	0.001	.25	.62 (2.7)	0.163	.10
Function	−5.43 (5.4)	<0.001	−.45	0.25 (6)	0.79	.02	3.02 (5.5)	0.001	.30	5.05 (5.8)	<0.001	.42	7.83 (6.1)	<0.001	.62	2.35 (3.2)	<0.001	.25
Awareness	1.48 (3.6)	0.018	.15	2.95 (5.1)	0.001	.33	4.46 (4.9)	<0.001	.50	1.08 (3.8)	0.102	.12	2.43 (4.1)	0.001	.29	1.47 (2.7)	<0.001	.20
Social	5.56 (1.9)	0.008	.28	9.8 (10.9)	<0.001	.55	10.39 (9.8)	<0.001	.57	3.71 (7.5)	0.006	.26	4.2 (4)	<0.001	.30	.57 (3.7)	0.335	.06

*$P < 0.05$ is significant; **ES = effect size: <0.2 = minimal change; 0.2–0.49 = small change; 0.5–0.8 = moderate change; >0.8 = large change.

However, women's QOL achieved a remarkable improvement in all 4 aspects in the same range with men after the surgery. This indicates that female QOL had more improvement. These findings offer support for some studies [21, 25]. Siow et al. suggested that improvement of self-confidence after surgery in women is more than men [30]. Nicodemo et al. using SF-36 reported higher mean score in emotional domain in female patient [31]. In contrast Choi et al. did not find association between gender and QOL [9]. This may be due to cultural differences.

Pahkala and Kellokoski suggested that patients who had mandibular setback were more satisfied than patients with skeletal class II that had mandibular advancement [32]. Our findings are in agreement with that study. In contrast Choi et al. showed that there was no significant difference in QOL scores between different dentofacial deformities in any time point after surgery [9]. More studies are necessary to clarify the relation between malocclusion type and changes QOL after orthognathic surgery.

According to results of previous studies patients undergoing surgery for dentofacial deformity are mostly satisfied with the surgical results [4, 19, 33–35]. Profit stated that almost all the patients that had gone under surgical procedures reported long term satisfaction (80–90% depend on deformity types). The same number of patients stated that according to their experience of surgery they have suggested others to such treatment and have been ready to experience it once again [19, 36]. The same results have been shown in the present study; patients reported high levels of satisfaction and improvement regarding surgical outcome and suggest the surgery to other people. Therefore, in aggregate, orthognathic surgery in patients with dentofacial deformity is considered beneficial from the patient's point of view. Smith and Cuningham evaluated willingness-to-pay for orthognathic surgery and came to the conclusion that patients with dentofacial deformity are willing to spend more than normal control and consider surgery as a good option in terms of cost-benefit. However a cost-benefit analysis study suggested comparing benefits and costs of orthognathic surgery in patients with dentofacial deformity [37].

This study has several limitations. More patients with longer follow-up and a survey before the institution of orthodontics would be useful to better correlate the results with lasting benefits obtained through orthognathic surgery.

In conclusion, orthognathic surgery causes significant improvement in patients' quality of life in Iranian patients. This improvement was seen in emotional, oral function, psychological, and social domains of quality of life. The maximum influence was in emotional and the least in functional aspect. Our study assessed quality of life in a limited period postoperatively and obviously there is a need for longitudinal studies in this area of healthcare services.

Acknowledgments

This study was granted by Isfahan University of Medical Sciences, Isfahan, Iran (no. 388488).

References

[1] M. Ong, "Spectrum of dentofacial deformities: a retrospective survey," *Annals Academy of Medicine Singapore*, vol. 33, no. 2, pp. 239–242, 2004.

[2] P. C. C. Leite, E. T. Camarini, G. J. Farah, and M. B. d. Silva, "Estudo epidemiológico das deformidades dentofaciais de Maringá/PR-1997–2003," *Pesquisa Brasileira em Odontopediatria e Clínica Integrada*, vol. 4, no. 3, pp. 217–220, 2005.

[3] R. J. Fonseca, R. D. Marciani, T. A. Turvey, and J. Scully, *Oral and Maxillofacial Surgery*, 2009.

[4] M. Modig, L. Andersson, and I. Wårdh, "Patients' perception of improvement after orthognathic surgery: Pilot study," *British Journal of Oral and Maxillofacial Surgery*, vol. 44, no. 1, pp. 24–27, 2006.

[5] A. Borzabadi-Farahani, F. Eslamipour, and I. Asgari, "A comparison of two orthodontic aesthetic indices.," *Australian orthodontic journal*, vol. 28, no. 1, pp. 30–36, 2012.

[6] A. Borzabadi-Farahani, A. Borzabadi-Farahani, and F. Eslamipour, "The relationship between the ICON index and the dental and aesthetic components of the IOTN index.," *World journal of orthodontics*, vol. 11, no. 1, pp. 43–48, 2010.

[7] Y. Sun and C. Jiang, "The impact of malocclusion on self-esteem of adolescents," *Chinese journal of stomatology*, vol. 39, no. 1, pp. 67–69, 2004.

[8] C. L. Soh and V. Narayanan, "Quality of life assessment in patients with dentofacial deformity undergoing orthognathic surgery—a systematic review," *International Journal of Oral and Maxillofacial Surgery*, vol. 42, no. 8, pp. 974–980, 2013.

[9] W. S. Choi, S. Lee, C. McGrath, and N. Samman, "Change in quality of life after combined orthodontic-surgical treatment of dentofacial deformities," *Oral Surgery, Oral Medicine, Oral Pathology, Oral Radiology and Endodontology*, vol. 109, no. 1, pp. 46–51, 2010.

[10] S. Lee, C. McGrath, and N. Samman, "Quality of life in patients with dentofacial deformity: a comparison of measurement approaches," *International Journal of Oral and Maxillofacial Surgery*, vol. 36, no. 6, pp. 488–492, 2007.

[11] M. T. Chew, "Spectrum and management of dentofacial deformities in a multiethnic Asian population," *Angle Orthodontist*, vol. 76, no. 5, pp. 806–809, 2006.

[12] K. K. Bui, D. J. Rinchuse, T. G. Zullo, and M. Cozzani, "Perception of facial attractiveness following modification of the nose and teeth," *International Orthodontics*, vol. 13, no. 2, pp. 195–209, 2015.

[13] Z. B. Al-Bitar, I. K. Al-Omari, H. T. Al-Ahmad, M. A. El Maaytah, and S. J. Cunningham, "A comparison of health-related quality of life between Jordanian and British orthognathic patients," *European Journal of Orthodontics*, vol. 31, no. 5, pp. 485–489, 2009.

[14] S. J. Cunningham, A. M. Garratt, and N. P. Hunt, "Development of a condition-specific quality of life measure for patients with dentofacial deformity: II. Validity and responsiveness testing," *Community Dentistry and Oral Epidemiology*, vol. 30, no. 2, pp. 81–90, 2002.

[15] S. J. Cunningham, A. M. Garratt, and N. P. Hunt, "Development of a conditionspecific quality of life measure for patients with dentofacial deformity: I. Reliability of the instrument," *Community Dentistry and Oral Epidemiology*, vol. 28, no. 3, pp. 195–201, 2000.

[16] A. B. de Almeida, I. C. G. Leite, C. A. Melgaço, and L. S. Marques, "Dissatisfaction with dentofacial appearance and

the normative need for orthodontic treatment: Determinant factors," *Dental Press Journal of Orthodontics*, vol. 19, no. 3, pp. 120–126, 2014.

[17] H. C. Gift and M. Redford, "Oral health and the quality of life," *Clinics in Geriatric Medicine*, vol. 8, no. 3, pp. 73–83, 1992.

[18] F. Cooke Macgregor, "Facial disfigurement: Problems and management of social interaction and implications for mental health," *Aesthetic Plastic Surgery*, vol. 14, no. 1, pp. 249–257, 1990.

[19] E. Motegi, J. P. Hatch, J. D. Rugh, and H. Yamaguchi, "Health-related quality of life and psychosocial function 5 years after orthognathic surgery," *American Journal of Orthodontics and Dentofacial Orthopedics*, vol. 124, no. 2, pp. 138–143, 2003.

[20] R. Scariot, D. J. da Costa, N. L. Barbosa Rebellato, P. R. Müller, and R. da Conceição Ferreira, "Epidemiological analysis of orthognathic surgery in a hospital in Curitiba, Brazil: Review of 195 cases," *Revista Espanola de Cirugia Oral y Maxilofacial*, vol. 32, no. 4, pp. 147–151, 2010.

[21] F. Bertolini, V. Russo, and G. Sansebastiano, "Pre- and post-surgical psycho-emotional aspects of the orthognathic surgery patient," *The International Journal of Adult Orthodontics and Orthognathic Surgery*, vol. 15, no. 1, pp. 16–23, 2000.

[22] E. Desforges, R. Mathis, A. Wilk et al., "The psychological impact of orthognathic surgery," *L' Orthodontie Française*, vol. 78, no. 2, pp. 113–121, 2007.

[23] N. Türker, A. Varol, K. Ögel, and S. Basa, "Perceptions of preoperative expectations and postoperative outcomes from orthognathic surgery: Part I: Turkish female patients," *International Journal of Oral and Maxillofacial Surgery*, vol. 37, no. 8, pp. 710–715, 2008.

[24] H. Sadek and G. Salem, "Psychological aspects of orthognathic surgery and its effect on quality of life in Egyptian patients," *Eastern Mediterranean Health Journal*, vol. 13, no. 1, pp. 150–159, 2007.

[25] L. Espeland, H. E. Høgevold, and A. Stenvik, "A 3-year patient-centred follow-up of 516 consecutively treated orthognathic surgery patients," *European Journal of Orthodontics*, vol. 30, no. 1, pp. 24–30, 2008.

[26] D. Nicodemo, M. D. Pereira, and L. M. Ferreira, "Self-esteem and depression in patients presenting angle class III malocclusion submitted for orthognathic surgery," *Medicina Oral, Patologia Oral y Cirugia Bucal*, vol. 13, no. 1, pp. E48–E51, 2008.

[27] T. Lazaridou-Terzoudi, H. A. Kiyak, R. Moore, A. E. Athanasiou, and B. Melsen, "Long-term assessment of psychologic outcomes of orthognathic surgery," *Journal of Oral and Maxillofacial Surgery*, vol. 61, no. 5, pp. 545–552, 2003.

[28] C. M. Flanary, G. M. Barnwell Jr., and J. M. Alexander, "Patient perceptions of orthognathic surgery," *American Journal of Orthodontics*, vol. 88, no. 2, pp. 137–145, 1985.

[29] O. T. Hunt, C. D. Johnston, P. G. Hepper, and D. J. Burden, "The psychosocial impact of orthognathic surgery: A systematic review," *American Journal of Orthodontics and Dentofacial Orthopedics*, vol. 120, no. 5, pp. 490–496, 2001.

[30] K. K. Siow, S. T. Ong, C. B. Lian, and W. C. Ngeow, "Satisfaction of orthognathic surgical patients in a Malaysian population.," *Journal of oral science*, vol. 44, no. 3-4, pp. 165–171, 2002.

[31] D. Nicodemo, M. D. Pereira, and L. M. Ferreira, "Effect of orthognathic surgery for class III correction on quality of life as measured by SF-36," *International Journal of Oral and Maxillofacial Surgery*, vol. 37, no. 2, pp. 131–134, 2008.

[32] R. H. Pahkala and J. K. Kellokoski, "Surgical-orthodontic treatment and patients' functional and psychosocial well-being," *American Journal of Orthodontics and Dentofacial Orthopedics*, vol. 132, no. 2, pp. 158–164, 2007.

[33] H. A. Kiyak, R. W. McNeill, R. A. West, T. Hohl, and P. J. Heaton, "Personality characteristics as predictors and sequelae of surgical and conventional orthodontics," *American Journal of Orthodontics*, vol. 89, no. 5, pp. 383–392, 1986.

[34] H. A. Kiyak, R. W. McNeill, and R. A. West, "The emotional impact of orthognathic surgery and conventional orthodontics," *American Journal of Orthodontics*, vol. 88, no. 3, pp. 224–234, 1985.

[35] R. W. Williams, H. C. Travess, and A. C. Williams, "Patients' experiences after undergoing orthognathic surgery at NHS hospitals in the south west of England," *British Journal of Oral and Maxillofacial Surgery*, vol. 42, no. 5, pp. 419–431, 2004.

[36] W. R. Proffit, H. W. Fields Jr., and D. M. Sarver, *Contemporary Orthodontics*, Elsevier Health Sciences, Amsterdam, Netherlands, 2014.

[37] A. S. A. Smith and S. J. Cunningham, "Which factors influence willingness-to-pay for orthognathic treatment?" *European Journal of Orthodontics*, vol. 26, no. 5, pp. 499–506, 2004.

21

The Influence of Sweet Taste Perception on Dietary Intake in Relation to Dental Caries and BMI in Saudi Arabian Schoolchildren

Heba Ashi,[1,2] Guglielmo Campus,[3,4] Heléne Bertéus Forslund,[5] Waleed Hafiz,[6] Neveen Ahmed,[7] and Peter Lingström[1,4]

[1]*Department of Cariology, Institute of Odontology, Sahlgrenska Academy, University of Gothenburg, Gothenburg, Sweden*
[2]*Department of Preventive Dentistry, Faculty of Dentistry, King Abdulaziz University, Jeddah, Saudi Arabia*
[3]*Department of Surgery, Microsurgery and Medicine, School of Dentistry, University of Sassari, Sassari, Italy*
[4]*WHO Collaborating Center for Epidemiology and Preventive Dentistry, Milan, Italy*
[5]*Department of Internal Medicine and Clinical Nutrition, Institute of Medicine, Sahlgrenska Academy, University of Gothenburg, Gothenburg, Sweden*
[6]*Department of Prosthodontics, North Jeddah Speciality Dental Center, Jeddah, Saudi Arabia*
[7]*Department of Pedodontics, Jeddah Speciality Dental Center, Jeddah, Saudi Arabia*

Correspondence should be addressed to Heba Ashi; heba.ashi@gmail.com

Academic Editor: Ali I. Abdalla

Objectives. The aim of the study was to evaluate the influence of sweet taste perception on dietary habits in Saudi schoolchildren. In addition, the relationship between dietary habits and both caries and BMI was studied. *Methods.* A cross-sectional observational study comprising 225 schoolchildren aged 13–15 years from Jeddah, Saudi Arabia, was conducted. The consumption frequency of certain food items was analysed from a beverage and snack questionnaire and a three-day estimated dietary record was obtained. The sweet taste perception level was determined as sweet taste threshold (TT) and sweet taste preference (TP). Children were grouped into low, medium, and high, according to their sweet taste perception level. ICDAS and DMFS indices were used for caries registration and anthropometric measurements using BMI were collected. *Results.* Sweet taste perception was found to be negatively correlated to the number of main meals and positively correlated to both snack and sweet intake occasions. Statistically significant differences were found between the TT and TP groups with regard to the number of main meals and sweet intake ($p \leq 0.01$). No significant correlation between the dietary variables and caries or BMI was found. *Conclusions.* The dietary habits and sweet intake were found to be influenced by the sweet taste perception level, while the relation between the dietary habits and the caries and BMI was found insignificant.

1. Introduction

A healthy diet is of significant importance for growth, development, and prevention from dietary-related diseases. There are different medical and oral conditions that are known to be related to dietary imbalance. These conditions include dental caries and obesity which are in turn known to affect general health [1–5].

Dietary habits and food intake have been found to be influenced by several factors. These factors include taste perception, which in turn can be affected by cultural and genetic factors [6–10]. In addition, the frequent consumption of a certain food type can change this perception to be habituated to the taste and increases the preference for this food item [11–13].

One of the main dietary items known for its unfavourable effect is sugar, and that when it is consumed in amounts above the recommended levels. A diet rich in sugar can affect the teeth at an early age and continues towards adolescence causing several oral problems such as dental caries [4, 5]. Both the amount and frequency of sugar consumption may have an adverse effect on the teeth [5, 14–16]. In addition, dietary habits such as frequent snacking have been found to be related to overweight, due to the high content of fat and sugars in snacks [1, 17]. Several studies have suggested that sugar intake is determined by several factors such as environmental and genetic factors [18–21].

Unhealthy dietary habits are common worldwide and especially in children. It has been found in many cultures that children do not follow the recommendations with regard to diet, and sometimes the dietary habits are at an acceptable level but still does not reach the optimum [22–24]. Regarding Saudi Arabia, poor dietary choices among schoolchildren have been reported, with regular sweet food and beverage consumption [25–27]. This can be attributed to the national increase in globalisation, westernisation, and economic and social revolution [28, 29].

The aim of this study was to evaluate the influence of sweet taste perception on dietary habits in Saudi schoolchildren aged 13–15 years. In addition, the relationship between dietary intake and caries, as well as BMI, was studied. Our aim was based on the hypothesis that sweet taste perception can affect children's dietary habits, which may in turn have an effect on both oral and general health.

2. Materials and Methods

2.1. Subjects and Study Design. The study was a cross-sectional observational investigation. It is a part of a broad multicenter study conducted in Italy, Mexico, and Saudi Arabia aimed to investigate the different taste perception level, dental caries, and BMI. Children from Jeddah, Saudi Arabia, who were included in the sample selected in the previous studies (33.6%) were further assessed regarding their dietary habits. This study included 225 children (114 boys/111 girls), aged 13–15 years, who were randomly selected from school lists entered into a computerized program. The boys and girls were selected from separate school lists as they were attending different schools. Children living in the country from six years of age were included in the survey. However, children with medical conditions or undergoing orthodontic treatment were excluded. In addition, any child with signs of flu at the time of the study was excluded, as flu can affect taste sense. The students were chosen using a computerized program and 1% of the population inserted into the program was randomly selected. A post hoc power analysis with a noncentrality parameter of 18, a critical χ^2 of 7.81, and a power (1-β err prob) of 0.96 was performed.

Ethical approval was obtained from the school of dentistry ethical committee at King Abdulaziz University (029-12). In addition, school entry and data collection permission was given by the Board of Education in Jeddah, Saudi Arabia. Parent's consent forms were signed prior to the start of the study and children were informed about the process of the data collection. Data collection was conducted in school settings and all the students were examined in their classrooms under natural light.

2.2. Estimated Food Record. Dietary information was collected via a three-day food and beverage diary presenting daily variations in intake. Participants were asked to report any food or drink consumed in terms of time and quantity from two weekdays and a day from the weekend. When possible, the event, whether it was regarded as breakfast, lunch, or dinner, was stated by the children.

The documents were handed to the participants at school and collected and reviewed by the main author and coauthor. The numbers of main meals (structured eating event), snacks (unstructured eating event and usually uncooked), and total intake occasions (sum of main meals and snacks intakes) were then retrieved and calculated from the dietary record. Any food and beverages consumed within 30 minutes were regarded as one intake event [30]. Subsequently, each event was classified as either a main meal or a snack, depending on the time and type of consumption. In addition, sweet intake frequency was assessed separately by counting all food and drinks containing sweet substances reported in the diary. No total energy intake evaluation was made.

2.3. Beverage and Snack Questionnaire. The food frequency questionnaire was adapted from the validated self-administered beverage and snack questionnaire [31, 32]. A total of 19 food and drink items (sugar-sweetened beverages, savoury snacks, and sweets) were included in the questionnaire. For data analysis, nine sweet-containing beverages and snacks were included (five beverages and four snacks). Students were asked to choose from seven options ranging from never (zero intake) to more than four times per day. Afterwards, a score was given to each option presented in the beverage and snack questionnaire (i.e., never or zero intake = 0, once a week = 1). The scores for the nine sweet items were then added for each participant and summed as a beverage sweet intake score (BS) and a snack sweet intake score (SS).

2.4. Sweet Taste Perception Test. The sweet taste perception level of the participant was determined using a modified version of Furquim et al. [33] method, originally described by both Nilsson and Holm [34] and Zengo and Mandel [35]. Two variables were to be described in relation to sweet taste perception; the first is the sweet taste threshold, defined as the first concentration at which the participants can identify the presence of sucrose and distinguish it from water and the second was the sweet taste preference, which is their preferred chosen solution that matches the level of sugar they might like in a drink. The participants tasted all ten different sucrose solutions with concentrations ranging from 1.62 to 821.52 gm/L. Between tasting the children rinsed with filtered water.

The solutions were tested in order of increasing concentration, after which children were asked to identify their sweet taste threshold level and sweet taste preference of the same solutions and mark the respective solution number on a sheet they were given. Instructions were given to use 10 ml of the offered solution, to guarantee exposing all the taste buds in the oral cavity for at least five seconds, and then to spit it out.

The children were subsequently grouped depending on the concentration chosen for the sweet taste preference (TP) and sweet taste threshold (TT) test, respectively. The children were regarded as "low," when they chose a solution in

Table 1: Mean and standard deviation (SD) for main meal, snack, total intake, and sweet intake in Saudi schoolchildren (boys, girls).

Variable	Boys (n = 114)		Girls (n = 111)		All (n = 225)		p value[(1)]
	Mean ± SD	Range	Mean ± SD	Range	Mean ± SD	Range	
Main meal	2.2 ± 0.7	1–3	2.5 ± 0.6	1–3	2.3 ± 0.7	1–3	0.003
Snack	2.2 ± 0.8	0–4	1.7 ± 0.7	0–3	1.9 ± 0.8	0–4	0.000
Total intake	4.4 ± 0.9	2–7	4.1 ± 0.8	3–6	4.2 ± 0.9	2–7	0.046
Sweet intake	2.8 ± 1.1	0–6	2.1 ± 1.4	0–5	2.4 ± 1.3	0–6	0.000

[(1)] p value: significance between boys and girls (independent t-test).

the range of 1.63–12.84 gm/L, "medium," when the chosen solution ranged from 25.67 to 102.69 gm/L, and "high," when the solution with a concentration of 205.38–821.52 gm/L was chosen.

2.5. Caries Registration. The number of decayed, missed, and filled tooth surfaces (DMFS) and the International Caries Detection and Assessment System (ICDAS) indices were used to diagnose caries. The DMFS index is defined as the sum and score of the total decayed, missed, and filled tooth surfaces of the subjects.

Regarding the ICDAS index, it constitutes scoring system of two digits (restoration code and tooth status). The second digit is the code for the tooth surface status scored from 1 to 6 with 1 presented as first visual change in enamel and 6 is distinctive lesion into dentine. The visible tooth change in enamel due to caries was defined as initial caries (ICDAS 1, 2, and 3) and any lesion reaching the dentine was manifest (ICDAS 4, 5, and 6).

All the children were examined in the classroom by the main author (HA) or one of the coauthors (WH). Disposable dental examination kits, gloves, and masks were used, according to WHO criteria. No radiographs were taken due to the school-setting nature of the study and examinations were performed under adequate natural light.

2.6. Anthropometric Measurements. Data on height (cm) and weight (kg) were obtained and body mass index (BMI; WHO BMI-for-age) [36–38] was evaluated for each study participant. Subsequently, BMI was calculated as body weight divided by height squared. Portable scales were used and the children were instructed to remove all shoes, socks, and heavy clothing when measured.

2.7. Statistical Analysis. The mean, standard deviation, and range for the variables were analysed using IMB® SPSS® (PASW version 23.0 IBM® Chicago, Ill, USA). The independent t-test was used to determine the differences between boys and girls. Differences between the sweet taste perception groups (low, medium, and high) were tested by one-way ANOVA. Regarding beverage and snack questionnaire, the BS and SS scores were considered as a dependent variable and used for multiple linear regression analysis. The relationship between variables was tested using Spearman's rank correlation. A p value of <0.05 was considered statistically significant.

3. Results

From the dietary record, it was found that the number of main meal events constitutes the largest part of the total daily intake events among Saudi children, followed by the snack intake events (Table 1). The majority of all eating and drinking occasions included the consumption of some sweet items (Table 1).

3.1. Sweet Taste Perception and Dietary Habits. An analysis of the correlation between sweet taste perception and dietary intake showed a significant yet weak to moderate negative correlation between the number of main meals and the sweet taste threshold and sweet taste preference, respectively ($p \leq 0.001$; $r = -0.228$ and $p \leq 0.001$; $r = -0.480$). In terms of the snack occasions and sweet intake occasions, a significant weak positive correlation was found for the sweet taste threshold ($p \leq 0.05$; $r = 0.169$ and $p \leq 0.001$; $r = 0.276$) and sweet taste preference, respectively ($p \leq 0.001$; $r = 0.286$ and $p \leq 0.001$; $r = 0.288$). No correlation was found between any of the three intake variables (number of main meals, snack events, and sweet intake events) and both caries and BMI, respectively.

In terms of the sweet taste threshold groups, the high sweet taste threshold group had the highest sweet intake and number of snack occasions and the lowest main meal frequency (Figure 1, Table 2). A statistically significant difference between the three groups was found for the number of main meals ($p \leq 0.01$) and sweet intake occasions ($p \leq 0.001$), (Table 2).

Similarly, regarding the grouping of children according to their sweet taste preference, statistically significant differences were found between the groups with regard to the number of main meals ($p \leq 0.001$) and sweet intake occasions ($p \leq 0.001$) (Table 3). In addition, the high sweet taste preference group was found to have a higher number of snacking and sweet intake occasions and the lowest number of main meals (Table 3).

3.2. Beverage and Snack Questionnaire. Fruit juice consumption showed a weak significant negative correlation to sweet taste threshold ($p \leq 0.05$; $r = -0.160$) and sweet taste

TABLE 2: Mean and standard deviation (SD) for main meal, snack, total intake, and sweet intake in Saudi schoolchildren according to TT (taste threshold) groups (low, medium, and high).

Variable	Low TT (n = 93)		Medium TT (n = 124)		High TT (n = 8)		p value[(1)]
	Mean ± SD	Range	Mean ± SD	Range	Mean ± SD	Range	
Main meal	2.5 ± 0.6	1–3	2.2 ± 0.7	1–3	2.0 ± 0.5	1–3	0.002
Snack	1.8 ± 0.7	1–3	2.0 ± 0.9	0–4	2.4 ± 0.9	1–3	0.063
Total intake	4.3 ± 0.8	3–6	4.2 ± 1.0	2–7	4.4 ± 1.2	3–6	0.675
Sweet intake	2.0 ± 1.3	0–5	2.7 ± 1.2	0–6	2.9 ± 1.6	1–5	<0.001

[(1)] p value: significance between TT groups (ANOVA).

TABLE 3: Mean and standard deviation (SD) for main meal, snack, total intake, and sweet intake in Saudi schoolchildren according to TP (taste preference) groups (low, medium, and high).

Variable	Low TP (n = 11)		Medium TP (n = 89)		High TP (n = 125)		p value[(1)]
	Mean ± SD	Range	Mean ± SD	Range	Mean ± SD	Range	
Main meal	3.0 ± 0.0	1–3	2.7 ± 0.5	2-3	2.0 ± 0.7	1–3	<0.001
Snack	1.8 ± 1.0	0–3	1.8 ± 0.6	1–3	2.1 ± 0.9	0–4	0.026
Total intake	4.8 ± 1.0	3–6	4.4 ± 0.7	3–6	4.1 ± 1.0	2–7	0.003
Sweet intake	2.4 ± 0.7	2–4	2.0 ± 1.3	0–5	2.8 ± 1.2	0–6	<0.001

[(1)] p value: significance between TP groups (ANOVA).

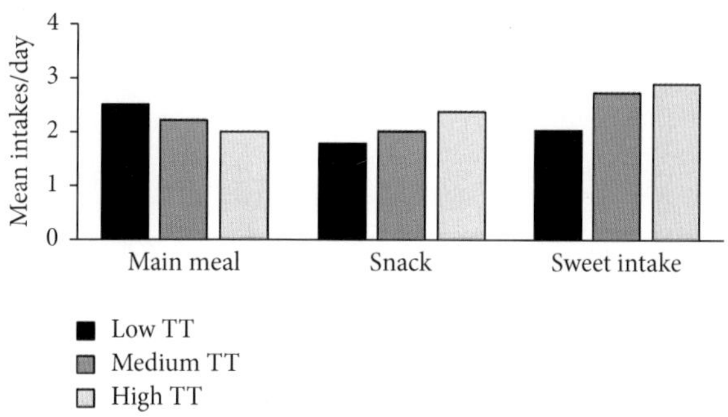

FIGURE 1: Mean value for main meal, snack, and sweet intake in sweet taste threshold groups. n = 225.

TABLE 4: Multiple linear regression analysis for factors associated with the beverage sweet intake score (BS).

Variables	B	Std. error	t	Sig.
TT	.001	.003	.434	.665
TP	.001	.001	1.402	.162
Sweet intake	.322	.093	3.470	.001
Snack	.116	.183	.638	.524
Main meals	–.322	.229	–1.406	.161
Gender	.813	.308	2.637	.009

preference, respectively ($p \leq 0.01$; $r = -0.232$) for all children. In addition, sports drink intake was moderately correlated to both sweet taste threshold and sweet taste preference ($p \leq 0.01$; $r = 0.295$; $p \leq 0.01$; $r = 0.342$). Regular soda showed weak positive correlation to sweet taste preference ($p \leq 0.05$; $r = 0.178$). Regarding snacks and sweet taste perception, sweet chocolates and gummies sweets showed a significant weak positive correlation to the sweet taste threshold ($p \leq 0.05$; $r = 0.151$) in all subjects.

Children who have a higher weekly intake of fresh juice had a lower BMI ($p \leq 0.05$; $r = -0.135$) and those with a higher intake of ice cream had a lower DMFS ($p \leq 0.05$; $r = -0.139$). None of the other food or drink items from the questionnaire showed any significant correlation with the dietary variables, BMI, or caries.

The BS was significantly associated with gender and sweet intake occasions (Table 4). Regarding SS, no significant association was found (data not shown). However, gender showed a borderline significance ($p = 0.059$, 95% CI = −0.044–2.34).

3.3. Gender Differences. A statistically significant difference was found between boys and girls for the number of main meals and snacking events ($p \leq 0.01$, resp., $p \leq 0.001$). The number of main meals was higher in girls, while the snacking occasions were found to be higher among boys (Table 1). However, boys reported a higher total number of intake occasions compared with girls (Table 1). Regarding sweet intake occasions, a higher intake was found among the boys ($p \leq 0.001$) (Table 1).

Statistically significant differences were found between boys and girls for the sweet taste threshold ($p \leq 0.001$), sweet taste preference ($p \leq 0.001$), and BMI ($p \leq 0.01$), with a higher mean value among boys (Table 5). Regarding the caries variables, girls had a higher mean value for initial lesions compared with boys ($p \leq 0.001$), while higher mean

Table 5: Mean and standard deviation (SD) for sweet taste threshold (TT), sweet taste preference (TP), BMI, initial, manifest lesions, and DMFS in Saudi schoolchildren (boys, girls).

Variable	Boys (n = 114)		Girls (n = 111)		All (n = 225)		p value$^{(1)}$
	Mean ± SD	Range	Mean ± SD	Range	Mean ± SD	Range	
TT (gm/L)	52.1 ± 58.7	1.6–410.8	22.9 ± 24.9	1.6–205.4	37.7 ± 47.5	1.6–410.8	0.000
TP (gm/L)	431.3 ± 316.3	1.6–821.5	205.1 ± 237.5	6.5–821.5	319.7 ± 302.1	1.6–821.5	0.000
BMI	25.1 ± 6.9	14.7–44.5	22.6 ± 4.8	12.6–37.7	23.9 ± 6.1	12.6 ± 44.5	0.002
Initial lesions	4.9 ± 4.6	0–21	8.6 ± 9.8	0–59	6.7–7.8	0–59	0.000
Manifest lesions	1.7 ± 3.6	0–24	0.9 ± 1.6	0–9	1.3 ± 2.8	0–24	0.025
DMFS	3.1 ± 4.5	0–25	2.9 ± 3.5	0–22	3.0 ± 4.0	0–25	0.679

$^{(1)}p$ values: significance between boys and girls (independent t-test).

values for DMFS and manifest lesions were found among boys (Table 5).

4. Discussion

In this study, the influence of sweet taste perception on dietary habits was evaluated as part of a multicenter study focusing on sweet taste perception in relation to different tested variables. The main hypothesis was supported by our findings, as the sweet taste threshold and preference were found to be directly related to both snack and sweet intake occasions and inversely related to the number of main meals. This is supported by Kourouniotis et al. [13], where the taste perception was found to affect diet and that subjects considering taste as an important factor in their food choices tend to consume more sweets and snacks with a high fat and sugar content.

Moreover, when children were categorised according to their sweet taste perception level, the group with the higher threshold and preference for sweets reported a higher number of sweet and snack intake occasions and a lower number of main meals. This could be due to the higher threshold for sweets over time, which leads to increased consumption in order to reach the preferred sweet taste and corresponds well to what was previously stated, "taste perception can result from a cumulative effect of lifetime exposure to certain food or taste" [13].

Children usually run a higher risk of adaptation to unhealthy dietary behaviours with an increase in sugar intake. Childhood is known to be a period with a high preference for sweets due to several factors, which may lead to food choices rich in calories [2, 20, 21, 39]. However, this sweet preference has been found to change with age, as less energy is needed [21].

The second hypothesis of the present study focused on the relationship between dietary patterns and caries. No significant relationship was found in this study between sweet intake occasions from the dietary record and any of the caries variables, despite the well-known relationship between sugar intake and caries [5, 14–16]. A possible explanation could be attributed to the cross-sectional design, where children's dietary assessment was conducted on a period of one week and thus reflects the present dietary habits with no adequate information of the past diet history. Meanwhile, caries is the net result of a longitudinal metabolic process that requires several factors contributing over time. Thus, the possible previous dietary factors affecting the children's caries level are not known in this study. However, in a previous study by our group, including the same children from Saudi Arabia, a relationship was found between sweet taste perception and DMFS.

Regarding the relationship between dietary patterns and BMI, no significant relationship was found in this study. However, a study by Washi and Ageib [17] stated that a significant relationship was reported between the number of meals and being overweight. Despite the fact that no relation was found in this study between the dietary habits and BMI or caries, it is well known from literature that both diseases can be affected by the dietary intake [1, 5, 14–17].

An association has been found in this study between the beverage sweet intake score (BS) and both the gender and sweet intake occasions and it can be attributed to the difference in behaviour presented in the population with regard to gender. This can also be seen when calculating the mean number of sweet intake occasions from the dietary records, where males reported a higher number of sweet intake occasions. Our findings may imply that the same dissimilarity can be seen between boys and girls in both the questionnaire and the food diary. Unhealthy habits in Saudi children have previously been discussed in the literature [25–27]. Due to the lifestyle and the cultural and environmental aspects in Saudi Arabia, the risk of an unhealthy lifestyle has previously been found especially high among females [27, 40–43]. In Saudi, fewer chances are offered for exercise, especially to females, which may cause an increased risk of obesity, as well as unhealthy dietary habits [43].

Moreover, differences between genders have been reported with regard to sweet taste perception. Females considered taste to be of great importance in food choices compared with males and this was linked to poor dietary habits [13, 43]. Conversely, our study revealed a difference in dietary pattern between boys and girls, with more positive habits among girls. Boys had a higher number of sweet and snack intake occasions and this is contrary to the findings in a study performed in Kuwait by Allafi et al. [44] where no differences between boys and girls were found with regard to sugar consumption. The differences found between boys and girls in the present study may be related to the higher reported sweet taste threshold and preference. In addition, higher BMI and DMFS values were found among the boys and this might also be related to the reported liking for sweets.

Regarding the beverage and snack questionnaire, the items with a sweet taste were included in the analysis, as this was the focus of our study. Children with a higher sweet taste threshold had a higher consumption of chocolates, gummy candies, and sports drink. A similar finding was made by Kourouniotis et al. [13], where more chocolates and sweets were consumed by those reporting taste as important. This could be explained by poor dietary choices being influenced by the high sweet taste threshold, so that more calories are consumed from sources other than proper cooked meals.

The children's perception of the importance of a healthy diet and why it should be adapted was not evaluated in this study, but it is of interest for further studies. It has previously been reported that only 11.3% of the children were concerned about general health, while the majority were concerned about looks and obesity [27].

The majority of children followed the instructions, but personal variations in presentation and reporting cannot be totally excluded. Even if the days reported in the dietary record were representative, the possibility cannot be excluded that certain food intakes were not identified. It is difficult to obtain an exact count of frequency in dietary records and especially at this age. Regarding the beverage and snack questionnaire, the exposure of a food item can be interpreted in different ways by different subjects. Items that were not listed in the questionnaire may have been consumed, as there are a limited number of items. In addition, limitations apply to any self-administered questionnaire and data should be handled with caution.

In a step towards a healthier lifestyle, Saudi Arabia banned carbonated drinks from school, but this did not apply to all sweetened beverages [28], as these drinks have been found to be linked to poor dietary choices [26]. In addition, special attention should be paid to children and adolescents, as this is the period in life where rapid growth, maturity, and lifelong habits may develop [17, 44].

5. Conclusions

Dietary habits and especially sweet intake in Saudi children were influenced by the sweet taste perception level, which may in turn have an adverse effect on health. However, no relation was found between the dietary habit and caries or BMI. Therefore, further longitudinal study design is recommended in this regard.

In addition, boys had poor dietary habits in comparison with girls, as well as a higher caries prevalence and BMI. This emphasises the effect of taste sense, as boys showed higher sweet taste perception than girls.

A healthier diet with a low sugar content is therefore of great importance for improved oral and general health. The recommendations are to try and control the food served at schools and public-health attention is needed to target children and adolescents to encourage them to adapt proper dietary habits and a healthier lifestyle. Further studies focusing on an analysis of actual energy intake in the diet are needed.

Acknowledgments

This study was conducted as part of a project supported by a scholarship from the Ministry of Higher Education, Saudi Arabia.

References

[1] K. Murakami and M. B. Livingstone, "Associations between meal and snack frequency and overweight and abdominal obesity in US children and adolescents from National Health and Nutrition Examination Survey (NHANES) 2003–2012," *British Journal of Nutrition*, vol. 115, no. 10, pp. 1819–1829, 2016.

[2] A. Lanfer, K. Knof, G. Barba et al., "Taste preferences in association with dietary habits and weight status in European children: Results from the IDEFICS study," *International Journal of Obesity*, vol. 36, no. 1, pp. 27–34, 2012.

[3] H.-C. Hung, K. J. Joshipura, R. Jiang et al., "Fruit and vegetable intake and risk of major chronic disease," *Journal of the National Cancer Institute*, vol. 96, no. 21, pp. 1577–1584, 2004.

[4] A. Alm, L. K. Wendt, G. Koch, D. Birkhed, and M. Nilsson, "Caries in adolescence—influence from early childhood," *Community Dentistry and Oral Epidemiology*, vol. 40, no. 2, pp. 125–133, 2012.

[5] E. Bernabé, M. M. Vehkalahti, A. Sheiham, A. Lundqvist, and A. L. Suominen, "The shape of the dose-response relationship between sugars and caries in adults," *Journal of Dental Research*, vol. 95, no. 2, pp. 167–172, 2016.

[6] J. A. Mennella, M. Y. Pepino, and D. R. Reed, "Genetic and environmental determinants of bitter perception and sweet preferences," *Pediatrics*, vol. 115, no. 2, pp. e216–e222, 2005.

[7] A. Drewnowski, S. A. Henderson, A. Levine, and C. Hann, "Taste and food preferences as predictors of dietary practices in young women," *Public Health Nutrition*, vol. 2, no. 4, pp. 513–519, 1999.

[8] A. Drewnowski, "Taste preferences and food intake," *Annual Review of Nutrition*, vol. 17, pp. 237–253, 1997.

[9] S. Opal, S. Garg, J. Jain, and I. Walia, "Genetic factors affecting dental caries risk," *Australian Dental Journal*, vol. 60, no. 1, pp. 2–11, 2015.

[10] E. Haznedaroğlu, M. Koldemir-Gündüz, N. Bakr-Coşkun et al., "Association of sweet taste receptor gene polymorphisms with dental caries experience in school children," *Caries Research*, vol. 49, no. 3, pp. 275–281, 2015.

[11] H. A. Jamel, A. Sheiham, R. G. Watt, and C. R. Cowell, "Sweet preference, consumption of sweet tea and dental caries; studies in urban and rural Iraqi populations," *International Dental Journal*, vol. 47, no. 4, pp. 213–217, 1997.

[12] M. A. McCrory, E. Saltzman, B. J. Rolls, and S. B. Roberts, "A twin study of the effects of energy density and palatability on

energy intake of individual foods," *Physiology and Behavior*, vol. 87, no. 3, pp. 451–459, 2006.

[13] S. Kourouniotis, R. S. J. Keast, L. J. Riddell, K. Lacy, M. G. Thorpe, and S. Cicerale, "The importance of taste on dietary choice, behaviour and intake in a group of young adults," *Appetite*, vol. 103, pp. 1–7, 2016.

[14] A. Sheiham and W. P. T. James, "A new understanding of the relationship between sugars, dental caries and fluoride use: implications for limits on sugars consumption," *Public Health Nutrition*, vol. 17, no. 10, pp. 2176–2184, 2014.

[15] P. Moynihan, "Sugars and dental caries: Evidence for setting a recommended threshold for intake," *Advances in Nutrition*, vol. 7, no. 1, pp. 149–156, 2016.

[16] M. A. Peres, A. Sheiham, P. Liu et al., "Sugar consumption and changes in dental caries from childhood to adolescence," *Journal of Dental Research*, vol. 95, no. 4, pp. 388–394, 2016.

[17] S. A. Washi and M. B. Ageib, "Poor diet quality and food habits are related to impaired nutritional status in 13- to 18-year-old adolescents in Jeddah," *Nutrition Research*, vol. 30, no. 8, pp. 527–534, 2010.

[18] L. Qi and Y. A. Cho, "Gene-environment interaction and obesity," *Nutrition Reviews*, vol. 66, no. 12, pp. 684–694, 2008.

[19] J. Overberg, T. Hummel, H. Krude, and S. Wiegand, "Differences in taste sensitivity between obese and non-obese children and adolescents," *Archives of Disease in Childhood*, vol. 97, no. 12, pp. 1048–1052, 2012.

[20] S. E. Coldwell, T. K. Oswald, and D. R. Reed, "A marker of growth differs between adolescents with high vs. low sugar preference," *Physiology and Behavior*, vol. 96, no. 4-5, pp. 574–580, 2009.

[21] A. Drewnowski, "Sensory control of energy density at different life stages," *Proceedings of the Nutrition Society*, vol. 59, no. 2, pp. 239–244, 2000.

[22] S. C. de Andrade, Á. N. Previdelli, C. L. G. Cesar, D. M. L. Marchioni, and R. M. Fisberg, "Trends in diet quality among adolescents, adults and older adults: A population-based study," *Preventive Medicine Reports*, vol. 4, pp. 391–396, 2016.

[23] R. Saulle, G. Del Prete, M. Stelmach-Mardas, M. De Giusti, and G. La Torre, "A breaking down of the mediterranean diet in the land where it was discovered. A cross sectional survey among the young generation of adolescents in the heart of cilento, Southern Italy," *Annali di Igiene*, vol. 28, no. 5, pp. 349–359, 2016.

[24] K. Handeland, M. Kjellevold, M. Wik Markhus et al., "A diet score assessing Norwegian adolescents' adherence to dietary recommendations—development and test-retest reproducibility of the score," *Nutrients*, vol. 8, no. 8, article 467, 2016.

[25] F. A. Quadri, H. Hendriyani, A. Pramono, and M. Jafer, "Knowledge, attitudes and practices of sweet food and beverage consumption and its association with dental caries among schoolchildren in Jazan, Saudi Arabia," *Eastern Mediterranean Health Journal*, vol. 21, no. 6, pp. 403–411, 2015.

[26] K. S. Collison, M. Z. Zaidi, S. N. Subhani, K. Al-Rubeaan, M. Shoukri, and F. A. Al-Mohanna, "Sugar-sweetened carbonated beverage consumption correlates with BMI, waist circumference, and poor dietary choices in school children," *BMC Public Health*, vol. 10, article 234, 2010.

[27] H. M. Al-Hazzaa, N. A. Abahussain, H. I. Al-Sobayel, D. M. Qahwaji, and A. O. Musaiger, "Physical activity, sedentary behaviors and dietary habits among Saudi adolescents relative to age, gender and region," *International Journal of Behavioral Nutrition and Physical Activity*, vol. 8, article 140, 2011.

[28] A. O. Musaiger, M. Al-Mannai, and N. Zagzoog, "Association between food intake frequency and obesity among adolescent girls in Saudi Arabia," *International Journal of Adolescent Medicine and Health*, vol. 26, no. 1, pp. 145–147, 2014.

[29] Y. Al-Nakeeb, M. Lyons, P. Collins et al., "Obesity, physical activity and sedentary behavior amongst British and Saudi youth: A cross-cultural study," *International Journal of Environmental Research and Public Health*, vol. 9, no. 4, pp. 1490–1506, 2012.

[30] T. A. Marshall, B. Broffitt, J. Eichenberger-Gilmore, J. J. Warren, M. A. Cunningham, and S. M. Levy, "The roles of meal, snack, and daily total food and beverage exposures on caries experience in young children," *Journal of Public Health Dentistry*, vol. 65, no. 3, pp. 166–173, 2005.

[31] M. L. Neuhouser, S. Lilley, A. Lund, and D. B. Johnson, "Development and validation of a beverage and snack questionnaire for use in evaluation of school nutrition policies," *Journal of the American Dietetic Association*, vol. 109, no. 9, pp. 1587–1592, 2009.

[32] C. Losasso, V. Cappa, M. L. Neuhouser, V. Giaccone, I. Andrighetto, and A. Ricci, "Students' consumption of beverages and snacks at school and away from school: a case study in the North East of Italy," *Frontiers in Nutrition*, vol. 2, article 30, 2015.

[33] T. R. D. Furquim, R. C. Poli-Frederico, S. M. Maciel, A. Gonini-Júnior, and L. R. F. Walter, "Sensitivity to bitter and sweet taste perception in schoolchildren and their relation to dental caries," *Oral Health and Preventive Dentistry*, vol. 8, no. 3, pp. 253–259, 2010.

[34] B. Nilsson and A.-K. Holm, "Taste thresholds, taste preferences, and dental caries in 15-year-olds," *Journal of Dental Research*, vol. 62, no. 10, pp. 1069–1072, 1983.

[35] A. N. Zengo and I. D. Mandel, "Sucrose tasting and dental caries in man," *Archives of Oral Biology*, vol. 17, no. 3, pp. 605–607, 1972.

[36] N. F. Butte, C. Garza, and M. de Onis, "Evaluation of the feasibility of international growth standards for school-aged children and adolescents," *Food and Nutrition Bulletin*, vol. 27, no. 4, supplement 5, pp. S169–S174, 2006.

[37] M. De Onis and T. Lobstein, "Defining obesity risk status in the general childhood population: Which cut-offs should we use?" *International Journal of Pediatric Obesity*, vol. 5, no. 6, pp. 458–460, 2010.

[38] WHO, *WHO. Growth Reference 5–19 Years*, World Health Organization, 2007.

[39] R. H. Mosli, A. L. Miller, K. E. Peterson, and J. C. Lumeng, "Sibling feeding behavior: Mothers as role models during mealtimes," *Appetite*, vol. 96, pp. 617–620, 2016.

[40] H. M. Al-Hazzaa, Y. Al-Nakeeb, and M. J. Duncan, "A cross-cultural comparison of health behaviors between Saudi and British adolescents living in urban areas: gender by country analyses," *International Journal of Environmental Research and Public Health*, vol. 10, no. 12, pp. 6701–6720, 2013.

[41] Y. Al-Nakeeb, M. Lyons, L. Dodd, and A. Al-Nuaim, "An investigation into the lifestyle, health habits and risk factors of young adults," *International Journal of Environmental Research and Public Health*, vol. 12, no. 4, pp. 4380–4394, 2015.

[42] R. M. Leech, S. A. McNaughton, and A. Timperio, "The clustering of diet, physical activity and sedentary behavior in children and adolescents: a review," *International Journal of Behavioral Nutrition and Physical Activity*, vol. 11, no. 1, article 4, 2014.

[43] H. Al-Sobayel, H. M. Al-Hazzaa, N. A. Abahussain, D. M. Qahwaji, and A. O. Musaiger, "Gender differences in leisure-time

22

Forensic Age Estimation of Chinese Malaysian Adults by Evaluating Occlusal Tooth Wear Using Modified Kim's Index

Chai Kit Lu, Margaret Chia Soo Yee, Spoorthi Banavar Ravi, and Rohit Pandurangappa

School of Dentistry, International Medical University, 126/Jalan 19/155B, Bukit Jalil, 57000 Kuala Lumpur, Malaysia

Correspondence should be addressed to Spoorthi Banavar Ravi; drspoorti@gmail.com

Academic Editor: Izzet Yavuz

Background and Objective. Evaluation of dental attrition is an easy and relatively accurate approach to estimating the age of an adult either ante- or postmortem for some specific population. Dental attrition represents a progressive physiological age change that can be measured using variety of indices to aid as an adjunct in forensic age estimation. Some of the previously proposed indices have their own practical limitations. This paper focuses on using modified Kim's criteria to score dental attrition to estimate the age of Chinese Malaysian adults and validate it. *Methodology.* Tooth wear was evaluated on 190 dental models of Chinese Malaysian adults (age range: 20–60 years) using modified Kim's index to custom-derive a population specific linear equation. The same equation was validated further on new 60 dental casts. *Results and Conclusion.* Regression analysis revealed good correlation between age and teeth wear and lower standard error of estimate. Test of regression on a test sample ($n = 30$ pairs, age range: 20–60 years) showed insignificant difference between predicted versus the actual age with statistically acceptable mean absolute difference. These data suggest that modified Kim's index can be used effectively in forensic age estimation.

1. Introduction

Establishing one's identity is an important aspect in any forensic casework. Numerous contributing factors like age, sex, population designation, and stature prediction help in reconstructing the identity. Among these factors, age estimation plays a vital role in such scenarios. This is especially true when the police or the investigators already have a putative age; a forensic age estimation that is close to the presumed age provides clarity in the line of investigation [1]. Since Gustafson's scoring system [2] for estimation of chronological age from human teeth, there have been several reports on improved methodologies [3–11] including digital techniques in this field [1]. However, some of these methods require tooth extraction and preparation of microscopic sections of teeth. Such invasive methods are not applicable to estimating the chronological age of a living person. Other noninvasive methods using radiographs wherein age is being predicted based on dental maturation [12] or the ratio between pulp chamber and the tooth have also been reported [13]. Kim et al., in the year 2000, originally proposed a system to objectively score the wear of the teeth of an adult individual [14]. Researchers [15, 16] have reported using this scoring system to estimate the age of an individual. Practical requirements such as presence of entire set of sound and healthy dentition for the system limit its usefulness. To overcome this, a proposed modification of the original Kim's system was used to assess its practical applicability, on a Chinese Malaysian population.

The aim of our study was to evaluate the validity of modified Kim's index as a practical clinical method of recording the degree of occlusal wear and estimating the chronological age.

2. Materials and Methods

The study was based on 250 randomly selected {125 pairs (95 pairs for the reference group and 30 pairs for the test group)} maxillary and mandibular full arch casts obtained from heterogeneous samples of males and females (53 males, 72 females) belonging to Chinese Malaysian origin, ranging in age from 20 to 60 years. The study samples were further divided into four groups (20–30 years, 31–40 years, 41–50 years, and 51–60 years). Age and gender distributions are

Table 1: Sample distribution across gender and different age group in the reference group.

Reference data set	n	Gender	
		M	F
Age group			
20–30	29	14	15
31–40	18	07	11
41–50	24	08	16
51–60	24	10	14
Total	95	38	57
Test data set	30	15	15
Total	125	53	72

Table 2: Modified Kim's index to score the teeth wear [14].

Score	Premolar	Molar
(0)	No visible wear	
(1)	1P/1L	1P/1L/2P/2L
(2)	2P/2L/1S/1B	3P/3L/4P/4L/1S/1B/2S/2B
(3)	2S/2B	3S/3B/4S/4B
(4)	Wear on more than 2/3 of occlusal surfaces	
(5)	1Pc/1Lc	1Pc/1Lc/2Pc/2Lc
(6)	2Pc/2Lc/1Sc/1Bc	3Pc/3Lc/4Pc/4Lc/1Sc/1Bc/2Sc/2Bc
(7)	2Sc/2Bc	3Sc/3Bc/4Sc/4Bc
(8)	Concavity on more than 2/3 of occlusal surfaces	
(9)	Filling, *caries, *crown (all teeth)	
(10)	Missing, stump of tooth, pontic, denture (all teeth)	

*If the extent of the filling materials or caries does not exceed 1/3 of the occlusal surface so that the degree of occlusal wear can be determined, the pertinent score should be given; P, point like wear facet less than ca. 1 mm in diameter; L, linear wear facet less than ca. 1 mm in width; S, surface like wear facet greater than ca. 1 mm in diameter; B, band like wear facet greater than ca. 1 mm in width or wear facet involving more than two surface like wear facets; "c" (concavity), the wear of dentin; in the situation where a tooth has several different degrees of occlusal wear, the highest degree should be selected as the occlusal wear score.

presented in Table 1. While randomly selecting the casts for the study, individuals having severe malocclusion that could affect the occlusal wear and edentulous casts were excluded from the study.

Only the posterior teeth (excluding third molars) were considered for tooth wear evaluation. Tooth wear score was categorised using 0–10 point scale based on the amount and pattern of tooth wear on the occlusal surface following the modified Kim's index, as given in Table 2. The full arch casts were evaluated by 2 examiners under regular room light using a magnifying glass. Two examiners scored the occlusal wear individually after a mutual calibration session. Twenty pairs of randomly selected casts were used to calibrate and evaluate the concordance between intraexaminer and interexaminer scoring method.

A total of 190 (95 pairs) full arch casts were evaluated first. The subjects were categorised into four groups (group 1 to group 4) based on their age as 21–30 years, 31–40 years, 41–50 years, and 51–60 years, respectively. All the casts were coded before their scoring to avoid any type of bias. After scoring the occlusal wear in all the 95 pairs of full arch casts, the casts were decoded to know the actual age and the gender. This sample of 95 pairs was referred to as "reference data set." The data generated from this group was used to derive a statistical linear regression equation. Further, the same equation was applied on later collected cases called "test data set" ($n = 30$ pairs) to predict the age of the subjects.

The difference between the actual age and the estimated age was calculated for every case in both the sets and the mean absolute difference (MAD) was calculated. This MAD (irrespective of the positive or the negative value) would represent the average magnitude of difference that was used as an average measure of accuracy. The differences in age prediction were calculated as to lie within ±3-, ±5-, and ±10-year range of the actual age, along with errors that are ≤10 years and ≥15 years as per Solheim and Sundnes [17] who have classified the former as "acceptable" and the latter as "unsatisfactory" in forensic age estimation.

2.1. Statistical Analysis. For all statistical evaluations, SPSS 2015 for windows was used (SPSS Inc., Chicago, IL: currently IBM corporation, New York). The statistical significance for all the tests were set at 0.05. To evaluate inter- and intraexaminer variability, interclass correlation coefficient (ICC) was employed. Gender difference in occlusal tooth wear scores between each tooth was evaluated using independent t-test. Correlation between occlusal tooth wear scores and the actual age was established using Karl Pearson correlation test. The regression analysis using the data from the reference data set provided a linear equation that when used would predict the age of the individual belonging to the test set based on the independent variables observed. In our study the age was the dependant variable and the teeth wear scores from 16 teeth (all premolars and molars) were independent variables. The equation derived was based on the statistical regression formula, $y = a + b(x)$. Multivariate regression analysis was followed as we had multiple independent variables.

$$\begin{aligned} Y = a &+ b_1x(14) + b_2x(15) + b_3x(16) + b_4x(17) \\ &+ b_5x(24) + b_6x(25) + b_7X(26) + b_8x(27) \\ &+ b_9x(34) + b_{10}x(35) + b_{11}x(36) + b_{12}x(37) \\ &+ b_{13}x(44) + b_{14}x(45) + b_{15}x(46) + b_{16}x(47). \end{aligned} \quad (1)$$

3. Results

The ICC scores of 0.97 ($P = 0.02$) and 0.95 ($P = 0.03$) showed very good concordance between the examiners. The mean occlusal wear scores of all teeth in the reference group were marginally higher in females than in males, but this difference was not statistically significant (3.62 versus 3.19, $P > 0.005$, Table 3). The mean wear scores of molars were significantly higher than the mean wear scores of premolars (3.88 versus 3.31, $P = 0.036$). Comparison of the mean occlusal wear scores among four different age groups in the reference data set group was statistically significant for all the teeth except teeth 24, 34, and 44. The mean wear scores of all the teeth across different age group showed a gradual increase

TABLE 3: Comparison of the mean occlusal wear scores of each tooth between males and females using independent t-test.

Tooth	Gender	N	Mean	Std. deviation	P value
14	Male	38	3.24	2.94	0.400
	Female	57	3.81	3.39	
15	Male	38	3.55	3.52	0.890
	Female	57	3.46	3.17	
16	Male	38	3.18	2.81	0.117
	Female	57	4.23	3.35	
17	Male	38	2.32	2.16	0.098
	Female	57	3.19	2.72	
24	Male	38	3.03	2.85	0.698
	Female	57	3.26	2.94	
25	Male	38	2.92	3.17	0.324
	Female	57	3.58	3.17	
26	Male	38	3.50	3.15	0.661
	Female	57	3.79	3.14	
27	Male	38	2.79	2.57	0.575
	Female	57	3.09	2.51	
34	Male	38	2.53	2.90	0.517
	Female	57	2.93	3.01	
35	Male	38	2.29	2.58	0.639
	Female	57	2.53	2.28	
36	Male	38	4.42	3.39	0.701
	Female	57	4.70	3.54	
37	Male	38	3.53	3.25	0.601
	Female	57	3.86	2.88	
44	Male	38	2.58	2.82	0.393
	Female	57	3.12	3.16	
45	Male	38	2.79	2.97	0.472
	Female	57	3.23	2.85	
46	Male	38	4.45	3.34	0.477
	Female	57	4.96	3.54	
47	Male	38	3.95	3.24	0.601
	Female	57	4.30	3.16	

with the age (Table 4). The correlation test revealed positive correlation between occlusal tooth wear scores and age with coefficient of determination (r^2) of 0.82 for males and 0.74 for females (Table 5). The standard errors *of age* were 7.37 and 7.26 for males and females, respectively. The degree of correlation was moderately positive between the tooth wear scores of all the teeth examined. The correlation coefficient values of all the molar teeth were higher than the premolars; the values were between 0.272 and 0.568 (Table 6, Figure 1).

Based on the regression analysis, a specific equation for age estimation was derived. This was based on $y = a + b(x)$, where the intercept (a) and the regression coefficient (b) for each tooth were derived as shown in Table 7. The complete equation derived for predicting the age was

$$\begin{aligned}\text{Predicted Age} = {} & 20.6 + 0.019\,(14) + 0.635\,(15) \\ & + 0.087\,(16) + 0.838\,(17) \\ & + 0.368\,(24) + 0.016\,(25) \\ & + 0.567\,(26) + 0.889\,(27) \\ & - 0.665\,(34) + 0.172\,(35) \\ & + 0.305\,(36) + 0.827\,(37) \\ & + 0.361\,(44) + 0.112\,(45) \\ & + 0.589\,(46) + 0.097\,(47).\end{aligned} \quad (2)$$

Further, by scoring all 16 teeth (independent variables: 14, 15, 16, 17, 24, 25, 26, 27, 34, 35, 36, 37, 44, 45, 46, and 47) the values were substituted in the equation to predict the age of an individual belonging to "test data set group." The accuracy of age prediction using the modified Kim's index was assessed by calculating the MAD as shown in Table 8. Predicted ages were within ±3 years and ±5 years of the actual age in 20% and 40% and 13.33 and 33.33% of males and females, respectively. Similarly, the number of subjects whose predicated age ranged within ±10 years was 66.66% for both males and females. Thirty-three percent of males and females had a prediction of their age to be >10 years of difference (Table 8). The mean absolute difference that truly represents the accuracy of the formula between the actual age and the predicted age was marginally higher in females than males, but it was not statistically significant. Table 9 shows the complete data and the age prediction of all the samples included in the reference group as well as the test group.

4. Discussion

Among all the types of regressive alterations affecting the teeth, attrition is the only change considered to be physiological that progressively increases with the advancing age. The rest are considered to be due to pathological process. Predicting the age of an individual based only on occlusal wear may not be an accurate estimate as the occlusal wear may be dependent on many factors [18] like dietary habits, mastication, pressure transmitted during mastication, number of teeth present, presence or absence of opposing teeth, presence of artificial teeth, geographic and environmental factors, parafunctional habits like bruxism, and factors like malocclusion. The relation between occlusal wear and aging was evaluated among indigenous Amazon population and suggested that tooth wear is a poor estimator of chronological age in the urban population; however it has a strong association with age for more remote indigenous populations [19]. However, some rare scenarios demand the forensic team to predict the age with limited available information. This may be due to cases like unknown illegal immigration, cases not permitting undertaking invasive samples, and so on. Predicting the age of an individual in such cases based on noninvasive methods like scoring occlusal wear can be an invaluable adjunct for the forensic team.

Table 4: Comparison of mean wear scores of each tooth across different age groups using ANOVA.

Tooth number	Age 21–30		31–40		41–50		51–60		ANOVA test F value	P value
	Mean	SD	Mean	SD	Mean	SD	Mean	SD		
14	2.17	2.82	3.29	2.78	4.38	3.17	4.75	3.43	3.839	0.012
15	1.50	1.85	2.47	1.86	5.58	3.55	4.63	3.61	11.065	0.000
16	1.77	1.61	2.65	2.46	5.50	3.26	5.50	3.23	13.089	0.000
17	1.03	0.96	2.41	1.78	3.50	2.52	4.75	2.79	14.960	0.000
24	2.37	3.18	2.76	2.74	3.58	2.34	4.04	2.93	1.817	0.150
25	1.37	1.88	2.88	2.48	4.92	3.60	4.46	3.15	8.696	0.000
26	1.57	0.86	2.88	2.49	4.83	3.23	5.71	3.51	12.946	0.000
27	1.30	0.92	3.06	2.54	3.29	1.94	4.67	3.14	10.626	0.000
34	1.73	2.96	2.65	2.87	3.50	2.93	3.42	2.75	2.192	0.094
35	1.00	0.87	2.29	2.22	3.29	2.46	3.46	2.89	7.321	0.000
36	2.30	2.45	3.53	2.76	5.75	3.27	7.04	3.14	13.798	0.000
37	1.50	0.82	3.41	2.68	5.29	3.11	5.17	3.24	13.095	0.000
44	1.83	2.91	2.71	2.82	3.38	2.93	3.92	3.06	2.479	0.066
45	1.17	0.91	3.24	2.99	3.96	2.84	4.38	3.37	8.294	0.000
46	2.87	2.61	3.12	2.38	5.21	3.12	7.83	3.09	15.852	0.000
47	2.13	2.08	3.59	3.11	5.63	3.12	5.63	2.99	9.809	0.000

Table 5: Karl Pearson's correlation coefficient (R), coefficient of determination (R^2), and standard error of the estimates for the collected data.

	Correlation coefficient (R)	R square	Std. error of the estimate
All (M & F)	0.806	0.649	8.176
Male (M)	0.908	0.824	7.377
Female (F)	0.864	0.747	7.264

Table 6: Correlation between actual age and tooth wear scores by Karl Pearson's correlation.

Tooth number	Correlation between age and tooth wear scores: Pearson correlation	P value
14	0.352	0.000
15	0.464	0.000
16	0.551	0.000
17	0.568	0.000
24	0.276	0.007
25	0.445	0.000
26	0.563	0.000
27	0.507	0.000
34	0.272	0.008
35	0.448	0.000
36	0.529	0.000
37	0.562	0.000
44	0.282	0.006
45	0.467	0.000
46	0.558	0.000
47	0.498	0.000

Table 7: The intercept and correlation coefficient (β coefficient) observed for multiple regression.

Constant (intercept)	20.6
β coefficient for each tooth	
14	0.019
15	0.635
16	0.087
17	0.838
24	0.368
25	0.016
26	0.567
27	0.889
34	0.665
35	0.172
36	0.305
37	0.827
44	0.361
45	0.112
46	0.589
47	0.097

Numerous systems or indices are available for evaluating the occlusal wear till date [14, 20–23]; however there is no universally accepted method. Kim et al. in the year 2000 presented their 0–8 point method of scoring or recording the occlusal wear and it was shown that their new system was a reliable and accurate method for age estimation [14]. Though Kim's system aims at evaluating the degree of occlusal wear, the system mandatorily requires sound and healthy teeth to be evenly considered. This becomes the biggest practical

TABLE 8: Comparison of accuracy of linear equation in predicting the age of the individuals of the test group.

Group	Mean wear scores	Predicted age that lies within the actual age range (in years)				MAD (in years)
Reference group		*±3*	*±5*	*±10*	*>10*	
Male (n = 38)	3.18	13.15% 5/38	28.93% 11/38	71.03% 27/38	26.31% 10/38	4.50
Female (n = 57)	3.62	21.05% 12/57	29.82% 17/57	70.17% 40/57	29.82% 17/57	8.10
Test group						
Male (n = 15)	4.67	20% 2/15	40% 6/15	66.66% 10/15	33.33% 5/15	8.14
Female (n = 15)	4.22	13.33% 2/15	33.33% 5/15	66.66% 10/15	33.33% 5/15	8.67

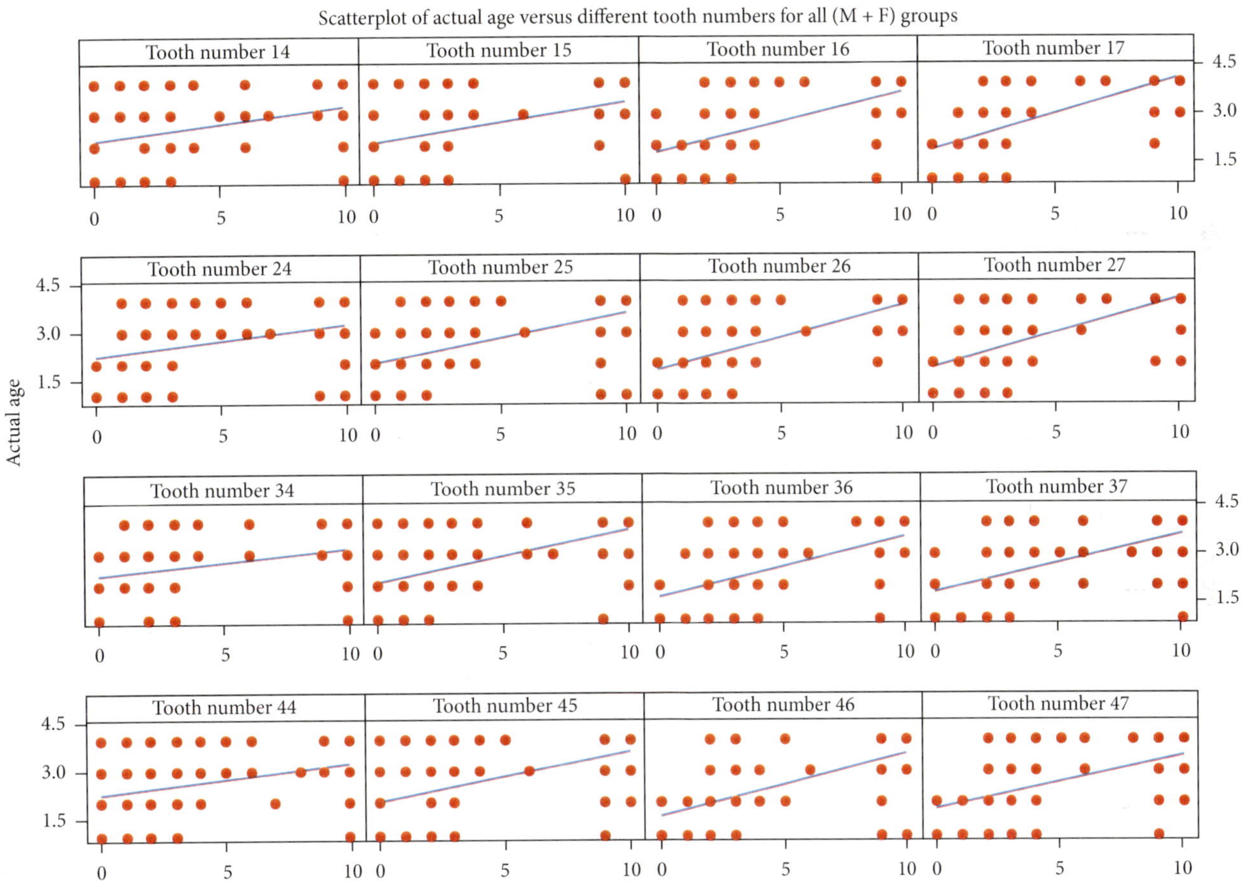

FIGURE 1: Scatter plot showing correlation of actual age with occlusal wear scores.

drawback as oral conditions like dental caries, fractures, and missing teeth are omnipresent in most populations worldwide. Clinicians would always prefer to have a system that is more versatile and that can be applied in widest of the conditions possible. To address this issue, Yun et al. [15] proposed a modification to the original Kim's index, where they included 2 additional points to the already existing 0–8 point scale (Table 2). The proposed modification had 0–10 point scale in evaluating the degree of occlusal wear. In the modified system, all of teeth except the 3rd molars are included and the system also scores for unsound, restored, and even the missing teeth. The basis for such additional points in their modification system is the observed good correlation between such oral conditions and aging. This has been validated on Korean population by a study conducted by Yun et al. [15]. The study by Vieira et al. [19] on indigenous Amazon population differs by saying that the results are population specific which is basically dependent upon their dietary habits. Hence our study aimed at evaluating the clinical validity of modified Kim's index in predicting the age of Chinese Malaysian population. More importantly, we modified the way the index was used. Instead of considering

TABLE 9: Master chart of the details regarding the data of the samples included for the study.

Subject number	Gender	Age group*	Actual age	Estimated age (Y)	Age difference	Groups**
(1)	F	1	24	27.664	3.664	2
(2)	F	1	23	33.887	10.887	4
(3)	F	3	50	52.215	2.215	1
(4)	M	3	41	46.115	5.115	3
(5)	M	1	25	33.018	8.018	3
(6)	F	1	24	30.552	6.552	3
(7)	F	1	24	30.455	6.455	3
(8)	M	1	23	37.889	14.889	4
(9)	M	1	23	30.033	7.033	3
(10)	M	2	33	34.775	1.775	1
(11)	F	2	35	26.546	−8.454	3
(12)	F	1	23	29.806	6.806	3
(13)	M	1	24	27.127	3.127	2
(14)	F	1	25	32.298	7.298	3
(15)	M	3	45	37.711	−7.289	3
(16)	M	1	22	30.326	8.326	3
(17)	M	3	49	42.981	−6.019	3
(18)	F	4	51	61.358	10.358	4
(19)	M	1	26	32.521	6.521	3
(20)	M	1	26	28.475	2.475	1
(21)	F	1	23	31.701	8.701	3
(22)	F	1	23	25.318	2.318	1
(23)	M	1	25	29.128	4.128	2
(24)	F	1	24	25.169	1.169	1
(25)	F	1	23	38.166	15.166	4
(26)	M	1	25	28.227	3.227	2
(27)	M	1	27	34.839	7.839	3
(28)	M	1	24	26.112	2.112	1
(29)	F	3	42	43.741	1.741	1
(30)	M	4	51	39.34	−11.66	4
(31)	F	1	23	27.22	4.22	2
(32)	F	3	47	54.247	7.247	3
(33)	F	1	21	48.486	27.486	4
(34)	M	3	46	49.175	3.175	2
(35)	F	1	27	44.471	17.471	4
(36)	M	2	39	45.959	6.959	3
(37)	F	1	24	34.068	10.068	4
(38)	F	4	57	82.351	25.351	4
(39)	F	4	51	42.457	−8.543	3
(40)	F	1	24	44.376	20.376	4
(41)	M	1	24	33.738	9.738	3
(42)	F	3	43	48.793	5.793	3
(43)	F	2	39	55.874	16.874	4
(44)	F	4	57	56.565	−0.435	1
(45)	M	1	23	25.135	2.135	1
(46)	F	3	43	53.165	10.165	4
(47)	M	1	23	28.464	5.464	3
(48)	F	4	60	48.014	−11.986	4
(49)	M	2	33	36.59	3.59	2
(50)	M	4	55	53.838	−1.162	1

TABLE 9: Continued.

Subject number	Gender	Age group*	Actual age	Estimated age (Y)	Age difference	Groups**
(51)	F	4	51	42.153	−8.847	3
(52)	M	1	24	32.671	8.671	3
(53)	M	4	57	48.133	−8.867	3
(54)	F	3	48	52.35	4.35	1
(55)	M	4	54	36.281	−17.719	4
(56)	M	3	43	55.636	12.636	4
(57)	F	2	40	44.089	4.089	2
(58)	M	3	42	58.93	16.93	4
(59)	F	3	44	48.023	4.023	2
(60)	M	4	60	45.443	−14.557	4
(61)	F	3	45	39.854	−5.146	3
(62)	F	2	35	43.245	8.245	3
(63)	M	4	57	51.838	−5.162	3
(64)	F	4	52	61.7	9.7	3
(65)	F	3	48	38.479	−9.521	3
(66)	M	4	51	47.52	−3.48	2
(67)	F	2	33	27.558	−5.442	3
(68)	F	2	32	26.427	−5.573	3
(69)	F	4	55	57.428	2.428	1
(70)	M	4	53	78.387	25.387	4
(71)	F	2	31	31.836	0.836	1
(72)	F	4	51	51.94	0.94	1
(73)	F	2	40	52.74	12.74	4
(74)	F	4	59	55.329	−3.671	3
(75)	F	3	50	62.75	12.75	4
(76)	F	2	38	48.489	10.489	4
(77)	F	2	32	35.668	3.668	2
(78)	F	2	38	39.207	1.207	1
(79)	F	2	35	49.73	14.73	4
(80)	F	3	50	59.302	9.302	3
(81)	F	3	42	52.317	10.317	4
(82)	M	4	56	61.646	5.646	3
(83)	F	2	33	39.608	6.608	3
(84)	F	3	47	45.104	−1.896	1
(85)	F	4	59	50.995	−8.005	3
(86)	F	4	57	66.936	9.936	3
(87)	M	3	44	63.697	19.697	4
(88)	F	4	57	62.015	5.015	3
(89)	M	2	39	53.772	14.772	4
(90)	M	2	34	44.133	10.133	4
(91)	F	4	52	52.702	0.702	1
(92)	F	3	46	51.89	5.89	3
(93)	F	3	43	61.303	18.303	4
(94)	M	4	60	71.593	11.593	4
(95)	M	3	49	56.861	7.861	3
(96)	F	2	36	37.881	1.881	1
(97)	F	4	60	44.366	−15.634	4
(98)	M	3	48	40.623	−7.377	3
(99)	M	4	56	47.26	−8.74	3
(100)	F	2	36	40.501	4.501	2
(101)	M	3	47	47.054	0.054	1

Table 9: Continued.

Subject number	Gender	Age group*	Actual age	Estimated age (Y)	Age difference	Groups**
(102)	M	4	58	37.511	−20.489	4
(103)	M	3	43	35.717	−7.283	3
(104)	M	4	57	47.256	−9.744	3
(105)	M	4	56	43.639	−12.361	4
(106)	M	4	52	41.936	−10.064	4
(107)	M	2	34	38.625	4.625	2
(108)	M	3	48	43.957	−4.043	2
(109)	M	3	46	42.507	−3.493	2
(110)	M	2	32	33.688	1.688	1
(111)	F	2	37	33.114	−3.886	2
(112)	F	4	57	41.291	−15.709	4
(113)	F	3	41	38.438	−2.562	3
(114)	F	3	44	38.076	−5.924	3
(115)	F	2	31	43.038	12.038	4
(116)	F	3	48	45.961	−2.039	1
(117)	F	4	54	44.933	−9.067	3
(118)	F	3	44	50.813	6.813	3
(119)	F	4	63	40.565	−22.435	4
(120)	M	4	60	44.287	−15.713	4
(121)	F	4	59	43.595	−15.405	4
(122)	M	4	51	48.068	−2.932	1
(123)	M	1	28	41.573	13.573	4
(124)	F	1	27	31.497	4.497	2
(125)	F	1	24	31.773	7.773	3

*Groupings for the age group considered. **Groupings for the age difference between the estimated age and the actual age. ±3 years, group 1; ±5 years, group 2; ±10 years, group 3; >10 years, group 4; subjects from serial numbers 1 to 95 are categorised as "reference group" and 96 to 125 are categorised as "test group."

all the teeth excluding third molars, we considered only the posterior teeth. This was based on the fact that posterior teeth are more prone for occlusal wear rather than the anterior teeth. Posterior teeth have a wider occlusal table making them more vulnerable than the anterior teeth. Previous studies [15, 16] report significantly higher wear among molars and premolars than the incisors and canines. Moreover, this approach will be practically more applicable when compared to using the original Kim's index for forensic applications.

In the present study, 250 (125 pairs) full arch casts were evaluated for occlusal wear. The degree of correlation was moderately positive between the tooth wear scores of all the teeth examined with the correlation coefficient values ranging from 0.272 and 0.568. This could be attributed to the fact that occlusal wear can have other confounding factors as explained by Johansson et al. [18], but nevertheless, the positive relation between aging and teeth wear scores is observed in our study as shown in the scatter plot diagrams. The results showed that the amount of occlusal wear was marginally higher in females than in males; this is in contrast to studies done by many researchers [15, 16]; however this difference was not statistically significant. This is in contrast to previous studies that report significantly higher attrition rates in males than in females [16]. This could be attributable to the dietary habits of the population studied. Our observations indicate similar dietary habits between the males and the females belonging to Chinese Malaysian population. Similarly higher degree of occlusal attrition was noted in older age group than the younger age groups. This is in accordance with previous studies [15, 16, 24, 25]. The mean wear scores of molars were found to be more than the mean occlusal wear scores of the premolars. This can be due to the fact that the molars bear more masticatory load than the premolars. The other reason for this could be due to the eruption sequence. First molars erupt significantly much earlier in the oral cavity than the premolars and hence are exposed earlier and for a longer duration to the physiological wear. This finding of our study is consistent with the previous reports [15, 16, 26–28]. Telang et al. conducted a study on a population of 120 Indians using the Kim's index [16]. The study predicted the age to be ±5 years in 70% and 68.3% and 50% and 50.1% to be ±3 years in males and females, respectively. These results are similar to the findings of our study. Similarly the findings of study done by Yun et al. on sample of 1092 randomly selected pairs also showed similar results [15]. No study previously described in the literature has evaluated occlusal wear and derived a population specific formula using regression analysis and had tested the same formula on a control "test data set group." In our study, we tested the derived formula on further collected cases called "test data set." The Mean absolute difference (MAD) between the predicted age and the actual age was within the acceptable range as described by Solheim and Sundnes [17] in 66.66%

in both males and females. The purpose of such an approach was to estimate the accuracy and practical applicability of the population specific formula in such forensic case work and not halt at an interpretation based correlation between teeth wear scores and the actual age. Moreover, Gorard [29] indicates that statistical estimates based on the standard error of estimate may give misleading interpretations and mentions that MAD is more appropriate in such cases and practical applications. When the predicted ages were compared with the actual age the difference between them was not statistically significant. The limitations of our study include limited number of sample of 250 pairs; a larger sample size might give a better regression formula with lower error rates.

In conclusion, we propose a method to evaluate occlusal wear using a modified index and this was shown to give a good age estimate even when tried on the test sample. These data suggest that the modified Kim's index can be used as an adjunct to quantify occlusal wear to predict the age of an adult individual. We do believe that there is still no universally acceptable method for evaluating occlusal wear; however the method of modifying the already existing index to be tailored to practical applicability renders it more useful than the original Kim's index.

Acknowledgments

This research was done under a financial grant (Project ID no. BDS I-01/13(11)2016) from the International Medical University, Kuala Lumpur, Malaysia.

References

[1] A. B. Acharya, "Forensic dental age estimation by measuring root dentin translucency area using a new digital technique," *Journal of Forensic Sciences*, vol. 59, no. 3, pp. 763–768, 2014.

[2] G. Gustafson, "Age determination on teeth," *The Journal of American Dental Association*, vol. 41, pp. 45–54, 1950.

[3] G. Dalitz, "Age determination of adult human remains by teeth examination," *Journal of the Forensic Science Society*, vol. 3, no. 1, pp. 11–21, 1962.

[4] W. R. Maples, "An improved technique using dental histology for estimation of adult age," *Journal of Forensic Sciences*, vol. 23, no. 4, pp. 764–770, 1978.

[5] A. B. Acharya and K. K. Kumar, "Age estimation in Indians from extracted unsectioned teeth," *Forensic Science International*, vol. 212, no. 1-3, pp. 275–e5, 2011.

[6] G. øilo, B. L. Dahl, G. Hatle, and A.-L. Gad, "An index for evaluating wear of teeth," *Acta Odontologica Scandinavica*, vol. 45, no. 5, pp. 361–365, 1987.

[7] B. L. Dahl, G. Øilo, A. Andersen, and O. Bruaset, "The suitability of a new index for the evaluation of dental wear," *Acta Odontologica Scandinavica*, vol. 47, no. 4, pp. 205–210, 1989.

[8] M. J. Roberts and K. M. Söderholm, "Comparison of three techniques for measuring wear of dental restorations," *Acta Odontologica Scandinavica*, vol. 47, no. 6, pp. 367–374, 1989.

[9] M. López-Nicolás, M. Canteras, and A. Luna, "Age estimation by IBAS image analysis of teeth," *Forensic Science International*, vol. 45, no. 1-2, pp. 143–150, 1990.

[10] V. K. Kashyap and N. R. Koteswara Rao, "A modified Gustafson method of age estimation from teeth," *Forensic Science International*, vol. 47, no. 3, pp. 237–247, 1990.

[11] K. L. Spalding, B. A. Buchholz, L.-E. Bergman, H. Druid, and J. Frisén, "Age written in teeth by nuclear tests," *Nature*, vol. 437, no. 7057, pp. 333-334, 2005.

[12] J. Jayaraman, N. M. King, G. J. Roberts, and H. M. Wong, "Dental age assessment: are Demirjian's standards appropriate for southern Chinese children?" *The Journal of Forensic Odonto-Stomatology*, vol. 29, no. 2, pp. 22–28, 2011.

[13] M. B. Jeevan, A. D. Kale, P. V. Angadi, and S. Hallikerimath, "Age estimation by pulp/tooth area ratio in canines: Cameriere's method assessed in an Indian sample using radiovisiography," *Forensic Science International*, vol. 204, no. 1-3, pp. 209–e5, 2011.

[14] Y. Kim, H. Kho, and K. Lee, "Age estimation by occlusal tooth wear," *Journal of Forensic Sciences*, vol. 45, no. 2, pp. 303–309, 2000.

[15] J.-I. Yun, J.-Y. Lee, J.-W. Chung, H.-S. Kho, and Y.-K. Kim, "Age estimation of Korean adults by occlusal tooth wear," *Journal of Forensic Sciences*, vol. 52, no. 3, pp. 678–683, 2007.

[16] L. A. Telang, K. Patil, and V. G. Mahima, "Age estimation of an Indian population by using the Kim's scoring system of occlusal tooth wear," *Journal of Forensic Dental Sciences*, vol. 6, pp. 16–24, 2014.

[17] T. Solheim and P. K. Sundnes, "Dental age estimation of Norwegian adults - A comparison of different methods," *Forensic Science International*, vol. 16, no. 1, pp. 7–17, 1980.

[18] A. Johansson, T. Haraldson, R. Omar, S. Kiliaridis, and G. E. Carlsson, "An investigation of some factors associated with occlusal tooth wear in a selected high-wear sample," *European Journal of Oral Sciences*, vol. 101, no. 6, pp. 407–415, 1993.

[19] E. P. Vieira, M. S. Barbosa, C. C. A. Quintão, and D. Normando, "Relationship of tooth wear to chronological age among indigenous Amazon populations," *PLoS ONE*, vol. 10, no. 1, Article ID e0116138, 2015.

[20] F. J. López-Frías, L. Castellanos-Cosano, J. Martán-González, J. M. Llamas-Carreras, and J. J. Segura-Egea, "Clinical measurement of tooth wear: Tooth wear indices," *Journal of Clinical and Experimental Dentistry*, vol. 4, no. 1, pp. 48–53, 2012.

[21] A. Johansson, T. Haraldson, R. Omar, S. Kiliaridis, and G. E. Carlsson, "A system for assessing the severity and progression of occlusal tooth wear," *Journal of Oral Rehabilitation*, vol. 20, no. 2, pp. 125–131, 1993.

[22] D. Bartlett, C. Ganss, and A. Lussi, "Basic Erosive Wear Examination (BEWE): A new scoring system for scientific and clinical needs," *Clinical Oral Investigations*, vol. 12, no. 1, pp. 65–68, 2008.

[23] P. F. Bardsley, "The evolution of tooth wear indices," *Clinical Oral Investigations*, vol. 12, pp. S15–S19, 2008.

[24] A. Hugoson, T. Bergendal, A. Ekfeldt, and M. Helkimo, "Prevalence and severity of incisal and occlusal tooth wear in an adult swedish population," *Acta Odontologica Scandinavica*, vol. 46, no. 5, pp. 255–265, 1988.

[25] M. A. Pigno, J. P. Hatch, R. C. M. Rodrigues-Garcia, S. Sakai, and J. D. Rugh, "Severity, distribution, and correlates of occlusal tooth wear in a sample of Mexican-American and European-American adults," *International Journal of Prosthodontics*, vol. 14, no. 1, pp. 65–70, 2001.

[26] O. Bernhardt, C. Schwahn, and G. Meyer, "Risk factors for high occlusal wear scores in a population-based sample: results of the study of health inPomerania (SHIP)," *International Journal of Prosthodontics*, vol. 17, pp. 333–339, 2004.

[27] S. P. Ramfjord and M. M. Ash, *Clinical Occlusion*, WB Sanders, Philadelphia, Pa, USA, 3rd edition, 1983.

[28] G. A. Zarb, C. L. Bolender, and G. E. Carlson, *Boucher's Prostodontic Treatment for Edentulous Patients*, Mosby, Singapore, 11th edition, 1997.

[29] S. Gorard, "Revisiting A 90-year-old debate: The advantages of the mean deviation," *British Journal of Educational Studies*, vol. 53, no. 4, pp. 417–430, 2005.

23

Oral Health of Lipjan Convicts: Kosovo Prison House

Luljeta Zajmi,[1] Agim Begzati ,[2] Milaim Sejdini,[3] Nora Berisha ,[3] and Lumnije Krasniqi[2]

[1] *Lipjan Correctional Center, Family Medicine Center Prishtina, Prishtina, Kosovo*
[2] *Department of Pediatric and Preventive Dentistry, University Dentistry Clinical Center of Kosovo, Prishtina, Kosovo*
[3] *Department of Orthodontics, University Dentistry Clinical Center of Kosovo, Prishtina, Kosovo*

Correspondence should be addressed to Agim Begzati; agim.begzati@uni-pr.edu

Academic Editor: Lia Rimondini

Objectives. The oral health services of the prison population are considered more complex than those of the general population. The aim of this study was to examine the oral health status (the DMFT index and OHI index) and to evaluate the relation between the oral health and risk factors of inmates of this population, thus identifying the dental health status of inmates by gender, age, and the duration of their sentence. *Materials and Methods.* Our study has included a total number of 150 inmates, of both genders, from Lipjan prison house in Kosovo. *Results.* Oral health condition of inmates in Lipjan prison house is severe; the average value of DMFT is 8.44: for minors 6.22, while for adults 9.55. The assessment of DMFT index within the recruited inmates in our study shows that the mean rate of oral cure was 3.21, while the mean extraction value and caries were 3.55 and 3.58, respectively. The mean plaque test value was 1.44. *Conclusion.* Based on this research, we have concluded that the oral health condition of the inmates in Lipjan prison is not good, due to the presence of different risk factors among them.

1. Introduction

Providing dental services within the prison environment can make dentists face up with many unique challenges, including concerns about the threats to personal security, inability to move freely, and the requirements to deliver dental services that, in many cases, require modernization [1]. The oral health services of the prison population are more comprehensive than those of the general population [2]. The strengthening of oral health services among the prison population is a priority determined specifically by the WHO taking into account the increased prevalence of oral disease and limitations of providing the oral health services in the prison conditions [3].

The most important principle for better dental services in prison houses is the oral health promotion and more effective commitments towards dental treatment [4].

The health system in prison houses is organized in order to respond to the health needs of convicts. Health care in prison houses includes the following: primary health care, clinical problems, infectious diseases, mental health in prisons, oral health, and special health requirements for female inmates.

So far, no scientific research has been conducted in terms of oral health in Kosovo prison houses, but in the routine annual reports performed in our country, the problem of limited oral health services within the general health evaluations in prison houses has been brought up. According to several published studies in other countries, we can see that the oral health of convicts is accompanied by several barriers compared to the general population [5, 6]. Osborn et al. stated that "oral health care in prisons is low; therefore, measures shall be taken to promote and improve oral health in prisons" [7]. "Inmates have poorer general and oral health than the nonprison population," concluded Heidari et al. [8]. Many people who suffer conviction are usually unemployed prior to their imprisonment, with poor financial incomes and lower social status. As it has been stated by this author, sixty-two percent ($n = 76$) of the study subjects were unemployed prior to their arrest, whereas the rest of them said that the most common previous employments were as a builder, a painter, a decorator, or in catering services [8].

In such circumstances, it is evident that their health in general is considerably neglected, especially oral health. Furthermore, the majority of convicts who enter prison suffer from poor oral health. Alcohol, tobacco smoking, and the use of drugs contribute to dental caries and oral mucosa disease [9]. According to the recently published data, the oral health condition of inmates is in a very severe condition [7, 8]. The need for dental services continues to grow with the increasing number of inmates. Current available literature indicates that the index of oral status amongst convicts is much worse than in the general population. Risk factors in prison houses increase due to the prevalence of drugs, tobacco, and low educational level. The drug addicts (e.g., heroin) mainly have xerostomia which precedes the rapid increase of caries lesions [10]. The inmates have had a few previous dental interventions; several convicts have physical and mental problems, and the majority experience anxiety when being examined by the dentist.

In a research conducted in 2003 in Australia, out of 789 inmates (657 males and 132 females), the average DMFT value was 20.4 [7]. In a research conducted in the USA, in a Correctional Service of Michigan, out of 251 males, within the inmates of 18–34 age groups, the DMFT value was 11.52 [11, 12].

In the outpatient department of Lipjan-Kosovo prison house, the dental clinic is supplied with all the necessary dental equipment, instruments, and materials, and it hires one general dentist.

Furthermore, this dental clinic has also been providing dental services to the convicts and detained subjects from other prison houses and detention centers such as Pristina and Prizren centers (Kosovo).

The aim of this descriptive epidemiologic study is to introduce the oral health status of the convicts in Lipjan prison (Kosovo).

The aim of this study was to examine the dental health status (the DMFT index) and to evaluate the relation between the oral health and the risk factors of inmates within this population. Moreover, the survey tends to identify the dental health status of the inmates by gender, age, and the duration of their sentence.

2. Materials and Methods

Our study involved a total number of 150 inmates, of both genders, from Lipjan prison house. Out of this number, 50 were juvenile male inmates, 50 were adult male inmates, and 50 were female inmates. The inmates were consecutively enrolled in order to reach the sample size of 150 individuals. For the comparison purposes of the results, we have divided the inmates/detainees by these respective age groups: 19–24 years old, 25–34 years old, and >35 years old. The patients were all informed about the purpose and the tasks of this research. The patients who refused to be examined have been replaced by other patients. The research did not include inmates and patients with chronic generalized parodontopathy, mobile prosthetic appliance users, remaining roots in both dental arches, and semi-impacted teeth.

The research included the following:

(1) The evaluation of dental health status with the DMFT index, amongst the convicts in the Lipjan prison house

(2) Separate DMFT structure specification for the number of carious/decayed teeth (D), extracted/missed (M) teeth, and filled (F) teeth

(3) Assessment of the oral hygiene using the plaque index and the tartar index

(4) Comparison of the values within the gender and the age of the inmates

(5) Assessment of the inmates' oral health depending on the duration of their sentence

(6) Proposal for the measures to improve the overall oral health

The assessment of the inmates' oral health has been conducted in the dental treatment center of the outpatient clinic of the Lipjan prison house, using dental mirrors, probes, and artificial light. An approval from the prison's directorate was obtained prior to the commencement of the research, and ethical principles of the Helsinki convention were implemented. The examination was carried out by the dentist working in the dental treatment center and professionally, with intra-examiner reliability of kappa = 0.95 based on the examination of 15 inmates of different ages, supported by the professors from the Faculty of Dentistry of the University of Prishtina, Kosovo. The manuscript has been approved by the ethical authority of Kosovo correctional service (08 No. 1249).

Data collection was completed utilizing questionnaires prepared for the purposes of this study that include the following data:

(i) General data (name and surname, birthplace, gender, age, nationality, education, smoking, drugs, alcohol, bruxism, breathing through the mouth, the sentence duration within the prison, teeth cleaning techniques, and brushing)

(ii) Data regarding the dental status—the presence of caries lesions, fillings, and extraction due to caries (DMFT index)

(iii) Assessment of the oral hygiene index

2.1. DMFT Index. DMFT index determination is conducted according to the presence of caries/decay (D), filling (F), and extraction (missing) due to the caries tooth (M). Decayed lesion cavity is defined as the presence of caries; it is visible for the eye, and there is a loss of transparency or dental probe stumble during easy probe.

2.2. Index of Oral Hygiene (OHI Index). Evaluation of oral hygiene index is determined by using the Green Vermilion index for dental plaque and tooth tartar.

2.3. Data Analysis. The introduction of the data is completed by using the tables and graphs. Data processing is conducted

Table 1: DMFT values according to the groups.

DMFT	Group: Juvenile inmates	Group: Adult inmates	Total
N	50	100	150
Mean	**6.22**	**9.55**	**8.65**
SD	4.65	6.21	5.54
Min	0	0	0
Max	26	28	28
Mann–Whitney U test	$U' = 1304$, $P = 0.712$	$U' = 5552$, $P = 0.177$	

Table 2: DMFT values for adult inmates according to their age group and gender.

Gender	DMFT	Age group/mean age: 19–24 (21.5 ± 1.7)	25–34 (28.7 ± 2.6)	35+ (40.2 ± 6.2)	Total
	N	14	22	14	50
F	Mean	6.21	7.18	13.64	**8.72**
	SD	6.13	5.34	6.46	6.56
	N	19	21	10	50
M	Mean	8.42	11.62	11.50	**10.38**
	SD	3.73	7.24	4.95	5.78
	N	**33**	**43**	**24**	**100**
Total	Mean	**7.48**	**9.35**	**12.75**	**9.55**
	SD	**4.93**	**6.65**	**5.86**	**6.21**

Table 3: Decay (D) value of the adult inmates according to the age group and gender.

Gender	D	Age group/mean age: 19–24 (21.5 ± 1.7)	25–34 (28.7 ± 2.6)	35+ (40.2 ± 6.2)	Total
	N	14	22	14	50
F	Mean	2.86	1.55	1.43	1.88
	SD	4.52	1.74	2.74	3.01
	N	19	21	10	50
M	Mean	3.95	5.00	3.60	4.32
	SD	2.84	4.76	2.50	3.71
	N	**33**	**43**	**24**	**100**
Total	Mean	**3.48**	**3.23**	**2.33**	**3.10**
	SD	**3.62**	**3.92**	**2.81**	**3.58**

with the statistical package Inst 3. The minimum and the maximum values were calculated from the statistical parameter index structure, arithmetic mean, and standard deviation. For the data testing, the Fisher exact test, χ^2 test, Mann–Whitney U test, and Kruskal–Wallis test were used, and the significant difference of $P < 0.05$ was used.

3. Results

3.1. DMFT Index Assessment Results. The research included 150 inmates who were divided into two groups of 50 juvenile inmates or 100 adult inmates. Table 1 shows the mean DMFT results for the whole number of examined inmates (8.65 (SD ± 5.54)). For juvenile inmates, the DMFT was 6.22 (SD ± 4.65), while it was 9.55 (SD ± 6.21) for adult inmates.

The average value of DMFT for adult inmates, according to their group age and gender, is presented in Table 2. The average DMFT of age group 19–24 years old was 7.48 (SD ± 4.93), that of 25–34 years old was 9.35 (SD ± 6.65), and that of 35+ years old was 12.75 (SD ± 5.86). The average value of DMFT for female inmates was 8.72 (SD ± 6 : 56). The DMFT average value of male inmates was 10.38 (SD ± 5.78).

Table 3 shows the average decayed teeth in the DMFT structure. The average value of decayed teeth (D) of the adult inmates between 19 and 24 years was 3.48 (SD ± 3.62); for those aged 25–34 years, the value was 3.23 (SD ± 3.92); and

Table 4: Missing (M) values of adult inmates according to age group and gender.

Gender	M	Age group/mean age 19–24 (21.5 ± 1.7)	25–34 (28.7 ± 2.6)	35+ (40.2 ± 6.2)	Total
	N	14	22	14	50
F	Mean	1.50	2.64	7.36	**3.64**
	SD	1.61	3.26	4.24	3.96
	N	19	21	10	50
M	Mean	2.74	3.52	4.90	**3.50**
	SD	2.42	3.34	3.67	3.13
	N	**33**	**43**	**24**	**100**
Total	Mean	**2.21**	**3.07**	**6.33**	**3.57**
	SD	**2.18**	**3.29**	**4.11**	**3.55**

Table 5: Filled (F) value of the adult inmates according to age group and gender.

Gender	F	Age group/mean age 19–24 (21.5 ± 1.7)	25–34 (28.7 ± 2.6)	35+ (40.2 ± 6.2)	Total
	N	14	22	14	50
F	Mean	2.00	3.05	4.86	**3.26**
	SD	1.75	3.88	3.48	3.42
	N	19	21	10	50
M	Mean	1.84	3.10	3.00	**2.60**
	SD	2.63	3.14	3.23	2.98
	N	**33**	**43**	**24**	**100**
Total	Mean	**1.91**	**3.07**	**4.08**	**2.93**
	SD	**2.27**	**3.50**	**3.44**	**3.21**

Table 6: DMFT, D, M, and F values according to the sentence duration.

Sentence duration	*N*	DMFT		D		M		F	
		Mean	SD	Mean	SD	Mean	SD	Mean	SD
Till 1 year	68	9.54	6.72	3.97	3.88	3.01	3.85	2.62	3.08
1–5 years	26	8.58	4.38	2.46	1.88	2.65	2.53	3.50	3.35
Over 5 years	6	6.83	4.45	0.33	0.52	2.50	3.33	4.00	4.00
Total	100	9.55	6.21	3.10	3.58	3.57	3.55	2.93	3.21
Kruskal–Wallis test		$P < 0.05$		$P < 0.05$		$P < 0.05$		$P < 0.05$	

for those aged 35+ years, it was 2.33 (SD ± 2.81). The average value of D of the female inmates was 1.88 (SD ± 3.01). The average value of D of the male inmates was 4.32 (SD ± 3.71).

The average value for extracted teeth (missing due to caries, M) is introduced in Table 4. This value for adult inmates between the ages of 19 and 24 years was 21.2 (SD ± 2.18), for those aged 25–34 years was 3.07 (SD ± 3.29), and for those aged 35+ years was 6.33 (SD ± 4.11). The average value of M of female inmates was 3.64 (SD ± 3.96). The average value of M of male inmates was 3.50 (SD ± 3.13).

Table 5 shows the average of treated teeth (filled, F). The average value of F for the adult inmates between the ages of 19 and 24 years was 1.91 (SD ± 2.27), for those of the age group 25–34 years was 3.07 (SD ± 3.50), and for those aged 35+ years was 4.08 (SD ± 3.44). The average value of F for female inmates was 3.26 (SD ± 3.42). The average value of F for the male inmates was 2.60 (SD ± 2.98).

DMFT index value results based on the sentence duration of the adult inmates are presented in Table 6. For adult inmates who had a sentence till 1 year, the DMFT was 9.54 (SD ± 6.72); for those sentenced from 1 to 5 years, the DMFT was 8.58 (SD ± 4.38); and for those sentenced for more than 5 years, it was 6.83 (SD ± 4.45). As shown in Table 6, in between values of DMFT, D, M, and F according to the sentence duration using Kruskal–Wallis test, we found a significant statistical difference for $P < 0.05$.

3.2. Oral Hygiene Index Results (Plaque Index). The average value of the dental plaque index/oral hygiene index (Table 7)

TABLE 7: Dental plaque index value of adult inmates according to their age group and gender.

Gender	Plaque index	Age group/mean age 19–24 (21.5 ± 1.7)	25–34 (28.7 ± 2.6)	35+ (40.2 ± 6.2)	Total
	N	14	22	14	50
F	Mean	1.43	1.23	1.50	**1.36**
	SD	0.65	0.61	0.85	0.69
	N	19	21	10	50
M	Mean	1.68	1.33	1.60	**1.52**
	SD	0.48	0.66	0.97	0.68
	N	**33**	**43**	**24**	**100**
Total	Mean	**1.58**	**1.28**	**1.54**	**1.44**
	SD	**0.56**	**0.63**	**0.88**	**0.69**

of adult inmates for the age groups of 19–24 years was 1.58 (SD ± 0.56), for those of the age group 25–34 years was 1.28 (SD ± 0.63), and for those aged 35+ years was 1.54 (SD ± 0.88). The average value of the dental plaque index for female inmates was 1.36 (SD ± 0.69). The average value of the dental plaque index for male inmates was 1.52 (SD ± 0.68).

OHI value results according to the sentence duration are presented in Table 8. The total plaque index value for adult inmates was 1.44 (SD ± 0.69), the tartar index value was 0.41 (SD ± 0.59), and the OHI value was 1.85 (SD ± 1.10). Based on calculated values introduced in Table 8 between the values of plaque index, the tartar tooth index, and OHI according to the sentence duration using Kruskal-Wallis test, we found an important statistical significance for $P < 0.05$.

3.3. The Harmful Habits of the Inmates. Out of the overall number of juvenile inmates, 60% were tobacco users and 10% of the juvenile inmates and 8% of the adult inmates stated that they drink alcohol.

Furthermore, 8% of the juvenile inmates stated that they use drugs. While among adult inmates, 16% stated "yes" for taking drugs. Bruxism is very common among inmates; about 50% have confirmed that grinding teeth is their habit. Oral breathing is more common among inmates. Thus, it is expressed in 28% of juvenile inmates and 19% of adult inmates.

4. Discussion

Inmates in jails and prisons are considered as a high-risk population and are exposed to a high prevalence of different communicable diseases, mental disease, and chronic diseases, and they are exposed to a higher risk for different infective diseases. Due to these circumstances at the prisons, this vulnerable group of the population does not have any favorable conditions for the maintenance of their oral health, and realistically, their oral health needs are higher compared to the general population [13].

Oral health conditions of Lipjan prison house inmates are severe, and the average value of DMFT is 8.44, for minors 6.22, while for adults 9.55. Higher value of DMFT is recorded for older inmates (+35 years old: 12.75).

TABLE 8: Plaque and tartar index values according to the sentence duration.

Sentence duration	*N*	Plaque index Mean	SD	Tartar index Mean	SD	Total OHI Mean	SD
Till 1 year	68	1.56	0.76	0.51	0.63	2.07	1.20
1–5 years	26	1.23	0.43	0.23	0.43	1.46	0.65
Over 5 years	6	1.00	0.00	0.00	0.00	1.00	0.00
Total	**100**	**1.44**	**0.69**	**0.41**	**0.59**	**1.85**	**1.10**
Kruskal-Wallis test		$P < 0.05$		$P < 0.05$		$P < 0.05$	

Comparing the oral health status of the inmates in Lipjan prison house with the oral health conditions in prisons around the world, there were no significant statistical differences.

A research similar to ours with an approximate mean of DMFT for adult inmates conducted in America, Correctional Service of Michigan, by Ormes, Carolyn, Thompson, and Brimm (1997) with a total number of 251 male inmates, for the age group 18–34 years, had the mean value of DMFT 11.52. We must note that most of these inmates were African-Americans [11, 14]. This mean DMFT is approximate with the DMFT of Lipjan male inmates being 10.55. High DMFT values (12.75) were found in the age group +35 years. Low DMFT (7.48) was found in the age group 19–24 years. But, we have found different values from the literature, sometimes very high; for example, in Australia, in a research conducted in 2003 on 789 inmates (657 males and 132 females) from 27 correctional centers in New South Wales, Australia, the mean DMFT value was 20.4 [7]. The mean DMFT index value of 340 inmates in South Africa reported by Naidoo et al. [15] was 15.45, while for 127 male Brazilian inmates the DMFT index value was 19.72 [16].

In Lipjan (Kosovo) prison, of 150 examined inmates, 50 were females, with the mean DMFT of 8.72. Compared to the data from the literature, these values are similar. In the research conducted for the purpose of determining the oral health of female inmates in the Correctional Department in New York City-Correction Department in Riker's Island Correctional Facility, out of the 183 inmates examined the DMFT mean value was 9.9 [17].

In our research, in order to determine the oral health of women in Lipjan prison house, we calculated a DMFT mean value of 8.5, and there was no significant difference compared to the female inmates in the Correctional Department of NY.

The evaluation of DMFT of inmates recruited in our study shows that the mean rate of oral cure was 3.21, while the mean extraction value and caries were 3.55 and 3.58, respectively. The main difference between our study and other results is that dental oral cure in our survey is 30%, while Ormes et al. [14] show a treatment success rate of over 60%.

During the comparison between the values of DMFT, D, M, and F and the sentence duration with the Kruskal–Wallis test, we have found that DMFT index values decrease with the increasing residence time in prison. Even though the value remains high, an improvement of oral health status has been noted. The data analysis according to the sentence duration shows that the number of treated teeth is the highest. Also, the plaque index is decreasing. This, as an overall result, is a consequence of active work of the prison dental clinic.

However, in our research through the OHI, the oral health status results as being in a quite severe condition. The total plaque index for adult inmates was 1.44. The author found some approximation between the data of the OHI of the inmates (1.96) and our data as well [18].

The data from the literature also reveal the negligence on oral hygiene: 97.4% of the subjects (inmates) needed oral hygiene instructions [19].

Bad habits such as smoking tobacco and the use of alcohol and drugs within the inmates were very commonly expressed. These bad habits can affect the overall situation of the oral health status of the inmates. The data from the literature also reveal a very high consumption of tobacco within the prison houses. In a study conducted by Akaji and Folaranmi, 52.2% of inmates were current smokers [20].

5. Conclusion and Recommendations

Based on this research, we have concluded that oral health conditions of the inmates in Lipjan prison house are not so good, due to the low structure of dental cure (approximately 30%) compared to the rate of dental extraction and dental caries (around 70% of DMFT structure).

Detention centers in Prishtina, Lipjan, and Prizren have no dental services; therefore, the inmates have to be transported to the dentist who works in Lipjan prison. This procedure in itself contains many difficulties. Detainees may be from different categories, including those of the high-risk category.

On the basis of this research, it is proved that the lack of dental services within the detention centers aggravates even more the already serious situation of the inmates' oral health. Taking into account the difficulties that a lot of doctors encounter in prisons, by security restrictions and by a large number of inmates, the need for further promotion of oral health in prisons is obvious.

The values of DMFT and OHI for inmates according to their sentence duration had some improvements. This means that the inmates who have remained in prison for a longer period of time, thanks to the available dental services, had experienced improvements of their oral health status.

We learn from the current available literature that the oral health condition of inmates is more serious than that within the general population. On the basis of this research, we found that there is a serious health condition within the inmates, but the serious oral health condition was evident in the general public as well.

The main aggravating factor of oral health for inmates is the low index of oral hygiene and then the bad habits of this population with direct impact on DMFT values, the plaque test, and the periodontal index. The presence of the dental clinic within the prison premises had resulted in an increased interest of inmates for dental treatment, for better oral hygiene, and alike. However, the DMFT and the plaque index values remain high, so inmates' health care should be more active.

5.1. Recommendations. There is a need for an increased awareness within our society of the wider population regarding oral health issues. Therefore, it is an imperative for the health care decision-makers to provide more dental services within the detention centers of our country and to further promote the oral health in prisons. The existence of full-service dental clinics within prisons will significantly affect the improvement of the convicts' health status.

Overall, the promotion of oral health in prisons, better health education, and the improvement of bad habits should be of top priority.

The measures at the central government level regarding the serious condition of the oral health of our inmates and of the general population need to be very serious and always in compliance with the WHO criteria.

Acknowledgments

The authors wish to thank the Prison Department Managers for their involvement and support in the actual study.

References

[1] C. G. A. Nobile, L. Fortunato, M. Pavia, and I. F. Angelillo, "Oral health status of male prisoners in Italy," *International Dental Journal*, vol. 57, no. 1, pp. 27–35, 2007.

[2] P. Neville, "Oral health among UK prisoners," *Perspectives in Public Health*, vol. 135, no. 4, pp. 176-177, 2015.

[3] R. Gray and S. Gregory, "Dental health in prisons," http://www.euro.who.int/__data/.../Prisons-and-Health,-12-Dental-health-in-prisons.pdf.

[4] P. Rouxel, D. Duijster, G. Tsakos, and R. G. Watt, "Oral health of female prisoners in HMP Holloway: implications for oral health promotion in UK prisons," *British Dental Journal*, vol. 214, no. 12, pp. 627–632, 2013.

[5] D. Mehlisch, "Oral health screening–a means to improve dental care in correctional institutions," *Journal of Prison & Jail Health*, vol. 6, no. 1, pp. 62–77, 1986.
[6] G. Barnes, T. Heid, W. Parker, J. Cole, and R. Fultz, "Dental care requirements of male inmates recently incarcerated in Texas department of corrections prisons," *Journal of Prison & Jail Health*, vol. 7, pp. 37–52, 1988.
[7] M. Osborn, T. Butler, and P. Barnard, "Oral health status of prison inmates—New South Wales, Australia," *Australian Dental Journal*, vol. 48, no. 1, pp. 34–38, 2003.
[8] E. Heidari, C. Dickinson, R. Wilson, and J. Fiske, "Oral health of remand prisoners in HMP Brixton, London," *British Dental Journal*, vol. 202, no. 2, p. E5, 2007.
[9] P. Barnard, *National Oral Health Survey Australia 1987-88: A Report of the First National Oral Health Survey of Australia*, Australian Government Publishing Service, Canberra, Australia, 1993.
[10] F. Di Cugno, C. Perec, and A. Tocci, "Salivary secretion and dental caries experience in drug addicts," *Archives of Oral Biology*, vol. 26, no. 5, pp. 363–367, 1981.
[11] W. S Ormes, *The Measurement of Dental Disease in a Correctional Setting-the Importance to Functional Service Delivery*, Western Michigan University, Kalamazoo, MI, USA, 1996.
[12] R. B. Greifinger, J. A. Bick, and J. Goldenson, *Public Health Behind Bars: From Prisons to Communities*, Springer, Berlin, Germany, 2007.
[13] H. M. Treadwell and M. E. Northridge, "Oral health is the measure of a just society," *Journal of Health Care for the Poor and Underserved*, vol. 18, no. 1, pp. 12–20, 2007.
[14] W. S. Ormes, D. Carlyon, W. F. Thompso, and M. Brim, "The measurement of dental disease in a correctional setting and its importance to functional service delivery," *Journal of Correctional Health Care*, vol. 4, no. 2, pp. 105–119, 1997.
[15] S. Naidoo, V. Yengopal, and B. Cohen, "A baseline survey: oral health status of prisoners–Western Cape," *Journal of the South African Dental Association*, vol. 60, no. 1, pp. 24–27, 2005.
[16] A. L. Cavalcanti, I. Rodrigues, I. de Melo Silveira et al., "Dental caries experience and use of dental services among Brazilian prisoners," *International Journal of Environmental Research and Public Health*, vol. 11, no. 12, pp. 12118–12128, 2014.
[17] V. Badner and R. Margolin, "Oral health status among women inmates at Rikers Island correctional facility," *Journal of Correctional Health Care*, vol. 1, no. 1, pp. 55–71, 1994.
[18] O. B. Braimoh, O. O. Sofola, and S. A. Okeigbemen, "Oral hygiene profile of inmates in a correctional home," *Annals of Biomedical Sciences*, vol. 11, no. 2, pp. 36–43, 2012.
[19] K. Singh, S. H. Bhandari, C. H. Anandani, P. Pani, S. H. Kansal, and H. Chaudhary, "Prevalence of periodontal diseases and oral hygiene practices among drug addicted inmates," *Journal of Oral Health and Dental Management*, vol. 13, no. 4, 2014.
[20] E. A. Akaji and N. Folaranmi, "Tobacco use and oral health of inmates in a Nigerian prison," *Nigerian Journal of Clinical Practice*, vol. 16, no. 4, pp. 473–477, 2013.

24

Survival and Success Rates of Different Shoulder Designs: A Systematic Review of the Literature

Marco Tallarico,[1,2] Marco Caneva,[3] Silvio Mario Meloni,[4] Erta Xhanari,[5] Yuki Omori,[3,6] and Luigi Canullo[2]

[1]*Implantology and Prosthetic Aspects, Master of Science in Dentistry Program, Aldent University, Tirana, Albania*
[2]*Private Practice, Rome, Italy*
[3]*ARDEC Academy, Ariminum Odontologica Srl, Rimini, Italy*
[4]*Dentistry Unit, University Hospital of Sassari, Sassari, Italy*
[5]*Private Practice, Tirana, Albania*
[6]*Department of Oral Implantology, Osaka Dental University, Hirakata, Osaka, Japan*

Correspondence should be addressed to Luigi Canullo; luigicanullo@yahoo.com

Academic Editor: Shinn-Jyh Ding

Objectives. To identify whether there is a relationship between different implant shoulder positions/orientations/designs and prosthetic and/or implant failures, biological or mechanical complications, radiographic marginal bone loss (MBL), peri-implant buccal recession (RC), aesthetic scores (Papilla Index, PES, and WES), and patient satisfaction after a minimum of 1 year function in the aesthetic zone, compared to the two-piece, conventional implant neck architecture. *Materials and Methods.* The systematic review was written according to the PRISMA guidelines. The search strategy encompassed the English literature from 1967 to September 2016 and was performed online (in the PubMed database of the U.S. National Library of Medicine, Embase, and the Cochrane Library) to identify relevant studies that met the inclusion criteria. The assessment of quality and risk of bias of the selected manuscripts was performed according to the guidelines provided by CONSORT and STROBE statements. *Results.* A total of 16 articles (7 randomized controlled trials, 4 observational comparative studies, and 5 systematic reviews) were selected to fulfill the inclusion criteria. A trend of higher implant failure and prosthetic complications were experienced in the one-piece group compared to the two-piece group, although no statistically significant differences were found. Higher marginal bone loss was found in the test group (one-piece, scalloped implants) compared to the control group (two-piece, flat implants). No comparative studies reporting data on sloped implants were found that fulfilled the inclusion and exclusion criteria of this systematic review. No differences were experienced between groups regarding aesthetic outcomes and patient satisfaction. *Conclusions.* There was sufficient evidence that different implant shoulder positions/orientations/designs (scalloped, sloped, and one piece) offer no benefit when compared to two-piece, conventional flat implants. Current evidence is limited due to the quality of available studies.

1. Introduction

Stability of the peri-implant soft and hard tissues is a prerequisite for a long-term aesthetic and function of implant-supported restoration [1]. In two-piece implants, early bone loss is observed after the connection of the abutment and delivery of final prosthesis, mostly due to the biologic width establishment [2–6]. This concept is being hypothesized as one of the most likely causes of early implant bone loss [2, 3]. The effect of surgical trauma, implant surface characteristics, macrodesign of the implant, and type of implant-abutment connection, as well as implant placement depth, soft tissue thickness, distance between adjacent implants, and abutment height, may all contribute to this process [4–6].

Traditionally, implants are two pieces, and they were placed in a two-step surgical procedure [7]. Two-piece designs can offer increased flexibility, with connections possible at the bone level, and wound closure can be easier.

In the 1980s [8], Schroeder and colleagues introduced an implant where the bone anchorage unit and contiguous transmucosal component were manufactured in a single unit. With one-piece implant designs, the transmucosal part is incorporated into the implants. This was an attempt to minimize crestal bone loss that reduces contamination of the implant-abutment junction. Furthermore, by using a one-piece implant, the second surgery procedure is avoided, as well as abutment connection/disconnection. The advantage of this procedure is to avoid the presence of a gap or micromovement at the implant-abutment junction for a beneficial effect on the peri-implant soft and hard tissues [9]. Nevertheless, compared with two-piece implants, they are much more difficult to place in the prosthetically driven position (height and angulation), which makes one-piece implants even more difficult to finalize. On the other hand, new implant and abutment designs have been proposed to minimize the crestal bone loss. Platform switching is done whenever an abutment is used that is smaller in diameter than the implant platform. This concept has been proposed as an effective prosthetic concept to reduce the amount of peri-implant bone loss around dental implants [10]. The concept of horizontal offset (platform switching) has made it possible to place implant shoulders at the crestal bone level with predictable minimal marginal bone resorption [10]. Scalloped and sloped implants represent other design changes that advocate for maintaining marginal bone levels [11–13]. The scalloped implant was designed with a modified platform that mirrors the natural cement-enamel junction of the anterior teeth and follows the anatomic contour of the anterior alveolar bone crest. The scalloped implants were developed with the intent of preserving interdental bony peaks, supporting the soft tissue, thereby maintaining or creating interimplant papillae [11, 12]. Recently, a dental implant with a sloped marginal contour and a height difference of the implant shoulder of approximately 1.5 mm has been developed with the aim of improving the congruence between the implant and the bone in extraction sites and sloped ridges [13].

The main objective of this systematic review was to compare the prosthetic and/or implant failures, biological or mechanical complications, radiographic marginal bone loss, peri-implant buccal recession, aesthetic scores, and patient satisfaction after at least 1 year of function, around single- or multiple-tooth implant-supported restorations in the aesthetic zone, on the two-piece, conventional implant neck architecture (flat implants with the same level on 360°) and one-piece, scalloped, or sloped implants.

2. Materials and Methods

This systematic review was written according to the Preferred Reporting Items for Systematic Reviews and Meta-Analyses (PRISMA) guidelines [14]. The focused question was to identify whether there is a relationship between different implant shoulder positions/orientations/designs (one piece, scalloped, and sloped) and prosthetic and/or implant failures, biological or mechanical complications, radiographic marginal bone loss, peri-implant buccal recession, aesthetic scores, and patient satisfaction after at least 1 year of function, compared to two-piece, flat implants with the same level on 360°. Initially, PICOS question (population (P), intervention (I), comparison (C), outcomes and study design (O), and study type (S)) defined the search strategy, where P = single and partial edentulous patients required an implant-supported restoration in the aesthetic zone; I = different implant shoulder positions/orientations/designs (scalloped, sloped, and one piece), after at least 1 year of function; C = two piece and same level on 360° (flat implants); O = prosthetic and/or implant failures, biological or mechanical complications, radiographic marginal bone loss (MBL), peri-implant buccal recession (BR), aesthetic scores (Papilla Index, PES, and WES), and patient satisfaction (patient questionnaire and VAS); and S = randomized controlled clinical trials (RCTs), case-control studies, and cohort studies.

2.1. Search Strategy. An initial search strategy that includes the English literature from 1967 to September 2016 was performed to identify relevant studies that met the inclusion criteria of this systematic review. The following databases were consulted: Embase (Excerpta Medica dataBASE), PubMed database of the U.S. National Library of Medicine, Grey Literature Database (New York Academy of Medicine Grey Literature Report), and the Cochrane Library. Screening was performed independently and simultaneously by two calibrated examiners (MT and SMM). The electronic databases were searched using the following terms: ((("dental implants"[Mesh] AND "dental implant abutment design"[Mesh]) OR "dental implant abutment interface"[All Fields]) OR (one[All Fields] AND piece[All Fields] AND implant[All Fields])) OR (("scalloped"[All Fields]) AND implant[All Fields]) OR (sloped[All Fields] AND implant [All Fields]) AND English[lang].

2.2. Eligibility Criteria. The following inclusion criteria were defined for the selection of articles:

(i) Written in English

(ii) Evaluate in their protocol the prosthetic and/or implant failures, biological or mechanical complications, radiographic marginal bone loss, peri-implant buccal recession, aesthetic scores, patient satisfaction, and/or the influence of the implant shoulder position/orientation/design on soft and hard tissue levels around single or multiple implants in the aesthetic zone with scalloped, sloped, and one-piece implants and a two-piece, conventional implant neck architecture (flat implants featured with the same level on 360°)

(iii) Randomized controlled clinical trials of implants of ≥1 year in function

(iv) Observational (prospective and retrospective) case-control studies of implants of ≥1 year in function

(v) Cross-sectional comparative studies of ≥1 year in function

(vi) Systematic reviews, narrative reviews, consensus statements, commentaries, or editorials

Articles were excluded if they were

(i) observational (prospective or retrospective) cohort studies without the control group;

(ii) in vitro studies;

(iii) finite element analyses;

(iv) animal studies;

(v) reports with <5 cases;

(vi) reports involving mini-implants, zirconia implants, or blade implants;

(vii) reports on implants of <1 year in function.

2.3. Data Extraction. The two calibrated reviewers screened all the data from the selected papers. Cohen's kappa values between examiners were calculated at both the stages of the research. Discrepancies were resolved by consensus, and a third examiner was consulted (LC). Articles without abstracts but with titles related to the objectives of this study were included, and their full texts were screened for possible eligibility. Reference lists of the selected articles, including published systematic reviews, were screened for possible additional papers.

The following outcome measures were analyzed when available: [1] prosthetic and/or implant failures leading to loss or removal of the prosthesis and/or implant [2], biological or mechanical complications [3], radiographic marginal bone loss (MBL) [4], peri-implant buccal recession (BR) [5], Papilla Index, pink aesthetic score (PES), and white aesthetic score (WES) [6], and patient satisfaction (patient questionnaire and VAS).

2.4. Assessment of Quality, Heterogeneity, and Risk of Bias of Individual Studies. The same reviewers assessed the quality of the included manuscripts, heterogeneity, and the risk of bias according to the guidelines provided by the CONSORT statement for the evaluation of randomized controlled trials (http://www.consort-statement.org) [15] and the STROBE statement for observational studies (http://www.strobe-statement.org), as well as the modified items from the Cochrane Collaboration's tool for assessing risk of bias [16]. The overall risk of bias was expressed as the percentage of negatively graded items [16]. Quality assessment was performed on the published full-text articles, independently by both reviewers. Disagreements between them were resolved upon discussion. An estimation of plausible risk of bias (low, moderate, or high) was completed for each selected study according to the Cochrane Handbook for Systematic Reviews of Interventions (version 5.1.0. http://www.cochrane.org/resources/handbook).

3. Results

3.1. Study Selection. A total of 945 potentially relevant titles and abstracts were found after the initial electronic and manual search. At this stage, 810 articles were excluded (% of agreement: 89.2%; Cohen's k: 0.35). Complete full-text manuscripts of the remaining 135 articles were evaluated, and 119 articles were excluded since they did not fulfill the inclusion criteria (% of agreement: 97.0; Cohen's k: 0.85), scoring an almost perfect agreement. Finally, a total of 16 articles that fulfilled the inclusion criteria of this systematic review were included in the qualitative analysis. Overall, data from 221 one-piece implants placed in 107 patients, 139 scalloped implants placed in 96 patients, and 366 flat implants (same level on 360°) placed in 207 patients were evaluated. No comparative studies reporting data on sloped implants that fulfilled the inclusion criteria were founded. Of the 16 selected studies, 7 were randomized controlled trials [9, 17–22], 4 were observational comparative studies (2 retrospective and 2 prospective) [23–26], and 5 were systematic reviews [27–31]. A diagram of the search strategy is shown in Figure 1.

Three pairs of manuscripts reported data from the same cohort of patients. Sanz Martin et al. [17] and Thoma et al. [18] published two manuscripts based on the same cohort of 60 patients, reporting volumetric soft tissue change and demographic and radiographic results, respectively. Van Nimwegen et al. [19] published a 5-year follow-up report on the 1-year report of Tymstra et al. [22]. Finally, den Hartog et al. published two manuscripts reporting data from single implants in the aesthetic zone with different neck designs. The first manuscript was published in 2011 and was aimed at reporting radiological and clinical outcome measures [20], while the second manuscript, published 2 years later, focused on the aesthetic outcomes from both professional's and patient's perception [21].

3.2. Risk of Bias. The 16 selected studies were published between 1993 and September 2016. None of the publications were associated with a low risk of bias, while five with a high risk of bias and six with a moderate risk of bias (Table 1). The included articles received minimum grading when written in agreement with the CONSORT/STROBE statement guidelines (0/11), evaluating submission to ethical committees (5/11), none or unclear randomization procedures (7/11), none or unclear allocation concealment (9/11), and blinding of participants/outcome assessors (0/11) (Table 1).

3.3. Prosthetic and/or Implant Failures and Biological or Mechanical Complications. Nine of the eleven clinical studies reported data on implant failure/success. Two studies regarding one-piece implants compared with two-piece implants scored a cumulative survival rate of 100% in both test and control groups [23, 26]. Thoma et al. [18] reported one implant failure in the one-piece group and none in the two-piece group. Duda et al. [24] reported 9 implant failures in the one-piece group (7 immediately loaded and 2 delayed loaded), while no implant failure was reported in the two-piece group. Most of these failures were experienced due to biological complications (peri-implantitis and lack of osseointegration). Conversely, Heijdenrijk et al. [9] reported 2 implant failures in the

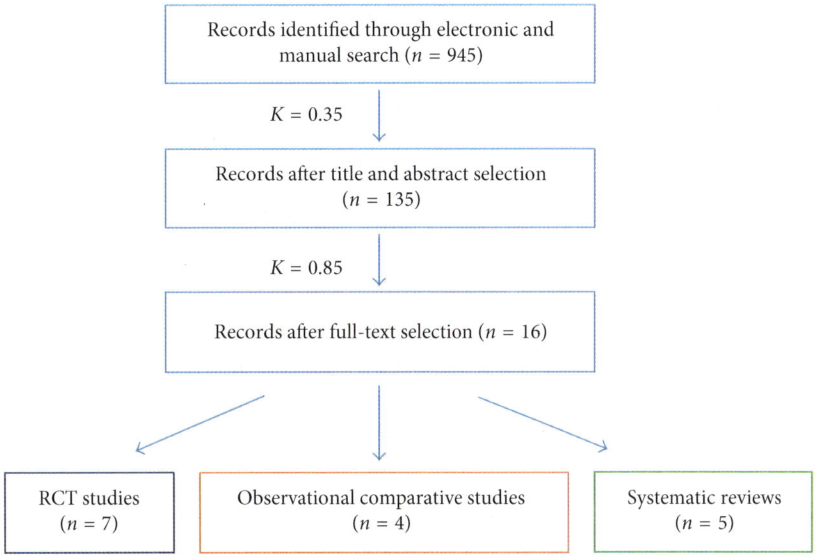

Figure 1: Flow chart.

two-piece implants compared to no failure in the one-piece group. All the implant failures were reported within the first year after function.

Three studies reported data from scalloped implants. den Hartog et al. [20, 21] reported only 1 implant failure in the control group (same level on 360°) compared with scalloped implants. Tymstra et al. [22] reported a cumulative survival rate of 100% in both groups at 1 year of follow-up, while Van Nimwegen et al. [19], over the same cohort of patients, reported 2 implant failures in the scalloped group, 4 years after their placement, due to extensive peri-implant bone loss.

Only one study included clinical complications as an outcome measure [23]. In this study, Ormianer et al. reported 8 porcelain fractures in the two-piece group and 4 in the one-piece group. Nevertheless, no statistically significant difference was found. All data are reported in Table 2. Finally, two systematic reviews of Barrachina-Díez et al. [27, 28] reported a high long-term survival rate but also high frequency of technical and biological complications in one-piece implants, both in one-part and two-part designs.

3.4. One-Piece versus Two-Piece Implants (MBL and BR). Sanz Martin et al. [17] and Thoma et al. [18] published two randomized controlled clinical trials on the same cohort of 60 patients (151 implants), aimed at assess the volumetric changes of the buccal soft tissues between baseline and 1 year after loading follow-up, [17] and to compare the clinical and radiographic outcomes using one-piece ($n = 65$; Straumann) and two-piece ($n = 86$; Nobel Biocare External Hex) dental implant systems [18]. These researches failed to find significant differences between the one- and two-piece implant types with regard to tissue thickness, crown height (CHC), and facial tissue volume (VC). Conversely, the two-piece group exhibited slightly less bone loss during the evaluated period. Differences between the two groups reached a statistical significance with less bone loss for the two-piece group.

Ormianer et al. [23] analyzed retrospectively one-piece ($n = 34$; Zimmer One-Piece, Zimmer Biomet) and two-piece ($n = 38$; Tapered Screw-Vent, Zimmer Biomet) implants placed in the mandible of the same patients ($n = 24$) according to a split-mouth design. After 5 years of function, marginal bone loss did not significantly differ between one- and two-piece dental implant systems (the mean MBL is not reported).

Duda et al. [24] in a retrospective comparative study evaluated clinical outcomes of immediate insertion and loading of one-piece implants (49 implants in 13 patients; Q-Implant; Trinon Titanium GmbH, Karlsruhe, Germany), compared to delayed loading of immediately placed one-piece implants (24 implants in 11 patients; Q-Implant; Trinon Titanium GmbH), and delayed placed two-piece nonsubmerged implants (39 implants in 10 patients; Q-Implant; Trinon Titanium GmbH). Mean MBL was 1.45 mm and 1.71 mm at the 5-year follow-up for one-piece implants with immediate loading and delayed loading, respectively. In case of two-piece implants, the mean MBL was 0.9 mm at the 3-year follow-up. The authors concluded that two-piece implants showed less MBL compared with one-piece implants in both the maxilla and mandible [24]. On the other hand, there was no statistical difference in MBL between immediate and delayed loaded one-piece implants, but immediate loaded implants showed more MBL in the maxilla [24].

Finally, Heijdenrijk et al. [9] in a randomized controlled trial with 5-year follow-up reported that the microgap at the implant-abutment interface in two-piece implants does not appear to have an adverse effect on the amount of peri-implant bone loss compared with one-piece implants [9]. All of the data are reported in Table 2.

3.5. Scalloped Implants (MBL and BR). Van Nimwegen et al. [19] randomly compared 20 patients with two adjacent implant-supported restorations delivered on scalloped implants ($n = 20$; NobelPerfect Groovy, Nobel Biocare) and implants with a flat

Table 1: Reporting quality of all selected full-text articles.

Author and year	Implant shoulder design	Study characteristics			Ethical board approval	Selection bias		Performance bias	Detection bias	Attrition bias	Reporting bias	Other sources of bias	Overall risk of bias
		Study design	Follow-up	CONSORT/ STROBE		Random sequence generation	Allocation concealment	Blinding of participants and personnel	Blinding of outcome assessors	Incomplete outcome data	Selective reporting		
Heijdenrijk et al. 2006 [9]	Scalloped	RCT	5 years	No	No	Unclear	Unclear	No	No	Medium risk	Low risk	Low risk	Medium risk
Sanz Martin et al. 2015 [17]*	One piece	RCT	1 year	No	Yes	Computer-generated list	No	No	Unclear	Low risk	Low risk	Low risk	Medium risk
Thoma et al. 2014 [18]*	One piece	RCT	1 year	No	Yes	Computer-generated list	No	No	No	Low risk	Low risk	Low risk	Medium risk
Van Nimwegen et al. 2015 [19]*	Scalloped	RCT	5 years	Unclear	No	Unclear	No	No	No	Low risk	Low risk	Low risk	High risk
den Hartog et al. 2011 [20]*	Scalloped	RCT	1 year	No	Yes	Randomization by minimization	Yes	No	No	Low risk	Low risk	Low risk	Medium risk
den Hartog et al. 2013 [21]*	Scalloped	RCT	1 year	No	Yes	Randomization by minimization	Yes	No	No	Low risk	Low risk	Low risk	Medium risk
Tymstra et al. 2011 [22]*	Scalloped	RCT	1 year	Unclear	No	Unclear	No	No	No	Low risk	Low risk	Low risk	High risk
Ormianer et al. 2016 [23]	One piece	Retrospective	5 years	No	No	Arbitrary	No	No	No	Low risk	Medium risk	Medium risk	High risk
Duda et al. 2016 [24]	One piece	Retrospective	3 years	No	No	No	No	No	No	Low risk	Medium risk	Medium risk	High risk
Khraisat et al. 2013 [25]	Scalloped	Prospective	3 years	No	Yes	No	No	No	No	Low risk	Low risk	Low risk	Medium risk
McAllister 2007 [26]	Scalloped/ one piece	Prospective	4 to 28 months	No	No	No	No	No	No	Medium risk	Medium risk	Medium risk	High risk

*Manuscripts that included the same cohort of patients.

Table 2: Results of the included studies.

Author and year		Patients/implants	Follow-up	Failed implants	Complications	MBL (mm)	BR	Papilla Index	PES/WES	Patient questionnaire/VAS
One-piece (test, T) versus two-piece (control, C) implants										
Heijdenrijk et al. 2006 [9]	T	20/40	5 years	0	NR	1.8	NR	NR	NR	NR
	C	20/40	5 years	1	NR	1.6	NR	NR	NR	NR
	C	20/40	5 years	1	NR	1.4	NR	NR	NR	NR
Sanz Martin et al. 2015 [17]*	T	30/65	1 year	NR	NR	NR	CHC: −0.17; VC: −0.03	NR	NR	NR
	C	30/86	1 year	NR	NR	NR	CHC: 0.02; VC: −0.12	NR	NR	NR
Thoma et al. 2014 [18]*	T	30/65	1 year	1	NR	0.27	NR	NR	NR	NR
	C	30/86	1 year	0	NR	0.05	NR	NR	NR	NR
Ormianer et al. 2016 [23]	T	24/34	5 years	0	4[ς]	NR	NR	NR	NR	NR
	C	24/38	5 years	0	8[ς]	NR	NR	NR	NR	NR
Duda et al. 2016 [24]	T	13/49[$]	5 years	7	NR	1.45	NR	NR	NR	NR
	T	11/24[°]	5 years	2	NR	1.71	NR	NR	NR	NR
	C	10/39	3 years	0	NR	0.9	NR	NR	NR	NR
One-piece (test, T) versus two-piece (control, C) scalloped implants										
McAllister 2007 [26]	T	9/9	18 months	0	NR	NR	NR	16 : 3; 2 : 2	NR	NR
	T	13/16	28 months	0	NR	NR	NR	25 : 3; 7 : 2	NR	NR
	C	NR/12	12 months	0	NR	NR	NR	NR	NR	NR
Scalloped (test, T) versus flat (control, C) implants										
Van Nimwegen et al. 2015 [19]*	T	20/40	5 years	2	2	3.4/2.4	NR	16, 32	NR	8.4
	C	20/40	5 years	0	0	1.5/1.3	NR	19, 38	NR	9.1
den Hartog et al. 2011 [20]*	T	31/31	18 months	0	NR	2.01	0.25	36 : 3; 41 : 2; 23 : 1	NR	NR
	C	31/31	18 months	1	NR	1.19	0.18	31 : 3; 53 : 2; 16 : 1	NR	NR
	C	31/31	18 months	0	NR	0.9	0.28	34 : 3; 45 : 2; 19 : 1	NR	NR
den Hartog et al. 2013 [21]*	T	31/31	18 months	0	NR	2.01	NR	NR	6.6/7.2	9.1
	C	31/31	18 months	1	NR	1.19	NR	NR	6.0/7.2	8.8
	C	31/31	18 months	0	NR	0.9	NR	NR	6.3/7.4	8.9
Tymstra et al. 2011 [22]*	T	20/40	1 year	0	NR	2.7/2.6	0.3	19, 38	NR	8.6
	C	20/40	1 year	0	NR	0.9	0.1	19, 38	NR	8.3
Khraisat et al. 2013 [25]	T	12/12	3 years	NR	NR	3.48/3.52	NR	NR	NR	NR
	C	12/12	3 years	NR	NR	1.35/1.27	NR	NR	NR	NR

*Manuscripts that included the same cohort of patients; [ς]porcelain fractures; [$]immediately loaded one-piece; [°]delayed loaded one-piece; NR: not reported; CHC: crown height changes in mm; VC: volume changes in mm.

platform ($n = 20$; NobelPerfect Groovy). This study is a 5-year follow-up on the 1-year preliminary report of Tymstra et al. [22]. More bone loss and more BoP with compromised interimplant papilla regeneration were found around scalloped implants. Nevertheless, the implant crown aesthetic index, as well as patient satisfaction, was not significantly different between the groups [19, 22].

den Hartog et al., in two similar randomized controlled trials with 18 months of follow-up [20, 21], evaluated the aesthetic outcome and the marginal bone level changes of anterior single-tooth implants with three different implant shoulder (neck) designs: a 1.5 mm machined implant neck (Replace Select Tapered, Nobel Biocare AB, Göteborg, Sweden), a rough implant neck with grooves (NobelReplace

Tapered Groovy, Nobel Biocare AB), and a scalloped rough implant neck with grooves (NobelPerfect Groovy, Nobel Biocare AB). Although there was a statistically significant difference in MBL between different implant shoulder designs (smooth neck 1.19 ± 0.82 mm, rough neck 0.90 ± 0.57 mm, and scalloped neck 2.01 ± 0.77 mm), there were no differences between groups regarding the PES/WES outcomes, as well as patient satisfaction. In a prospective comparative study, Khraisat et al. [25] evaluated MBL and soft tissues around single implants with the scalloped shoulder design (Nobel Perfect, Nobel Biocare) and a smooth collar of 1.5 mm, within 3 years of function. The mean MBLs around scalloped implants were compared to MBLs around conventional flat platform 3.75 mm diameter TiUnite surface implants with external hex (MK III RP, Nobel Biocare), after both 1 and 3 years of function. The results of the present prospective study demonstrated that scalloped implants did not maintain marginal bone levels. All of the data are reported in Table 2.

Data from other reviews provide insufficient evidence about the efficacy of scalloped implant designs in the stability of peri-implant tissues [30, 31]. On the other hand, favorable results regarding scalloped implants were reported by Prasad et al. [29].

3.6. One-Piece versus Two-Piece Scalloped Implants. Consecutively, restored one-piece (NobelPerfect One-Piece) and two-piece (NobelPerfect, Nobel Biocare) scalloped dental implants were radiographically and clinically compared in a study of McAllister [26]. Radiographic evaluation of 16 two-piece scalloped implants and 9 one-piece scalloped implants revealed enhanced interproximal bone levels compared to a nonscalloped conventional flat-top implant design. Based on the Jemt system for interproximal soft tissue level evaluation, 78% of the two-piece implants scored 3 and 22% scored 2 and 89% of the one-piece implants scored 3 and 11% scored 2. The authors concluded that enhanced interproximal tissue preservation from scalloped implant designs may lead to more predictable aesthetic dental implant restorations in the anterior maxilla. All of the data are reported in Table 2.

3.7. Sloped Implants (MBL and BR). No comparative studies reporting data on sloped implants were found that fulfilled the inclusion and exclusion criteria of this systematic review.

3.8. Aesthetic Outcomes (Papilla Index, PES, and WES) and Patient Satisfaction. Four studies reported no differences in aesthetic outcomes between scalloped and flat implants [19–22]. Tymstra et al. [22] and Van Nimwegen et al. [19] evaluated the soft tissues around the adjacent implants and the neighbouring teeth using the Papilla Index according to Jemt [32]. den Hartog et al. [20, 21] analyzed the volume of the interproximal papilla using the Papilla Index in the first study [20] and two objective aesthetic indexes, pink aesthetic score/white aesthetic score (PES/WES) and implant crown aesthetic index (ICAI), in the second study [21]. Three of them reported outcomes on patient satisfaction, using the patient questionnaire or VAS, scoring no differences between groups [19, 21, 22]. All the data are reported in Table 2.

4. Discussion

The aim of this systematic review was to identify whether there is a relationship between different implant shoulder positions/orientations/designs in the anterior dentition and prosthetic and/or implant failures, biological or mechanical complications, radiographic marginal bone loss, peri-implant buccal recession, aesthetic scores, and patient satisfaction after a minimum of 1-year function. The types of the implant analyzed were one-piece implants, compared with two-piece implants, and scalloped and sloped implants, compared with the conventional implant neck architecture (flat implants with the same level on 360°).

The results of the present systematic review indicate that different implant shoulder positions (scalloped, sloped, and one piece) seem to offer no benefit when compared to conventional, two-piece, flat implants.

A trend of higher implant failure and prosthetic complications were experienced in the one-piece group compared to the two-piece group, even if no statistically significant differences were found. This is in agreement with two systematic reviews by the same author [27, 28] which concluded that, despite high long-term prosthetic survival rates, technical and biological complications are frequent in one-piece implants independently by the loading protocols, implant surfaces, or type of edentulism.

One-piece implants are generally placed in a nonsubmerged approach. This means that implant placement is performed in a single surgical procedure, with no need for surgical reopening. Compared to a two-stage procedure, this approach is more comfortable for the patient, due to the fewer number of surgeries, and reduces the healing period. Implant shoulder placed at the level of the soft tissue offers many advantages since it is easily accessible for procedures such as impression taking and represents an excellent basis for cemented implant restorations [17, 18]. Moreover, due to its design, one-piece implants have their transmucosal surface unaltered during all of the prosthetic procedures since abutment reconnection is avoided (one-piece, one-part implants) or it is performed at the supramucosa or marginal mucosa level (one-piece, two-part implants). This avoids trauma to the soft tissue, which could result in a more apical position of the connective tissue and be responsible for additional marginal bone resorption.

A clinical study by Heijdenrijk et al. [9] evaluated the feasibility of using a two-piece implant system in a nonsubmerged procedure compared to the two-piece implant system placed in the traditional submerged procedure and one-piece implants placed in a nonsubmerged procedure. After 5 years of functioning, no association was found between the level of the microgap and the amount of bone loss, suggesting that two-piece implants used in a nonsubmerged procedure may be as predictable as when used in a submerged procedure or as one-piece implants [9].

Three studies included in this review reported differences in MBL between one- and two-piece implants. Thoma et al.

[18] and Duda et al. [24] reported higher MBL in the one-piece implants, whilst Ormianer et al. [23] reported no differences between groups. Sanz Martin et al. [17] assessed the volumetric changes of the buccal soft tissue between baseline and 1 year of loading between one- and two-piece dental implants. This research failed to find significant differences between the one- and two-piece implant types with regard to tissue thickness, crown height, and facial tissue volume.

The concept of scalloped implants was introduced to maintain the alveolar ridge and the peri-implant soft tissue contour by mimicking the scalloped shape of natural topography of the healthy marginal bone contour [12]. The long-term results showed stable soft tissues around the scalloped implants in spite of some loss of marginal bone support in relation to the originally intended marginal bone level [33].

The primary aesthetic goal of the scalloped implant design is to avoid the dark, triangular space known as the "black triangle." This space appears when bone remodeling results in loss of osseous support for the papillae [34]. The aesthetic concern is increased when a patient presents an alveolar morphotype, with a pronounced scalloped profile of the hard and soft tissues. This can be further complicated by the gingival display of a high smile line [34]. A five-year randomized controlled trial [19] was realized as follow-up of a 1-year report [22] to evaluate peri-implant soft and hard tissue of two adjacent implant-support restorations in the aesthetic region using a scalloped or flat platform. More bone loss and compromised interimplant papilla regeneration were obtained around scalloped implants, indicating that scalloped implants do not offer benefits in the aesthetic region [19, 22]. The other articles included in this review [20, 21, 25] comparing scalloped implants with the conventional implant neck architecture reported higher marginal bone loss in the test group (scalloped implants) compared to implants with the same level on 360°. Other than MBL, Khraisat [25] also analyzed the soft tissue level around scalloped single implants compared to conventional rough surface implants with external hex in the aesthetic zone over a 3-year period. The Jemt system was used to clinically assess sizes of the mesial and distal interproximal papillae, showing that soft tissue height was not consistently maintained around the scalloped area of the implants. Different results were obtained in a study of McAllister [26] where consecutively restored one- and two-piece scalloped implants were radiographically and clinically compared to a flat-top implant with similar implant geometry regarding taper and thread design. Enhanced interproximal hard and soft tissue preservation was obtained for scalloped implants leading to predictable aesthetic restorations in the anterior maxilla. The authors concluded that interproximal soft tissue levels may be enhanced by maintaining the crestal bone level and avoiding interproximal soft tissue attachment manipulation during abutment connection.

No comparative studies were found that fulfilled the inclusion and exclusion criteria of the sloped implants' systematic review. Nevertheless, the available data provide encouraging results for sloped implants in preserving the bone crest and the interplant papilla [13]. Placing an implant in a healed alveolar ridge with differences in height between the buccal and lingual bone crest will not allow the buccal part of the marginal portion of the implant to be completely invested in the bone, resulting in a risk of aesthetic complications [13]. In a prospective multicenter study, non-submerged implants (OsseoSpeed Profile implants; Astra Tech AB, Molndal, Sweden) were placed in a recipient site with a buccal-lingual bone height discrepancy of 2.0–5.0 mm, and the sloped part of the device was located at the buccal and most apical position of the preparation. Sixteen weeks later, bone level alterations were 0.02 mm lingually and 0.30 mm buccally, and at the 1-year reexamination, the average change in interproximal bone levels was 0.54 mm. The authors concluded that sloped implant placement in an alveolar ridge with a sloped marginal configuration resulted in minor remodeling, preserving discrepancies between buccal and lingual bone levels [13].

5. Conclusions

(i) Although no statistically significant differences were found, a trend of higher implant failure and prosthetic complications were experienced in the one-piece group compared to the two-piece group.

(ii) A trend of higher marginal bone loss was found in the test group compared to the control group. This trend is moderate when comparing one-piece versus two-piece implants and high when comparing scalloped versus flat implants.

(iii) Although no studies were found comparing sloped versus flat implants, preliminary results may encourage future studies.

(iv) No differences were experienced between groups regarding aesthetic outcomes and patient satisfaction.

There was sufficient evidence that different implant shoulder positions/orientations/designs (scalloped, sloped, and one piece) offer no benefit when compared to two-piece, conventional flat implants. Current evidence is limited due to the quality of available studies. Marginal bone loss seems to be affected by the implant neck design, while aesthetics and patient satisfaction appear to be independent. Further studies, designed as randomized controlled clinical trials reported according to the CONSORT statement, are needed.

References

[1] T. Albreksson, G. Zarb, P. Worthington, and A. R. Eriksson, "The long-term efficacy of currently used dental implants: a review and proposed criteria of success," *International Journal of Oral and Maxillofacial Implants*, vol. 1, no. 1, pp. 11–25, 1986.

[2] T. J. Oh, J. Yoon, C. E. Misch, and H. L. Wang, "The causes of early implant bone loss: myth or science?," *Journal of Periodontology*, vol. 73, no. 3, pp. 322–333, 2002.

[3] D. L. Cochran, J. S. Hermann, R. K. Schenk, F. L. Higginbottom, and D. Buser, "Biologic width around titanium implants: a histometric analysis of the implanto-gingival junction around unloaded and loaded nonsubmerged implants in the canine mandible," *Journal of Periodontology*, vol. 68, no. 2, pp. 186–198, 1997.

[4] N. Elian, M. Bloom, M. Dard, S. C. Cho, R. D. Trushkowsky, and D. Tarnow, "Effect of interimplant distance (2 and 3 mm) on the height of interimplant bone crest: a histomorphometric evaluation," *Journal of Periodontology*, vol. 82, no. 12, pp. 1749–1756, 2011.

[5] D. P. Tarnow, S. C. Cho, and S. S. Wallace, "The effect of inter-implant distance on the height of inter-implant bone crest," *Journal of Periodontology*, vol. 71, no. 4, pp. 546–549, 2000.

[6] A. Pozzi, E. L. Agliardi, M. Tallarico, and A. Barlattani, "Clinical and radiological outcomes of two implants with different prosthetic interfaces and neck configurations: randomized, controlled, split-mouth clinical trial," *Clinical Implant Dentistry and Related Research*, vol. 16, no. 1, pp. 96–106, 2014.

[7] M. Tallarico, A. Vaccarella, and G. C. Marzi, "Clinical and radiological outcomes of 1- versus 2-stage implant placement: 1-year results of a randomised clinical trial," *European Journal of Oral Implantology*, vol. 4, no. 1, pp. 13–20, 2011.

[8] A. Schroeder, B. Maeglin, and F. Sutter, "ITI (Internationales Team fur orale Implantologie) type-F hollow cylinder implant for denture retention in the edentulous jaw," *Schweizerische Monatsschrift für Zahnheilkunde*, vol. 93, no. 9, pp. 720–733, 1983.

[9] K. Heijdenrijk, G. M. Raghoebar, H. J. Meijer, B. Stegenga, and W. A. van der Reijden, "Feasibility and influence of the microgap of two implants placed in a non-submerged procedure: a five-year follow-up clinical trial," *Journal of Periodontology*, vol. 77, no. 6, pp. 1051–1060, 2006.

[10] L. Canullo, M. Caneva, and M. Tallarico, "Ten-year hard and soft tissue results of a pilot double-blinded randomized controlled trial on immediately loaded post-extractive implants using platform-switching concept," *Clinical Oral Implants Research*, vol. 28, no. 10, pp. 1195–1203, 2016.

[11] J. Y. Kan, K. Rungcharassaeng, G. Liddelow, P. Henry, and C. J. Goodacre, "Periimplant tissue response following immediate provisional restoration of scalloped implants in the esthetic zone: a one-year pilot prospective multicenter study," *Journal of Prosthetic Dentistry*, vol. 97, no. 6, pp. S109–S118, 2007.

[12] P. S. Wohrle, "Nobel perfect esthetic scalloped implant: rationale for a new design," *Clinical Implant Dentistry and Related Research*, vol. 5, no. 1, pp. 64–73, 2003.

[13] R. Noelken, M. Donati, J. Fiorellini et al., "Soft and hard tissue alterations around implants placed in an alveolar ridge with a sloped configuration," *Clinical Oral Implants Research*, vol. 25, no. 1, pp. 3–9, 2014.

[14] D. Moher, A. Liberati, J. Tetzlaff, D. G. Altman, and The PRISMA Group, "Preferred reporting items for systematic reviews and meta-analyses: the PRISMA statement," *PLoS Medicine*, vol. 6, no. 7, p. e1000097, 2009.

[15] K. F. Schulz, D. G. Altman, D. Moher, and CONSORT Group, "CONSORT 2010 statement: updated guidelines for reporting parallel group randomised trials," *European Journal of Oral Implantology*, vol. 8, pp. 129–140, 2015.

[16] J. P. T. Higgins, D. G. Altman, P. C. Gøtzsche et al., "The Cochrane Collaboration's tool for assessing risk of bias in randomised trials," *BMJ*, vol. 343, no. 2, p. d5928, 2011.

[17] I. Sanz Martin, G. I. Benic, C. H. Hämmerle, and D. S. Thoma, "Prospective randomized controlled clinical study comparing two dental implant types: volumetric soft tissue changes at 1 year of loading," *Clinical Oral Implants Research*, vol. 27, no. 4, pp. 406–411, 2015.

[18] D. S. Thoma, I. Sanz Martin, G. I. Benic, M. Roos, and C. H. Hämmerle, "Prospective randomized controlled clinical study comparing two dental implant systems: demographic and radiographic results at one year of loading," *Clinical Oral Implants Research*, vol. 25, no. 2, pp. 142–149, 2014.

[19] W. G. Van Nimwegen, G. M. Raghoebar, K. Stellingsma, N. Tymstra, A. Vissink, and H. J. Meijer, "Treatment outcome of two adjacent implant-supported restorations with different implant platform designs in the esthetic region: a five-year randomized clinical trial," *International Journal of Prosthodontics*, vol. 28, no. 5, pp. 490–498, 2015.

[20] L. den Hartog, H. J. Meijer, B. Stegenga, N. Tymstra, A. Vissink, and G. M. Raghoebar, "Single implants with different neck designs in the aesthetic zone: a randomized clinical trial," *Clinical Oral Implants Research*, vol. 22, no. 11, pp. 1289–1297, 2011.

[21] L. den Hartog, G. M. Raghoebar, J. J. Slater, K. Stellingsma, A. Vissink, and H. J. Meijer, "Single-tooth implants with different neck designs: a randomized clinical trial evaluating the aesthetic outcome," *Clinical Implant Dentistry and Related Research*, vol. 15, no. 3, pp. 311–321, 2013.

[22] N. Tymstra, G. M. Raghoebar, A. Vissink, L. den Hartog, K. Stellingsma, and H. J. Meijer, "Treatment outcome of two adjacent implant crowns with different implant platform designs in the aesthetic zone: a 1-year randomized clinical trial," *Journal of Clinical Periodontology*, vol. 38, no. 1, pp. 74–85, 2011.

[23] Z. Ormianer, M. Duda, J. Block, and S. Matalon, "One- and two-piece implants placed in the same patients: clinical outcomes after 5 years of function," *International Journal of Prosthodontics*, vol. 29, no. 6, pp. 608–610, 2016.

[24] M. Duda, S. Matalon, I. Lewinstein, N. Harel, J. Block, and Z. Ormianer, "One piece immediately loaded implants versus 1 piece or 2 pieces delayed: 3 years outcome," *Implant Dentistry*, vol. 25, no. 1, pp. 109–113, 2016.

[25] A. Khraisat, A. Zembic, R. E. Jung, and C. H. Hammerle, "Marginal bone levels and soft tissue conditions around single-tooth implants with a scalloped neck design: results of a prospective 3-year study," *International Journal of Oral & Maxillofacial Implants*, vol. 28, no. 2, pp. 550–555, 2013.

[26] B. S. McAllister, "Scalloped implant designs enhance interproximal bone levels," *International Journal of Periodontics & Restorative Dentistry*, vol. 27, no. 1, pp. 9–15, 2007.

[27] J. M. Barrachina-Díez, E. Tashkandi, S. Stampf, and W. Att, "Long-term outcome of one-piece implants. Part I: implant characteristics and loading protocols. A systematic literature review with meta analysis," *International Journal of Oral & Maxillofacial Implants*, vol. 28, no. 2, pp. 503–518, 2013.

[28] J. M. Barrachina-Díez, E. Tashkandi, S. Stampf, and W. Att, "Long-term outcome of one-piece implants. Part II: prosthetic outcomes. A systematic literature review with meta-analysis," *International Journal of Oral & Maxillofacial Implants*, vol. 28, no. 6, pp. 1470–1482, 2013.

[29] D. K. Prasad, M. Shetty, N. Bansal, and C. Hegde, "Crestal bone preservation: a review of different approaches for successful implant therapy," *Indian Journal of Dental Research*, vol. 22, pp. 317–323, 2011.

[30] M. Bateli, W. Att, and J. R. Strub, "Implant neck configurations for preservation of marginal bone level: a systematic review," *International Journal of Oral and Maxillofacial Implants*, vol. 26, no. 2, pp. 290–303, 2011.

[31] S. Bishti, J. R. Strub, and W. Att, "Effect of the implant-abutment interface on peri-implant tissues: a systematic review," *Acta Odontologica Scandinavica*, vol. 72, no. 1, pp. 13–25, 2014.

[32] T. Jemt, "Regeneration of gingival papillae after single-implant treatment," *International Journal of Periodontics and Restorative Dentistry*, vol. 17, no. 4, pp. 326–333, 1997.

[33] S. Paul and U. Held, "Immediate supracrestal implant placement with immediate temporization in the anterior dentition: a retrospective study of 31 implants in 26 patients with up to 5.5-years follow-up," *Clinical Oral Implants Research*, vol. 24, no. 6, pp. 710–717, 2013.

[34] R. Noelken, F. Oberhansl, M. Kunkel, and W. Wagner, "Immediately provisionalized OsseoSpeed™ Profile implants inserted into extraction sockets: 3-year results," *Clinical Oral Implants Research*, vol. 27, no. 6, pp. 744–749, 2016.

25

Knowledge and Practices on Periodontal Health among Adults, Misungwi, Tanzania

John Michael Nyorobi,[1] Lorna Celia Carneiro,[2] and Msafiri Nicodemus Kabulwa[3]

[1]*Dental Unit, Misungwi District Hospital, P. O. Box 8, Misungwi, Mwanza, Tanzania*
[2]*Department of Restorative Dentistry, Muhimbili University of Health and Allied Sciences, P. O. Box 65451, Dar es Salaam, Tanzania*
[3]*Oral Health Section, Ministry of Health, Community Development, Gender, Elderly and Children, P. O. Box 743, Dodoma, Tanzania*

Correspondence should be addressed to Lorna Celia Carneiro; carneiro2@hotmail.com

Academic Editor: Carlos A. Munoz-Viveros

The level of knowledge and practices on periodontal health of 388 adults in Misungwi District, Tanzania, was assessed. Analysis included frequency distributions and the chi-square test at a p value of 0.05. Many more participants were males ($n = 197$; 50.8%) and of younger age group ($n = 215$; 55.4%) and having seven years of education ($n = 257$; 66.2%). Higher number of participants reported owning a mobile phone ($n = 289$; 74.5%) and a radio ($n = 298$; 76.8%), while few ($n = 45$; 11.6%) had their houses connected to electricity. Study participants who were males ($n = 101$; 51.3%), had more than seven years of schooling ($n = 67$; 72.3%), who owned a mobile phone ($n = 143$; 49%), owned a radio ($n = 144$; 48.3%), and resided in houses having electricity ($n = 37$; 82.2%) were statistically significantly more knowledgeable on periodontal health when compared to their counterparts. A statistical significant difference was seen in oral health practices conducive to periodontal health among those who were males ($n = 133$; 67.0%), having more than seven years of education ($n = 78$; 83.0%), owning a mobile phone ($n = 189$; 65.4%), owning a radio ($n = 195$; 65.4%), and residing in house having electricity ($n = 35$; 77.8%). This study observed that participants who were males, owned a mobile phone, owned a radio, resided in houses having electricity, and having more than seven years of education were more knowledgeable and had more conducive oral health practices on periodontal health.

1. Introduction

Periodontal disease is a chronic disease that affects one or more components of the periodontium and is a growing burden to people, healthcare systems, and societies across the world [1]. It refers to the inflammatory processes that occur in the tissues surrounding the teeth in response to bacterial accumulations (dental plaque) [2]. Gingivitis and periodontitis are a continuum of the same inflammatory process [3], and while gingivitis is the presence of gingival inflammation without loss of connective tissue attachment, periodontitis is the presence of gingival inflammation at sites where there has been apical migration of the epithelial attachment onto the root surfaces accompanied by loss of connective tissue and the alveolar bone [4].

Periodontal disease has been associated with self-reported signs and symptoms-like "swollen gums," "sore gums," "receding gums," "loose teeth," "drifting teeth," "bad breath," and "toothache" [5]. Furthermore, severe periodontitis, which may result in tooth loss [6], is found in 5–20% of most adult populations worldwide [7].

The prevalence of periodontal disease in a population is dependent on risk characteristics like age, sex, education, geographic and environmental status, oral hygiene practices, and social characteristics [8]. In addition, dental awareness, oral health, and oral health-related behaviors have been reported to be influenced also by the socioeconomic status [9], and the link between periodontal disease and socio-economic status has been reported [10]. Socioeconomic status associated with the health status of an individual including oral health has been assessed using various indicators such as owning a television, refrigerator, mobile phone, bicycle, car, utensils, access to utilities (electricity and water), and housing characteristics (materials used for floor, number of rooms, and quality of toilets) [11]. It has been further documented that higher income enables people to afford better housing and permit increased access to healthcare and offers the opportunity to adopt appropriate oral health practices [12].

So as to maintain oral health and prevent the occurrence of periodontal diseases in a population, it is essential that there be acquisition of adequate oral health knowledge together with instilling of appropriate self-care practices [13]. Moreover, prevention of and early intervention into periodontal disease are critical, and successful management of periodontal disease depends on the capacity of patient's oral self-care practices [14, 15]. The single most important step an individual can take to reduce plaque accumulation and the consequent risk of plaque-associated diseases, such as periodontitis, is perhaps routinely performing tooth brushing [16]. With regard to frequency of tooth brushing, a previous study demonstrated that individuals who cleaned their teeth at least twice a day exhibited less visible plaque, as compared with those who cleaned their teeth less than once a day or never [17]. However, the benefit of toothpaste in removing plaque during brushing has been controversial [18].

In Tanzania, dental plaque has been reported to be prevalent among adolescents [19] and adults [20], and it is estimated that, on average, at the age of 40 to 49 years, each Tanzanian has lost at least one tooth because of advanced periodontal disease, and after the age of 50, the problem becomes more marked [21]. To address this, an oral health policy to promote primary, secondary, and tertiary levels of oral healthcare to Tanzanians through community involvement particularly in the rural areas was developed [22].

A previous study on oral health issues for the elderly in Tanzania reported that people aged 40+ years, who live in the rural areas, are at a higher risk of destructive periodontal disease, and it was recommended that oral health education, focusing on behavior change, should be initiated from childhood [23].

Identifying the level of oral health knowledge and practices on periodontal health can assist in planning preventive strategies towards reducing periodontal disease. This study therefore aimed at determining the level of knowledge and practices on periodontal health among adults of Misungwi District in Tanzania.

2. Materials and Methods

Misungwi District in Mwanza Region in Tanzania has 4 divisions, 20 wards, 78 villages, and 40,364 households, with a total population of 316,687 people [24]. Using multistage stratified cluster random sampling, two of the four divisions within Misungwi District were selected. Subsequently, in each division, one ward was selected, and from each ward, two villages were chosen. From each village, ten households are grouped and referred to as ten cells, and in each village, 25 ten cells were visited. Adults present in each household within a ten cell were informed of the purpose of the study by the local administrative authority following which consent was obtained. Participants excluded from the study were those below 18 years of age, adults who were nonresidents of Misungwi, and those who were either mentally challenged or sick.

Following consent, a structured self-administered questionnaire that was translated into Kiswahili was used to gather the necessary information from the study participants. The questionnaire was divided into four sections, namely, sociodemographic information, socioeconomic status indicators, assessment of the level of knowledge, and assessment of practices on periodontal health. Pretesting to establish meaning and clarity of the questionnaire was done using a randomly selected group of forty people from one of the villages (Buhunda). Following testing, words and sentences that appeared not clear were rectified and retesting of the questionnaire was done. Reproducibility of the answers ranged between 90 and 100% indicating adequate reliability of the questionnaire.

Sociodemographic information included details on age (young adults-18–34 years and middle aged to elderly adults-35–74 years), sex (male and female), and level of education (not gone to school, seven years of education, and more than seven years of education).

Socioeconomic status indicators included information on owning a radio (yes = 1 or no = 0) or mobile phone (yes = 1 or no = 0) or having electricity in household (yes = 1 or no = 0).

Level of knowledge on periodontal health was assessed using 6 questions (knowledge on types of oral diseases, presentation of the gum disease, causes of gum disease, effects of gum disease, prevention of gum disease, and harmful effects to the gum due to smoking). Responses to the questions were itemized and coded following which incorrect responses were awarded a zero mark, and correct responses were awarded a mark of one. A count of correct responses to all questions was done, and a subject was regarded as being knowledgeable if three or more of the six questions were correctly answered and not knowledgeable if less than three of the questions were correctly answered.

Level of oral health practice on periodontal health was assessed using 5 questions, namely, use of toothpaste for brushing (yes = 1 or no = 0), time spent during tooth brushing (less than two minutes during tooth brushing, and two or more minutes during tooth brushing), frequency of tooth brushing (once a day or two or more times a day), having attended a dental health facility (yes = 1 or no = 0), and practice of smoking (yes = 1 or no = 0). Responses to the five questions were counted, and participants who scored 3 or more were considered to have practices conducive for periodontal health, while participants who scored below three were regarded as having practices not conducive for periodontal health.

Data processing was done using Statistical Package of the Social Sciences, IBM™, version 17.0 of 2016 (Chicago, IL, USA). Independent variables were sociodemographic details (age, sex, and level of education) and socioeconomic status indicators (owning a radio or mobile phone or having electricity), while dependent variables were questions on oral health knowledge and practices towards periodontal health. Data analysis included frequency distribution and cross tabulation. Frequency distributions of respondent's responses to the questions on knowledge and practice were generated. The chi-square test was performed to identify associations between independent and dependent variables, and a p value of 0.05 was used to determine the level of statistical significance.

Prior to conducting the study, a Research clearance Certificate Number CREC/039/2013 was obtained from the Catholic University of Health and Allied Sciences (CUHAS)/Bugando Medical Centre (BMC) Research Ethical Committee (CREC) and used to obtain permission from the Regional and District authorities of Misungwi.

3. Results

A total of 388 adults participated in this study with an age ranging from 18 to 74 years and median age of 32 ± 0.58 years. With regard to sociodemographic details, there were slightly more males (50.8%) than females and young adults under the age of 35 years (55.4%). Participants who had not gone to school were the minority ($n = 37$; 9.6%), while those who had seven years of education were the majority ($n = 257$; 66.2%). The remaining participants had more than seven years of education ($n = 94$; 24.2%). On assessment of socioeconomic status indicators, about three-quarters ($n = 289$; 74.5%) owned mobile phones and 76.8% ($n = 298$) owned a radio, while only few ($n = 45$; 11.6%) had their houses connected to electricity. Owning of a mobile phone and radio among those who had not gone to school was 4.4% and 7.2%, respectively. About half ($n = 190$; 49.0%) of the participants could mention any oral disease, 68.6% ($n = 266$) could mention signs and symptoms of periodontal diseases, and about a quarter ($n = 103$; 26.5%) could mention causes of gum diseases, while 32% ($n = 124$) and 29.6% ($n = 115$) could mention effects and prevention of gums diseases, respectively. About a third ($n = 129$; 33.2%) were aware on the harmful effects of smoking on gum diseases. Majority of the participants used toothpaste during brushing their teeth ($n = 321$; 82.7%) and reported to spend two minutes or more during tooth brushing ($n = 336$; 86.6%), while less than half ($n = 180$; 46.4%) brushed their teeth two or more times a day. A little more than a third ($n = 154$; 39.7%) had ever attended a dental health facility, and a minority ($n = 59$; 15.2%) reported that they smoke (Table 1).

Table 2 shows the distribution of the participant's level of knowledge on periodontal health by sociodemographic and socioeconomic variables. Compared to females, male participants were more knowledgeable ($n = 101$; 51.3%) on periodontal health, and the difference was statistically significant (p value = 0.018). With regard to age, there was no statistical significant difference (p value = 0.082) between level of knowledge on periodontal health of young adults ($n = 106$; 49.3%) when compared to middle aged to elderly participants ($n = 70$; 40.5%). Study participants who had

Table 1: Frequency distribution of the study participants' oral health knowledge and oral health practices on periodontal health by sociodemographic and socioeconomic variables ($n = 388$).

	Number (n)	Percentage (%)
Sociodemographic variables		
Sex		
Male	197	50.8
Female	191	49.2
Age group		
18–34	215	55.4
35+	173	44.6
Level of education		
Not gone to school	37	9.6
Seven years of education	257	66.2
More than seven years of education	94	24.2
Socioeconomic variables		
Owning a cell phone		
Yes	289	74.5
No	99	25.5
Owning a radio		
Yes	298	76.8
No	90	23.2
House having electricity		
Yes	45	11.6
No	343	88.4
Oral health knowledge		
Can they mention types of oral diseases?		
Yes	190	49.0
No	198	51.0
Can they mention signs and symptoms of periodontal diseases?		
Yes	266	68.6
No	122	31.4
Can they mention causes of gum diseases?		
Yes	103	26.5
No	285	73.5
Can they mention effects of gum diseases?		
Yes	124	32.0
No	264	68.0
Can they mention prevention of gum of diseases?		
Yes	115	29.6
No	273	70.4
Awareness on harmful effects of smoking on gums		
Yes	129	33.2
No	259	66.8
Oral health practice		
Use of toothpaste during teeth brushing		
Yes	321	82.7
No	67	17.3
Time spent during tooth brushing		
Less than two minutes	52	13.4
Two minutes or more	336	86.6
Frequency of tooth brushing		
Less than twice a day	208	53.6
Twice or more a day	180	46.4
Ever attended dental health facility?		
Yes	154	39.7
No	234	60.3
Do you smoke?		
Yes	59	15.2
No	329	84.8

TABLE 2: Distribution of the participant's level of knowledge on periodontal health by sociodemographic and socioeconomic variables.

		Level of oral health knowledge		p value
		Not knowledgeable	Knowledgeable	
Sociodemographic variables				
Sex	Male	96 (48.7%)	101 (51.3%)	0.018
	Female	116 (60.7%)	75 (39.3%)	
Age (years)	18–34	109 (50.7%)	106 (49.3%)	0.082
	35+	103 (59.3%)	70 (40.5%)	
Level of education	Not gone to school	30 (81.1%)	7 (18.9%)	0.0001
	Seven years of education	156 (60.7%)	101 (39.3%)	
	More than seven years of education	26 (27.7%)	68 (72.3%)	
Socioeconomic variables				
Owning a cell phone	Yes	146 (50.5%)	143 (49.5%)	0.005
	No	66 (66.7%)	33 (33.3%)	
Owning a radio	Yes	154 (51.7%)	144 (48.3%)	0.033
	No	58 (64.4%)	32 (35.6%)	
Houses having electricity	No	204 (59.5%)	139 (40.5%)	0.0001
	Yes	8 (17.8%)	37 (82.2%)	

more than seven years of schooling were statistically significantly more knowledgeable ($n = 68$; 72.3%) on periodontal health when compared to their counterparts (p value = 0.0001). Participants residing in houses having electricity ($n = 37$; 82.2%) had a statistically significantly higher (p value = 0.0001) level of knowledge on periodontal health when compared to participants residing in houses not connected to electricity ($n = 139$; 40.5%). Participants owning a mobile phone ($n = 143$; 49.5%) were statistically significantly more knowledgeable on periodontal health than those who did not own mobile phones ($n = 33$; 33.3%) with a p value of 0.005. Compared to those who did not own a radio ($n = 32$; 35.6%), the ones who owned it ($n = 144$; 48.3%) were statistically significantly more knowledgeable on periodontal health (p value = 0.033).

Table 3 shows the distribution of the participant's level of oral health practices on periodontal health by sociodemographic and socioeconomic variables. Proportionately, there were more male ($n = 133$; 67.0%) compared to female ($n = 108$; 56.5%) participants who had conducive oral health practices ($p = 0.034$). Participants aged 18–34 years ($n = 132$; 61.4%) and those aged 35 years and above ($n = 108$; 62.4%) showed no statistical significant differences in their oral health practices ($p = 0.835$). A high statistical significant difference (p value = 0.0001) was seen in oral health practices conducive to periodontal health among participants who did not go to school ($n = 18$; 48.6%), with seven years of education ($n = 144$; 56.0%), and those with more than seven years of education ($n = 78$; 83.0%). Practices conducive to oral health were statistically significantly different ($p = 0.014$) among participants who owned ($n = 189$; 65.4%) or did not own a cell phone ($n = 51$; 51.5%). Owning a radio ($p = 0.008$) or living in houses with electricity ($p = 0.019$) was seen to be a contributing factor towards practices conducive to oral health.

4. Discussion

This study assessed the level of knowledge and practices on periodontal health among adults of Misungwi District in Tanzania using a representative sample of selected clusters of households. These findings are adequate to give some insights into the level of knowledge and practices on periodontal health of adults in Misungwi, Tanzania, and provide baseline data for planning purposes.

With regard to sociodemographic findings of this study, majority of participants were males (50.8%) and of the younger age group (55.4%) and having seven years of education (66.2%). Studies conducted in Tanzania [25] and Brazil [26] also reported similar findings. Being a developing country, it is expected that the number of young adults compared to older adults in Tanzania will be higher. Furthermore, the higher number of participants with seven years of education could be a reflection of the government efforts to make primary school free and accessible to all [27]. The higher number of males in this study is contrary to findings reported in another study conducted among adults in Tanzania [28]. This difference could be attributed to the differences in study design and sample size.

When we assessed the socioeconomic status as reflected in the 2012 Tanzanian Census (19), the prevalence of the mobile phone and radio ownership was high at 74.5 and 76.8%, respectively, while the percentage of households with a connection to electricity was low at 11.6%.

It is speculated that income generated from either employment, farming, or other business together with reasonable purchasing costs could have enabled the owning of a mobile phone or radio by participants. Furthermore, electricity to the majority of the population in Tanzania is still a challenge and similar to findings reported in this study, and it has been reported that only few households in Tanzania currently have electricity [29]. It is speculated that the few participants who had electricity in their houses had their houses close to an already installed electrical system and hence were able to obtain electricity for a nominal fee.

Assessment of the study participant's knowledge on periodontal health showed that many more could mention signs and symptoms of periodontal diseases (68.6%) compared to mentioning of any oral disease (49.0%), causes

Table 3: Distribution of the participant's level of oral health practices on periodontal health by sociodemographic and socioeconomic variables.

		Level of oral health practices		p value
		Not acceptable	Acceptable	
Sociodemographic variables				
Sex	Male	65 (33.0%)	132 (67.0%)	0.034
	Female	83 (43.5%)	108 (56.5%)	
Age (years)	18–34	83 (38.6%)	132 (61.4%)	0.835
	35+	65 (37.6%)	108 (62.4%)	
Level of education	Not gone to school	19 (51.4%)	18 (48.6%)	0.001
	Seven years of education	113 (44.0%)	144 (56.0%)	
	More than seven years of education	16 (17.0%)	78 (83.0%)	
Socioeconomic variables				
Owning a cell phone	Yes	100 (34.6%)	189 (65.4%)	0.014
	No	48 (48.5%)	51 (51.5%)	
Owning a radio	Yes	103 (34.6%)	195 (65.4%)	0.008
	No	45 (50.0%)	45 (50.0%)	
House having electricity	Yes	10 (22.2%)	35 (77.8%)	0.019
	No	138 (40.2%)	205 (59.8%)	

(26.5%), effects (32%), and prevention (29.6%), while about a third (33.2%) were aware on the harmful effects of smoking on periodontal disease. These findings are comparable to a study conducted in Finland [30]. Contrastingly in the United Kingdom [31] and Kuwait [32], a higher proportion of study participants were knowledgeable on effects of smoking rather than on signs and symptoms of periodontal diseases. Personal experience and observation by participants could have contributed to the reported higher level of knowledge on signs and symptoms of periodontal disease in this study.

Assessed oral health practices on periodontal health by participants reported that the majority (82.7%) used toothpaste and spend two minutes or more during tooth brushing (86.6%) while less than half (46.4%) brushed their teeth two or more times a day. The use of toothpaste by majority was also reported by Kikwilu et al. [33]. Similar to results of this study, the general consensus amongst oral healthcare professionals is that individuals should spend at least 2 minutes brushing their teeth with an effective technique at least twice a day [34]. The proportion of participants (39.7%) who reported the practice of having attended a dental health facility in the present study was similar to other studies done in Tanzania [25, 35] and different to reports from developed countries like Germany [36] and USA [37]. Furthermore, smoking practiced by a few (15.2%) participants in this study was similar to results of the standardized estimate of smoking reported in Tanzania by the World Health Organization [38]. The reported oral health practices could be attributed to marketing strategies employed to ensure that toothpaste is readily available at a reasonable cost, lack of availability of a health facility or not having the means to access the service, and personal or social choices made by few who smoke.

Study participants who were males (51.3%), had more than seven years of education (72.8%), residing in houses having electricity (82.2%), and who owned a radio (48.3%) were statistically significantly more knowledgeable on periodontal health when compared to their counterparts.

Tanzanian males were significantly more knowledgeable about periodontal disease than their female counterparts, which is in agreement with the findings of a previous study conducted in India (34) but in contrast to the results of a Nigerian study (35).

The significant statistical difference in oral health knowledge observed between male and female may be due to inequalities in the opportunity to education within communities which favors males more than females. Furthermore, inequalities in educational opportunities for females could have been contributed to by tradition and culture which favored early marriage of females and early drop out from school due to getting pregnant. It is anticipated that this difference will be decreased in the coming years as the government has made efforts to make primary school free and accessible to all [27].

A highly statistical significant difference (p value = 0.0001) was seen in oral health practices conducive to periodontal health between participants who had not gone to school, with seven years of education, and those with more than seven years of education (83.0%). Other studies [39, 40] have also reported the level of education as a strong determinant of oral hygiene practices. Furthermore, the level of education was suggested as a potential risk indicator for oral health practices [41, 42]. Being educated probably gives one the foundation and basis of understanding and the ability to make decisions with regard to practices conducive to oral health.

Owning a radio ($p = 0.008$), a mobile phone ($p = 0.014$), or living in houses with electricity ($p = 0.019$) was seen to be a contributing factor towards practices conducive to oral health. The observed findings could have been contributed to by participants having adequate knowledge on oral health that heightened the observed practices. In addition, the observed oral healthcare practices could have been enabled by the interlinking of the various socioeconomic variables. Furthermore, ownership of the mobile phones or radios can be used in future as a means of assessment of knowledge and practices on oral health within a community.

5. Conclusions

Participants in this study who were males, owned a mobile phone, owned a radio, resided in houses having electricity, and having more than seven years of education were more knowledgeable and had more conducive oral health practices on periodontal health. These findings can be used to develop strategies for oral health promotion and control of periodontal diseases in the country.

Acknowledgments

The authors would like to acknowledge the Catholic University of Health and Allied Sciences (CUHAS)/Bugando Medical Centre (BMC) Research Ethical Committee (CREC) for providing the ethical clearance to conduct this study. Sincere gratitude is also extended towards the Misungwi District authorities and participants for their acceptance to participate in this study. Misungwi district authority provided the necessary funding to conduct this study.

References

[1] R. G. Watt and P. E. Petersen, "Periodontal health through public health--the case for oral health promotion," *Periodontology 2000*, vol. 60, no. 1, pp. 147–155, 2012.

[2] W. J. Loesche and N. S. Grossman, "Diagnosis and treatment periodontal disease as a specific, albeit chronic infection," *Clinical Microbiology Reviews*, vol. 14, no. 4, pp. 727–752, 2001.

[3] D. F. Kinane and R. Attström, "Advances in the pathogenesis of periodontitis. Group B consensus report of the fifth European Workshop in Periodontology," *Journal of Clinical Periodontology*, vol. 32, no. 6, pp. 130-131, 2005.

[4] G. C. Armitage, "Periodontal diagnoses and classification of periodontal diseases," *Periodontology 2000*, vol. 34, no. 1, pp. 9–21, 2004.

[5] I. Needleman, C. McGrath, P. Floyd, and A. Biddle, "Impact of oral health on the life quality of periodontal patients," *Journal of Clinical Periodontology*, vol. 31, no. 6, pp. 454–457, 2004.

[6] B. L. Pihlstrom, B. S. Michalowicz, and N. W. Johnson, "Periodontal diseases," *The Lancet*, vol. 366, no. 9499, pp. 1809–1820, 2005.

[7] P. E. Petersen, D. Bourgeois, H. Ogawa, S. Estupinan-Day, and C. Ndiaye, "The global burden of oral diseases and risks to oral health," *Bulletin of the World Health Organization*, vol. 83, no. 9, pp. 661–669, 2005.

[8] Y. A. Aljehani, "Risk factors of periodontal disease: review of the literature," *International Journal of Dentistry*, vol. 2014, Article ID 182513, 9 pages, 2014.

[9] P. E. Petersen, "Global policy for improvement of oral health in the 21st century--implications to oral health research of World Health Assembly 2007, World Health Organization," *Community Dentistry and Oral Epidemiology*, vol. 37, no. 1, pp. 1–8, 2009.

[10] S. S. Kadtane, "Periodontal health status of different socio-economic groups in out-patient department of TMDC and RC, moradabad, India," *Journal of Clinical and Diagnostic Research*, vol. 8, no. 7, pp. ZC61–ZC64, 2014.

[11] J. Smits and R. Steendijk, "The international wealth index (IWI)," *Social Indicators Research*, vol. 122, no. 1, pp. 65–85, 2015.

[12] T. US Department of health and human services, *Oral Health in America: A Report of the Surgeon General*, National Institute of Dental and Craniofacial Research, Bethesda, MD, USA, 2000.

[13] R. Deinzer, W. Micheelis, N. Granrath, and T. Hoffmann, "More to learn about: periodontitis-related knowledge and its relationship with periodontal health behaviour," *Journal of Clinical Periodontology*, vol. 36, no. 9, pp. 756–764, 2009.

[14] H. Löe, "Oral hygiene in the prevention of caries and periodontal disease," *International Dental Journal*, vol. 50, no. 3, pp. 129–139, 2000.

[15] P. Axelsson, B. Nyström, and J. Lindhe, "The long-term effect of a plaque control program on tooth mortality, caries and periodontal disease in adults: results after 30 years of maintenance," *Journal of Clinical Periodontology*, vol. 31, no. 9, pp. 749–757, 2004.

[16] C. N. J. Egelberg, "Role of mechanical dental plaque removal in prevention and therapy of caries and periodontal diseases," in *Proceedings of European Workshop on mechanical plaque control*, pp. 190–247, Berne, Switzerland, May 1998.

[17] K. B. Hill, B. Chadwick, R. Freeman, I. O'Sullivan, and J. J. Murray, "Adult Dental Health Survey 2009: relationships between dental attendance patterns, oral health behaviour and the current barriers to dental care," *British Dental Journal*, vol. 214, no. 1, pp. 25–32, 2013.

[18] T. Y. Eid Ma, "A clinical trial on the effectiveness of professional tooth-brushing using dentifrice and water," *Odontostomatol Trop*, vol. 14, no. 2, pp. 9–12, 1991.

[19] L. C. Carneiro and M. N. Kabulwa, "Dental caries, and supragingival plaque and calculus among students, tanga, Tanzania," *ISRN Dentistry*, vol. 2012, article 245296, 6 pages, 2012.

[20] P. T. Lembariti B.S, J. E. Frenken, Prevalence and severity of periodontal conditions among adults in urban and rural Morogoro, Tanzania," *Community Dentistry and Oral Epidemiology*, vol. 16, no. 4, pp. 240–243.

[21] Ministry of Health and Social Welfare, *Oral Health. Guide for Health Care Providers at Reproductive and Child Health Clinic*, Central Oral Health Unit, Dar es Salaam, Tanzania, 2003.

[22] Ministry of Health and Social Welfare, *Policy Guidelines for Oral Health Care in Tanzania Dar es Salaam*, Ministry of Health and Social Welfare, Dar es Salaam, Tanzania, 2010.

[23] N. M. C. Luhanga, "Geriatric oral health issues in Africa: Tanzanian perspective," *International Dental Journal*, vol. 51, no. 3, pp. 219–227, 2001.

[24] 2012 Population and Housing Census Population Distribution by, 2013.

[25] E. N. Kikwilu, J. R. Masalu, F. K. Kahabuka, and A. R. Senkoro, "Prevalence of oral pain and barriers to use of emergency oral care facilities among adult Tanzanians," *BMC Oral Health*, vol. 8, no. 1, pp. 1–7, 2008.

[26] M. de L. C. Bonfim, F. F. Mattos, E. F. e Ferreira, A. C. V. Campos, and A. M. D. Vargas, "Social determinants of health and periodontal disease in Brazilian adults: a cross-sectional study," *BMC Oral Health*, vol. 13, no. 1, p. 22, 2013.

[27] R. Rajani and G. Omondi, *The Primary Education Development Plan (PEDP), A Summary*, HakiElimu Working Paper Series No. 6, p. 1, 2003.

[28] S. K. Singh, O. S. Stanslaus, and H. V. Aroon, "Occurrence of dental caries among the adults attending a regional referral hospital in Tanzania," *Journal of Orofacial Research*, vol. 4, no. 1, pp. 30–34, 2014.

[29] World Bank, *Increasing Electricity Access in Tanzania to Reduce Poverty*, http://www.worldbank.org/en/.../increasing-electricity-access-in-tanzania-to-reduce-poverty.

[30] A. J. Markkula and H. Murtomaa, "Conceptions of Finnish people about the etiology and prevention of dental caries and periodontal disorders," *Community Dentistry and Oral Epidemiology*, vol. 5, no. 3, pp. 108–115, 1977.

[31] M. Terrades, W. A. Coulter, H. Clarke, B. H. Mullally, and M. Stevenson, "Summary of: patients' knowledge and views about the effects of smoking on their mouths and the involvement of their dentists in smoking cessation activities," *British Dental Journal*, vol. 207, no. 11, pp. 542-543, 2009.

[32] K. F. Al-Shammari, M. A. Moussa, J. M. Al-Ansari, and Y. S. Al-Duwairy, "Dental patient awareness of smoking effects on oral health: comparison of smokers and nonsmokers," *Journal of Dentistry*, vol. 34, no. 3, pp. 173–178, 2006.

[33] E. N. Kikwilu, J. E. Frencken, and J. Mulder, "Utilization of toothpaste and fluoride content in toothpaste manufactured in Tanzania," *Acta Odontologica Scandinavica*, vol. 66, no. 5, pp. 293–299, 2008.

[34] A. Gallagher, "The effect of brushing time and dentifrice on dental plaque removal in vivo," *Journal of Dental Hygiene*, vol. 83, no. 3, pp. 111–116, 2009.

[35] J. R. Masalu, E. N. Kikwilu, F. K. Kahabuka, A. R. Senkoro, and I. A. Kida, "Oral health related behaviors among adult Tanzanians: a national pathfinder survey," *BMC Oral Health*, vol. 9, no. 1, pp. 1–9, 2009.

[36] F. Erdsiek, D. Waury, and P. Brzoska, "Oral health behaviour in migrant and non-migrant adults in Germany: the utilization of regular dental check-ups," *BMC Oral Health*, vol. 17, no. 1, pp. 5–7, 2017.

[37] T. P. Wall, M. Vujicic, and K. Nasseh, "Recent trends in the utilization of dental care in the United States," *Journal of Dental Education*, vol. 76, no. 8, pp. 1020–1027, 2012.

[38] WHO, *World Health Organization Report on the Global Tobacco Epidemic, Country Profile: United Republic of Tanzania*, pp. 1–2, vol. II, World Health Organization, Geneva, Switzerland, 2007.

[39] M. Chen, R. M. Andersen, D. E. Barmes, M. H. Leclerq, and C. S. Lyttle, *Comparing oral health care systems: a second international collaborative study*, World Health Organization, Geneva, Switzerland, 1997.

[40] P. E. Petersen, *Inequalities in Oral Health: The Social Context for Oral Health*, Quintessence, London, UK, 2007.

[41] Y. Jiang, C. A. Okoro, J. Oh, and D. L. Fuller, "Sociodemographic and health-related risk factors associated with tooth loss among adults in Rhode Island," *Preventing Chronic Disease*, vol. 10, article 110285, 2013.

[42] J. B. Park, K. Han, Y. G. Park, and Y. Ko, "Association between socioeconomic status and oral health behaviors: the 2008-2010 Korea national health and nutrition examination survey," *Experimental and Therapeutic Medicine*, vol. 12, no. 4, pp. 2657–2664, 2016.

26

Importance of Mechanical Periodontal Therapy in Patients with Diabetes Type 2 and Periodontitis

Priscilla Naiff,[1] Valéria Carneiro,[2] and Maria do Carmo Guimarães[2]

[1]*Ph.D. Student, Faculty of Health Sciences, University of Brasilia, Distrito Federal, Brazil*
[2]*Ph.D. Professor at Periodontics Division, University of Brasilia, Distrito Federal, Brazil*

Correspondence should be addressed to Priscilla Naiff; pri_naiff@yahoo.com

Academic Editor: Maha El Tantawi

Periodontitis is an infectious and inflammatory disease of high prevalence worldwide and constitutes a significant oral health problem. It can lead to tooth loss. In addition, the local inflammatory process can cause the release of inflammatory mediators in the bloodstream and, consequently, contribute to the emergence of systemic effects as cardiovascular and diabetic complications. The purpose of this mini review is to alert health professionals about the risk that periodontitis represents for the onset or exacerbation of complications in individuals with type 2 diabetes mellitus and to emphasize that the mechanical treatment of periodontal disease and reestablishment of oral health are essential for the metabolic control of these patients. The periodontal therapy may help to reduce the risk of systemic complications in diabetes patients. Proper dental management should be suggested by health professionals, mainly from physicians to their patients, in order to improve the health conditions in these individuals.

1. Introduction

Diabetes mellitus (DM) is a metabolic disease in which the body does not produce insulin or cannot use it properly. There is an estimative that there are about 422 million people with DM worldwide [1].

The two main forms of the disease are type 1 (DM1) and type 2 (DM2) diabetes. Besides, other forms are also described in the literature, such as gestational diabetes, as well as other specific types of DM such as those associated with genetic disorders, among other factors. However, DM1 and DM2 affect most of the population, where 90% of the disease's cases are concentrated in type 2 [2].

In type 1 DM, beta-pancreatic cells are mistakenly attacked by the human's immune system. So, insufficient or no insulin is released. Consequently, glucose stays in the blood instead of being used as energy by the body [2].

Because most of the studies about the relation of DM and periodontitis are related to DM2 and this is the most prevalent type of diabetes, this review will approach the aspects only involved in the treatment of periodontitis in Diabetes mellitus type 2 patients.

DM2, a global public health problem, consists of a heterogeneous group of metabolic disorders that presents chronic hyperglycemia as a result of defects in the action or the insulin secretion. DM2 results from a combination of insulin resistance and inadequate compensatory response to insulin secretion, leading to a relative deficiency in the release of this hormone [3]. Insulin is the only hormone responsible for the reduction of blood glucose and is produced and released by the β-cells of the pancreatic islets of Langerhans [4].

The major complications of diabetes are microangiopathy, nephropathy, neuropathy, macrovascular disease, and delayed wound healing. Periodontitis is considered the sixth complication of DM [2].

Periodontitis is a primarily infectious and inflammatory disease caused by anaerobic bacteria (*Porphyromonas gingivalis, Treponema denticola, Prevotella intermedia, Prevotella nigrescens, Eikenella corrodens, Aggregatibacter actinomycetemcomitans*, among others) in association or not with other periodontopathogens, in dental biofilm. It affects teeth's protection and support tissues as gingiva and alveolar bone and can lead to dental mutilation [1, 5].

Periodontitis has been recently very strongly associated with the role of an overreactive immune system in the critical point of the periodontal disease development [6, 7]. Periodontopathogens stimulate, among other inflammatory mediators, the production of cytokines as interleukin 1 beta (IL1-β), interferon gamma (IFN-γ), tumor necrosis factor-alpha (TNF-α), and chemokines (CXCL-1, CXCL-8, CCL-5) by gingival epithelium, adhesion molecules, increased permeability of the gingival capillaries, and chemotaxis of neutrophils from the junctional epithelium to the gingival sulcus. This initial response, with the production of specific cytokines and chemokines, promotes the migration of an inflammatory infiltrate composed of perivascular T cells and monocytes to the connective tissue [6, 7]. If the cellular immune response fails to control the infection, recruitment of B cells that differentiate into plasma cells occurs. Plasma cells produce immunoglobulins (antibodies) that may confer protection to periodontal tissues, control the infectious process, or induce deleterious effects, leading to the destruction of connective tissue and promoting reabsorption of the alveolar bone. The effectiveness of this response varies between individuals and demonstrates importance in determining disease susceptibility [6].

Nowadays is well established the relationship between the progression of periodontitis and several factors, such as the presence of the periodontal pathogens, high levels of proinflammatory cytokines (IFN-γ and TNF-α), matrix metalloproteinases (MMP) and prostaglandin E_2 (PGE_2), and low levels of inflammation's inhibitory cytokines (IL-10), transforming growth factor beta (TGF-β), and tissue inhibitors of MMP (TIMP) [6, 8].

The susceptibility and extent of tissue destruction appear to be determined by the complex cytokine balance produced by the presence of numerous associations between periodontal microorganisms. When the host's response is exacerbated, it can lead to tissue damage, causing loss of periodontal support [6, 7].

Systemic diseases, such as diabetes, can also interfere with the periodontal condition, turning the prognosis of the associated diseases unfavorable [9]. Intravascular dissemination of microorganisms and their products throughout the body may occur because of the inflammation in the periodontal tissues. The total surface area of this periodontal inflammatory field is estimated to be the size of the palm of the hand. Immediate medical intervention should be done if one lesion of this size was on the skin. However, periodontitis is frequently ignored by health professionals, even though it may be associated with a range of systemic diseases and conditions [10].

The association of periodontitis with DM has been investigated and studies have shown that there is a definite correlation between both [11]. It can be observed that individuals with diabetes and inadequate glycemic control are more likely to develop severe periodontal disease and that periodontitis may interfere in the glycemic control of these individuals [12, 13].

2. Mechanisms of Action

Patients with uncontrolled diabetes can present with micro- or macrovascular complications. The prevalence of both complications occurs according to the type and duration of DM. Microvascular defects affect most intricately vascularized organs, as the retina (retinopathy), kidney (nephropathy), and peripheral nerves (neuropathy). The macrovascular defects affect large blood vessels, and consequently, some noble organs as the heart (cardiovascular disease), brain (cerebrovascular disease), and the peripheral arteries (peripheral vascular disease) [14]. Vascular disorders are usually progressive. The main problem in uncontrolled diabetes is the activation of the immune system that leads to micro- and macroangiopathies and other immune reactions contributing to all major organs failure. For example, nephropathy, begins insidiously, but over time, may contribute significantly to morbidity and mortality, resulting in severe damage to the organs. Cardiovascular diseases (CVDs) also account for increased morbidity and mortality in DM2 patients [15].

CVD usually occurs about two decades earlier among DM2 patients than in those without the disease [16, 17]. About 70% of individuals with DM2 die of CVD [18]. The combination of the duration of diabetes (>15 years) and prior CVD was associated with a 30-fold increased risk of fatal CVD [19].

Several factors can explain the mechanisms of periodontal destruction due to DM. Initially, the hyperglycemia state can directly favor the growth of periodontal pathogens, hinder or prejudice cellular functions and, consequently, host defenses. One pathogenic consequence of hyperglycemia in diabetes is an insufficiency in detoxification of reactive carbonyl compounds. Reactive carbonyl increases due to oxidative and nonoxidative reactions where carbohydrates and lipids lead proteins to chemical modification and then, at a late stage, to oxidative stress and tissue damage. This chronic and accelerated chemical modification of proteins is associated with the AGEs (advanced glycation end products) hypothesis which proposes that by increasing concentration of glucose in diabetes alters the structure and function of tissue proteins, contributing and precipitating the development of diabetic complications [20].

The immunological mechanisms mediating the effect of periodontitis on the control of diabetes have moderated level of support in the current literature. Most studies demonstrate that circulating proinflammatory mediators as TNF-α, CRP, and mediators of oxidative stress are elevated in patients with both diseases and these subjects tend to demonstrate higher dyslipidemia, reduced beta cell function, and elevated oxidative stress (that may act synergistically in worsening cardiovascular complications in diabetes) than patients with diabetes alone. Probably these mediators affect the control of DM, but there is no sufficient information from animal studies to support this possibility [21].

There is also a substantial increase in mediators as proinflammatory cytokines and secretion of collagen-degrading enzymes. Diabetes, through the formation of AGEs, can indirectly alter the union of the extracellular matrix, as well as cellular activities, amplifying inflammatory reactions, and decreasing cellular viability, which leads to deterioration of the healing process and potential change in periodontal tissues [22].

On the other hand, the mechanisms by which periodontitis promotes metabolic dysfunction are not yet fully understood. It is believed that in response to endotoxins such as lipopolysaccharide (LPS) produced by periodontal microorganisms, there is an augment in the production of proinflammatory cytokines, chemokines, reactive oxygen species (ROS), and C-reactive protein (CRP) that can alter lipid metabolism and insulin resistance, leading to hyperlipidemia and hyperglycemia [22]. Additionally, TNF-α has been identified as a potent insulin receptor blocker [23].

In severe untreated periodontitis, the ulcerated epithelium of the periodontal pockets has an estimated surface area of 8 to 20 cm^2 [24]. This inflamed and ulcerated subgingival epithelial area of periodontal pockets constitutes a vast portal of entry for periodontopathogenic bacteria, their products, endotoxins such as LPS, and stimulated inflammatory mediators to reach the systemic circulation [25, 26].

Periodontal microorganisms as well as their antigens, when systemically dispersed, can cause significant systemic inflammation and contribute to DM complications. Leukocytes, endothelial cells, and hepatocytes respond to virulence factors with the secretion of proinflammatory mediators such as cytokines, chemokines, ROS, and CRP. If excessive, ROS release by phagocytes can reach circulation and cause systemic oxidative stress. CRP is a protein mainly produced by the liver as result of increased levels of TNF-α and IL-6 in the inflammatory process [27]. Cardiovascular disease has CRP as an independent predictor of its occurrence [28].

Data from a systematic review [29] concluded that human studies, animal experiments, and ex vivo cell culture studies provide evidence for elevated levels of interleukin-6 and interleukin-1β in periodontal tissues and crevicular fluid in patients with DM and periodontitis compared to systemically healthy patients.

Animal models with type 2 diabetes mellitus suggest that TNF-α plays an essential role in prolonging periodontal inflammation [29] and in the development of insulin resistance [23]. This mediator reduces the expression of glucose transporter type 4 (GLUT4) which is an insulin-regulated glucose transporter. TNF-α also induces serine phosphorylation of insulin receptor substrate-1 (IRS-1) that acts as an inhibitor of insulin receptor and down streams the signaling of phosphatidylinositol-3 kinase activation [23].

The increased release of proinflammatory cytokines (IL-1β, IL-6, and TNF-α), an altered RANKL/osteoprotegerin ratio, interactions between advanced glycation end products and their receptors, increased production of reactive oxygen species, and increased interaction between endothelial cells and leukocytes play a crucial role in the two-way relationship between diabetes and periodontitis. These complex changes, resulting from the presence of diabetes, modify the local inflammatory reaction in the periodontium, leading to a proinflammatory state in the gingival tissue and microcirculation [29]. With continued exposure, soluble antigens react with specific circulating antibodies to form immune complexes that amplify inflammation at the sites of deposition. Likewise, proinflammatory mediators, produced locally in the inflamed gingival tissues, can reach the systemic circulation. Proinflammatory cytokines in the circulation induce leukocytosis and acute phase proteins (e.g., CRP). In this context, the increase in the number of white blood cells is associated with an augmented risk of coronary heart disease, cardiovascular disease (CVD), atherosclerosis, thrombosis, and myocardial ischemia. This increase may be caused by the inflammatory nature of chronic infections such as periodontitis [30, 31].

Periodontitis may cause bacteremia and enhance atherosclerotic plaque formation because some microorganisms related to periodontal diseases were detected in atherosclerotic plaques [32, 33, 34]. However, other oral pathogens as *Streptococcus mutans* also have been found in atheromatous plaque samples [35]. Thus, it seems that the disruption of epithelial integrity from periodontal pockets may also provide a point of entry for nonperiodontal pathogens, as those usually found in caries-affected teeth.

Periodontal bacteria, as *P. gingivalis,* or their products can also interact with platelets (direct or *via* the vascular endothelium) and promote prothrombotic effects [36].

Proinflammatory cytokines, which have been reported to be associated with periodontitis, are also involved in atherothrombogenesis [37, 38]. Furthermore, periodontitis patients present many similar risk factors to those with CVD including age, lower socioeconomic status, and smoking [39]. This suggests that periodontitis and CVD may share common etiological pathways and that the association between both is plausible.

Periodontitis is a risk factor for atherosclerosis through endothelial activation. Bacterial products (LPS, outer membrane vesicles, or fimbriae), cytokines, and chemokines resulted from the infectious and inflammatory periodontal process fall into the bloodstream and may stimulate a superregulation of endothelial cell surface receptors in addition to the expression of adhesion on vascular endothelium. This promotes chemotaxis for circulating monocytes. These cells adhere to the activated endothelium. Due to molecular mimicry, immunoglobulins against specific bacterial proteins act as autoantibodies and induce apoptosis in the endothelium. The monocytes then migrate into the subendothelial space and differentiate into macrophages. There, they pick up oxidized low-density lipoprotein (LDL) and become foam cells. Apoptosis of LDL-loaded macrophages results in the accumulation of lipids in the subendothelial space, contributing to the formation of atheromatous plaques. In addition, invading periodontal pathogens induce the proliferation of smooth muscle cells in the formation of the intima and neointima. The extracellular matrix development and the extravasation of T lymphocytes result in the formation of a fibrous envelope covering the atheroma. The fibrous cap and its prothrombotic components are exposed after endothelial cell apoptosis. The enzymatic degradation of the extracellular matrix results in plaque rupture with consequent exposure of its prothrombotic components and formation of thrombi, leading to vessel occlusion. Clinically, this manifest as acute myocardial infarction, in the case of an occluded coronary artery, or a stroke in the case of an occluded cerebral vessel [40].

On the other hand, complications of DM2 because of periodontitis can be prevented or diminished if periodontal disease is treated. Studies have demonstrated that mechanical periodontal therapy can promote the reduction of inflammation's markers in the bloodstream (CRP, IL-6, among others) [41, 42, 43].

3. Importance of the Diagnosis of Periodontitis and Periodontal Debridement

Periodontal diseases have been associated with a reduced glycemic control in diabetes. Periodontitis increases the risk for the diabetes incidence in nondiabetic patients [21] as well as increases insulin resistance in patients with DM and disease complications, including mortality [44, 45].

The implications of periodontitis in the oral environment and maintenance of affected teeth, by themselves, would justify the relevance of seeking the complete understanding of its etiopathogenesis and, from this, implement active forms of individualized therapy. However, in addition to the implications of the disease in oral health, its meaning reaches systemic proportions, whose mechanisms are still not precise.

The effect of periodontitis on the control of DM type 2 has been studied, and there is indirect evidence to support biological mechanisms mediating this effect as reduced pancreatic islets β-cell function, elevated oxidative stress, and dyslipidemia. People with DM and periodontitis usually have elevated circulating proinflammatory mediators, like TNF-α, IL-6, CRP, and reactive oxygen species (ROS) that can interfere with diabetes metabolic control [44] and may act synergistically in worsening cardiovascular complications in diabetes [45].

Mechanical periodontal therapy involves the removal of bacterial agents from periodontium, supra, and subgingival calculus, by scaling and root planning with periodontal curettes or ultrasonic devices. It is the conventional treatment for periodontitis for resolution of inflammation from periodontal tissues and consequently, control of periodontal disease [46].

There is considerable evidence that nonsurgical periodontal treatment reduces oxidative stress, C-reactive protein level, and proinflammatory cytokines (i.e., tumor necrosis factor-alpha, interleukin-1β, and interleukin-6) [21, 42, 47, 48].

To monitor the success of the treatment of periodontal disease and the resolution of inflammation before and after therapy, besides radiographic examination, the oral clinical examination must include some essential periodontal indexes which are analyzed with the aid of a periodontal probe. The parameters usually analyzed are probing depth (PD), clinical attachment level (CAL), visible plaque index (PI), and gingival bleeding on probing (BOP) index [49].

In fact, if periodontitis truly has measurable effects on general health, treatment of this infection may alter the severity of the outcomes, with the resolution of inflammation.

The importance of periodontal treatment is not only to promote the reduction of local clinical inflammation, but it has also been associated with a subsequent decrease in serum levels of IL-6, TNF-α, CRP, and ROS [50–55]. This evidence supports the mechanistic link between periodontitis and diabetes through inflammatory mediators.

It is important to emphasize that diabetes can interfere with the homeostatic interaction between microorganisms and host at periodontal sites, where host immune response to diabetes can trigger a destructive inflammatory pathway against previously well-tolerated microorganisms. Experimental models demonstrate that the development of periodontitis in diabetic rats involves a high expression of proinflammatory cytokines (TNF-α, IL-1β, IL-6) and destructive tissue factors as advanced glycation end products (AGEs) without significant changes in commensal oral microbiota [56].

Patients with DM2 usually have glycated hemoglobin HbA1C elevation in serum, so current studies have shown that periodontal therapy can improve the control of HbA1C levels in patients with both diseases. Periodontal treatment can also successfully reduce circulating levels of TNF-α, CRP in patients with DM associated with periodontitis [57, 58]; however, research about the impact of successful long-term periodontal treatment does not exist and should be done. The magnitude of reported HbA1C reductions ranges from 0.27% to 0.48% at 3-4 months following periodontal therapy [58], which means the same quantity of short-term HbA1C reduction obtained to that often achieved by adding a second medication to a pharmacological regimen [59]. If such decreases can be sustained over the longer term after periodontal therapy, it may contribute to reduced morbidity and mortality associated with DM.

It is challenging to estimate the social cost of the morbidities related to patients living with diabetes. Many individuals are unable to continue their work activities because of chronic complications of the disease or remain with some limitations in their professional performance, causing significant losses regarding productivity. Thus, the control of periodontal disease in patients with DM through mechanical debridement (scaling and root planning) is crucial and may lead to better metabolic control and, consequently, to the improvement of the quality of life of these people.

It is of extreme relevance that health-care professionals, as physicians, to be aware of periodontitis and its implications for glycemic control and complications in individuals with diabetes. Diagnosis of periodontitis should be an integral part of a diabetes care visit. A periodontal examination should be done as part of their ongoing management of DM by a dentist. Even without diagnosed periodontitis initially, an annual periodontal review is recommended. All patients with DM should be provided with oral health education as part of their overall educational program [21].

In the other hand, dentists should pay attention in identifying both prediabetes and undiagnosed diabetes mellitus because periodontitis could increase the risk of many diabetes complications as retinopathy, nephropathy, neuropathic foot ulceration, cardiovascular diseases and mortality [60].

In conclusion, periodontitis and diabetes establish a two-way pathway, and each one, if untreated, could promote or exacerbate complications of each other. Periodontal screening must be part of the overall clinical examination of patients with diabetes and, if diagnosed, periodontal disease must be treated appropriately to avoid or exacerbate diabetes complications besides improving glycemic control in these individuals.

Additional Points

Clinical Significance. To alert health professionals about the relation of diabetes mellitus and periodontitis and encourage them to conduct a multidisciplinary treatment/assistance.

Acknowledgments

Priscilla Naiff was supported by Amazonas State Research Support Foundation (FAPEAM). The authors acknowledge the National Council of Scientific and Technological Development (CNPQ), the Federal District Research Support Foundation (FAPDF), and SABIN laboratory for the financial support related to the research project developed by the postgraduation program in Health Sciences of the University of Brasilia (UnB), according to the Ph.D. thesis of Priscilla Farias Naiff, the main author of this article.

References

[1] World Health Organization, *Global Report on Diabetes*, World Health Organization, Geneva, Switzerland, 2016.

[2] A. M. Karande, R. Khandeparkar, and C. S. Vergeese, "Interrelationship between diabetes mellitus and periodontal disease based on their molecular mechanisms," *Journal of Advanced Medical and Dental Sciences Research*, vol. 5, pp. 24–32, 2017.

[3] A. Milech, A. P. Angelucci, A. Golbert et al., *Diretrizes da Sociedade Brasileira de Diabetes 2015-2016*, Sociedade Brasileira de Diabetes, AC Farmacêutica, São Paulo, Brazil, 2016.

[4] C. Dai, M. Brissova, Y. Hang, C. Thompson, G. Poffenberger, and A. Shostak, "Islet-enriched gene expression and glucose-induced insulin secretion in human and mouse islets," *Diabetologia*, vol. 55, no. 3, pp. 707–718, 2012.

[5] A. Jindal, N. Agarwal, D. Sakalle, and P. Dushyant, "Diabetes mellitus and periodontitis—a two way relationship," *PJSR*, vol. 10, pp. 91–94, 2017.

[6] P. J. Ford, J. Gamonal, and G. Seymour, "Immunological differences and similarities between chronic periodontitis and aggressive periodontitis," *Periodontology 2000*, vol. 53, pp. 111-123, 2010.

[7] P. F. Naiff, P. P. Orlandi, and M. C. Dos-Santos, "Imunologia da periodontite crônica," *Scientia Amazonia*, vol. 1, pp. 28–36, 2012.

[8] O. Andrukhov, C. Ulm, H. Reischl, P. Nguyen, M. Matejka, and X. Rausch-Fan, "Serum cytokine levels in periodontitis patients in relation to the bacterial load," *Journal of Periodontology*, vol. 82, no. 6, pp. 885–892, 2011.

[9] J. Lindhe, T. Karring, and N. P. Lang, *Tratado de Periodontia Clínica e Implantologia Oral*, Guanabara Koogan, Rio de Janeiro, Brazil, 6th edition, 2018.

[10] G. U. Mohangi, S. Singh-Rambirich, and A. Volchansky, "Periodontal disease: mechanisms of infection and inflammation and possible impact on miscellaneous systemic diseases and conditions," *SADJ*, vol. 68, pp. 464–467, 2013.

[11] M. Soory, "Chronic periodontitis as a risk marker for systemic diseases with reference to cardiometabolic disorders: common pathways in their progression," *Immunology and Immunogenetics Insights*, vol. 2, pp. 7–21, 2010.

[12] S. Guzman, M. Karima, H. Y. Wang, and T. E. van Dyke, "Association between interleukin—1 genotype and periodontal disease in a diabetic population," *Journal of Periodontology*, vol. 74, no. 8, pp. 1183–1190, 2003.

[13] C. Tsai, C. Hayes, and G. W. Taylor, "Glycemic control of type 2 diabetes and severe periodontal disease in the US adult population," *Community Dentistry and Oral Epidemiology*, vol. 30, no. 3, pp. 182–192, 2002.

[14] A. D. Deshpande, M. Harris-Hayes, and M. Schootman, "Epidemiology of diabetes and diabetes-related complications," *Physical Therapy*, vol. 88, no. 11, pp. 1254–1264, 2008.

[15] J. B. Meigs, "Epidemiology of type 2 diabetes and cardiovascular disease: translation from population to prevention: the Kelly West award lecture 2009," *Diabetes Care*, vol. 33, no. 8, pp. 1865–1871, 2010.

[16] V. Lundberg, B. Stegmayr, K. Asplund, M. Eliasson, and F. Huhtasaari, "Diabetes as a risk factor for myocardial infarction: population and gender perspectives," *Journal of Internal Medicine*, vol. 241, no. 6, pp. 485–492, 1997.

[17] S. M. Haffner, S. Lehto, T. Ronnemaa, K. Pyorala, and M. Laakso, "Mortality from coronary heart disease in subjects with type 2 diabetes and in non-diabetic subjects with and without prior myocardial infarction," *New England Journal of Medicine*, vol. 339, no. 4, pp. 229–234, 1998.

[18] M. Laakso and S. Lehto, "Epidemiology of macro vascular disease in diabetes," *Diabetes Reviews*, vol. 5, pp. 294–315, 1997.

[19] F. B. Hu, M. J. Stampfer, C. G. Solomon et al., "The impact of diabetes mellitus on mortality from all causes and coronary heart disease in women: 20 years of follow-up," *Archives of Internal Medicine*, vol. 161, no. 14, pp. 1717–1723, 2001.

[20] M. Brownlee, "Advanced protein glycosylation in diabetes and aging," *Annual Review of Medicine*, vol. 46, no. 1, pp. 223–234, 1993.

[21] M. Sanz, A. Ceriello, M. Buysschaert et al., "Scientific evidence on the links between periodontal diseases and diabetes: consensus report and guidelines of the joint workshop on periodontal diseases and diabetes by the International Diabetes Federation and the European Federation of Periodontology," *Diabetes Research and Clinical Practice*, vol. 137, pp. 231–241, 2018.

[22] P. Chang and L. P. Lim, "Interrelationships of periodontitis and diabetes: a review of the current literature," *Journal of Dental Sciences*, vol. 7, no. 3, pp. 272–282, 2012.

[23] M. S. H. Akash, K. Rehman, and A. Liaqat, "Tumor necrosis factor-alpha: role in development of insulin resistance and pathogenesis of type 2 diabetes mellitus," *Journal of Cellular Biochemistry*, vol. 119, no. 1, pp. 105–110, 2018.

[24] P. P. Hujoel, B. A. White, R. I. Garcia, and M. A. Listgarten, "The dentogingival epithelial surface area revisited," *Journal of Periodontal Research*, vol. 36, no. 1, pp. 48–55, 2001.

[25] B. G. Loos, J. Craandijk, F. J. Hoek, P. M. Wertheim-van Dillen, and U. van der Velden, "Elevation of systemic markers

related to cardiovascular diseases in the peripheral blood of periodontitis patients," *Journal of Periodontology*, vol. 71, no. 10, pp. 1528–1534, 2000.

[26] B. G. Loss, "Systemic markers of inflammation in periodontitis," *Journal of Periodontology*, vol. 76, no. 11-s, pp. 2106–2115, 2005.

[27] I. G. Ursărescu, M. A. Martu-Stefanache, S. M. Solomon et al., "The assessment of Il-6 and RANKL in the association between chronic periodontitis and osteoporosis," *Revista De Chimie*, vol. 67, pp. 386–389, 2016.

[28] P. M. Ridker, "Clinical application of C-reactive protein for cardiovascular disease detection and prevention," *Circulation*, vol. 107, no. 3, pp. 363–369, 2003.

[29] S. K. Sonnenschein and J. Meyle, "Local inflammatory reactions in patients with diabetes and periodontitis," *Periodontology 2000*, vol. 69, no. 1, pp. 221–254, 2015.

[30] W. T. Y. Loo, Y. Yue, C. B. Fan et al., "Comparing serum levels of cardiac biomarkers in cancer patients receiving chemotherapy and subjects with chronic periodontitis," *Journal of Translational Medicine*, vol. 10, no. 1, pp. 1–7, 2012.

[31] G. J. Linden, A. Lyons, and F. A. Scannapieco, "Periodontal systemic associations: review of the evidence," *Journal of Clinical Periodontology*, vol. 40, pp. S8–S19, 2013.

[32] B. Chiu, "Multiple infections in carotid atherosclerotic plaques," *American Heart Journal*, vol. 138, no. 5, pp. S534–S536, 1999.

[33] J. Haraszthy, M. Zambon, M. Trevisan, and R. Zeid, "Identification of periodontal pathogens in atheromatous plaques," *Journal of Periodontology*, vol. 71, no. 10, pp. 1554–1560, 2000.

[34] E. Lalla, I. Lamster, M. Hofmann et al., "Oral infection with a periodontal pathogen accelerates early atherosclerosis in apolipoprotein E-null mice," *Arteriosclerosis, Thrombosis, and Vascular Biology*, vol. 23, no. 8, pp. 1405–1411, 2003.

[35] K. Nakano, H. Inaba, R. Nomura et al., "Detection of cariogenic *Streptococcus mutans* in extirpated heart valve and atheromatous plaque specimens," *Journal of Clinical Microbiology*, vol. 44, no. 9, pp. 3313–3317, 2006.

[36] L. K. Jennings, "Mechanisms of platelet activation: need for new strategies to protect against platelet-mediated atherothrombosis," *Thrombosis and Haemostasis*, vol. 102, no. 8, pp. 248–257, 2009.

[37] P. Ridker, C. Hennekens, J. Buring, and N. Rifai, "C-reactive protein and other markers of inflammation in the prediction of cardiovascular disease in women," *New England Journal of Medicine*, vol. 342, no. 12, pp. 836–843, 2000.

[38] P. Ridker and J. Silvertown, "Inflammation, C-reactive protein, and atherothrombosis," *Journal of Periodontology*, vol. 79, no. 8s, pp. 1544–1551, 2008.

[39] J. Beck and S. Offenbacher, "Oral health and systemic disease: periodontitis and cardiovascular disease," *Journal of Dental Education*, vol. 62, no. 10, pp. 859–870, 1998.

[40] M. Kebschull, R. T. Demmer, and P. N. Papapanou, ""Gum bug, leave my heart alone!"-epidemiologic and mechanistic evidence linking periodontal infections and atherosclerosis," *Journal of Dental Research*, vol. 89, no. 9, pp. 879–902, 2010.

[41] F. D'Aiuto, D. Ready, and M. S. Tonetti, "Periodontal disease and C-reactive protein-associated cardiovascular risk," *Journal of Periodontal Research*, vol. 39, no. 4, pp. 236–241, 2004.

[42] F. D'Aiuto, M. Parkar, G. Andreou et al., "Periodontitis and systemic inflammation: control of the local infection is associated with a reduction in serum inflammatory markers," *Journal of Dental Research*, vol. 83, no. 2, pp. 156–160, 2004.

[43] A. C. Leite, V. M. Carneiro, and M. C. Guimarães, "Effects of periodontal therapy on C-reactive protein and HDL in serum of subjects with periodontitis," *Revista Brasileira de Cirurgia Cardiovascular*, vol. 29, no. 1, pp. 69–77, 2014.

[44] B. L. Mealey and L. F. Rose, "Diabetes mellitus and inflammatory periodontal diseases," *Current Opinion in Endocrinology, Diabetes and Obesity*, vol. 15, no. 2, pp. 135–141, 2008.

[45] C. H. Peng, Y. S. Yang, K. C. Chan, E. Kornelius, J. Y. Chiou, and C. N. Huang, "Periodontal treatment and the risks of cardiovascular disease in patients with type 2 diabetes: a retrospective cohort study," *Internal Medicine*, vol. 56, no. 9, pp. 1015–1021, 2017.

[46] AAP, The American Academy of Periodontology, *Proceedings of the World Workshop in Clinical Periodontics*, AAP, Chicago, IL, USA, 1989.

[47] M. S. Tonetti and T. E. Van Dyke, "Periodontitis and atherosclerotic cardiovascular disease: consensus report of the joint EFP/AAP workshop on periodontitis and systemic diseases," *Journal of Periodontology*, vol. 84, no. 4-s, pp. S24–S29, 2013.

[48] Y. W. Fu, X. X. Li, H. Z. Xu, Y. Q. Gong, and Y. Yang, "Effects of periodontal therapy on serum lipid profile and proinflammatory cytokines in patients with hyperlipidemia: a randomized controlled trial," *Clin Oral Investig*, vol. 20, no. 6, pp. 1263–1269, 2016.

[49] J. Ainamo and I. Bay, "Problems and proposals for recording gingivitis and plaque," *International Dental Journal*, vol. 25, pp. 229–235, 1975.

[50] F. D'Aiuto, M. Parkar, G. Andreou, P. M. Brett, D. Ready, and M. S. Tonetti, "Periodontitis and atherogenesis: causal association or simple coincidence?," *Journal of Clinical Periodontology*, vol. 31, no. 5, pp. 402–411, 2004.

[51] P. M. Duarte, M. da Rocha, E. Sampaio et al., "Serum levels of cytokines in subjects with generalized chronic and aggressive periodontitis before and after non-surgical periodontal therapy: a pilot study," *Journal of Periodontology*, vol. 81, no. 7, pp. 1056–1063, 2010.

[52] T. Nakajima, T. Honda, H. Domon et al., "Periodontitis-associated up-regulation of systemic inflammatory mediator level may increase the risk of coronary heart disease," *Journal of Periodontal Research*, vol. 45, no. 1, pp. 116–122, 2010.

[53] H. P. C. Artese, A. M. Foz, M. D. S. Rabelo et al., "Periodontal therapy and systemic inflammation in type 2 diabetes mellitus: a meta-analysis," *PLoS One*, vol. 10, no. 5, Article ID e0128344, 2015.

[54] S. Gopalakrishnan, T. Ramakrishnan, P. Harinath, J. Moses, V. Shankarram, and S. Raj, "Effects of non-surgical periodontal therapy on plasma level of reactive oxygen metabolites and glycemic status in type-2 diabetic patients with chronic periodontitis," *Biosciences, Biotechnology Research Asia*, vol. 14, no. 1, pp. 357–365, 2017.

[55] A. F. Stadler, P. D. Angst, R. M. Arce, S. C. Gomes, R. V. Oppermann, and C. Susin, "Gingival crevicular fluid levels of cytokines/chemokines in chronic periodontitis: the meta-analysis," *Journal of Clinical Periodontology*, vol. 43, no. 9, pp. 727–745, 2016.

[56] M. Claudino, G. Gennaro, T. M. Cestari, C. T. Spadella, G. P. Garlet, and G. F. Assis, "Spontaneous periodontitis development in diabetic rats involves an unrestricted expression of inflammatory cytokines and tissue destructive factors in the absence of major changes in commensal oral microbiota," *Experimental Diabetes Research*, vol. 2012, p. 10, 2012.

[57] P. N. Madianos and P. A. Koromantzos, "An update of the evidence on the potential impact of periodontal therapy on diabetes outcomes," *Journal of Clinical Periodontology*, vol. 45, no. 2, pp. 188–195, 2018.
[58] D. Polak and L. Shapira, "An update of the evidence for pathogenic mechanisms that may link periodontitis and diabetes," *Journal of Clinical Periodontology*, vol. 45, no. 2, pp. 150–166, 2018.
[59] B. M. Mishriky, D. M. cummings, and R. J. Tanenberg, "The efficacy and safety of DPP4 inhibitors compared to sulfonylureas as add-on therapy to metformin in patients with Type 2 diabetes: a systematic review and meta-analysis," *Diabetes Research and Clinical Practice*, vol. 109, no. 2, pp. 378–388, 2015.
[60] P. Sharma, T. Dietrich, C. J. Ferro, P. Cockwell, and I. L. C. Chapple, "Association between periodontitis and mortality in stages 3–5 chronic kidney disease: NHANES III and linked mortality study," *Journal of Clinical Periodontology*, vol. 43, no. 2, pp. 104–113, 2016.

27

Cumulative Success Rate of Short and Ultrashort Implants Supporting Single Crowns in the Posterior Maxilla: A 3-Year Retrospective Study

Giorgio Lombardo,[1] Jacopo Pighi,[1] Mauro Marincola,[2] Giovanni Corrocher,[1] Miguel Simancas-Pallares,[2,3] and Pier Francesco Nocini[1]

[1]*School of Dentistry, Department of Surgery, Dentistry, Paediatrics and Gynaecology (DIPSCOMI), University of Verona, Verona, Italy*
[2]*Dental Implant Unit, University of Cartagena, Cartagena, Colombia*
[3]*Research Department, Faculty of Dentistry, University of Cartagena, Cartagena, Colombia*

Correspondence should be addressed to Miguel Simancas-Pallares; msimancasp@unicartagena.edu.co

Academic Editor: Luigi Canullo

Aim. To determine cumulative success rate (CSR) of short and ultrashort implants in the posterior maxilla restored with single crowns. *Patients and Methods.* We performed a retrospective study in 65 patients with 139 implants. 46 were ultrashort and 93 short. Implants were placed with a staged approach and restored with single crowns. Success rate, clinical and radiographic outcomes, and crown-to-implant ratio (CIR) were assessed after three years. Statistical analysis was performed by descriptive and inferential statistics. A log-binomial regression model where the main outcome was implant success was achieved. Coefficients and 95% confidence intervals were reported. Analyses were performed with Stata 13.2 for Windows. *Results.* 61.54% of patients were female and mean overall age was 51.9 ± 11.08 years old. Overall CSR was 97.1% (95% CI: 92.4–98.9): 97.9 and 95.1% for short and ultrashort, respectively (P value: 0.33). Four implants failed. Covariates were not associated with CSR (P value > 0.05). Regression model showed coefficients correlated with implant success for ultrashort implants (0.87) and most of covariates but none were statistically significant (P values > 0.05). *Conclusions.* Our results suggest that short and ultrashort implants may be successfully placed and restored with single crowns in the resorbed maxillary molar region.

1. Introduction

The partially edentulous posterior maxilla bone quality is often poorly characterized by large marrow spaces and reduced both vertical and horizontal bone volumes due to the severe atrophy, increased sinus pneumatization, and also iatrogenic prosthesis. Patients with extremely atrophic upper posterior maxilla require major surgical sinus lift procedures [1] or even zygomatic implants to be successfully restored and then recover their oral function [2–5]. These options are clinically challenging, because of the increased patient morbidity and also the greater chance of intra- and postoperative complications [6, 7]. Likewise, the development of innovative implant designs and surface textures in cases of intermediate atrophy suggests the use of short implants as minimally invasive treatment options in these cases [8].

The definition of a short implant in scientific literature has been a historical debate. At first, "short" implants were defined as those with <11 mm in length [9, 10], 10 mm [11, 12], 8 mm [13], and 6 mm [14], and ultimately "extra-short" implants were defined as those with a ≤5 mm intrabony length [15]. However, the most recent European Consensus Conference on short, angulated, and diameter-reduced implants defined short implants as those with ≤8 mm in length and ≥3.75 mm in diameter, standard implants as those >8 mm in length and ≥3.75 mm in diameter, and ultrashort implants as those <6 mm in length [16]. Also they stated that short implants are used primarily to avoid bone augmentation procedures and they are applicable if vertical bone volume is limited by other anatomical structures such as maxillary sinus or the mandibular canal, but there is sufficient alveolar ridge width to use ≥3.75 mm diameter implants [16].

Short implants were historically associated with lower survival rates and with unpredictable long-term outcomes [17–20], but, currently due to their design improvement, scientific evidence suggests that short implants (>6 but ≤8 mm) have similar survival rates compared to standard implants (>8 mm) [15]. Splinted restorations were highly recommendable in the posterior area of the jaw in order to avoid unfavorable strains over the prosthesis [21], but further studies showed the success of nonsplinted short implants supporting single restorations, offering a comfortable prosthetic approach including better emergence profiles and oral hygiene access compared to other fixed partial prostheses options [22].

Several types of connections between the implant and its prosthetic abutment are commercially available. Screw-retained hexagonal (internal and external) or locking-taper have been subjected to research in the past [23]. Screw-retained systems exhibits greater rate of complications due to instability at the implant-abutment interface (IAI), poor accuracy of thread coupling, and the presence of microgap allowing microbial colonization at the IAI leading to higher rates of biological complications. To deal with this, the locking-taper connection was introduced. It is defined as a tapered connection with an angle connection <1.5 degrees on both components [24]. Major advantages of the locking-taper connection include increased mechanical stability with no micromovements or microgaps at the IAI, thus leading to fewer rates of biological and prosthetic complications. Numerous studies have shown the high survival rates of dental implants with this type of connection [23, 25, 26].

To the best of our knowledge most of these studies focused mainly on 8 mm length implant clinical outcomes, but the scientific evidence for 5 or 6 mm length implants supporting single crowns in the posterior jaw is scarce, thus leaving no clinical recommendations at this time for its clinical usage. So our aim was to determine cumulative success rates of 5 and 6 mm length implants in the posterior jaw restored with single crowns.

2. Materials and Methods

2.1. Study Design and Sample. We performed a retrospective study in 65 patients who had at least one 5, 6, or 8 mm length Bicon™ dental implant (Bicon Dental Implants, Boston, MA, USA) placed between January 2012 and December 2013 at the University of Verona Dental Clinic. One hundred thirty-nine dental implants were placed overall. Sample was selected by a convenience sampling according to the inclusion criteria described below.

2.2. Inclusion Criteria. Patients with ASA I or II status who voluntarily agreed to participate, aged > 18 years old, being partially edentulous in the posterior area of the maxilla, with a residual ridge that allowed insertion of ≤8 mm length implants, with 3 months of healing after tooth extraction and having at least one 8, 6, or 5 mm Bicon implant in length, and restored with single crowns with at least 3 years of function were included. Amongst all of the 139 implants, 52 were 8 mm, 46 were 6 mm, and 41 were 5 mm in length.

The study was conducted in accordance with the Helsinki statement, and all patients signed a written informed consent form. Also the University of Verona Institutional Review Board approved the protocol.

2.3. Preoperative Steps. Before implant placement, all patients received clinical examinations regarding periodontal diseases, caries, and soft tissue status and, if needed, dentate subjects were periodontally treated in order to obtain good oral health before implant placement. Also complete radiographic evaluation including panoramic and periapical radiographs with parallelism technique was obtained. When more than one implant was needed, surgical templates were delivered. All of the patients were prescribed Amoxicillin plus Clavulanate (Augmentin, GlaxoSmithKline SpA, Verona, Italy) one hour before the implant placement to prevent systemic or local infections.

2.4. Surgical Procedure. Local infiltrative anesthesia was used. 2% Xylocaine (Dentsply Pharmaceutical, York, PA, USA) was used to complete the surgical procedure.

Intrasulcular incisions were performed by using a N°15 blade in a Bard-Parker scalpel. Full thickness flap was obtained in the area and then this surgical protocol was followed for implant placement; we began with pilot (2 mm diameter) drilling to achieve cortical perforation. Initial pilot drilling length (3-4 mm) was determined upon residual bone height (RBH) measurement. This high-speed drill (1100 Revolutions Per Minute (RPMs)) was used with external saline irrigation and had a cutting edge at the apical portion. RBH aimed to determine also implant selection, but final pilot drilling length was calculated by adding 3 mm to the selected implant length. Once pilot drilling was performed, a periapical X-ray was obtained in order to control vertical and horizontal positions with regard to the adjacent anatomical structures.

The following steps were achieved with latch reamers (LRs) at 50 RPMs without external irrigation. LRs were used to widen the osteotomy, but length was always set at the computed final drilling length (by adding 3 mm to the desired implant length). LRs are designed with a 0.5 mm diameter progressive increase and were used until the final implant diameter was reached. Due to the fact that the LRs did not need external irrigation and have low RPMs, we collected autogenous bone from the latch reaming process. This bone was stored in a Silicone Dappen Dish during the procedure. Then the selected implant (Bicon Dental Implants, Boston, MA, USA) was manually inserted into the osteotomy through the healing plug. Healing plug was carefully removed and then, with a seating tip mounted into a straight handle, we seated the implant into the osteotomy. Healing plug was cut ensuring that no sharp edges were present and could irritate soft tissue. Then we placed harvested bone over the implant shoulder.

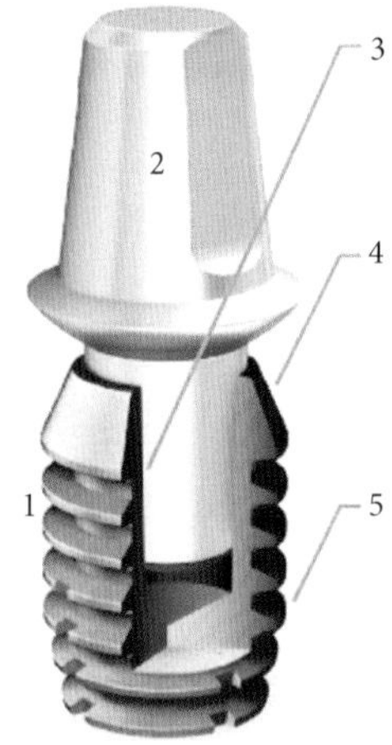

FIGURE 1: Schematic drawing of the Bicon dental implant system and its macrogeometric features. 1 represents the short root-plateau form implant body; 2 represents the abutment; 3 represents the 1.5° internal connection (locking-taper); 4 indicates the convergent crest module (sloping shoulder); and 5 represents the implant *plateaus*.

Single suture with polyglycolid acid (Vicryl, ACE Surgical Supply Co., Brockton, MA, USA) was used to close the incisions. After implant insertion, immediate postoperative X-ray was performed. The patient received postoperative and homecare instructions as well as antibiotic and analgesic prescriptions to avoid infections and pain/swelling, respectively.

After a 4-to-6-month healing period, the implants were uncovered, temporary abutments were placed, flaps were readapted, and sutures were placed around the temporary abutments. After 3 weeks of soft tissue healing, definitive impressions were taken and within 2 weeks definitive ceramic or composite single crown restorations were delivered. At each recall appointment and when needed, occlusal adjustments were made and the prosthetic restorations were checked for loosening, chipping, or other prosthetic complications.

2.5. Implant System. We used a locking-taper (Morse taper or Morse cone) dental implant system (Bicon Dental Implants, Boston, MA, United States) designed in 1985. Besides the aforementioned clinical advantages of a locking-taper connection with proven bacterial seal [27], this implant has a convergent crest module, platform switching, and a root-form plateau design (Figure 1). Regarding its surface, Integra-Ti™ (grit-blasted and acid-etched) and Integra-CP™ (Hydroxylapatite treated or covered by Hydroxyapatite) are commercially available.

2.6. Follow-Up Examination. After 3 years, patients were recalled for radiographic and clinical examinations. Peri-implant tissues and prostheses were also assessed. Figure 2 depicts a case of two upper posterior-placed implants at the tooth numbers 14 and 15 with porcelain-fused-to-metal restorations. Number 14 was a 5.0 × 8.0 mm and number 15 a 5.0 × 5.0 mm implant, respectively.

2.7. Study Variables. All of the implants had the same diameter (5 mm), but three different lengths were included (5, 6, or 8 mm). The major predictor variable was implant length classified as short (S) (≤8 mm in length) or ultrashort (US) (<6 mm in length) according the proposed criteria of the European Consensus Conference on short, angulated, and diameter-reduced implants [16].

The main outcome was the cumulative success rate (CSR). Secondary variables (covariates) included the following: sex, age, smoking history, NSAIDs consumption, and clinical-related parameters such as implanted tooth type, history of periodontal disease on the treated site, and implant surface. Prosthetic-related covariates were type of restorative material and crown-to-implant ratio.

2.8. Crown-to-Implant Ratio (CIR) Determination. At first, crown height (in mm) was measured on the radiograph immediately after prosthetic loading as the most occlusal point to the implant-abutment interface (IAI) [28]. Then crown-to-implant ratios were calculated by dividing the digital length of the crown over the implant length and were dichotomized as >2 or <2 units.

Vertical distortion occurs equally in the crown and in the implant on the radiograph; and because the crown-to-implant ratio is not dependent on absolute values, the effect of vertical distortion on a ratio is then minimal [29].

2.9. Study Outcomes

2.9.1. Primary Outcome: Cumulative Success Rate. Expressed as CSR was the primary outcome variable in our study. Failure was defined as the need of implant removal. Also implant failures were classified in two types: early (or initial) and late that occurred before and after implant loading (crown insertion), respectively.

2.9.2. Secondary Outcomes: Biological and Prosthetic Complications. Biological complications included mucositis (swollen soft tissue and bleeding on probing without bone loss) and peri-implantitis (swollen tissues, bleeding on probing, bone loss, and peri-implant pocket depth > 5 mm) [30].

Prosthetic complications were considered as crown detachment, chipping, or material fracture. However, prosthesis failure was defined as the need to remake the crown due to fracture or loosening.

2.10. Statistical Analysis. We first performed univariate analysis through descriptive statistics. For qualitative variables, we computed proportions and 95% confidence intervals. However, to analyze quantitative data, we first tested normality assumptions by using the Shapiro-Wilks test. If normality criteria were met, we reported mean and standard deviation; otherwise median and interquartile range (IQR) were reported.

In bivariate analysis, we compared proportions using χ^2 or Fisher's exact test, but, to compare means across groups, we used Student's t-test or the Mann–Whitney test, considering if normality assumption and homoscedasticity criteria were met (Levene's test).

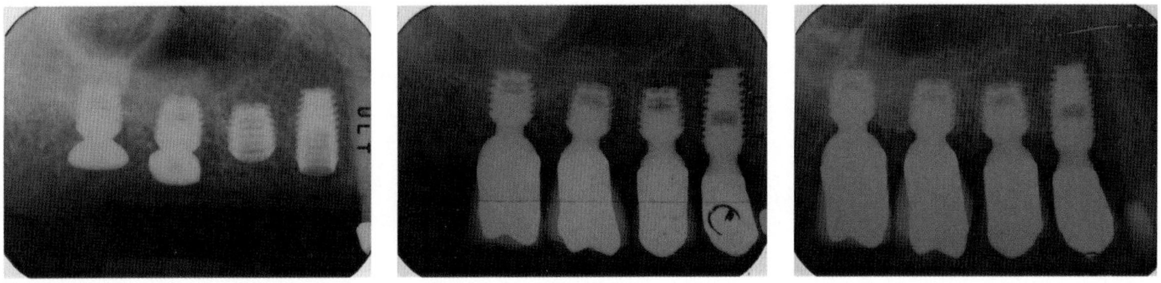

(a) (b) (c)

Figure 2: (a) Immediate postoperative radiography of premolar implants placed at the upper posterior maxilla (premolars); internal sinus lift cases were not included in this study. (b) Immediate X-ray obtained at crown insertion. (c) X-ray obtained at three-year follow-up showing the implant-restoration success.

Finally, for multivariate analysis, we created a generalized linear model (log-binomial regression) model where the outcome (β) was the implant success rate due to the high rate of the outcome [31]. Major predictors were defined a priori being those with biological plausibility. From this model we reported standardized coefficients and 95% confidence intervals. Marginal probability predictions were also estimated for each group of implant length (short or ultrashort). Statistical analysis was performed using Stata v.13.2 for Windows (StataCorp, College Station, TX, USA).

3. Results

Amongst the 65 patients, 61.5% were females. Overall mean age was 51.9 ± 11.08 years old. Most of the patients were nonsmokers (75.38%), ASA status II (52.31%), and non-NSAIDs consumers. Most of the implanted sites were located in the molar area, coated by the Integra-CP surface and restored using porcelain (porcelain-fused-to-metal (PFM) Technique).

When we analyzed sample distribution according to length definition (short or ultrashort), we only found statistical significance for patients having history of periodontal disease on the implanted site (58.46%), implanted tooth type (molars: 51.8%), and also type of restorative material (porcelain: 76.26%). Overall mean follow-up time was 32.69 ± 15.62 months. Table 1 presents uni- and bivariate demographic and clinical-related outcomes.

Our overall cumulative success rate was 97.12% (95% CI: 92.49–98.92). Among the 139 implants, 4 implants failed: 3 due to peri-implantitis and the other one due to no osseointegration (early failure). When we analyzed failures according to implant length, implanted tooth type, restorative material, and also periodontal status before implantation, we found they were equally distributed amongst groups (P values > 0.05). Nonetheless, most of the failed implants were Integra-CP coated (4 implants) with crown-to-implant ratio > 2 (2 implants). Bivariate analysis for the cumulative success rate is presented in Table 2 showing no statistical significance of the aforementioned parameters with the cumulative success rates (P values > 0.05).

Table 3 shows the descriptive statistics for length definition distribution of the successes and failures according implanted tooth type, implant surface, restorative material, CIR, and also periodontal status before implantation.

Finally, we entered covariates into the log-binomial regression model and coefficients with 95% CI are presented in Table 4. Implant success increases with ultrashort implants in male patients with ASA status I, mostly consuming NSAIDs, and implants covered by Integra-CP. Regarding prosthetic covariates, success increases with crowns made by ceromer and with CIR > 2. On the other hand, failures increases in periodontally compromised patients. However, none of these parameters were statistically significant (P value > 0.05).

Probability prediction after regression indicated that overall probability of success for short and ultrashort implants are 96.24 and 94.39%, respectively. Finally, according to CIR (>2), probability of success for short and ultrashort implants was 95.64 and 93.51%, respectively.

4. Discussion

Placed implants in augmented bone in both mandible and maxilla simultaneously or after a staged 6-month period from lateral sinus floor elevation procedure were shown to provide high survival rates [32]. However, these associated procedures are highly invasive and often associated with a high rate of complications such as membrane perforation, sinusitis, and total or partial loss of the grafted material [33–37].

This led to an increase usage of short implants especially in the posterior area of the lower jaw. Also a large number of studies including systematic and narrative reviews suggest that short implants could be considered an alternative treatment to advanced bone augmentation techniques with significantly less complications rates and higher patient's satisfaction [38]. However, several of these reviews clustered short implants outcomes supporting different types of restoration, so the evidence about clinical outcomes of short

Table 1: Overall placed implants according to studied covariates. Also distribution of placed implants according to implant length is presented in this table.

Variable	Overall		Short		Ultrashort		*P* value
	n	%	*n*	%	*n*	%	
Sex							
Female	40	61.54	26	65.00	14	56.00	0.46
Male	25	38.46	14	35.00	11	44.00	
Age	51.90 ± 11.08		51.07 ± 10.38		53.24 ± 12.22		0.44
Smoking history							
Yes	16	24.62	7	17.50	9	36.00	0.09
No	49	75.38	33	82.50	16	64.00	
ASA status							
I	31	47.69	21	52.50	10	40.00	0.32
II	34	52.31	19	47.50	15	60.00	
NSAIDs consumption							
Yes	5	7.69	2	5.00	3	12.00	0.36
No	60	92.31	38	95.00	22	88.00	
History of periodontal disease							
Yes	38	58.46	19	47.50	19	76.00	0.02*
No	27	41.54	21	52.50	6	24.00	
Implanted tooth type							
Premolar	67	(48.20)	56	(57.14)	11	(26.83)	0.00*
Molar	72	(51.80)	42	(42.86)	30	(73.17)	
Implant surface							
Integra-CP	117	87.31	80	84.21	37	94.87	
HA-coated	12	8.96	10	10.53	2	8.96	0.29
Integra-Ti	5	3.73	5	5.26	0	3.73	
Restorative material							
Ceromer	33	(23.74)	18	(18.37)	15	(36.59)	0.02*
Porcelain	106	(76.26)	80	(81.63)	26	(63.41)	

*Statistically significant differences between groups. Age is presented as mean ± standard deviation.

implants supporting single crowns in the posterior maxilla is scarce [39, 40].

To the best of our knowledge, there is only one comprehensive systematic review aimed to evaluate the prognosis of the posterior area restoration with single crowns supported by short implants [41]. In this review, even when authors did not find differences between ≤6 and >7 but in ≤8 mm implants in length, they hypothesized that this might be due to the small sample of the 6 mm and 5 mm length implants included, and if, with a larger sample size of the 6 mm and 5 mm implants, the meta-regression analysis results should be different, finding statistically significant differences between implants ≤8 mm and >8 mm in length.

Recently, Lai et al. [42] in a 5–10-year study followed 231 short Straumann implants supporting single crowns. 110 implants were placed in the maxilla and found that the 6 and 8 mm length implants showed, respectively, a cumulative survival rate of 97 and 98.5%, with no differences in regard to the implanted jaw. Gulje et al. examined 41 patients randomly allocated to receive an 11 mm implant in combination with maxillary sinus floor elevation surgery or to receive a 6 mm implant without any grafting in the posterior maxilla. At the 12-month evaluation implant, survival was 100% in both groups [43]. Schincaglia et al. [44] and Bechara et al. [45], in two studies with similar designs, reported a cumulative survival rate of 100% for the 6 mm implants after 1 and 3 years, respectively. Even when we performed a mid-term (three years) follow-up, our results are also comparable to those at long-term (ten years) follow-up. Mangano et al., on a prospective clinical study including 215 short (8 mm) implants also supporting single crowns in the posterior region of the jaws, showed an implant-based cumulative survival rate of 98.5% [46], also highlighting the clinical applicability of short implants.

Our results show that overall cumulative success rates for short and ultrashort implants was 97.9% and 95.1%, respectively (*P* value = 0.58), thus being equivalent. These results are also consistent with previous evidence about short implants supporting single crowns in the posterior maxilla and, as a matter of fact, not only short but also

TABLE 2: Bivariate analysis of the success rate according to study included covariates.

Variable	Overall		P value
	Success n (%)	Failure n (%)	
Implant length			
Short	96 (97.96)	2 (2.04)	0.33
Ultrashort	39 (95.12)	2 (4.88)	
Implanted tooth type			
Premolar	65 (97.01)	2 (2.99)	1.00
Molar	70 (97.22)	2 (2.78)	
Implant surface			
Integra-CP	113 (96.58)	4 (3.42)	
Hydroxyapatite (HA) coating	12 (100)	0 (0.00)	1.00
Integra-Ti	5 (100)	0 (0.00)	
Restorative material			
Ceromer	31 (93.94)	2 (6.06)	0.23
Ceramic	104 (98.11)	2 (1.89)	
Crown-to-implant ratio			
<2 Units	71 (98.61)	1 (1.39)	0.60
>2 Units	63 (96.92)	2 (3.08)	
Periodontal status before implantation			
Periodontally compromised	36 (94.74)	2 (5.26)	1.00
Nonperiodontally compromised	25 (92.59)	2 (7.41)	

TABLE 3: Descriptive analysis of the success rate according to study groups.

Variable	Short		Ultrashort	
	Success n (%)	Failure n (%)	Success n (%)	Failure n (%)
Implanted tooth type				
Premolar	55 (57.29)	1 (50.00)	10 (25.64)	1 (50.00)
Molar	41 (42.70)	1 (50.00)	29 (74.35)	1 (50.00)
Implant surface				
Integra-CP	78 (83.87)	2 (100)	35 (94.59)	2 (100)
HA-coated	10 (10.75)	0 (0.00)	2 (5.40)	0 (0.00)
Integra-Ti	5 (5.37)	0 (0.00)	0 (0.00)	0 (0.00)
Restorative material				
Ceromer	18 (18.75)	0 (0.00)	13 (33.33)	2 (100)
Ceramic	78 (81.25)	2 (100)	26 (66.66)	0 (0.00)
Crown-to-implant ratio				
<2 Units	66 (69.47)	1 (50.00)	5 (12.82)	0 (0.00)
>2 Units	29 (30.52)	1 (50.00)	34 (87.17)	1 (100)
Periodontal status before implantation				
Periodontally compromised	20 (52.63)	1 (50.00)	5 (21.73)	1 (50.00)
Nonperiodontally compromised	18 (47.36)	1 (50.00)	18 (78.26)	1 (50.00)

ultrashort implants can support single crowns and remain as a successful treatment in the atrophic posterior maxilla, even with high C/I ratios (>2). It is important to note that the prevalence of crowns with CIR > 2 (47.4%) was higher than the previously published in the literature. Moreover when we analyzed success rates of short and ultrashort implants according to CIR, we did not find any statistical significance, thus suggesting that either short or ultrashort implants could be restored with single crowns having CIR > 2. Besides this, the multivariate analyses show the positive effect of CIR > 2 on the implant success rate (coefficient = 0.79). Even when our study only included dental implants restored by means of single crowns, our results are also comparable with those of Mangano et al., who showed a high CSR (97,2%), for

Table 4: Standardized coefficients derived from log-binomial regression and 95% confidence intervals for factors associated with success rate.

Variable	Estimates Coefficients	95% CI	*P* value
Implant length			
Ultrashort	0.87	1.05–2.79	0.37
Sex			
Male	0.47	−1.42–2.36	0.62
ASA status			
I	0.09	−1.80–1.99	0.92
NSAIDs consumption			
Yes	1.38	−0.68–3.45	0.19
Implant surface			
Integra-CP	14.85	−4318.28–4348.00	
HA-coated	−14.19	−3787.47–3759.08	0.99
Integra-Ti	−13.88	−5171.07–5143.29	
Restorative material			
IACs (ceromer)	1.16	−0.75–3.08	0.23
Crown-to-implant ratio			
>2 units	0.79	−1.58–3.17	0.51
Periodontal status before implantation			
Periodontally compromised	−0.34	−2.23–1.55	0.72

standard (>10 mm) implants restored using fixed prosthesis with follow-up periods as high as 20 years [47].

Urdaneta et al. evaluated 326 short and ultrashort implants with the same implant design supporting single-tooth crowns with a mean C/IR of 1.6 (ranging from 0.79 to 4.95) and found that after 6 years (70.7 months) of follow-up a CIR up to 4.95 did not lead to an increased risk of implant failures, crown failures, or crown fractures [26]. Malchiodi et al., in a prospective study on 259 tapered truncated cone shaped implants with 5, 7, 9, or 12 mm in length, reported that 36% of the implants presented a C/I ratio >2, showing a CSR of 95.6% [48] being comparable to our results (96.9%). Anitua et al. [49], in a retrospective study with a mean follow-up of 28.9 months, reviewed the clinical outcomes of 128 short implants being mostly restored with bridges or splinted crowns and found a CSR of 100%. Only 42 out of the 128 implants (32.8%) had a >2 CIR. Recently, Mangano et al. [50], in a 5-year prospective study, followed 68 6.5 mm long implants in 51 patients. Twenty-nine out of the 65 implants (72%) were restored by means of single crowns. Twenty-five percent (17 out of 68) of the implants had at baseline CIR ≥ 2 and 3 failures were reported, all in the >2 CIR group.

Current scientific evidence demonstrates that implant design can play a determining role to allow higher clinical performance [51], and it is assumed to be particularly true for short implants. Moreover our results support these facts for ultrashort implants. Results from finite element analysis studies show that different implant bodies and abutment connection types may influence peri-implant bone stresses and abutment micromovement, determining the threshold values of tensile and shear stresses that cause resorption of cortical bone, thus affecting implant success rate [52].

Features like a reverse conical neck design, the locking-taper implant-abutment connection, and a plateau root form body are associated with low occlusal stress concentration on the buccal bone and limited harmful abutment micromovement inside the connection [52]. Furthermore, the locking-taper feature inhibits the bacterial leakage at the implant-abutment connection level [27], thus providing numerous benefits in terms of healing and osseointegration, leading to a better biomechanical fixation [53]. From a biomechanical standpoint, a locking-taper connection is mechanically more stable than external-hexagon or butt-joint implant-abutment connections. While the rate of biological and prosthetic complications related to screw-retained systems is high, locking-taper implants demonstrates minimizing all these problems. Also this type of implant-abutment connection can also withstand large lateral forces [54]. Thanks to the Morse taper principle, the high friction between the surfaces of two equal conical parts links them altogether. This phenomenon is known as "cold welding," since both surfaces undergo a kind of interpenetration and fusion between their asperities as result of contact pressure. This means that both implant and abutment virtually create a single body; so compared to screw-retained systems, stress distribution is homogeneous through the unit [24].

All these facts that aim to elucidate the high CSR from our study are also well supported in scientific evidence from systematic reviews [55]. Implant placement in a subcrestal (submerged) fashion and the usage of an implant with convergent crest module, represented by the sloping shoulder geometry, enhance the platform switching (PS) to occur. This PS allows an increase in residual crestal alveolar bone volume around the neck of the an implant, repositions the papilla to a more esthetic and apposite level, reduces mechanical stress in the crestal alveolar bone area, and assists in enhancing the vascular supply to hard and soft tissue in case of reduced interdental space.

Even when our study was able to demonstrate the high cumulative success rate and low fate of biological complications, some limitations are evident such as the relatively small sample size, the mid-term follow-up, and imbalanced distribution across groups (short versus ultrashort). These factors might partially explain our nonstatistically significant associations presented here.

5. Conclusions

Results from our study suggest the adequate clinical performance of short and ultrashort implants. After 3 years of loading, the clinical applicability of these implants with locking-taper connection, sloping shoulder, and plateau-form which are supporting single crowns in the posterior maxilla is evident. Since we did not find any statistical difference between groups, even according to CIR, this is the first evidence to hypothesize that short and ultrashort implants are clinically equivalent and could be used either on premolar or on molar areas. However, in most cases where residual bone height in the molar area is limited, ultrashort implants are recommended for implant-supported restorations.

Acknowledgments

This paper is supported by Department of Surgery, Dentistry, Paediatrics and Gynaecology (DIPSCOMI). University of Verona.

References

[1] B. E. Pjetursson, W. C. Tan, M. Zwahlen, and N. P. Lang, "A systematic review of the success of sinus floor elevation and survival of implants inserted in combination with sinus floor elevation: part I: lateral approach," *Journal of Clinical Periodontology*, vol. 35, Supplement 8, pp. 216–240, 2008.

[2] G. Lombardo, A. D'Agostino, L. Trevisiol et al., "Clinical, microbiologic and radiologic assessment of soft and hard tissues surrounding zygomatic implants: a retrospective study," *Oral Surgery, Oral Medicine, Oral Pathology and Oral Radiology*, vol. 122, no. 5, pp. 537–546, 2016.

[3] P. F. Nocini, L. Trevisiol, A. D'Agostino, G. Zanette, V. Favero, and P. Procacci, "Quadruple zygomatic implants supported rehabilitation in failed maxillary bone reconstruction," *Oral and Maxillofacial Surgery*, vol. 20, no. 3, pp. 303–308, 2016.

[4] A. D'Agostino, P. Pasquale, F. Ferrari, L. Trevisiol, and N. P. Francesco, "Zygoma implant-supported prosthetic rehabilitation of a patient after subtotal bilateral maxillectomy," *Journal of Craniofacial Surgery*, vol. 24, no. 2, pp. e159–e162, 2013.

[5] P. F. Nocini, A. D'agostino, L. Chiarini, L. Trevisiol, and P. Procacci, "Simultaneous le fort I osteotomy and zygomatic implants placement with delayed prosthetic rehabilitation," *Journal of Craniofacial Surgery*, vol. 25, no. 3, pp. 1021–1024, 2014.

[6] P. Boffano and T. Forouzanfar, "Current concepts on complications associated with sinus augmentation procedures," *Journal of Craniofacial Surgery*, vol. 25, no. 2, pp. e210–e212, 2014.

[7] A. D'Agostino, L. Trevisiol, V. Favero, M. Pessina, P. Procacci, and P. F. Nocini, "Are zygomatic implants associated with maxillary sinusitis?" *Journal of Oral and Maxillofacial Surgery*, vol. 74, no. 8, pp. 1562–1573, 2016.

[8] A. Y. Alqutaibi and F. Altaib, "Short dental implant is considered as a reliable treatment option for patients with atrophic posterior maxilla," *Journal of Evidence-Based Dental Practice*, vol. 16, no. 3, pp. 173–175, 2016.

[9] F. das Neves, D. Fones, S. Bernardes, C. do Prado, and A. Neto, "Short implants-an analysis of longitudinal studies," *The International Journal of Oral & Maxillofacial Implants*, vol. 21, no. 1, pp. 86–93, 2006.

[10] F. P. Strietzel and P. A. Reichart, "Oral rehabilitation using Camlog screw-cylinder implants with a particle-blasted and acid-etched microstructured surface. Results from a prospective study with special consideration of short implants," *Clinical Oral Implants Research*, vol. 18, no. 5, pp. 591–600, 2007.

[11] M. Morand and T. Irinakis, "The challenge of implant therapy in the posterior maxilla: providing a rationale for the use of short implants.," *The Journal of oral implantology*, vol. 33, no. 5, pp. 257–266, 2007.

[12] G. Tawil and R. Younan, "Clinical evaluation of short, machined-surface implants followed for 12 to 92 months," *The International Journal of Oral & Maxillofacial Implants*, vol. 18, no. 6, pp. 894–901, 2003.

[13] F. Renouard and D. Nisand, "Impact of implant length and diameter on survival rates," *Clinical Oral Implants Research*, vol. 17, supplement 2, pp. 35–51, 2006.

[14] M. Srinivasan, L. Vazquez, P. Rieder, O. Moraguez, J.-P. Bernard, and U. C. Belser, "Efficacy and predictability of short dental implants (<8 mm): a critical appraisal of the recent literature," *International Journal of Oral and Maxillofacial Implants*, vol. 27, no. 6, pp. 1429–1437, 2012.

[15] D. Nisand and F. Renouard, "Short implant in limited bone volume," *Periodontology 2000*, vol. 66, no. 1, pp. 72–96, 2014.

[16] J. Neugebauer, H. Nickenig, and J. Zöller, "Update on short, angulated an diameter-reduced implants," in *Proceedings of the 11th European Consensus Conference (EuCC '16)*, pp. 1–9, European Association of Dental Implantologists, Bonn, Germany, February, 2016.

[17] O. Bahat, "Branemark system implants in the posterior maxilla: clinical study of 660 implants followed for 5 to 12 years," *International Journal of Oral and Maxillofacial Implants*, vol. 15, no. 5, pp. 646–653, 2000.

[18] S. Winkler, H. F. Morris, and S. Ochi, "Implant survival to 36 months as related to length and diameter," *Annals of periodontology*, vol. 5, no. 1, pp. 22–31, 2000.

[19] L. Pierrisnard, F. Renouard, P. Renault, and M. Barquins, "Influence of implant length and bicortical anchorage on implant stres distribution," *Clinical Implant Dentistry and Related Research*, vol. 5, no. 4, pp. 254–262, 2003.

[20] D. Weng, Z. Jacobson, D. Tarnow, M. B. Hurzeler, O. Faehn, and F. Sanavi, "A prospective multicenter clinical trial of 3i machined-surface implants: results after 6 years of follow-up," *The International Journal of Oral & Maxillofacial Implants*, vol. 18, no. 3, pp. 417–423, 2003.

[21] B. R. Rangert, R. M. Sullivan, and T. M. Jemt, "Load factor control for implants in the posterior partially edentulous segment," *International Journal of Oral and Maxillofacial Implants*, vol. 12, no. 3, pp. 360–370, 1997.

[22] G. S. Solnit and R. L. Schneider, "An alternative to splinting multiple implants: use of the ITI system," *Journal of Prosthodontics*, vol. 7, no. 2, pp. 114–119, 1998.

[23] K. O. Demiralp, N. Akbulut, S. Kursun, D. Argun, N. Bagis, and K. Orhan, "Survival rate of short, locking taper implants with a plateau design: a 5-year retrospective study," *BioMed Research International*, vol. 2015, Article ID 197451, 8 pages, 2015.

[24] G. Sannino and A. Barlattani, "Mechanical evaluation of an implant-abutment self-locking taper connection: finite element analysis and experimental tests," *The International Journal of Oral & Maxillofacial Implants*, vol. 28, no. 1, pp. e17–e26, 2013.

[25] F. Mangano, A. Macchi, A. Caprioglio, R. L. Sammons, A. Piattelli, and C. Mangano, "Survival and complication rates of fixed restorations supported by locking-taper implants: a prospective study with 1 to 10 years of follow-up," *Journal of Prosthodontics*, vol. 23, no. 6, pp. 434–444, 2014.

[26] R. A. Urdaneta, S. Daher, J. Leary, K. M. Emanuel, and S. K. Chuang, "The survival of ultrashort locking-taper implants," *The International Journal of Oral & Maxillofacial Implants*, vol. 27, no. 3, pp. 644–654, 2012.

[27] S. Dibart, M. Warbington, M. F. Su, and Z. Skobe, "In vitro evaluation of the implant-abutment bacterial seal: the locking taper system," *International Journal of Oral and Maxillofacial Implants*, vol. 20, no. 5, pp. 732–737, 2005.

[28] R. J. Blanes, J. P. Bernard, Z. M. Blanes, and U. C. Belser, "A 10-year prospective study of ITI dental implants placed in the posterior region. II: influence of the crown-to-implant ratio and different prosthetic treatment modalities on crestal bone loss," *Clinical Oral Implants Research*, vol. 18, no. 6, pp. 707–714, 2007.

[29] H. Birdi, J. Schulte, A. Kovacs, M. Weed, and S.-K. Chuang, "Crown-to-implant ratios of short-length implants," *The Journal of Oral Implantology*, vol. 36, no. 6, pp. 425–433, 2010.

[30] M. Sanz, I. L. Chapple, and Working Group 4 of the VEWoP, "Clinical research on peri-implant diseases: consensus report of working group 4," *Journal of Clinical Periodontology*, vol. 39, Supplement 12, pp. 202–206, 2012.

[31] T. Skov, J. Deddens, M. R. Petersen, and L. Endahl, "Prevalence proportion ratios: estimation and hypothesis testing," *International Journal of Epidemiology*, vol. 27, no. 1, pp. 91–95, 1998.

[32] A. Aloy-Prosper, D. Peñarrocha-Oltra, M. Penarrocha-Diago, and M. Penarrocha-Diago, "The outcome of intraoral onlay block bone grafts on alveolar ridge augmentations: a systematic review," *Medicina Oral, Patologia Oral y Cirugia Bucal*, vol. 20, no. 2, pp. e251–e258, 2015.

[33] W. C. Tan, N. P. Lang, M. Zwahlen, and B. E. Pjetursson, "A systematic review of the success of sinus floor elevation and survival of implants inserted in combination with sinus floor elevation Part II: Transalveolar technique," *Journal of Clinical Periodontology*, vol. 35, Supplement 8, pp. 241–254, 2008.

[34] H.-L. Chan and H.-L. Wang, "Sinus pathology and anatomy in relation to complications in lateral window sinus augmentation," *Implant Dentistry*, vol. 20, no. 6, pp. 406–412, 2011.

[35] H.-W. Lee, W.-S. Lin, and D. Morton, "A retrospective study of complications associated with 100 consecutive maxillary sinus augmentations via the lateral window approach," *International Journal of Oral and Maxillofacial Implants*, vol. 28, no. 3, pp. 860–868, 2013.

[36] O. Camps-Font, G. Burgueno-Barris, R. Figueiredo, R. E. Jung, C. Gay-Escoda, and E. Valmaseda-Castellon, "Interventions for dental implant placement in atrophic edentulous mandibles: vertical bone augmentation and alternative treatments. a meta-analysis of randomized clinical trials," *Journal of Periodontology*, vol. 87, no. 12, pp. 1444–1457, 2016.

[37] F. G. Draenert, P. W. Kammerer, M. Berthold, and A. Neff, "Complications with allogeneic, cancellous bone blocks in vertical alveolar ridge augmentation: prospective clinical case study and review of the literature," *Oral Surgery, Oral Medicine, Oral Pathology and Oral Radiology*, vol. 122, no. 2, pp. e31–e43, 2016.

[38] B. Pommer, G. Mailath-Pokorny, R. Haas, D. Busenlechner, R. Furhauser, and G. Watzek, "Patients' preferences towards minimally invasive treatment alternatives for implant rehabilitation of edentulous jaws," *European journal of oral implantology*, vol. 7, Supplement 2, pp. S91–109, 2014.

[39] D. S. Thoma, J. Cha, and U. Jung, "Treatment concepts for the posterior maxilla and mandible: short implants versus long implants in augmented bone," *Journal of Periodontal & Implant Science*, vol. 47, no. 1, p. 2, 2017.

[40] C. A. A. Lemos, M. L. Ferro-Alves, R. Okamoto, M. R. Mendonça, and E. P. Pellizzer, "Short dental implants versus standard dental implants placed in the posterior jaws: a systematic review and meta-analysis," *Journal of Dentistry*, vol. 47, pp. 8–17, 2016.

[41] L. A. Mezzomo, R. Miller, D. Triches, F. Alonso, and R. S. A. Shinkai, "Meta-analysis of single crowns supported by short (<10 mm) implants in the posterior region," *Journal of Clinical Periodontology*, vol. 41, no. 2, pp. 191–213, 2014.

[42] H.-C. Lai, M.-S. Si, L.-F. Zhuang, H. Shen, Y.-L. Liu, and D. Wismeijer, "Long-term outcomes of short dental implants supporting single crowns in posterior region: a clinical retrospective study of 5–10 years," *Clinical Oral Implants Research*, vol. 24, no. 2, pp. 230–237, 2013.

[43] F. L. Gulje, G. M. Raghoebar, A. Vissink, and H. J. Meijer, "Single crowns in the resorbed posterior maxilla supported by either 6-mm implants or by 11-mm implants combined with sinus floor elevation surgery: a 1-year randomised controlled trial," *European Journal of Oral Implantology*, vol. 7, no. 3, pp. 247–255, 2014.

[44] G. P. Schincaglia, D. S. Thoma, R. Haas et al., "Randomized controlled multicenter study comparing short dental implants (6 mm) versus longer dental implants (11–15 mm) in combination with sinus floor elevation procedures. Part 2: Clinical and radiographic outcomes at 1 year of loading," *Journal of Clinical Periodontology*, vol. 42, no. 11, pp. 1042–1051, 2015.

[45] S. Bechara, R. Kubilius, G. Veronesi, J. T. Pires, J. A. Shibli, and F. G. Mangano, "Short (6-mm) dental implants versus sinus floor elevation and placement of longer (≥10-mm) dental implants: a randomized controlled trial with a 3-year follow-up," *Clinical Oral Implants Research*, 2016.

[46] F. G. Mangano, J. A. Shibli, R. L. Sammons, F. Iaculli, A. Piattelli, and C. Mangano, "Short (8-mm) locking-taper implants supporting single crowns in posterior region: a prospective clinical study with 1-to 10-years of follow-up," *Clinical Oral Implants Research*, vol. 25, no. 8, pp. 933–940, 2014.

[47] C. Mangano, F. Iaculli, A. Piattelli, and F. Mangano, "Fixed restorations supported by Morse-taper connection implants: a retrospective clinical study with 10–20 years of follow-up," *Clinical Oral Implants Research*, vol. 26, no. 10, pp. 1229–1236, 2015.

[48] L. Malchiodi, A. Cucchi, P. Ghensi, D. Consonni, and P. F. Nocini, "Influence of crown-implant ratio on implant success rates and crestal bone levels: a 36-month follow-up prospective study," *Clinical Oral Implants Research*, vol. 25, no. 2, pp. 240–251, 2014.

[49] E. Anitua, L. Pinas, and G. Orive, "Retrospective study of short and extra-short implants placed in posterior regions: influence of crown-to-implant ratio on marginal bone loss," *Clinical Implant Dentistry and Related Research*, vol. 17, no. 1, pp. 102–110, 2015.

[50] F. Mangano, I. Frezzato, A. Frezzato, G. Veronesi, C. Mortellaro, and C. Mangano, "The effect of crown-to-implant ratio on the clinical performance of extra-short locking-taper implants," *Journal of Craniofacial Surgery*, vol. 27, no. 7, pp. 675–681, 2016.

[51] K.-J. Lee, Y.-G. Kim, J.-W. Park, J.-M. Lee, and J.-Y. Suh, "Influence of crown-to-implant ratio on periimplant marginal bone loss in the posterior region: a five-year retrospective study," *Journal of Periodontal and Implant Science*, vol. 42, no. 6, pp. 231–236, 2012.

[52] Y. Yamanishi, S. Yamaguchi, S. Imazato, T. Nakano, and H. Yatani, "Influences of implant neck design and implant-abutment joint type on peri-implant bone stress and abutment micromovement: three-dimensional finite element analysis," *Dental Materials*, vol. 28, no. 11, pp. 1126–1133, 2012.

[53] P. G. Coelho, M. Suzuki, M. V. M. Guimaraes et al., "Early bone healing around different implant bulk designs and surgical techniques: a study in dogs," *Clinical Implant Dentistry and Related Research*, vol. 12, no. 3, pp. 202–208, 2010.

[54] K. Gotfredsen, T. Berglundh, and J. Lindhe, "Bone reactions adjacent to titanium implants subjected to static load: a study in the dog," *Clinical Oral Implants Research*, vol. 12, no. 1, pp. 1–8, 2001.

[55] C. M. Schmitt, G. Nogueira-Filho, H. C. Tenenbaum et al., "Performance of conical abutment (Morse Taper) connection implants: a systematic review," *Journal of Biomedical Materials Research A*, vol. 102, no. 2, pp. 552–574, 2014.

28

Ridge Preservation Procedures after Tooth Extractions: A Systematic Review

Gabriella Balli,[1] Andreas Ioannou,[1] Charles A. Powell,[2] Nikola Angelov,[1] Georgios E. Romanos,[3,4] and Nikolaos Soldatos[1]

[1]*Department of Periodontics and Dental Hygiene, School of Dentistry, University of Texas Health Science Center at Houston, Houston, TX, USA*
[2]*Department of Surgical Dentistry, Division of Periodontics, School of Dental Medicine, University of Colorado, Anschutz Medical Campus, Aurora, CO, USA*
[3]*Department of Periodontology, Stony Brook University School of Dental Medicine, Stony Brook, NY, USA*
[4]*Department of Oral Surgery and Implant Dentistry, Johann Wolfgang Goethe University of Frankfurt, Frankfurt, Germany*

Correspondence should be addressed to Nikolaos Soldatos; nikolaos.k.soldatos@uth.tmc.edu

Academic Editor: Chia-Tze Kao

Background. The purpose of this systematic review was to accurately assess the procedural success of ridge preservation technique through the application of strict inclusion and exclusion criteria. *Data Sources.* A methodical search of PubMed of the US National Library of Medicine and the Cochrane Central Register of Controlled Trials was conducted for applicable articles. Only randomized controlled trials comparing ridge preservation treatment with a nongrafting control, ten-subject minimum sample size, and three or more months of follow-up were included in our study. *Types of Studies Reviewed.* In a screening between January 1980 and September 2017, articles meeting predetermined criteria were further examined in a qualitative data analysis. A thorough search of the databases provided 1876 articles. Of these records, 174 were assessed for eligibility through the systematic employment of inclusion and exclusion criteria. *Results.* Two records were appropriate for further data analysis. One study used a mixture of a deproteinized cancellous bovine bone and porcine collagen fibers in a block form (DBB/CF), while the other study used leukocyte-platelet-rich fibrin (L-PRF). The use of DBB/CF reduced the magnitude of vertical bone resorption, yet the study showed high risk of bias. The use of L-PRF reduced the magnitude of both the horizontal and vertical crestal bone resorption; however, the low sample size created wide standard deviations between the test and control groups. Inherent weaknesses were present in both studies. Through methodical analysis of both records, the dissimilarities prevented the conduction of a meta-analysis. *Implications of Key Findings.* Within the limitations of this systematic review, L-PRF reduced the magnitude of vertical and horizontal bone resorption, which places L-PRF as a potential material of choice for ridge preservation procedures. *Conclusions.* Within the limitations and weaknesses of both studies, the use of DBB/CF prevented the vertical crestal bone resorption while the L-PRF prevented both the horizontal and vertical crestal bone resorption. More randomized controlled clinical trials are needed to eliminate all the confounding factors, which bias the outcome of ridge preservation techniques.

1. Introduction

With the advent of implant dentistry, there has been an increased emphasis placed on preserving and maintaining the implant-bearing environment. Disruption to the oral environment by tooth extraction can compromise the integrated tissue morphology, inducing healing mechanisms similar to those of new tissue formation [1]. Two very important components for the socket integrity (bundle bone and periodontal ligament fibers) vanish by the 14th day after extraction [1]. Schropp et al. determined that major changes of an extraction site are occurring within 12 months, during which time a 50% (5–7 mm) reduction of alveolar ridge width can be observed, with two-thirds of this reduction occurring within the first three months [2]. These changes at the extraction site may be due to the loss of periodontal ligament fibers, bundle bone, and loss of blood supply. These morphologic changes pose significant challenges in restorative treatment, as soft tissue recession and buccal plate resorption define the anatomical profile of the socket and may narrow the viable treatment options [3]. Elian et al. [3] have classified sockets following extraction into three simplified socket types: Type I sockets, intact with normal levels of facial soft tissue and buccal plate bone, provide anatomical predictability with implant placement leading to esthetically satisfying results; Type II sockets with normal facial soft tissue appearance yet partially missing buccal plate bone creates the greatest challenge in proper diagnosis; and Type III sockets exhibit reduced facial soft tissue and buccal plate bone, thus requiring guided bone regeneration to reconstruct insufficient tissues. Repairing socket defects to create an anticipated foundation for implant placement is the rationale behind the surgical technique of ridge preservation [3]. According to the American Academy of Periodontology Glossary of Periodontal Terms, ridge preservation is a surgical procedure aimed at preventing ridge collapse and preserving ridge dimension after tooth extraction, typically done for purposes of implant site development [4].

Allograft, xenograft, and alloplastic materials, along with the autogenous bone, have been utilized in preserving the alveolar ridge to maximize implant outcomes [5]. During postextraction healing, vertical and horizontal bone loss is expected, yet the use of grafting materials can provide dimensional stability to the alveolar ridge [6, 7].

In a study performed by Araújo et al., deproteinized cancellous bovine bone and porcine collagen fibers in a block form (DBB/CF) placed in fresh extraction sites proved to be effective in offsetting hard tissue reduction with approximately 3% reduction in the cross-sectional area of the grafted alveolar ridges, as compared to nongrafted sites with roughly 25% of reduction [8]. Araújo and Lindhe differentiated the xenograft bone from the autologous bone, as the autologous bone was unsuccessful in the formation of a new bone and the prevention of ridge resorption after extraction [9]. Cardaropoli et al. compared an extraction control to sockets grafted with a DBB/CF. The DBB/CF provided horizontal ridge width loss of 0.71 mm with ridge preservation, compared to 4.04 mm width loss with spontaneous healing, irrespective of the buccal bone thickness [7].

In a study performed by Iasella et al., the use of mineralized freeze-dried bone allograft (FDBA) resulted in a 1.2 ± 0.9 mm loss of horizontal ridge width, when compared to a control, untreated extraction socket (2.6 ± 2.3 mm). In addition, this study showed a gain of vertical ridge height of 1.30 ± 2.00 mm in the FDBA group indicating that ridge preservation has the capacity to provide necessary bone volume for implant placement [6]. To augment the bone grafting process through space maintenance and preventing migration of surrounding soft tissue into the socket, resorbable and nonresorbable membranes are used [10, 11]. Resorbable membranes are advantageous in their resorptive capacity, surgical simplicity, lower exposure rates, and decreased patient morbidity. However, these membranes can compromise the healing environment with their variable resorption rates, need for tenting screws to prevent collapse, incomplete resorption, associated material memory, and potential movement amplified by the membrane microenvironment [10]. The most common resorbable membrane used is a collagen membrane, designed to match the properties of the periodontal connective tissues [10, 11]. These membranes act as a scaffold to amplify tissue flap thickness, promoting primary wound closure by chemotaxis of periodontal ligament and gingival fibroblasts, and encourage wound healing through hemostasis and maintenance of membrane integrity [11]. Prolonged resorption rates, linearly related to the degree of cross-linking, adequately prevent apical migration of the epithelium as the membrane remains intact during epithelial proliferation [11].

Various ridge preservation techniques are presented in the literature. Amongst these methods, the "ice cream cone" technique has been acceptable for cases of buccal plate defects (Type I and II sockets), after extraction [3, 12]. As confirmed by Tan-Chu et al., the "ice cream cone" technique performed with bone allograft and resorbable collagen membrane restored the buccal plate with a small ridge width reduction of 1.32 mm, proving the success of this procedure [12]. Jiang et al. suggested a pressure-bearing microtitanium stent to preserve the contour of the extraction socket [13]. The microtitanium stent, even with its distortion, is acceptable in preserving the alveolar ridge, yet the stent fails to act as a barrier membrane [13]. SocketKAP™ and SocketKAGE™ prefabricated devices have also been studied for their effectiveness in ridge preservation [14, 15].

Local and systemic patient factors can compromise the definitive outcome. Smoking has been associated with dimensional reduction of postextraction sockets, where a 0.5 mm bone loss is expected in smokers as compared to nonsmokers [16]. As ridge preservation continues to evolve, there is an increased demand for appropriate assessment of procedural success, which is difficult without omission of all possible confounding factors.

This systematic review aims at eliminating these confounding factors through the development of criteria based on the study design, method of obtaining study results, number of subjects enrolled per study, and systemic factors of subjects. In addition, this systematic review aims at answering the focus question, If extraction and ridge preservation with the use of biologic materials can influence the magnitude of horizontal and vertical bone resorption, compared to spontaneous healing in patients needing extraction and ridge preservation?

2. Materials and Methods

2.1. Search Strategy. Our methodology followed the materials and methods of a previous systematic review from Kotsakis et al. [17]. The PRISMA (Preferred Reporting Items for Systematic Reviews and Meta-Analyses) guidelines for reporting a systematic review were followed [18]. Two electronic databases, PubMed of the US National Library of

Medicine and the Cochrane Central Register of Controlled Trials, were methodically searched for applicable articles, in the English language.

Selected key words "*ridge preservation*," "*alveolar ridge preservation*," and "*socket preservation*" were applied, and results were individually screened in a follow-up equal or greater to three months, between January 1980 and September 2017.

In addition to the electronic search, manual searching of selected journal titles was performed: *Journal of Periodontology, Journal of American Dental Association, Journal of Clinical Periodontology, The International Journal of Oral and Maxillofacial Implants, The International Journal of Periodontics and Restorative Dentistry, Clinical Implant Dentistry and Related Research, Clinical Oral Implants Research, and Implant Dentistry.*

At the first phase of selection, the titles and abstracts of all articles found through the electronic and manual searches were screened, independently, by two reviewers (Gabriella Balli and Nikolaos Soldatos). When studies met the inclusion criteria or when data from the abstracts were insufficient to determine eligibility, the full article was obtained. Following the initial phase of selection, the two reviewers scrutinized the full text articles of all relevant studies for final inclusion. If there was disagreement between the two reviewers, consensus was achieved by discussion with a third reviewer (Andreas Ioannou).

2.2. PICOS. The criteria for inclusion of studies for this review were organized by the PICOS (Population, Intervention, Control, Outcome, Setting, and Study design) approach as follows: Population—subjects in the included trials must have been humans undergoing the ridge preservation procedure; Intervention—the intervention of interest was ridge preservation; Control—randomized control studies; Outcome—dimensional changes of the ridge on the site of interest with the help of the CBCT was set as the primary outcome variable; Setting—university, hospital, and private practice; and Study designs—randomized control clinical trials.

2.3. Eligibility Criteria. Studies were filtered to include randomized controlled trials, comparing ridge preservation treatment with a nongrafting control, ten-subject minimum sample size, and three or more months of follow-up. Cone beam computed tomography (CBCT) was used to obtain study results, before and after rendered treatment. The population of interest was narrowed to healthy human subjects aged 18 years and older.

3. Results

A PRISMA flow diagram was developed to display the search results (Figure 1) [18]. The literature search of both databases provided a total of 2,411 studies. Through the manual search, five supplementary studies were added. After the duplicates were removed, 1,876 papers were available for screening. Of the 1,876 articles retrieved, 1702 articles were excluded because they employed guided bone regeneration techniques rather than ridge preservation. Full-text articles were obtained for the 174 remaining articles. One hundred and seventy-two studies were excluded because the subjects were smokers or with significant systemic diseases, including uncontrolled diabetes mellitus, diseases affecting bone metabolism, and those with periodontal or endodontic lesions. Two articles met the inclusion criteria for qualitative data analysis.

The studies included in the final review are displayed in Table 1 [19, 20]. Pang et al. included sixty patients in a randomized controlled clinical study. The authors performed ridge preservation with a mixture of a DBB/CF and a collagen membrane. The flap management involved two vertical releasing incisions on the mesial and distal areas, respectively. The test group was divided on two buccal defect levels: level A (defects between 3 and 5 mm from the crest) and level B (defects 5 mm or more). The control group consisted of spontaneous healing sockets. A CBCT was used preoperatively and postoperatively to measure the bone levels between the groups. The patients were followed up for 6 months postoperatively. Regarding the changes in the vertical dimension, both level A and level B test groups had statistically significant less bone loss compared to the control groups (*level A*: test, -1.53 ± 0.26 mm; control, -2.92 ± 0.31 mm) (*level B*: test, -2.48 ± 0.22 mm; control, -3.17 ± 0.37 mm). The horizontal dimensions did not show significant differences over the control and test groups in both the levels (*level A*: test, -2.87 ± 0.25 mm; control, -3.26 ± 0.44 mm) (*level B*: test, -3.05 ± 0.18 mm; control, -3.82 ± 0.33 mm). In both the groups, the implants were placed and measured through the ISQ system. Three months postoperatively, the ISQ numbers did not differ significantly between the groups [19].

Temmerman et al. included twenty-two patients in a randomized controlled clinical study. Two to three leukocyte-platelet-rich fibrins (L-PRF) were placed in the sockets of the test groups. The control groups were left to heal spontaneously. The patients were followed up for 3 months postoperatively. The test and control groups were divided to horizontal and vertical resorption sites as well as buccal and lingual surfaces. Moreover, the horizontal groups were subdivided to 3 more groups: 1, 2, and 5 mm below the crest (HW-1, HW-3, and HW-5). The buccal surface of the horizontal dimension showed statistically significant bone resorption at the control group compared to the test group, at HW-1 and HW-3 levels (*HW-1*: control, -3.3 ± 2.6 mm; test, -1.2 ± 2.6 mm) (*HW-3*: control, -1.0 ± 1.1 mm; test, -0.8 ± 0.9 mm). The lingual surface of the horizontal dimension showed statistically significant bone resorption at the control group, compared to the test group only at the HW-1 level (*HW-1*: control, -2.0 ± 2.6 mm; test, -0.3 ± 1.9 mm). The buccal aspect of the vertical dimension presented statistically significant bone resorption on the control group, compared to the test group (control: -1.6 ± 1.2 mm; test: -0.1 ± 1.6 mm) [20].

Both the studies were evaluated for risk of bias based on van Tulder et al., Boutron et al., and the Cochrane Handbook of Systematic Reviews of Interventions, Chapter 8 (version

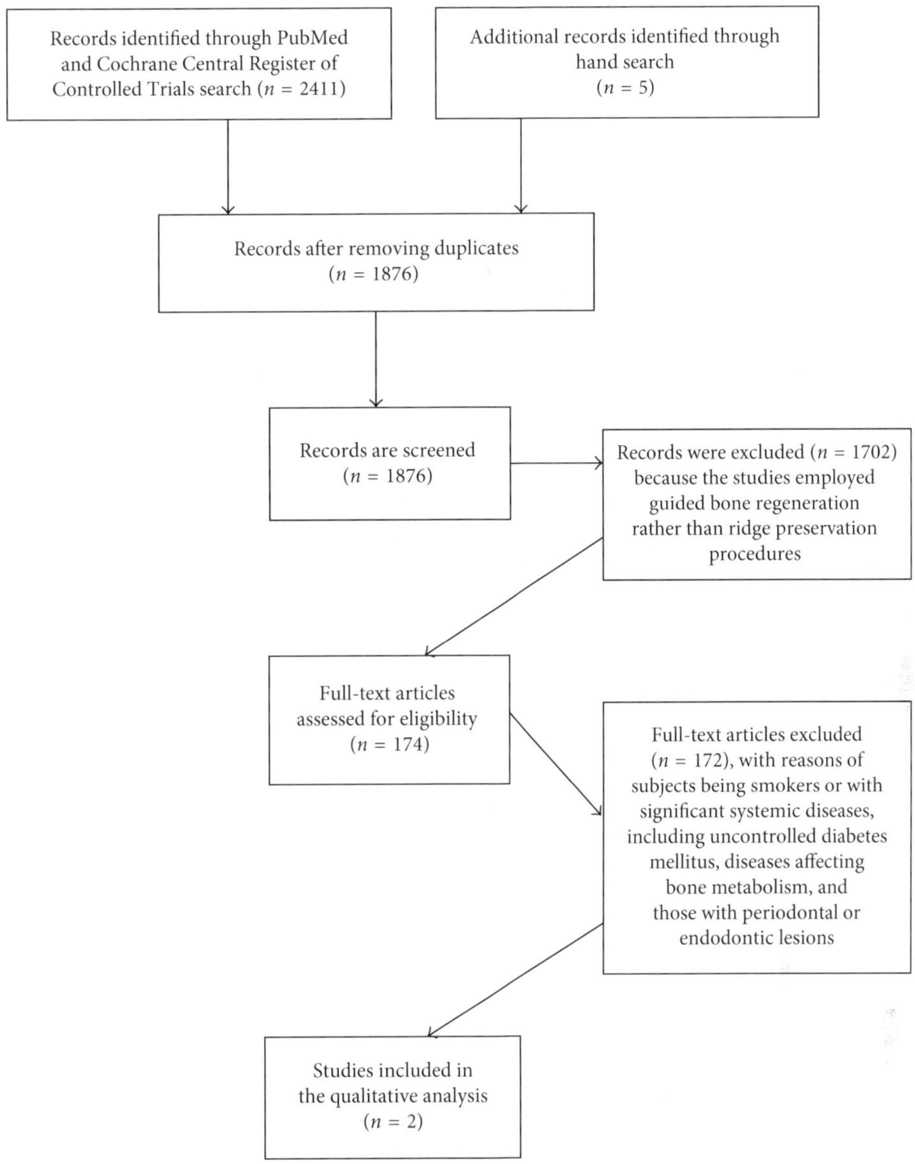

FIGURE 1: The PRISMA flow diagram.

5.1, updated on March 2011) [21, 22]. Pang et al. showed higher risk of bias (Table 2) [19].

4. Discussion

When screening for applicable articles, this systematic review limited the population of interest by age, health, and lifestyle factors. In former systematic reviews, many of the appropriate articles contained subjects with a smoking habit [16, 23]. A systematic review published in 2009, by Van der Weijden et al., highlights one limitation of their review as the heterogeneity amongst the selected studies, stemming from differences in evaluation parameters, reasons for extraction, study designs, and study populations, amongst others. This systematic review failed to control the smoking habit amongst the study populations, which is a known confounding variable on postextraction healing, as the authors noted [16]. However, our systematic review strictly excluded studies, which included individuals with a smoking habit. This exclusion criterion functioned to eliminate the effects of smoking on the dimensional stability of the extraction socket.

In addition to confounding population variables, many studies in selected systematic reviews were not segregated by socket location, reasons for extraction, or measurement approach [5, 23]. Measurement data gathered from acrylic stents, titanium pins, and cast models, along with the use of assorted surgical protocols, proved to be inconsistent and unreliable. Similar to the systematic review by Van der Weijden et al., a 2012 systematic review published by Vignoletti et al. also included studies with subjects possessing a smoking habit along with a lack of outcome measurement standardization. In the Vignoletti et al. study, the array of measurement methods resulted in the need for

Table 1: The studies included in the final review.

Study	Pang et al. [19]	Temmerman et al. [20]
Methods	Randomized controlled clinical trial	Randomized controlled clinical split mouth trial
Participants	60 patients	22 patients
Surgical considerations	Extraction with two vertical releasing incisions (mesial/distal) plus collagen membrane with DBB collagen sponge	Extraction plus 2-3 PRF
Intervention	*Test group*: deproteinized collagen bovine bone covered with collagen membrane *Control group*: spontaneous healing *Level A buccal defects*: between 3 and 5 mm *Level B buccal defects*: 5 mm or more	*Test group*: leukocyte-platelet-rich fibrin *Control group*: spontaneous healing
Measurement method	CBCT/ISQ	CBCT
Follow-up	6 months postoperatively	3 months postoperatively
Outcome	*Vertical resorption*: (i) Level A (*control group*): -2.92 ± 0.31 mm (ii) Level A (*test group*): -1.53 ± 0.26 mm (iii) Level B (*control group*): -3.17 ± 0.37 mm (iv) Level B (*test group*): -2.48 ± 0.22 mm *Horizontal resorption*: (i) Level A (*control group*): -3.26 ± 0.44 mm (ii) Level A (*test group*): -2.87 ± 0.25 mm (iii) Level B (*control group*): -3.82 ± 0.33 mm (iv) Level B (*test group*): -3.05 ± 0.18 mm *Mean ISQ test group:* Immediately after implant placement: 62.33–63.40 1 month postoperatively: 60 3 months postoperatively: 72 *Mean ISQ control group:* 1 month postoperatively:– 3 months postoperatively: 70	*Vertical resorption (lingual):* -0.7 ± 0.8 mm (control group) -0.3 ± 1.2 mm (L-PRF group) *Vertical resorption (buccal):* -1.6 ± 1.2 mm (control group) -0.1 ± 1.6 mm (L-PRF group) *Horizontal resorption (lingual):* *(Control group)* HW-1 mm: -2.0 ± 2.6 mm HW-3 mm: -0.2 ± 0.3 mm HW-5 mm: -0.1 ± 0.3 mm *(Test group)* HW-1 mm: -0.3 ± 1.9 mm HW-3 mm: -0.1 ± 0.3 mm HW-5 mm: -0.0 ± 0.1 mm *Horizontal resorption (buccal):* *(Control group)* HW-1 mm: -3.3 ± 2.6 mm HW-3 mm: -1.0 ± 1.1 mm HW-5 mm: -0.5 ± 0.7 mm *(Test group)* HW-1 mm: -1.2 ± 2.6 mm HW-3 mm: -0.8 ± 0.9 mm HW-5 mm: -0.5 ± 0.6 mm
Secondary outcome	Level B (control group): implants could not be placed in 3 patients	L-PRF group: 94.7% socket fill Control group: 63.3% socket fill

Table 2: The risk of bias for both studies.

Study	Pang et al. [19]	Temmerman et al. [20]
Random sequence generation	High risk	Low risk
Allocation concealment	High risk	Low risk
Blinding of participants	High risk	Low risk
Blinding of personnel/care providers	High risk	High risk
Detection bias	High risk	High risk
Incomplete outcome data	Low risk	Low risk
Selective reporting	Low risk	Low risk
Group similarity at the baseline	High risk	High risk
Cointerventions	Low risk	Low risk
Compliance	Low risk	Low risk
Intention-to-treat analysis	Low risk	Low risk
Timing of outcome assessments	Low risk	Low risk
Other biases	High risk	High risk

subgroup analysis in order to determine the effect of measurement methods on study outcomes [23]. Juxtaposing the methodology of Vignoletti et al., our systematic review accounts for the bias induced by variable measurement methods by standardizing the evaluation of study outcomes by the inclusion of the CBCT. CBCT was introduced in the 1990s and was used to display a three-dimensional image of the jaws to identify anatomical structures such as the maxillary sinus, the inferior alveolar nerve, and the length and the resorption of roots [24]. CBCT has shown to be more accurate compared to the conventional two-dimensional radiographic methods like periapical and panoramic X-rays [25–27]. The average amount of distortion expressed as percentages are 14% for periapical X-rays, 23.5% for panoramic X-rays, and 1.8% for the CBCT's [25]. However, the problem of the CBCT is the radiation, which is higher compared to the conventional radiographic methods [24]. Significant dose reduction can be achieved by reducing the field of view to the area of interest [25].

Published in 2015, a systematic review by Jambhekar et al. contained similar limitations to other systematic reviews as measurement methods, and anatomic socket location was not consisted between the selected studies. In addition to these limitations, 6 of the 32 selected studies utilized allograft for socket preservation, which can induce bias, as this grafting material was unavailable in certain areas outside of the United States due to legal restrictions of the cadaver bone use, as discussed by the authors as well [5]. In our study, we did not exclude any type of biomaterial. The strict inclusion and exclusion criteria created a framework for this systematic review, which assisted in reducing the intrinsic bias and confounding variables that can mask the outcome of the ridge preservation technique. The studies utilized in this systematic review were filtered to include randomized controlled clinical trials, comparing ridge preservation treatment with a nongrafting control, ten-subject minimum sample size, three or more months of follow-up, and the use of CBCT as the method of evaluation. Our methodology allowed us to reduce effects of broad study designs and heterogeneous evaluation techniques.

Two studies were included for the final review [19, 20]. Pang et al. divided equally 60 patients into 2 groups; level A group was defined as having a buccal bone defect between 3 and 5 mm, while level B group as more than 5 mm. The use of DBB/CF was advantageous to spontaneous healing only for reducing the magnitude of vertical crestal resorption. The weaknesses of this study are the lack of power analysis, the lack of histology, the use of vertical releasing incisions in the test group, and the inclusion of defects more than 5 mm, since they require guided bone regeneration, rather than ridge preservation [19]. Temmerman et al. used L-PRF as a socket filling material in the test group and spontaneous healing in the control group. Horizontal and vertical bone resorption on both buccal and lingual aspects was evaluated with the use of CBCT, preoperatively and 3 months postoperatively. The horizontal bone resorption was measured in three different levels below the crest (HW-1, HW-3, and HW-5). The use of L-PRF was advantageous to spontaneous healing as far as reducing the magnitude of horizontal bone loss, both in lingual and buccal dimensions at the HW-1 level and the vertical bone loss on the buccal aspect. Although the results at the HW-1 level show statistical significance, the sample size is low, ending up in very wide standard deviations between the test and control groups. Weaknesses of this study are the lack of histology, the unequal distribution of sites between the maxilla and mandible, and the small sample size [20]. Procedure complications were noted in both studies. Pang et al. reported three sites which regenerated bone, not sufficient for implant placement, while Temmerman et al. demonstrated two sites from the control group that had to be retreated [19, 20].

Meta-analysis is typically utilized to combine results for further projection of evidence favoring the use of ridge preservation. A significant weakness in this type of statistical analysis is the source of heterogeneity amid the selected studies [16]. The weighted mean difference (WMD) should be interpreted carefully as clinical discrepancies within the selected studies may collude the statistic. Vignoletti et al. ran a meta-analysis, coupled with subgroup analysis and metaregression in attempts to assess moderator variable influence. However, this meta-analysis was unable to draw conclusions concerning the implant-related outcomes due to inadequate data [23]. In the present systematic review, authors were unable to conduct a meta-analysis as the two selected studies were dissimilar and were deemed unsuitable for combined extension of the data. The results obtained by statistical analysis in selected systematic reviews acknowledged a lack of evidence as to which biomaterials and surgical procedures should be deemed the "gold standard" in ridge preservation.

5. Conclusions

Within the limitations and weaknesses of both studies, the use of DBB/CF reduced the magnitude of vertical bone resorption, while the L-PRF reduced the magnitude in both the horizontal and vertical crestal bone resorption. More randomized controlled clinical trials are needed to eliminate all confounding factors, which bias the outcome of ridge preservation techniques.

Disclosure

The study was presented as a poster presentation at the Academy of Osseointegration 2018 Annual Meeting, February 28–March 3, Los Angeles, CA, under the title "Ridge Preservation Procedures after Tooth Extractions. A Systematic Review and Decision Tree."

References

[1] G. Cardaropoli, M. Araujo, and J. Lindhe, "Dynamics of bone tissue formation in tooth extraction sites: an experimental study in dogs," *Journal of Clinical Periodontology*, vol. 30, no. 9, pp. 809–818, 2003.

[2] L. Schropp, A. Wenzel, L. Kostopoulos, and T. Karring, "Bone healing and soft tissue contour changes following single tooth extraction: a clinical and radiographic 12-month prospective study," *International Journal of Periodontics and Restorative Dentistry*, vol. 23, no. 4, pp. 313–323, 2003.

[3] N. Elian, S. C. Cho, S. Froum, R. B. Smith, and D. P. Tarnow, "A simplified socket classification and repair technique," *Practical Procedures & Aesthetic Dentistry*, vol. 19, no. 2, pp. 99–104, 2007.

[4] American Academy of Periodontology, *Glossary of Periodontal Terms*, American Academy of Periodontology, Chicago, IL, USA, 2001.

[5] S. Jambhekar, F. Kernen, and A. S. Bidra, "Clinical and histological outcomes of socket grafting after flapless tooth extraction: a systematic review of randomized controlled clinical trials," *Journal of Prosthetic Dentistry*, vol. 113, no. 5, pp. 371–382, 2015.

[6] J. Iasella, H. Greenwell, R. Miller et al., "Ridge preservation with freeze dried bone allograft and a collagen membrane compared alone for implant site development: a clinical and histologic study in humans," *Journal of Periodontology*, vol. 74, no. 7, pp. 990–999, 2003.

[7] D. Cardaropoli, L. Tamagnone, A. Roffredo, and L. Gaveglio, "Relationship between the buccal bone plate thickness and the healing of post-extraction sockets with/without ridge preservation," *International Journal of Periodontics and Restorative Dentistry*, vol. 34, no. 2, pp. 214–217, 2014.

[8] M. Araújo, J. Costa da Silva, A. F. de Mendonca, and J. Lindhe, "Ridge alterations following grafting of fresh extraction sockets in man: a randomized clinical trial," *Clinical Oral Implants Research*, vol. 26, no. 4, pp. 407–412, 2015.

[9] M. Araújo and J. Lindhe, "Socket grafting with the use of autologous bone: an experimental study in the dog," *Clinical Oral Implants Research*, vol. 22, no. 1, pp. 9–13, 2011.

[10] N. Soldatos, P. Stylianou, V. Koidou, N. Angelov, R. Yukna, and G. E. Romanos, "Limitations and options using resorbable versus non-resorbable membranes for successful guided bone regeneration," *Quintessence International*, vol. 48, no. 2, pp. 131–147, 2017.

[11] P. Bunyaratavej and H.-L. Wang, "Collagen membranes: a review," *Journal of Periodontology*, vol. 72, no. 2, pp. 215–229, 2001.

[12] J. Tan-Chu, F. Tuminelli, K. Kurtz, and D. Tarnow, "Analysis of buccolingual dimensional changes of the extraction socket using the "Ice cream cone" flapless grafting technique," *International Journal of Periodontics and Restorative Dentistry*, vol. 34, no. 3, pp. 399–403, 2014.

[13] X. Jiang, Y. Zhang, B. Chen, and Y. Lin, "Pressure bearing device affects extraction socket remodeling of maxillary anterior tooth: a prospective clinical trial," *Clinical Implant Dentistry and Related Research*, vol. 19, no. 2, pp. 296–305, 2016.

[14] H. Zadeh, A. Abdelamid, M. Omran, N. Bakhshalian, and D. Tarnow, "An open randomized controlled clinical trial to evaluate ridge preservation and repain using SocketKAP™ and Socket KAGE™: part 1-three-dimensional volumetric soft tissue analysis of study casts," *Clinical Oral Implants Research*, vol. 27, no. 6, pp. 640–649, 2016.

[15] A. Abdelamid, M. Omran, N. Bakhshalian, D. Tarnow, and H. Zadeh, "An open randomized controlled clinical trial to evaluate ridge preservation and repair using SocketKAP™ and Socket KAGE™: part 2-three-dimensional alveolar bone volumetric analysis of CBCT imaging," *Clinical Oral Implants Research*, vol. 27, no. 6, pp. 631–639, 2016.

[16] F. Van der Weijden, F. Dell' Acqua, and D. E. Slot, "Alveolar bone dimensional changes of post-extraction sockets in humans: a systematic review," *Journal of Clinical Periodontology*, vol. 36, no. 12, pp. 1048–1058, 2009.

[17] G. A. Kotsakis, A. L. Ioannou, J. E. Hinrichs, and G. E. Romanos, "A systematic review of observational studies evaluating implant placement in the maxillary jaws of medically compromised patients," *Clinical Orthopaedics and Related Research*, vol. 17, no. 3, pp. 598–609, 2015.

[18] D. Moher, A. Liberati, J. Tetziaff et al., "The PRISMA statement for reporting systematic reviews and meta-analyses of studies that evaluate health care interventions: explanation and elaboration," *PLoS Medicine*, vol. 6, no. 7, article e1000100, 2009.

[19] C. Pang, Y. Ding, K. Hu, H. Zhou, R. Qin, and R. Hou, "Influence of preservation of the alveolar ridge on delayed implants after extraction of teeth with different defects in the buccal bone," *British Journal of Oral and Maxillofacial Surgery*, vol. 54, no. 2, pp. 176–180, 2016.

[20] A. Temmerman, J. Vandessel, A. Castro et al., "The use of leucocyte and platelet rich fibrin in socket management and ridge preservation: a split-mouth randomized, controlled clinical trial," *Journal of Clinical Periodontology*, vol. 43, no. 11, pp. 990–999, 2016.

[21] M. van Tulder, A. Furlan, C. Bombardier, and L. Bouter, "Updated method guidelines for systematic reviews in the Cochrane collaboration back review group," *Spine*, vol. 28, no. 12, pp. 1290–1299, 2003.

[22] I. Boutron, C. Estellat, and P. Ravaud, "A review of blinding in randomized controlled trials found results inconsistent and questionable," *Journal of Clinical Epidemiology*, vol. 58, no. 12, pp. 1220–1226, 2005.

[23] F. Vignoletti, P. Matesanz, D. Rodrigo et al., "Surgical protocols for ridge preservation after tooth extraction: a systematic review," *Clinical Oral Implants Research*, vol. 23, pp. 22–38, 2012.

[24] M. Bornstein, W. Scarfe, V. Vaughn, and R. Jacobs, "Cone beam computed tomography in implant dentistry: a systematic review focusing on guidelines, indications and radiation dose risks," *International Journal of Oral & Maxillofacial Implants*, vol. 29, pp. 55–77, 2014.

[25] M. Sonick, J. Abrahams, and R. Faiella, "A comparison of the accuracy of periapical, panoramic, and computerized tomographic radiographs in locating the mandibular canal," *International Journal of Oral & Maxillofacial Implants*, vol. 9, pp. 455–460, 1994.

[26] K. Kobayashi, S. Shimoda, Y. Nakagawa, and A. Yamamoto, "Accuracy in measurement of distance using limited CBCT," *International Journal of Oral & Maxillofacial Implants*, vol. 19, no. 2, pp. 228–231, 2004.

[27] H. Pinsky, S. Dyda, R. Pinsky, K. Misch, and D. Sarment, "Accuracy of three-dimensional measurements using cone-beam ct," *Dentomaxillofacial Radiology*, vol. 35, no. 6, pp. 410–416, 2006.

29

Oral Cancer Knowledge Assessment: Newly Graduated versus Senior Dental Clinicians

Gisele Pavão Spaulonci, Ricardo Salgado de Souza, Vanessa Gallego Arias Pecorari, and Luciano Lauria Dib

Paulista University (UNIP), Indianópolis, SP, Brazil

Correspondence should be addressed to Gisele Pavão Spaulonci; giselepavao@terra.com.br

Academic Editor: Silvio Abati

The present study assessed the level of dentists' knowledge regarding oral cancer in the city of São Paulo, Brazil. A questionnaire was used to compare the level of knowledge among newly graduated and senior clinicians. A total of 20,154 e-mails were correctly delivered to the dentists registered in the database of the Regional Dentistry Council of São Paulo, and 477 (2.36%) responses were received. This sample consisted of 84 newly graduated clinicians and 105 senior clinicians. For the statistical analysis, the chi-square test and the logistic regression analysis were performed with $\alpha = 0.05$, and the results were described herein. According to their knowledge level, the results were statistically different between the groups, since 19% of the newly graduated clinicians were evaluated with knowledge grade A (excellent) in comparison to 6.7% of the senior clinicians. In spite of the results indicated that newly graduated clinicians' knowledge regarding oral cancer was 2.1 times higher, 34.5% of the professionals in this group had regular or poor knowledge on the subject, and several questions relating to clinical characteristics and risk factors indicated that there still exist some knowledge gaps, demonstrating that there is a need for further studies and information activities addressing oral cancer.

1. Introduction

Oral cancer is considered a worldwide public health problem. It is the sixth most frequent type of cancer, and two out of three cases occur in developing countries [1, 2]. The Brazilian National Cancer Institute (INCA) had estimated the occurrence of 11,140 new cases of oral cancer in men and 4,350 in women in 2016 [3]. According to this estimation, the south and southeast regions would be the most affected, with the highest incidence rates [3].

The most prevalent type of cancer is the squamous cell carcinoma [3–5]. It is considered to have poor prognosis [6], with a five-year survival rate in 50 to 60% of cases [1, 6, 7]. It is worth mentioning that there has not been notable prognosis improvement in the recent decades [5–7].

The patients' survival rate and the functional consequences are related to the disease staging at the time of diagnosis [8]. The early detection and the immediate treatment of oral cancer may reduce the mortality rates [1, 2, 5, 9–11]. However, studies have demonstrated that two out of three cancers are diagnosed in advanced stages (III and IV) [2, 10, 12–14]. This delay in diagnosis is due to factors related to patients [13–15], health profissionais [13, 14], and the health system, as the late diagnosis has also been associated with the difficult access to specialized services, especially for people who live away from large centers [15].

The shortage of dental professionals and dental schools in Brazil may be ruled out as a possible factor for this delay [16], given that there are currently more than 280,000 professionals and 220 dental schools in the country [17].

The oral cancer may be identified at an early stage by means of visual and tactile examinations, and the dentists are key role health professionals in counselling patients about early detection of this disease [18]. The preventive role of these professionals relies on the fact that they have the greatest chances to identify asymptomatic lesions through routine examinations and to diagnose the disease before it starts unfolding, revealing its devastating consequences [19]. This fact emphasizes the importance of assessing the clinical professional knowledge regarding oral cancer risk factors and its diagnostic procedures.

Studies have been carried out in several parts of the world, indicating dentists' poor or lacking knowledge regarding oral cancer [2, 14, 18, 20–25]. In Brazil, some studies have been performed using a questionnaire previously published in the study of Dib et al. [19], which, at that time, demonstrated the low level of professional knowledge on this theme [8, 26–29].

Previous studies in countries like Yemen and Canada have suggested that newly graduated professionals had more knowledge in comparison to senior professionals [4, 25]. The hypothesis of the present study is that there may be differences in dentists' knowledge due to the number of years of professional experience or seniority. However, there are doubts whether newly graduated dentists have more knowledge than seniors for being closer to their university experience period or whether the most experienced professionals know more for having more clinical practice years. In addition, it should be taken into consideration that professionals with 30 years of experience or more have received information from the studies carried out in the 1980s, which have indicated cancer aspects that are similar to those found in current studies [30–32].

In Brazil, there are no studies that have assessed these differences justified by the time of experience with regard to oral cancer knowledge. Therefore, the objective of the present study was to assess dentists' knowledge about oral cancer by means of a literature-validated questionnaire (Figure 1) and to compare the knowledge level among two groups of professionals: junior or newly graduated (0 to 5 years of professional practice) versus senior dental clinicians (above 30 years of experience).

2. Materials and Methods

The present study was approved by the Research Ethics Committee of Paulista University (UNIP), São Paulo, Brazil (approval report 1,543,946-CAAE 54493716.8.0000.5512).

A cross-sectional observational study was carried out, where the database of the Regional Dentistry Council of São Paulo was accessed, which contained 28,671 listed professionals at the time of questionnaire submission, out of which 25,321 had their e-mails listed in their profile within the council database.

A questionnaire validated by Dib et al. [19] was modified and uploaded for online accessing using the Survey Monkey online platform (Survey Monkey Brazil Internet Ltd., São Paulo, Brazil) (Figure 1). The e-mails with the invitation to participate in the study along with the web link to access the questionnaire and a published consent form were distributed on July 2016 to the 25,321 listed dentists.

Out of all e-mails sent, 5,167 were not received due to outdated profile information or incorrect e-mail addresses in the profiles, and 20,154 e-mails were correctly received. After allowing one month for responses, the received data were fed into an Excel spreadsheet. The participation was anonymous, and no personal identification from the participants was registered.

The questionnaire consisted of 39 items divided into three parts (Figure 1). The first part covered the participants' general characteristics regarding their clinical practice related to the disease and interest in the topic. Values were not attributed to the responses in the first part. The second part addressed the knowledge about the clinical characteristics of oral cancer occurrence through six questions. Each question was worth one point. The third part consisted of 17 questions regarding risk factors, along with the question about oral cancer identification and diagnosis stage and time, totalling four points (Figure 1).

Grades were attributed to each participant according to their knowledge level. The applied criteria were A (excellent) for those who scored from 9 to 10 points; B (good) for those who scored from 7 to 8.99 points; C (regular) for those who scored from 5 to 6.99 points; and D (poor) for those who scored below 4.99 points.

The variables "age" and "seniority" (Figure 1) were categorized to perform the cross-tabulation of the questions and compared according to the junior and senior dental clinicians' knowledge level.

The statistical analysis was carried out in two stages. First, the univariate test was performed using Pearson's chi-square test with $\alpha = 0.20$ to detect possible associations of the responses according to the time of formation. Subsequently, a multiple logistic regression analysis was performed with $\alpha = 0.05$, with the dependent variable being the appropriate level of knowledge (A and B) in function of the independent variables (age, gender, time of experience, graduation institution, self-assessment of knowledge, level of confidence in performing diagnostic procedures, training at the university, qualification, and if attended a course on oral cancer) to obtain the odds ratios and the confidence intervals. The SPSS 22 statistical program was used (Statistical Package for Social Sciences, IBM™, Chicago, USA).

3. Results

A total of 20,154 e-mails were sent; however, only 477 of them were replied, representing a response rate of 2.36%. The participants were grouped according to practice seniority in order to compare 84 newly graduated dental clinicians with 105 senior dental clinicians. With this, the sample corresponded to 189 participants (Tables 1–6).

There was a statistical difference in the variable "gender" according to seniority in the comparison between the two groups (Table 1). The percentage of junior female dental clinicians was 78.6%, whereas the percentage of senior female dental clinicians was 57.1% (Table 1).

Regarding the knowledge level, there was a statistical difference according to the participants' seniority. Among the newly graduated dental clinicians, 19% obtained grade A (excellent), whereas only 6.7% of the senior dental clinicians obtained the same grade (Table 1).

The assessment of the variable "qualification" (Figure 1) showed that the results were also statistically different according to seniority (Table 1). Among the junior dental clinicians, 55.9% reported being general dental practitioners,

* 1. Age:
( )

* 2. Gender:
( ) Male
( ) Female

* 3. Time of experience:
( )

* 4. Undergraduation institution:
( ) Public
( ) Private

* 5. What is your highest qualification (general practitioner, specialist, Master's degree, Ph.D.) and in which area?

* 6. What is your self-assessment of your level of oral cancer knowledge?
( ) Excellent
( ) Good
( ) Fair
( ) Poor

* 7. Do you perform a dental examination to detect oral cancer in the first appointment of your patients?
( ) Yes
( ) No

* 8. Explain why you do not perform oral cancer examination.
( ) I perform the examination
( ) I do not know how to do it
( ) I do not think it is necessary
( ) I do not receive payment for the examination

* 9. When you detect malignancy suspected lesions, how do you refer the cases?
( ) I perform the diagnostic procedures
( ) Dental surgeons specialized in stomatology
( ) Physicians
( ) Dental schools
( ) Specialized hospitals
( ) When it is not the main patients' complaint, I wait until they ask for guidance

* 10. Which is the most common type of oral cancer?
( ) Lymphoma
( ) Squamous cell carcinoma
( ) Kaposi's sarcoma
( ) Ameloblastoma
( ) Adenoma of salivary glands
( ) I do not know

* 11. Which is the most frequent anatomical region for oral cancer?
( ) Tongue
( ) Oral floor
( ) Gingiva
( ) Palate
( ) Jugal mucosa
( ) I do not know

* 12. Among the mentioned issues, which is the most common aspect in patients with initial oral cancer?
( ) Abundant salivation
( ) Painless ulcer
( ) Hard nodule
( ) Intense pain
( ) I do not know

Figure 1: Continued.

∗ 13. Which is the predominant age group with oral cancer occurrence?
( ) Less than 18 years
( ) 18 to 39 years
( ) More than 40 years
( ) I do not know

∗ 14. When the most characteristic cervical lymph node metastases in oral cancer are palpated, they are:
( ) Hard, painful, with mobility
( ) Hard, painless, with or without mobility
( ) Soft, painful, with mobility
( ) Soft, painless, with or without mobility
( ) I do not know

∗ 15. According to epidemiological data, which oral cancer stage is most frequently diagnosed in Brazil?
( ) Pre-malignant
( ) Early
( ) Advanced
( ) I do not know

∗ 16. Which of the following conditions is more commonly associated to oral cancer?
( ) Leukoplakia
( ) Pemphigus vulgaris
( ) Stomatitis
( ) Candidiasis
( ) Geographic tongue
( ) I do not know

In questions 17 to 33 answer whether or not you consider the condition mentioned as a risk factor for oral cancer

∗ 17. Use of injectable drugs:
( ) Yes
( ) No

∗ 18. Having previously had other types of cancer:
( ) Yes
( ) No

∗ 19. Consumption of alcohol:
( ) Yes
( ) No

∗ 20. Use of tobacco:
( ) Yes
( ) No

∗ 21. Family history of cancer:
( ) Yes
( ) No

∗ 22. Emotional stress:
( ) Yes
( ) No

∗ 23. Lower consumption of fruit and vegetables:
( ) Yes
( ) No

∗ 24. Oral sex:
( ) Yes
( ) No

∗ 25. Poorly fitting dentures:
( ) Yes
( ) No

Figure 1: Continued.

* 26. Poor dental status:
    ( ) Yes
    ( ) No

* 27. Consumption of spicy food:
    ( ) Yes
    ( ) No

* 28. Poor oral hygiene:
    ( ) Yes
    ( ) No

* 29. Direct infection:
    ( ) Yes
    ( ) No

* 30. Sun exposure:
    ( ) Yes
    ( ) No

* 31. Hot beverages and food:
    ( ) Yes
    ( ) No

* 32. Obesity:
    ( ) Yes
    ( ) No

* 33. HPV infection:
    ( ) Yes
    ( ) No

* 34. Do you consider your patients sufficiently informed about oral cancer (prevention and diagnosis)?
    ( ) Yes
    ( ) No
    ( ) I do not know

* 35. What is your level of confidence in performing diagnostic procedures to detect oral cancer?
    ( ) High
    ( ) Low
    ( ) I do not know

* 36. Do you consider that the university provided training on oral cancer examination during your undergraduate program?
    ( ) Yes
    ( ) No
    ( ) I do not know

* 37. When was the last time you attended a continuing education course on oral cancer?
    ( ) Last year
    ( ) During the last two years.
    ( ) More than two years.
    ( ) Never
    ( ) I do not remember.

* 38. Are you interested in attending a continuing education course on oral cancer in the future?
    ( ) Yes
    ( ) No
    ( ) I am not sure.

* 39. According to your opinion, what is the level of importance of the dental surgeon in the prevention and early diagnosis of oral cancer?
    ( ) High
    ( ) Medium
    ( ) Fair
    ( ) Low
    ( ) I do not know

Figure 1: Questionnaire applied to assess oral cancer knowledge (Survey Monkey Brazil Internet Ltd.).

Table 1: Distribution of the number and percentages of responses regarding dentists' general characteristics according to responders' seniority.

Categorical	Variables	Dental clinicians		Total (%)	p
		Junior	Senior		
Grade obtained	A (excellent)	16 (19%)	7 (6.7%)	23 (12.2%)	**0.025***
	B (good)	39 (46.4%)	44 (41.9%)	83 (43.9%)	
	C (regular)	20 (23.8%)	40 (38.1%)	60 (31.7%)	
	D (poor)	9 (10.7%)	14 (13.3%)	23 (12.2%)	
Gender	Female	66 (78.6%)	60 (57.1%)	126 (66.7%)	**0.002***
	Male	18 (21.4%)	45 (42.9%)	63 (33.3%)	
Institution	Public	29 (34.5%)	44 (41.9%)	73 (38.6%)	0.300
	Private	55 (65.5%)	61 (58.1%)	116 (61.4%)	
Qualification	General practitioner	47 (55.9%)	22 (21%)	69 (36.5%)	**≤0.001***
	Specialist	32 (38.1%)	59 (56.2%)	91 (48.1%)	
	Master's degree	5 (6%)	16 (15.2%)	21 (11.1%)	
	PhD	0 (0)	8 (7.6%)	8 (4.2%)	
		84 (44.4%)	**105 (55.6%)**	**189 (100%)**	

Note. *p values lower than 0.05 indicate statistically significant results.

Table 2: Distribution of the number and percentages of responses to specific questions about oral cancer knowledge according to responders' seniority.

Variables	Categories	Dental clinicians		Total (%)	p
		Junior	Senior		
Most common cancer	Squamous cell carcinoma	57 (67.9%)	68 (64.8%)	125 (66.1%)	0.655
	Other	27 (32.1%)	37 (35.2%)	64 (33.9%)	
Most frequent anatomical region	Tongue	50 (59.5%)	53 (50.5%)	103 (54.5%)	0.215
	Other	34 (40.5%)	52 (49.5%)	86 (45.5%)	
Most common aspect in initial cancer	Painless ulcer	72 (85.7%)	90 (85.7%)	162 (85.7%)	1.000
	Other	12 (14.3%)	15 (14.3%)	27 (14.3%)	
Most common age group	More than 40 years old	75 (89.3%)	92 (87.6%)	167 (88.4%)	0.723
	Other	9 (10.7%)	13 (12.4%)	22 (11.6%)	
Most characteristic regional lymph node metastasis	Hard, painless, with or without mobility	58 (69%)	73 (69.5%)	131 (69.3%)	0.944
	Other	26 (31%)	32 (30.5%)	58 (30.7%)	
Diagnostic status in Brazil	Advanced	64 (76.2%)	87 (82.9%)	151 (79.9%)	0.256
	Other	20 (23.8%)	18 (17.1%)	38 (20.1%)	
Most common condition associated with cancer	Leukoplakia	62 (73.8%)	79 (75.2%)	141 (74.6%)	0.823
	Other	22 (26.2%)	26 (24.8%)	48 (25.4%)	
		84 (44.4%)	**105 (55.6%)**	**189 (100%)**	

Note. p values lower than 0.05 indicate statistically significant results; other = one of the incorrect answers.

38.1% declared themselves specialists, and 6% had a Master's degree. On the other hand, among the senior dental clinicians, 56.2% reported being specialists, 21% were general dental practitioners, 15.2% had a Master's degree, and 7.6% held PhDs (Table 1). There was no statistical difference in the responses from both groups regarding the knowledge about the clinical characteristics of oral cancer (Table 2).

With regard to the risk factors of oral cancer development (Figure 1), there was a statistical difference between the two groups of professionals in the responses relating to "low consumption of fruit and vegetables," "poor fitting of dentures," "poor dental status," "poor oral hygiene," and "consumption of hot beverages and food" (Table 3).

Table 4 shows the response frequencies according to the factors related to attitudes toward oral cancer diagnosis and the perception about the topic according to the participants' seniority.

The multiple logistic regression analysis results indicated that the oral cancer knowledge of junior dental clinicians was 2.1 times higher in comparison to the senior dental clinicians' knowledge (OR = 2.1; 1.1–3.9 95% CI; $p = 0.024$) (Table 6). In addition, it was found that the professionals who had graduated from public institutions were 2.3 times

TABLE 3: Distribution of the number and percentages of responses to specific questions addressing the knowledge about risk factors of oral cancer according to responders' seniority.

Variables	Categories	Dental clinicians		Total (%)	*p*
		Junior	Senior		
Injected drug use	Yes	29 (34.5%)	30 (28.6%)	59 (31.2%)	0.380
	No	55 (65.5%)	75 (71.4%)	130 (68.8%)	
Had other types of cancer previously	Yes	70 (83.3%)	83 (79%)	153 (81%)	0.456
	No	14 (16.7%)	22 (21%)	36 (19%)	
Alcohol consumption	Yes	81 (96.4%)	105 (100%)	186 (98.4%)	0.051
	No	3 (3.6%)	0 (0)	3 (1.6%)	
Tobacco consumption	Yes	84 (100%)	105 (100%)	189 (100%)	—
	No	0 (0)	0 (0)	0 (0)	
Family history of cancer	Yes	80 (95.2%)	100 (95.2%)	180 (95.2%)	1.000
	No	4 (4.8%)	5 (4.8%)	9 (4.8%)	
Emotional stress	Yes	47 (56%)	71 (67.6%)	118 (62.4%)	0.100
	No	37 (44%)	34 (32.4%)	71 (37.6%)	
Lower consumption of fruit and vegetables	Yes	26 (31%)	50 (47.6%)	76 (40.2%)	**0.020***
	No	58 (69%)	55 (52.4%)	113 (59.8%)	
Oral sex	Yes	43 (51.2%)	62 (59%)	105 (55.6%)	0.280
	No	41 (48.8%)	43 (41%)	84 (44.4%)	
Poorly fitting dentures	Yes	51 (60.7%)	98 (93.3%)	149 (78.8%)	**≤0.001***
	No	33 (39.3%)	7 (6.7%)	40 (21.2%)	
Poor dental status	Yes	37 (44%)	80 (76.2%)	117 (61.9%)	**≤0.001***
	No	47 (56%)	25 (23.8%)	72 (38.1%)	
Consumption of spicy food	Yes	20 (23.8%)	36 (34.3%)	56 (29.6%)	0.117
	No	64 (76.2%)	69 (65.7%)	133 (70.4%)	
Poor oral hygiene	Yes	34 (40.5%)	68 (64.8%)	102 (54%)	**≤0.001***
	No	50 (59.5%)	37 (35.2%)	87 (46%)	
Direct infection	Yes	9 (10.7%)	19 (18.1%)	28 (14.8%)	0.156
	No	75 (89.3%)	86 (81.9%)	161 (85.2%)	
Sun exposure	Yes	76 (90.5%)	86 (81.9%)	162 (85.7%)	0.094
	No	8 (9.5%)	19 (18.1%)	27 (14.3%)	
Hot beverages and food	Yes	34 (40.5%)	78 (74.3%)	112 (59.3%)	**≤0.001***
	No	50 (59.5%)	27 (25.7%)	77 (40.7%)	
Obesity	Yes	14 (16.7%)	17 (16.2%)	31 (16.4%)	0.930
	No	70 (83.3%)	88 (83.8%)	158 (83.6%)	
HPV infection	Yes	71 (84.5%)	97 (92.4%)	168 (88.9%)	0.088
	No	13 (15.5%)	8 (7.6%)	21 (11.1%)	
		84 (44.4%)	**105 (55.6%)**	**189 (100%)**	

Note. **p* values lower than 0.05 indicate statistically significant results.

more aware about oral cancer (OR = 2.3; 1.2–4.3 95% CI; $p = 0.013$). The participants who performed self-assessment and reported having satisfactory oral cancer knowledge (excellent or good) were 2.2 times more likely to have higher knowledge level (OR = 2.2; 1.2–4.2 95% CI; $p = 0.013$) in comparison to the participants who reported regular or poor knowledge level (Table 6).

4. Discussion

Studies assessing dentists' knowledge, opinions, and practices relating to the prevention and early detection of oral cancer have been carried out in several countries [2, 4, 10, 11, 18, 20–25, 33–40]. The use of Internet and e-mails to obtain information has increased in recent years [2, 20, 41]. No articles have been found in Brazil with regard to the assessment of the dentists' oral cancer knowledge level considering and comparing their practice seniority, that is, newly graduated professionals versus senior professionals.

In contrast to the response rate observed in this study, in a Japanese study [20], which used the same electronic platform and sent 131 questionnaires, the response rate was 62.6%, represented by the 82 e-mails in response to the research. A Spanish study with 1,000 sent e-mails had 795

Table 4: Distribution of the number and percentages of responses about attitudes toward diagnosis of cancer and perception about this issue according to responders' seniority.

Variables	Categories	Dental clinicians		Total (%)	p
		Junior	Senior		
Self-assessment of knowledge	Excellent/good	46 (54.8%)	54 (51.4%)	100 (52.9%)	0.648
	Regular/poor	38 (45.2%)	51 (48.6%)	89 (47.1%)	
Performs cancer exam in the 1st appointment	Yes	66 (78.6%)	90 (85.7%)	156 (82.5%)	0.199
	No	18 (21.4%)	15 (14.3%)	33 (17.5%)	
Reason for not performing the exam	Performed the exam	67 (79.8%)	88 (83.8%)	155 (82%)	0.551
	I do not know how to do it	8 (9.5%)	11 (10.5%)	19 (10.1%)	
	I do not think it is necessary	6 (7.1%)	5 (4.8%)	11 (5.8%)	
	I do not receive fees	3 (3.6%)	1 (1%)	4 (2.1%)	
Referral of suspicious lesions	Stomatology	53 (63.1%)	73 (69.5%)	126 (66.7%)	**0.007***
	Myself	13 (15.5%)	19 (18.1%)	32 (16.9%)	
	Dental school	15 (17.9%)	3 (2.9%)	18 (9.5%)	
	Specialized hospital	2 (2.4%)	6 (5.7%)	8 (4.2%)	
	Physician	1 (1.2%)	4 (3.8%)	5 (2%)	
Confidence level	High	26 (31%)	40 (38.1%)	66 (34.9%)	0.407
	Low	55 (65.5%)	59 (56.2%)	114 (60.3%)	
	I do not know	3 (3.6%)	6 (5.7%)	9 (4.8%)	
Training at the university	Yes	59 (70.2%)	46 (43.8%)	105 (55.6%)	**≤0.001***
	No	25 (29.8%)	55 (52.4%)	80 (42.3%)	
	I do not know	0 (0)	4 (3.8%)	4 (2.1%)	
Attended a course on oral cancer	Last year	17 (20.2%)	13 (12.4%)	30 (15.9%)	**0.006***
	Two years ago	24 (28.6%)	20 (19%)	44 (23.3%)	
	More than two years ago	19 (22.6%)	52 (49.5%)	71 (37.6%)	
	Never	14 (16.9%)	12 (11.4%)	26 (13.8%)	
	I do not remember	10 (11.9%)	8 (7.6%)	18 (9.5%)	
		84 (44.4%)	**105 (55.6%)**	**189 (100%)**	

Note. *p values lower than 0.05 indicate statistically significant results.

acknowledged as received and 340 (42.7%) responded questionnaires [2]. In contrast, another Brazilian study [27] sent 5,000 questionnaires via e-mail and the response rate was 1.4%, suggesting that the Brazilian professional population may be less partaking in scientific research, especially with respect to the elected method of data collection.

Therefore, it is natural to envision that Brazilian dentists have little interest in the subject. However, one possible explanation for the low response rate in the present study could be the excessive circulating advertising or spam and the ease with which they can be ignored or discarded [2]. However, the authors agree with López-Jornet et al. [2] when they say that this sort of communication is faster and easier to manage, in addition to being less costly. Therefore, new efforts and resources should be made for e-mails to be taken into consideration in future research so that important contents do not go unnoticed.

Nevertheless, despite these limitations of the low response rate, the number of participants (477) represents an expressive sample in comparison to the ones found in literature [2, 4, 10, 18, 20, 22–24, 27–29, 36, 42]. Therefore, the present study provides significant information about the knowledge of dentists in São Paulo that may contribute to new projects.

According to the dentists' obtained knowledge level grades, there was a statistical difference between newly graduated clinicians and senior dental clinicians (Table 1). Among junior dental clinicians, 19% obtained grade A (excellent) in comparison to 6.7% of senior dental clinicians. The results of the logistic regression analysis indicated that the knowledge level of junior dental clinicians was 2.1 times higher (OR = 2.1; 1.1–3.9 95% CI; p = 0.024) (Table 6). This result is similar to that of other studies [4, 25].

Although there was a significant difference between the two groups, the data analysis allowed to observe that there are many concepts that are still not well-defined amongst professionals of both groups, showing that there is much to be discussed on means to stimulate oral cancer knowledge building.

In the question about the anatomical region of higher oral cancer prevalence (Figure 1), 45.5% of participants did not know the answer (Table 2). Rocha-Buelvas et al. [24] revealed that only a few professionals knew the most frequent locations of oral malignance. This is disturbing because if the professionals do not have the adequate knowledge about the most frequent locations of oral cancer development, then the injury may go unnoticed during

TABLE 5: Distribution of the number and percentages of responses relating to the dentists' general characteristics according to their self-assessment of oral cancer knowledge.

Variables	Categories	Self-assessment of the level of knowledge about oral cancer		Total (%)	*p*
		Satisfactory	Unsatisfactory		
Institution	Public	43 (43%)	30 (33.7%)	73 (38.6%)	0.190
	Private	57 (57%)	59 (66.3%)	116 (61.4%)	
Time of experience	Junior dental clinicians	46 (46%)	38 (42.7%)	84 (44.4%)	0.648
	Senior dental clinicians	54 (54%)	51 (57.3%)	105 (55.6%)	
Qualification	General practitioner	35 (35%)	34 (38.2%)	69 (36.5%)	0.648
	Graduated[1]	65 (65%)	55 (61.8%)	120 (63.5%)	
Training at the university	Yes	66 (66%)	39 (43.8%)	105 (55.6%)	**0.002***
	No/I do not know	34 (34%)	50 (56.2%)	84 (44.4%)	
Attended a course on oral cancer	Two years ago	53 (53%)	21 (23.6%)	74 (39.2%)	**≤0.001***
	More than two years ago/never	47 (47%)	68 (76.4%)	115 (60.8%)	
Grades obtained	A-B (excellent/good)	67 (67%)	39 (43.8%)	106 (56.1%)	**≤0.001***
	C-D (regular/poor)	33 (33%)	50 (56.2%)	83 (43.9%)	
		100 (52.9%)	**89 (47.1%)**	**189 (100%)**	

Note. *p values lower than 0.05 indicate statistically significant results. [1]The "Graduated" category refers to the participants that reported having specialization, Master's degree, and/or PhD.

TABLE 6: Association of the general characteristics and clinical practice of the dentists relating to the level of knowledge about oral cancer according to attributed grades (A = excellent; B = good).

Characteristics	Categories	Grades obtained (A = excellent; B = good)		
		Number (%)	OR (95% CI)	*p*
Self-assessment of knowledge	Satisfactory	100 (52.9%)	2.2 (1.2–4.2)	**0.013***
	Unsatisfactory	89 (47.1%)		
Time of experience	Junior dental clinicians	84 (44.4%)	2.1 (1.1–3.9)	**0.024***
	Senior dental clinicians	105 (55.6%)		
Graduation institution	Public	73 (38.6%)	2.3 (1.2–4.3)	**0.013***
	Private	116 (61.4%)		
Attended a course on oral cancer	Two years ago	74 (39.2%)	1.5 (0.8–2.9)	0.234
	More than two years ago or never	115 (60.8%)		

Note. *p values lower than 0.05 indicate statistically significant results. The time when the responder attended a course on oral cancer was an adjustment variable for the multiple logistic regression analysis.

a routine examination and, thus, the disease diagnosis may be delayed or ignored.

Our study revealed that one-third of the respondents do not know about regional metastases (Table 2), which coincides with a study conducted in New York, USA [21]; other studies found that less than 40% of dentists have reported that they palpated the patients' lymph nodes during the complete examination of oral cavities [11, 43]. These data highlight the need to improve the professionals' level of knowledge about clinical characteristics and cancer screening, giving that lymph node palpation often aids in the diagnosis of the disease during its asymptomatic stage.

The questions regarding the risk factors of the disease (tobacco, alcohol, and HPV) (Figure 1) were properly answered by the groups of professionals (Table 3), in opposition to a Japanese study [20], in which alcohol and HPV were poorly identified as risk factors for oral cancer. It is possible that the results of these studies are due to massive campaigns about the dangers of cigarettes and alcohol.

An interesting aspect was the controversy about the trauma of poor denture fitting (Figure 1), since 60.7% of junior clinicians and 93.3% of senior clinicians reported that it was a risk factor (Table 3), demonstrating that, despite the statistical difference, more than 60% of the professionals took this controversial issue into consideration. Although from the scientific perspective, the injuries caused by poor denture fitting do not cause cancer, these chronic injuries alter the oral environment and mask the symptoms, and initial lesions may not be properly diagnosed. Therefore, the professionals should eliminate these traumatic factors in the maintenance of oral health.

In the current study, 54% of respondents answered that poor oral hygiene (Figure 1) is a risk factor for oral cancer (Table 3). However, the role of poor oral hygiene is controversial, and this study corroborates with the observations from Oji and Chukwuneke [44], considering that only a major prospective study would provide appropriate information to scientifically clarify its impact in oral cancer genesis.

The low consumption of fruit and vegetables (Figure 1) was considered as a risk factor for oral cancer by 40.2% of professionals (Table 3). It is believed that eating fruit and vegetables may reduce the risk of cancer, including oral cancer, because they play an important part as a protective factor. Shivappa et al. [45] suggested a positive interaction between a proinflammatory diet with alcohol consumption and smoking in association with oral cancer. However, Dholam and Chouksey [46] found that a diet as a risk factor for oral cancer was not statistically significant. Moreover, this study agrees with Scully's [5] research that randomized clinical trials are needed to explore the effectiveness of dietary supplementation as chemoprevention to reduce the risk of oral cancer.

It is worth mentioning the importance appointed by the professionals regarding emotional stress (Figure 1). This issue was reported as a risk factor for oral cancer by 62.4% of dentists (Table 3). A recent study found an increased risk of oral cancer in patients who had suffered emotional stress. However, according to Dholam and Chouksey [46], emotional stress is a modern life symptom, and it may be responsible for delays in diagnosis due to work and family-related commitments, which probably generate patients' negligence toward their symptoms, but emotional stress would not be the core cause of oral cancer. Prospective studies with oral cancer patients would be necessary, excluding those who have scientifically proven risk factors, such as tobacco and alcohol consumption, and/or genetic factors, to show whether emotional stress alone could cause the disease.

The assessment of the variable "oral sex" (Figure 1) indicated a considerable number of positive responses, being a risk factor for 55.6% of professionals (Table 3). Nevertheless, these results may be a confounding factor because they probably associate oral sex with the possibility of HPV infection, which is strongly related to oral cancer [3, 7, 47]. Therefore, it is essential to provide patients with information about HPV and regarding the importance of preventive methods during sexual intercourse, in addition to the possibility of vaccination as a method to prevent virus infection.

Considering the attitudes for the diagnosis of suspected lesions (Figure 1), 17.9% of junior dental clinicians reported that they usually referred these cases to dental schools, compared to 2.4% of senior dental clinicians (Table 4). These results may be due to the fact that recent graduates feel more familiar with those institutions, possibly due to their recent undergraduation.

When asked about oral cancer screening training during the undergraduation (Figure 1), 70.2% of the junior clinicians reported having received training, compared to 43.8% of senior clinicians (Table 4). This means that almost 30% of the professionals were not properly trained, demonstrating that much needs to be improved in that aspect, considering the importance and seriousness of the matter. A study conducted in Spain [2] found that dentists, who were trained on oral cancer during their undergraduation, were more likely to agree that they had updated knowledge. This finding corroborates with the ones of the present study, since 66% of the participants that "rated themselves with satisfactory knowledge level" (excellent or good) reported that they had been trained for the examination of oral cancer during their undergraduation studies ($p = 0.002$) (Table 5). In addition, logistic regression analysis indicated that they were 2.2 times more likely to have greater knowledge about the disease (OR = 2.2; 1.2–4.2 95% CI; $p = 0.013$) (Table 6).

The logistic regression analysis indicated that dentists who graduated from public institutions had 2.3 times more knowledge about oral cancer in comparison to private institutions' graduates (OR = 2.3; 1.2–4.3 95% CI; $p = 0.013$) (Table 6), demonstrating that specific studies on the analysis of the curriculum of public and private universities may be object of further research.

Considering participation in "continuing education courses on oral cancer" (Figure 1), 39.2% of the professionals had attended a course on oral cancer in the previous year or in the last two years (Table 4). This result is disturbing since the knowledge acquired during undergraduation tends to weaken with the absence of further knowledge support or updates [23]. Also, in the present study, 53% of the participants that reported satisfactory knowledge level (excellent or good) had attended a course on oral cancer in the last two years ($p \leq 0.001$) (Table 5), coinciding with the study carried out by Hertrampf et al. [36], which found that the perceptions and practice relating to early detection of oral cancer had improved, particularly in the group of dentists that had attended further educational courses, emphasizing that these programs improved dental professionals' competence, findings in agreement with other studies [10, 23–25]. In Spain, the professionals who had benefited from continuing education courses were 3.5 times more likely to perform biopsies in suspicious lesions and twice as likely to give advice about alcohol consumption to patients [48], demonstrating the positive effect of further studies and professional updates.

Therefore, it is necessary that the professionals have greater interest in continuing education courses so that their knowledge and skills may be updated, contributing to the oral cancer prevention and minimizing practical failures regarding cancer screening, providing, when necessary, early disease detection.

The results of the present study demonstrated that although the junior dental clinicians had a knowledge level 2.1 times higher compared to senior dental clinicians (Table 6), there is still lack of knowledge about some topics related to risk factors and clinical characteristics of the disease.

Probably, as these results may be explained by the fact that the information obtained by newly graduated clinicians was more updated, or due to the lack of practice in the area, more experienced dentists were not interested in the subject. Further studies conducted with a larger number of professionals are required to confirm the results of this study.

5. Conclusion

Within the limitations of the study due to the low percentage of responses, we can conclude that, among the studied population, the newly graduated clinicians had a 2.1 times higher knowledge level in comparison to dentists who had more than 30 years of practice experience. However, when several factors regarding the knowledge of the risk factors and diagnostic procedures were individually assessed, the results indicated high rates of incorrect answers, demonstrating that there is room for further studies in the area and for oral cancer information activities. Therefore, oral cancer aspects must be emphasized so that more people, clinicians, and patients become interested in the topic. This goal may be achieved through clarification campaigns, dental school's program improvement, and the encouragement of professionals in attending continuing education courses for better qualification. New studies must be performed to compare our results.

References

[1] J. Seoane, P. Alvarez-Novoa, I. Gomez et al., "Early oral cancer diagnosis: the Aarhus statement perspective. A systematic review and meta-analysis," *Head & Neck*, vol. 38, no. 1, pp. E2182–E2189, 2016.

[2] P. López-Jornet, F. Camacho-Alonso, and F. Molina-Miñano, "Knowledge and attitudes about oral cancer among dentists in Spain," *Journal of Evaluation in Clinical Practice*, vol. 16, no. 1, pp. 129–133, 2010.

[3] Brasil. Ministério da Saúde. Instituto Nacional de Câncer, "Incidência de câncer no Brasil: estimativa 2016. Rio de janeiro: INCA.estimativa-2016–v11.pdf," January 2017. http://www.inca.gov.br/estimativa/2016/estimativa-2016-v11.pdf.

[4] N. A. Alaizari and S. A. Al-Maweri, "Oral cancer: knowledge, practices and opinions of dentists in Yemen," *Asian Pacific Journal of Cancer Prevention*, vol. 15, no. 14, pp. 5627–5631, 2014.

[5] C. Scully, "Oral cancer aetiopathogenesis; past, present and future aspects," *Medicina Oral Patología Oral y Cirugia Bucal*, vol. 16, no. 3, pp. e306–e311, 2011.

[6] J.-M. Seoane-Romero, I. Vázquez-Mahía, J. Seoane, P. Varela-Centelles, I. Tomás, and J.-L. López-Cedrún, "Factors related to late stage diagnosis of oral squamous cell carcinoma," *Medicina Oral Patología Oral y Cirugia Bucal*, vol. 17, no. 1, pp. e35–e40, 2012.

[7] C. Carreras-Torras and C. Gay-Escoda, "Techniques for early diagnosis of oral squamous cell carcinoma: systematic review," *Medicina Oral Patología Oral y Cirugia Bucal*, vol. 20, no. 3, pp. e305–e315, 2015.

[8] S. N. Andrade, L. V. Muniz, J. M. A. Soares, A. L. F. Chaves, and R. I. M. A. Ribeiro, "Câncer de boca: avaliação do conhecimento e conduta dos dentistas na atenção primária à saúde," *Revistas*, vol. 71, no. 1, pp. 42–47, 2014.

[9] C. L. Tax, S. K. Haslam, M. Brillant, H. J. Doucette, J. E. Cameron, and S. E. Wade, "Oral cancer screening: knowledge is not enough," *International Journal of Dental Hygiene*, vol. 15, no. 3, pp. 179–186, 2015.

[10] J. Seoane-Lestón, J. Velo-Noya, S. Warnakulasuriya et al., "Knowledge of oral cancer and preventive attitudes of Spanish dentists. Primary effects of a pilot educational intervention," *Medicina Oral Patología Oral y Cirugia Bucal*, vol. 15, no. 3, pp. e422–e426, 2010.

[11] K. V. Vijay Kumar and V. Suresan, "Knowledge, attitude and screening practices of general dentists concerning oral cancer in Bangalore city," *Indian Journal of Cancer*, vol. 49, no. 1, pp. 33–38, 2012.

[12] A. L. N. Francisco, M. V. Furlan, P. M. Peresi et al., "Head and neck mucosal melanoma: clinicopathological analysis of 51 cases treated in a single cancer centre and review of the literature," *International Journal of Oral and Maxillofacial Surgery*, vol. 45, no. 2, pp. 135–140, 2016.

[13] P. Güneri and J. B. Epstein, "Late stage diagnosis of oral cancer: components and possible solutions," *Oral Oncology*, vol. 50, no. 12, pp. 1131–1136, 2014.

[14] F. Esmaelbeigi, M. Hadji, I. Harirchi, R. Omranipour, M. vand Rajabpour, and K. Zendehdel, "Factors affecting professional delay in diagnosis and treatment of oral cancer in Iran," *Archives of Iranian Medicine*, vol. 17, no. 4, pp. 253–257, 2014.

[15] F. B. Sousa, M. R. de Freitas e Silva, C. P. Fernandes, P. G. de Barros Silva, and A. P. N. N. Alves, "Oral cancer from a health promotion perspective: experience of a diagnosis network in Ceará," *Brazilian Oral Research*, vol. 28, no. 1, pp. 1–8, 2014.

[16] E. Traebert and J. Traebert, "Oral cancer in Brazil: dentists' lack of technical knowledge," *Brazilian Oral Research*, vol. 29, no. 1, pp. 1-2, 2015.

[17] Brasil. Conselho Federal de Odontologia, "Estatísticas. Quadro_estatistico_faculdade.pdf," November 2016, http://cfo.org.br/wp-content/uploads/2009/10/quadro_estatistico_faculdade.pdf.

[18] G. Colella, G. M. Gaeta, A. Moscariello, and I. F. Angelillo, "Oral cancer and dentists: knowledge, attitudes, and practices in Italy," *Oral Oncology*, vol. 44, no. 4, pp. 393–399, 2008.

[19] L. L. Dib, R. S. Souza de, and N. Tortamano, "Avaliação do conhecimento sobre câncer bucal entre alunos de odontologia, em diferentes unidades da Universidade Paulista," *Journal of Health Science Institute*, vol. 23, no. 4, pp. 287–295, 2005.

[20] S. Haresaku, M. Makino, S. Sugiyama, T. Naito, and R. J. Mariño, "Comparison of practices, knowledge, confidence, and attitude toward oral cancer among oral health professionals between Japan and Australia," *Journal of Cancer Education*, 2016.

[21] S. Gajendra, G. D. Cruz, and J. V. Kumar, "Oral cancer prevention and early detection: knowledge, practices, and opinions of oral health care providers in New York State," *Journal of Cancer Education*, vol. 21, no. 3, pp. 157–162, 2006.

[22] M. Greenwood and R. J. Lowry, "Primary care clinicians' knowledge of oral cancer: a study of dentists and doctors in the North East of England," *British Dental Journal*, vol. 191, no. 9, pp. 510–512, 2001.

[23] M. Pentenero, A. Chiecchio, and S. Gandolfo, "Impact of academic and continuing education on oral cancer knowledge, attitude and practice among dentists in north-western Italy," *Journal of Cancer Education*, vol. 29, no. 1, pp. 151–157, 2014.

[24] A. Rocha-Buelvas, C. Hidalgo-Patiño, G. Collela, and I. Angelillo, "Oral cancer and dentists: knowledge, attitudes and practices in a South Colombian context," *Acta Odontológica Latinoamericana*, vol. 25, no. 2, pp. 155–162, 2012.

[25] J. B. Clovis, A. M. Horowitz, and D. H. Poel, "Oral and pharyngeal cancer: knowledge and opinions of dentists in British Columbia and Nova Scotia," *Journal of Canadian Dental Association*, vol. 68, no. 7, pp. 415–420, 2002.

[26] T. M. N. de Morais, *Câncer de Boca: Avaliação do Conhecimento dos Cirurgiões Dentistas Quanto Aos Fatores de Risco e Procedimentos de Diagnóstico*, M.S. thesis, São Paulo: Universidade de São Paulo, Faculdade de Odontologia, Dental Graduate Program, São Paulo, Brazil, 2003.

[27] A. C. B. S. Cimardi and A. P. S. Fernandes, "Câncer bucal: a prática e a realidade clínica dos cirurgiões-dentistas de Santa Catarina," *RFO UPF*, vol. 14, no. 2, pp. 99–104, 2009.

[28] M. M. L. Falcão, T. D. B. Alves, V. S. Freitas, and T. C. B. Coelho, "Conhecimento dos cirurgiões-dentistas em

relação ao cancer bucal," *RGO*, vol. 58, no. 1, pp. 27–33, 2010.

[29] M. L. Alvarenga, M. G. Couto, A. Ribeiro, R. C. M. Milagres, M. R. Messora, and L. T. Kawata, "Avaliação do conhecimento dos cirurgiões-dentistas quanto ao câncer bucal," *RFO UPF*, vol. 17, no. 1, pp. 31–35, 2012.

[30] S. T. Ildstad, D. J. Tollerud, M. E. Bigelow, and J. P. Remensnyder, "A multivariate analysis of determinants of survival for patients with squamous cell carcinoma of the head and neck," *Annals of Surgery*, vol. 209, no. 2, pp. 237–241, 1989.

[31] A. Mashberg and A. M. Samit, "Early detection, diagnosis, and management of oral and oropharyngeal cancer," *Cancer Journal for Clinicians*, vol. 39, no. 2, pp. 67–88, 1989.

[32] L. L. Dib, D. S. Pinto, L. C. Sanvitto, H. Contesini, V. Lombardo, and E. Franco, "Determinantes de sobrevida em câncer de boca: fatores sócio-demográficos e anatômicos," *Revista Brasileira de Cirurgia de Cabeça e Pescoço*, vol. 14, no. 1, pp. 1–9, 1990.

[33] C. Maybury, A. M. Horowitz, and H. S. Goodman, "Outcomes of oral cancer early detection and prevention statewide model in Maryland," *Journal of Public Health Dentistry*, vol. 72, no. 1, pp. S34–S38, 2012.

[34] E. Applebaum, T. N. Ruhlen, F. R. Kronenberg, C. Hayes, and E. S. Peters, "Oral cancer knowledge, attitudes and practices: a survey of dentists and primary care physicians in Massachusetts," *Journal of the American Dental Association*, vol. 140, no. 4, pp. 461–467, 2009.

[35] A. M. Horowitz, P. Siriphant, A. Sheikh, and W. L. Child, "Perspectives of Maryland dentists on oral cancer," *Journal of the American Dental Association*, vol. 132, no. 1, pp. 65–72, 2001.

[36] K. Hertrampf, H.-J. Wenz, M. Koller, S. Grund, and J. Wiltfang, "Early detection of oral cancer: dentists' opinions and practices before and after educational interventions in Northern-Germany," *Journal of Cranio-Maxillofacial Surgery*, vol. 41, no. 8, pp. 201–207, 2013.

[37] L. L. Patton, J. R. Elter, J. H. Southerland, and R. P. Strauss, "Knowledge of oral cancer risk factors and diagnostic concepts among North Carolina dentists. Implications for diagnosis and referral," *Journal of the American Dental Association*, vol. 136, no. 5, pp. 602–610, 2005.

[38] O. Kujan, A. J. Duxbury, A. M. Glenny, N. S. Thakker, and P. Sloan, "Opinions and attitudes of the UK's GDPs and specialists in oral surgery, oral medicine and surgical dentistry on oral cancer screening," *Oral Diseases*, vol. 12, no. 2, pp. 194–199, 2006.

[39] J. A. Yellowitz, A. M. Horowitz, T. F. Drury, and H. S. Goodman, "Survey of U.S. dentists' knowledge and opinions about oral pharyngeal cancer," *Journal of the American Dental Association*, vol. 131, no. 5, pp. 653–661, 2000.

[40] A. Y. Alami, R. F. El Sabbagh, and A. Hamdan, "Knowledge of oral cancer among recently graduated medical and dental professionals in Amman, Jordan," *Journal of Dental Education*, vol. 77, no. 10, pp. 1356–1364, 2013.

[41] E. Daley, V. Dodd, R. DeBate et al., "Prevention of HPV-related oral cancer: assessing dentists' readiness," *Public Health*, vol. 128, no. 3, pp. 231–238, 2014.

[42] J. C. Leão, P. Góes, C. B. Sobrinho, and S. Porter, "Knowledge and clinical expertise regarding oral cancer among Brazilian dentists," *International Journal of Oral and Maxillofacial Surgery*, vol. 34, no. 4, pp. 436–439, 2005.

[43] Ö. Kebabcıoğlu and F. N. Pekiner, "Assessing oral cancer awareness among dentists," *Journal of Cancer Education*, 2017.

[44] C. Oji and F. Chukwuneke, "Poor oral hygiene may be the sole cause of oral cancer," *Journal of Maxillofacial and Oral Surgery*, vol. 11, no. 4, pp. 379–383, 2012.

[45] N. Shivappa, J. R. Hébert, V. Rosato, W. Garavello, D. Serraino, and C. La Vecchia, "Inflammatory potential of diet and risk of oral and pharyngeal cancer in a large case-control study from Italy," *International Journal of Cancer*, vol. 141, no. 3, pp. 471–479, 2017.

[46] K. P. Dholam and G. C. Chouksey, "Squamous cell carcinoma of the oral cavity and oropharynx in patients aged 18-45 years: a case-control study to evaluate the risk factors with emphasis on stress, diet, oral hygiene, and family history," *Indian Journal of Cancer*, vol. 53, no. 2, pp. 244–251, 2016.

[47] S. De Santis, M. C. Spinosi, J. Cambi, C. Bengala, and S. Boccuzzi, "Oropharyngeal squamous cell carcinoma and HPV. Systematic review on overall management," *Journal of Stomatology, Oral and Maxillofacial Surgery*, vol. 118, no. 2, pp. 103–108, 2017.

[48] J. Seoane, P. Varela-Centelles, I. Tomás, J. Seoane-Romero, P. Diz, and B. Takkouche, "Continuing education in oral cancer prevention for dentists in Spain," *Journal of Dental Education*, vol. 76, no. 9, pp. 1234–1240, 2012.

30

Application of D-Amino Acids as Biofilm Dispersing Agent in Dental Unit Waterlines

Ruchanee Salingcarnboriboon Ampornaramveth,[1] **Nilada Akeatichod**,[1,2] **Jesita Lertnukkhid**,[1] **and Nichakorn Songsang**[1,3]

[1]*Research Unit on Oral Microbiology and Immunology, Department of Microbiology, Faculty of Dentistry, Chulalongkorn University, Bangkok, Thailand*
[2]*Pakhum Hospital, Buriram, Thailand*
[3]*Trat Hospital, Trat, Thailand*

Correspondence should be addressed to Ruchanee Salingcarnboriboon Ampornaramveth; ruchanee.a@chula.ac.th

Academic Editor: Carlos A. Munoz-Viveros

Aim and Purpose. Biofilms in dental unit waterlines (DUWLs) are extremely difficult to eliminate. Aim of this study is to evaluate the efficacy of a mixture of four D-amino acids on biofilm dispersion in DUWLs. *Materials and Methods.* A mixture of four D-amino acids (D-methionine, D-tryptophan, D-leucine, and D-tyrosine, 10 mM each), distilled water (control), and 0.1 M hydrochloric acid (HCl) was used in the experiment. In laboratory, pieces of DUWLs covered with biofilms were submerged in different solutions for 5 days, flushed, and measured OD^{600} of the dispersed biofilms. Remnants of biofilms on the DUWLs were evaluated by SEM. In clinic, fifteen DCUs were incubated with test and control solutions, flushed, and measured OD^{600} of the dispersed biofilms. Microbial count of DUWL output water was enumerated twice a week for four weeks. *Results.* There was a slight, but not significant, increase in OD^{600} of flushing water in D-amino acids group. D-amino acids effectively reduced bacterial plaque as demonstrated by SEM. Incubation with D-amino acids significantly reduced biofilms especially after the first day of flushing. Bacterial count in DUWL output water was significantly reduced after treatment with D-amino acids. *Conclusion.* D-amino acids are applicable as biofilm dispersing agents in DUWLs.

1. Introduction

Biofilms, the term for a community of microorganisms, are resistant to physical and chemical stresses. Biofilms can be found in any aquatic environment including pipelines of medical devices [1]. In dentistry, dental unit waterlines (DUWLs) consist of narrow (approximately 2–3 mm internal diameter) plastic tubes, and they deliver cooling water for dental equipment [1]. DUWLs are prone to biofilm formation which results in a heavily contaminated water output. This problem has been first identified almost 50 years ago and is still of significant concern since several reports indicate biofilm-related infection for both normal and immunocompromised patients [1, 2].

Numerous approaches have been introduced to decrease the presence of DUWL biofilms. These include both nonchemical and chemical methods. Regarding a nonchemical strategy, which includes flushing, drying, and applying an antimicrobial filter, using deionized, distilled, or even sterile water appears not to affect existing biofilms [1, 2]. The application of chemical agents has been proven to be effective [3–6]. Since regrowth of biofilms takes only a short period of time, a continuous chemical treatment is necessary. However, chemical agents can have an adverse effect on the patient's oral tissues, dental chair unit (DCU) components, as well as dental restorative materials. This is, in particular, the case for residual agents present in DUWL output water, which enter the patient's oral cavity and may even be swallowed or inhaled from aerosols generated by dental instruments [7]. Nowadays, searching a better approach for the elimination of pathogenic bacterial biofilms is still a very relevant issue in the field of infection control and prevention.

Amino acids (except glycine) can occur in two isomeric forms; these are called L- and D-forms. Only L-amino acids are produced by cells and incorporated into proteins. Therefore, most natural amino acids are in the L-form. D-amino acids are found in the cell walls of bacteria, but not in their proteins. D-amino acids have been proposed to be stress signaling and are released during depletion of nutrients to trigger the dispersion of "old" biofilms [8]. These D-amino acids help bacteria adapt to environmental challenges by modulating the structure and composition of peptidoglycans which are one of the major components in the bacterial cell wall [8–10].

D-amino acids are also involved in inhibition of bacterial biofilm formation and dispersion. Kolodkin-Gal et al. demonstrated that D-amino acids could disperse *B. subtilis* biofilm by affecting the function of amyloid fibers. When noncanonical D-amino acids incorporate into peptidoglycan, they interfere with the anchoring of amyloid fibers that normally assists in holding the biofilms together [11]. Bucher et al. reported D-leucine (D-Leu) as a noncanonical D-amino acid which competes with D-alanine (D-Ala) for the fifth pentapeptide of *B. subtilis* cell wall and interferes with transpeptidation and transglycosylation. The disturbance of the composition of the bacterial cell wall specifically interferes with biofilm formation [12]. D-amino acids including D-tyrosine (D-Tyr), D-methionine (D-Met), D-FFtophan (D-Tryp), and D-leucine (D-Leu) can prevent pellicle formation [13]. The minimal inhibitory concentration (MIC) of these D-amino acids that could inhibit biofilm formation depends on the type of D-amino acid. Testing these amino acids individually revealed that the MIC of D-Met was 2 mM, of D-Tryp was 5 mM, of D-Tyr was 3 μM, and of D-Leu was 8.5 mM. D-Tyr proved to be the most effective among the four. Nonetheless, the mixture of all four amino acids is more effective than D-Tyr alone. As for the dispersion of biofilms, D-Tyr (3 μM) or a mixture of D-Tyr, D-Met, D-Tryp, and D-Leu (2.5 nM each) breakdowns the biofilm pellicle of *B. subtilis* [13]. Not only this type of biofilm was affected but D-amino acids can also affect *Staphylococcus aureus* and *Pseudomonas aeruginosa* biofilms [13–16].

Recently, several studies have proposed D-amino acids as candidate molecules to be applied as a biofilm dispersing agent in endodontic treatment. Rosen et al. demonstrated that D-Leu was effective in inhibiting *E. faecalis* biofilms grown on human dentin slabs [17]. Zilm et al. demonstrated that a mixture of D-amino acids containing D-Leu, D-Met, D-Tyr, and D-Tryp significantly reduced biofilm formation of *E. faecalis*. The inhibitory effect of D-amino acids on biofilm formation was concentration dependent. The authors of this study, therefore, proposed D-amino acids as a novel biofilm inhibitor in endodontic treatment [18].

These effects of D-amino acids on biofilm dispersion together with their safety support their use as a candidate for the removal of biofilms in DUWLs. Therefore, the present study aims to investigate the efficacy of D-amino acid mixtures on the removal of biofilm in DUWLs.

2. Material and Methods

2.1. Efficacy of D-Amino Acid Mixture on Dispersing Biofilm on DUWLs In Vitro. DUWLs covered with biofilm, as was judged by eye, were obtained from in-use dental chair units (DCUs) and cut into small pieces with a length of 2.5 cm. A mixture of four D-amino acids, consisting of D-methionine (D-Met; #M9375, Sigma-Aldrich, St. Louis, MO), D-tryptophan (D-Tryp; #T9753, Sigma–Aldrich, St. Louis, MO), D-leucine (D-Leu; #L0027, TCI, Tokyo, Japan), and D-tyrosine (D-Tyr; TCI, Tokyo, Japan), was prepared by dissolving them in 0.1 M hydrochloric acid (HCl) to get a final concentration of 10 mM (each). In a preliminary set of experiments, we assessed that 10 mM was the most effective concentration of D-amino acids to be used for the removal of a biofilm.

The DUWLs were submerged in 4 mL of one of the following three solutions: (i) distilled water (negative control), (ii) D-amino acids, and (iii) 0.1 M HCl (dissolvent control). The samples were incubated at room temperature for 5 days before each sample was rinsed 3 times with 1 mL of distilled water. The dispersed biofilm from each sample was collected to sonicate and to measure the OD at 600 nm. The DUWL samples were then fixed with 2.5% glutaraldehyde for 24 hours and washed with 1 mL of PBS for 3 times. They were then dehydrated, critical-point dried, gold-sputter coated, and examined using a scanning electron microscopy (JSM-5410 LV; JEOL, Tokyo, Japan) at a magnification of ×2000. Biofilms found inside the reservoir bottle of DCUs were also incubated with test and control solutions for 5 days, flushed, and visualized with SEM.

2.2. Efficacy of D-Amino Acid Mixture on Dispersing Biofilm on DUWLs in a Clinical Setting. Fifteen dental chair units (DCUs) were randomly divided into 3 groups of 5 DCUs each: distilled water (negative control), D-amino acids, and 0.1 M HCl (dissolvent control). The study used DCUs of the dental school during summer break; a period during which the DCUs were not in use. Before the start of the experiment, water from the DUWLs was collected to evaluate the initial bacterial CFUs. The water samples were sonicated for 5 minutes to disperse clumps of microorganisms. Then, a serial ten-fold dilution was performed before plating a 100 μL of each sample onto R2A agar plates, and these were then incubated at 35°C. The baseline CFUs were assessed after 7 days of incubation. In the D-amino acids and HCl groups, the water supplying the DCUs was replaced with a mixture of D-amino acids or 0.1 M HCl, respectively.

In order to limit the amount of D-amino acid used in each DCUs, the minimum amount of water that completely flushed to the outlet of the waterline was determined by flushing diluted gentian violet into the DUWL. Fifty-five mL of the tested solution was determined as an appropriate amount to completely fill up the waterlines with testing solution. The test solutions were left in the tubing of DUWLs for 5 days. After 5 days of incubation, the waterlines were repeatedly flushed with 1.6 liters of water every other day for

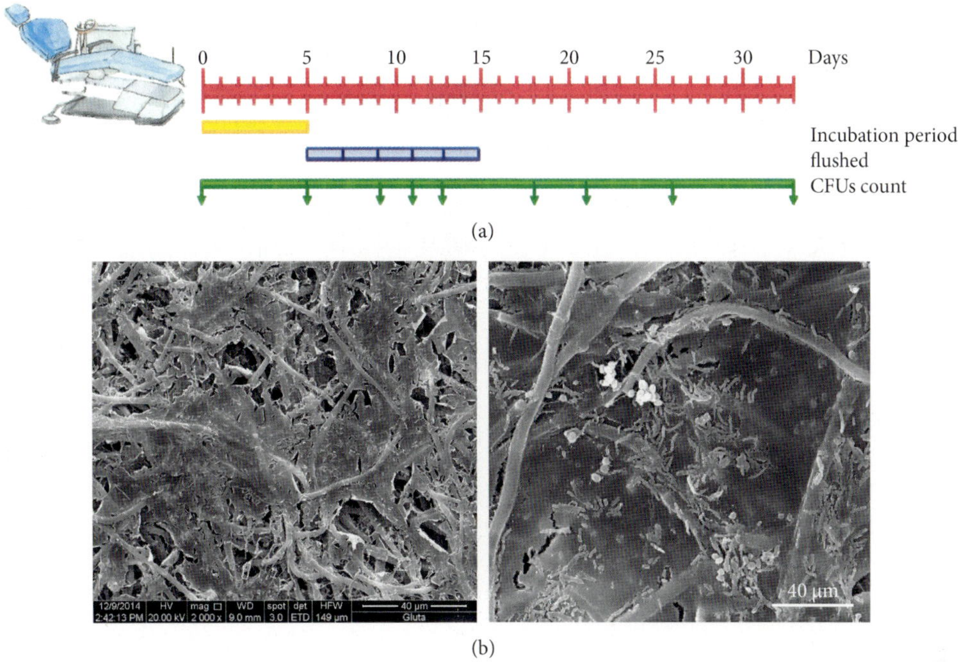

Figure 1: Scheme of the experimental time line (a). Incubation period: DUWLs were incubated with different solutions for 5 days (yellow bar). Flushed: DUWLs were flushed, every other day, with 1.6 L water (blue bar). Flushing water was collected to measure the dispersed biofilms by OD. CFU count: Time point at which water samples were collected for bacterial CFU counts (green bar with arrow). SEM image of biofilm mass on the inner surface of DUWLs (b). Magnification ×2000 (left image); A higher magnification image is shown on the right side.

10 days and the flushing water was collected to measure the OD at 600 nm. After flushing, 25 mL of water from each unit was collected and sonicated for 5 minutes. The samples were diluted ten-fold, plated on R2A agar, and incubated at 35°C for 7 days. The bacterial CFUs were then counted. Bacterial contamination in DCU output water samples was evaluated twice a week repeatedly for 4 weeks (Figure 1).

All data were analyzed using SPSS 18. The Kruskal–Wallis test and the Mann–Whitney U test were used for both in vitro and clinical experiments. Significance was set at p values < 0.05.

3. Results

Biofilm mass was shown to cover the inner surface of DUWLs as shown by SEM (Figure 1(b)). After 5 days of incubation, the biofilms on the inner surface of the tubes were seen to become loosened, some were even detached in the D-amino acids and HCl groups (Figure 2(a)). Fragments of biofilm collected in rinsing water were used to measure OD at 600 nm. There was a trend of an increase of OD of dispersed biofilms in the D-amino acids group compared with control, though this did not prove to be statistically significant (Figure 2(b)). Evaluation by SEM showed DUWL biofilms consisting of bacterial plaque on top of which smear-like structures were seen (Figure 3). Treatment the DUWL with D-amino acid mixtures was able to disperse the bacterial plaque that covered the biofilm (Figure 3(a)). Biofilms dispersing effects were also found on biofilms on the inner surfaces of water reservoir bottle of the DCUs that were incubated with D-amino acids for 5 days (Figure 3(b)).

In the clinical setting, the highest OD of dispersed biofilms was observed on the first day of flushing in the group treated with the D-amino acid mixture (Figure 4). After treating the DUWL with control and test solutions, bacterial contamination recovered from DCU output water was analyzed twice a week for approximately 4 weeks (Figure 5). A statistically significant lower number of average CFUs was found in the DUWL treated with D-amino acids compared with the distilled water control group (Figure 6).

4. Discussion

Our results demonstrated that a mixture of D-amino acids consisting of D-methionine, D-tryptophan, D-leucine, and D-tyrosine at a final concentration of each amino acid of 10 mM was effective in dispersing biofilm in DUWLs. This cleaning effect was found both in an in vitro setting and in a clinical setting. SEM analysis revealed that bacterial biofilms inside the DUWL were eliminated after incubation with the D-amino acid mixture for 5 days. Treatment of the DUWLs with the D-amino acid mixture also significantly reduced bacterial contamination in output water of DCUs. In previous studies, the efficiency of D-amino acids in dispersing biofilms has been demonstrated in vitro with single species biofilms or microbial aggregates formed by mixed cultures [13, 14, 19]. Our study is, for the first time, proposing a clinical application of a mixture of D-amino acids in the removal of biofilms in medical devices like DCUs.

Many methods both mechanical and chemical have been utilized to reduce bacterial contamination in dental unit waterlines, but none of these methods were able to disperse

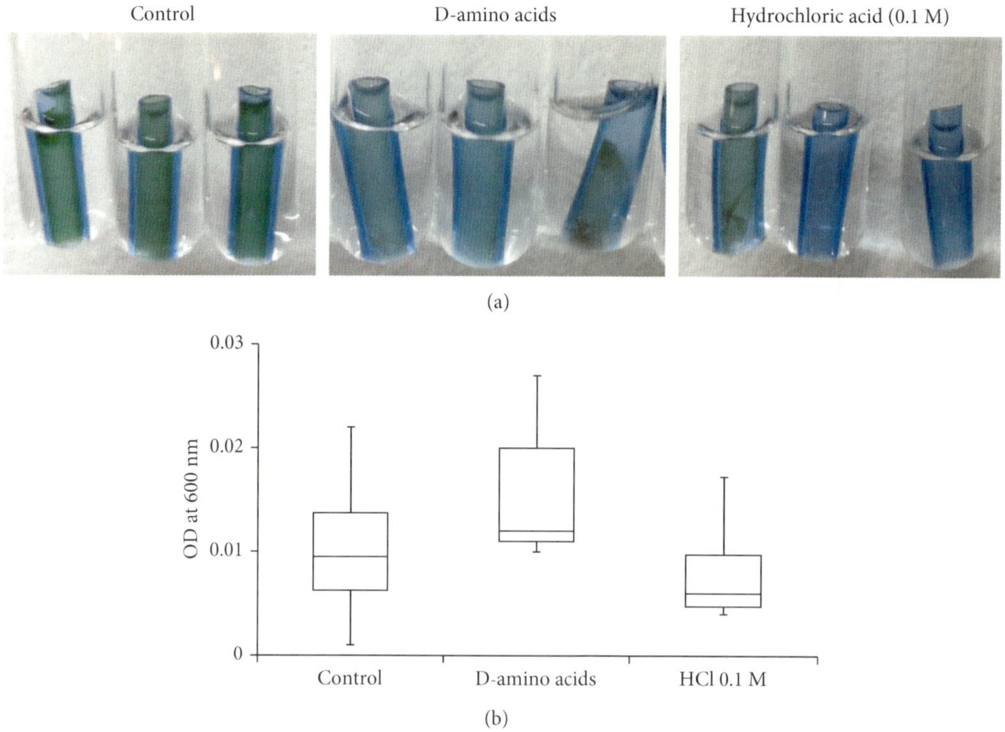

FIGURE 2: 2.5 mm pieces of DUWL tube after incubation with distilled water, D-amino acids mixture (10 mM each), or 0.1 M hydrochloric acid (dissolvent control) for 5 days (a). Optical density at 600 nm (OD^{600}) of dispersed biofilms in flushing water collected after the 2.5 mm pieces of DUWLs were incubated with distilled water, D-amino acids mixture (10 mM each), or 0.1 M HCl (dissolvent control) for 5 days (b).

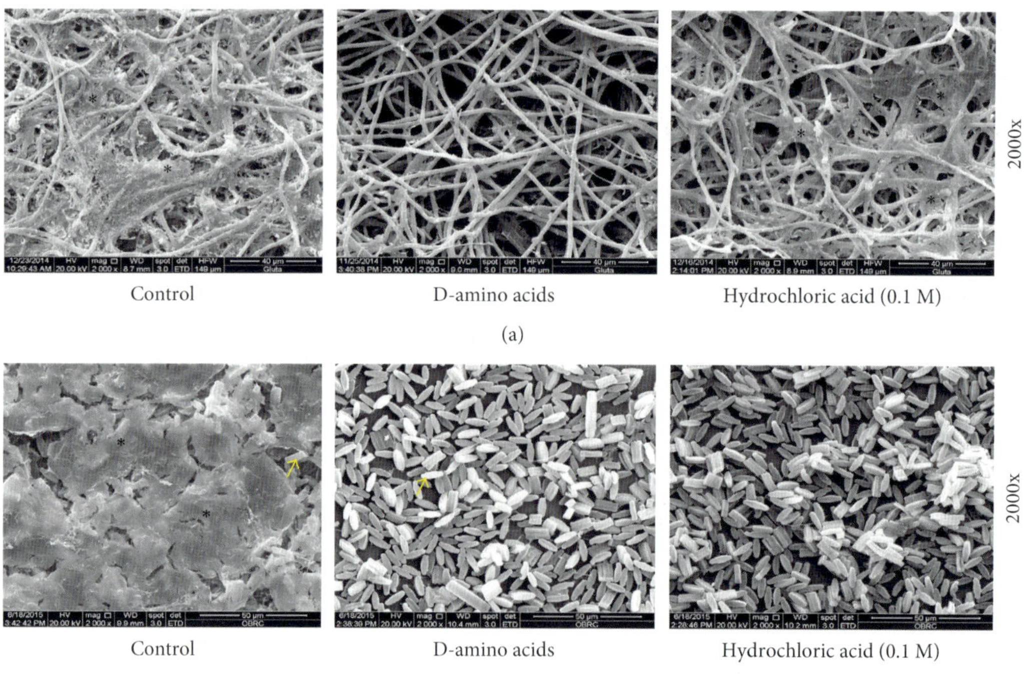

FIGURE 3: Scanning electron microscopy revealed the presence of biofilms inside DUWLs (a) and reservoir bottle of DCUs (b) after incubation with distilled water, D-amino acids mixture (10 mM each), or 0.1 M hydrochloric acid (dissolvent control) for 5 days and subsequently flushed with distilled water. Bacterial biofilm on top of the underlying structure was eliminated in the D-amino acid groups. *Bacterial biofilm. Arrow indicates surface texture of water reservoir bottle.

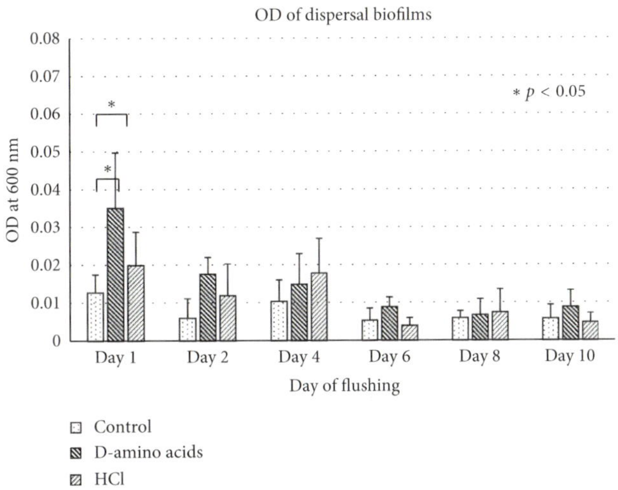

FIGURE 4: Optical density at 600 nm of dispersed biofilms in flushing water collected after the DUWLs of DCUs were incubated with distilled water (control), D-amino acids mixture (D-amino acids, 10 mM each), or 0.1 M HCl for 5 days. The DUWLs were flushed every other day for 10 days, and the flushing water was collected to measure the OD^{600} of dispersed biofilms. *Statistically different at $p < 0.05$.

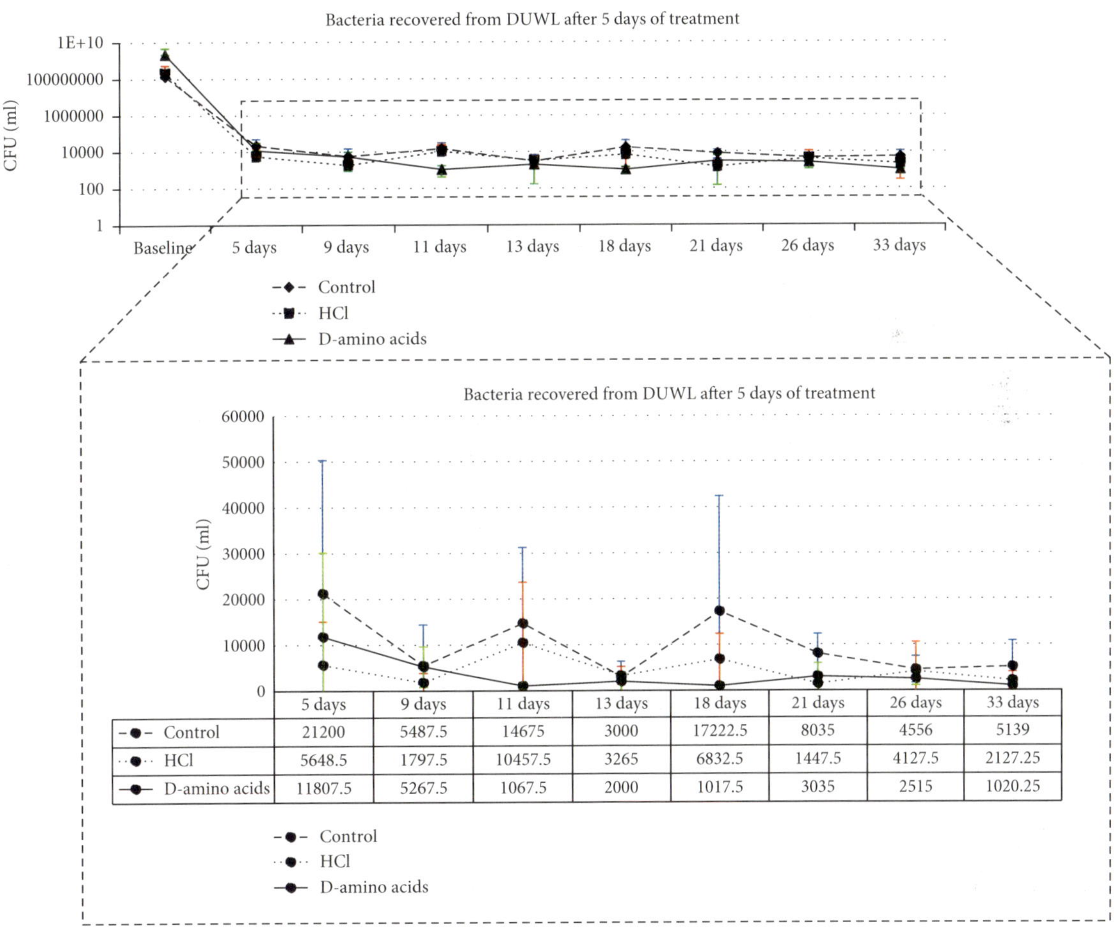

	5 days	9 days	11 days	13 days	18 days	21 days	26 days	33 days
Control	21200	5487.5	14675	3000	17222.5	8035	4556	5139
HCl	5648.5	1797.5	10457.5	3265	6832.5	1447.5	4127.5	2127.25
D-amino acids	11807.5	5267.5	1067.5	2000	1017.5	3035	2515	1020.25

FIGURE 5: Bacterial contamination in DCU output water collected every 2-3 days for 4 weeks after the DUWLs were flushed with distilled water (control), D-amino acids mixture (D-amino acids, 10 mM each), or 0.1 M hydrochloric acid (HCl) for 5 days. A treatment of the DUWLs with D-amino acids reduced bacterial contamination in dental unit output water more than was seen in the control and HCl group.

the existing biofilms in the complex tubing system of DUWLs. The efficiency of controlling bacterial contamination in DUWLs depends solely on chemical or physical methods of destroying or removing planktonic bacteria. Thus, the effectiveness of D-amino acid in the removal of existing biofilms in the complex dental unit tubing system

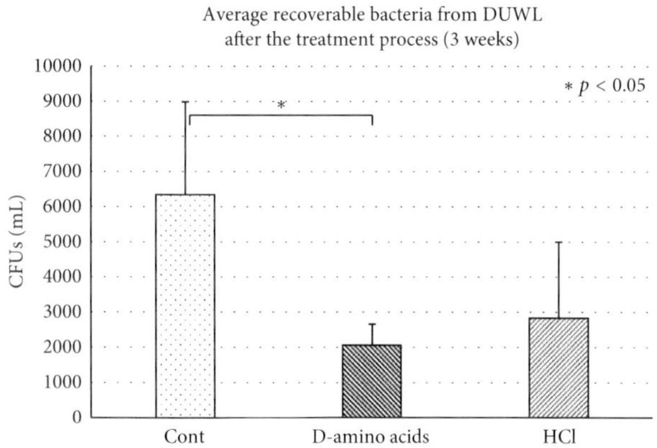

FIGURE 6: The average bacterial count in output water of the DCUs collected during the last 3 weeks after treatment of the DUWLs with distilled water (control), D-amino acids mixture (D-amino acids, 10 mM each), or 0.1 M HCl for 5 days. *Statistically different at $p < 0.05$.

appears to be an attractive way to remove biofilms from the inner parts of medical devices.

Our findings demonstrate the efficiency of D-amino acids in this process. It should be noted that also treatment of the waterlines with HCl alone partially removed biofilms. This effect might be due to the acidity of hydrochloric acid and its effect on biofilm dispersion [20, 21]. According to Tam et al., biofilm detachment of *Streptococcus mutans* occurs more rapidly as the pH drops [21]. However, HCl might corrode the metal part of the dental tubing system if it is used at a high concentration for a longer period. Although the recommended diluent for D-amino acids is 0.1 M HCl, a diluent with a neutral pH might be more suitable.

The concentration of D-amino acid mixture used in our study is slightly higher than the one used in previous studies [13, 14]. Yet, Hochbaum et al. reported a dose-dependent effect of D-amino acids with a minimum concentration of 10 mM to disperse the *Staphylococcus aureus* biofilm [14]. Kolodkin-Gal et al. proposed 3 μM of D-tyrosine or a mixture of D-Tyr, D-Met, D-Tryp, and D-Leu (2.5 nM each) to disrupt the *B. subtilis* biofilm [13]. The concentrations of D-amino acids used in previous studies were effective against single species biofilms. In our study, a more complex model of naturally occurring biofilms was utilized, and therefore, a higher concentration of D-amino acids was employed.

Besides a biofilm-dispersing property, D-amino acids have also been demonstrated to inhibit or slow down the growth of biofilms [16, 22, 23]. However, there are some contradicting data regarding the efficacy of D-amino acids on inhibiting biofilm formation. Some studies demonstrated that the effect of D-amino acids was rather strain specific [15, 22, 24, 25]. One of the possible mechanisms by which D-amino acids act on biofilms was proposed to trigger the disassembly of matrix-associated amyloid fibers (see Introduction). This effect was observed in *B. subtilis* biofilms which are known to produce this type of matrix [8, 13]. However, also with organisms that do not seem to produce amyloid fibers, for example, *S. aureus* and *P. aeruginosa*, D-amino acids appear to trigger the disassembly of biofilms. The exact mechanisms involved in how D-amino acids disperse biofilms need further examination [8, 26].

5. Conclusion

A mixture of D-amino acids was shown to partly remove biofilms in dental unit waterlines. This study, therefore, proposes the use of such a mixture as a new approach to decontaminate bacterial biofilms in dental unit waterlines.

Acknowledgments

This work was supported by the Asia Research Center at Chulalongkorn University. The authors would like to express their sincere gratitude to Professor Vincent Everts from the Department of Oral Cell Biology, Academic Centre for Dentistry Amsterdam (ACTA), University of Amsterdam and Vrije Universiteit Amsterdam, for his contribution in editing the English grammar and giving some fruitful comments on the manuscript.

References

[1] M. J. O'Donnell, M. A. Boyle, R. J. Russell, and D. C. Coleman, "Management of dental unit waterline biofilms in the 21st century," *Future Microbiology*, vol. 6, no. 10, pp. 1209–1226, 2011.

[2] S. K. Garg, S. Mittal, and P. Kaur, "Dental unit waterline management: historical perspectives and current trends," *Journal of Investigative and Clinical Dentistry*, vol. 3, no. 4, pp. 247–252, 2012.

[3] L. L. Coan, E. A. Hughes, J. C. Hudson, and C. J. Palenik, "Sampling water from chemically cleaned dental units with detachable power scalers," *Journal of Dental Hygiene*, vol. 81, no. 4, p. 80, 2007.

[4] W. Zhang, O. Onyango, Z. Lin, S. S. Lee, and Y. Li, "Evaluation of Sterilox for controlling microbial biofilm contamination of dental water," *Compendium of Continuing Education in Dentistry*, vol. 28, no. 11, pp. 586–588, 2007.

[5] L. Montebugnoli, G. Dolci, D. A. Spratt, and R. Puttaiah, "Failure of anti-retraction valves and the procedure for between patient flushing: a rationale for chemical control of dental unit waterline contamination," *American Journal of Dentistry*, vol. 18, no. 4, pp. 270–274, 2005.

[6] S. M. Lin, K. K. H. Svoboda, A. Giletto, J. Seibert, and R. Puttaiah, "Effects of hydrogen peroxide on dental unit biofilms and treatment water contamination," *European Journal of Dentistry*, vol. 5, no. 1, pp. 47–59, 2011.

[7] D. G. Kadaifciler and A. Cotuk, "Microbial contamination of dental unit waterlines and effect on quality of indoor air," *Environmental Monitoring and Assessment*, vol. 186, no. 6, pp. 3431–3444, 2014.

[8] F. Cava, H. Lam, M. A. de Pedro, and M. K. Waldor, "Emerging knowledge of regulatory roles of D-amino acids in bacteria," *Cellular and Molecular Life Sciences*, vol. 68, no. 5, pp. 817–831, 2011.

[9] P. Horcajo, M. A. de Pedro, and F. Cava, "Peptidoglycan plasticity in bacteria: stress-induced peptidoglycan editing by

noncanonical D-amino acids," *Microbial Drug Resistance*, vol. 18, no. 3, pp. 306–313, 2012.

[10] H. Lam, D.-C. Oh, F. Cava et al., "D-amino acids govern stationary phase cell wall remodeling in bacteria," *Science*, vol. 325, no. 5947, pp. 1552–1555, 2009.

[11] Y. Oppenheimer-Shaanan, N. Steinberg, and I. Kolodkin-Gal, "Small molecules are natural triggers for the disassembly of biofilms," *Trends in Microbiology*, vol. 21, no. 11, pp. 594–601, 2013.

[12] T. Bucher, Y. Oppenheimer-Shaanan, A. Savidor, Z. Bloom-Ackermann, and I. Kolodkin-Gal, "Disturbance of the bacterial cell wall specifically interferes with biofilm formation," *Environmental Microbiology Reports*, vol. 7, no. 6, pp. 990–1004, 2015.

[13] I. Kolodkin-Gal, D. Romero, S. Cao, J. Clardy, R. Kolter, and R. Losick, "D-amino acids trigger biofilm disassembly," *Science*, vol. 328, no. 5978, pp. 627–629, 2010.

[14] A. I. Hochbaum, I. Kolodkin-Gal, L. Foulston, R. Kolter, J. Aizenberg, and R. Losick, "Inhibitory effects of D-amino acids on *Staphylococcus aureus* biofilm development," *Journal of Bacteriology*, vol. 193, no. 20, pp. 5616–5622, 2011.

[15] Z. Sanchez, A. Tani, and K. Kimbara, "Extensive reduction of cell viability and enhanced matrix production in *Pseudomonas aeruginosa* PAO1 flow biofilms treated with a D-amino acid mixture," *Applied and Environmental Microbiology*, vol. 79, no. 4, pp. 1396–1399, 2013.

[16] K. S. Brandenburg, K. J. Rodriguez, J. F. McAnulty et al., "Tryptophan inhibits biofilm formation by *Pseudomonas aeruginosa*," *Antimicrobial Agents and Chemotherapy*, vol. 57, no. 4, pp. 1921–1925, 2013.

[17] E. Rosen, I. Tsesis, S. Elbahary, N. Storzi, and I. Kolodkin-Gal, "Eradication of *Enterococcus faecalis* biofilms on human dentin," *Frontiers in Microbiology*, vol. 7, p. 2055, 2016.

[18] P. S. Zilm, V. Butnejski, G. Rossi-Fedele, S. P. Kidd, S. Edwards, and K. Vasilev, "D-amino acids reduce *Enterococcus faecalis* biofilms in vitro and in the presence of antimicrobials used for root canal treatment," *PLoS One*, vol. 12, no. 2, article e0170670, 2017.

[19] X. Si, X. Quan, Q. Li, and Y. Wu, "Effects of D-amino acids and norspermidine on the disassembly of large, old-aged microbial aggregates," *Water Research*, vol. 54, pp. 247–253, 2014.

[20] P. Uppuluri, A. K. Chaturvedi, A. Srinivasan et al., "Dispersion as an important step in the *Candida albicans* biofilm developmental cycle," *PLoS Pathogens*, vol. 6, no. 3, p. e1000828, 2010.

[21] K. Tam, N. Kinsinger, P. Ayala, F. Qi, W. Shi, and N. V. Myung, "Real-time monitoring of *Streptococcus mutans* biofilm formation using a quartz crystal microbalance," *Caries Research*, vol. 41, no. 6, pp. 474–483, 2007.

[22] S. A. Leiman, J. M. May, M. D. Lebar, D. Kahne, R. Kolter, and R. Losick, "D-amino acids indirectly inhibit biofilm formation in *Bacillus subtilis* by interfering with protein synthesis," *Journal of Bacteriology*, vol. 195, no. 23, pp. 5391–5395, 2013.

[23] W. T. Kao, M. Frye, P. Gagnon, J. P. Vogel, and R. Chole, "D-amino acids do not inhibit *Pseudomonas aeruginosa* biofilm formation," *Laryngoscope Investigative Otolaryngology*, vol. 2, no. 1, pp. 4–9, 2017.

[24] C. J. Sanchez Jr., K. S. Akers, D. R. Romano et al., "D-amino acids enhance the activity of antimicrobials against biofilms of clinical wound isolates of *Staphylococcus aureus* and *Pseudomonas aeruginosa*," *Antimicrobial Agents and Chemotherapy*, vol. 58, no. 8, pp. 4353–4361, 2014.

[25] C. J. Sanchez Jr., E. M. Prieto, C. A. Krueger et al., "Effects of local delivery of D-amino acids from biofilm-dispersive scaffolds on infection in contaminated rat segmental defects," *Biomaterials*, vol. 34, no. 30, pp. 7533–7543, 2013.

[26] A. Jayaraman and T. K. Wood, "Bacterial quorum sensing: signals, circuits, and implications for biofilms and disease," *Annual Review of Biomedical Engineering*, vol. 10, no. 1, pp. 145–167, 2008.

Evaluation of Marginal Misfit of Metal Frameworks Welded by Gas-Torch, Laser, and Tungsten Inert Gas Methods

Wilson Matsumoto,[1] Paula Pastana Beraldo,[2] Rossana Pereira de Almeida,[1] Ana Paula Macedo,[1] Beatriz Roque Kubata,[1] and Takami Hirono Hotta[1]

[1]*Department of Dental Materials and Prosthodontics, Dental School of Ribeirão Preto, University of São Paulo, Ribeirão Preto 14040-904, Brazil*
[2]*Private Practice, Ribeirão Preto 14025-010, Brazil*

Correspondence should be addressed to Wilson Matsumoto; wmatsumoto@forp.usp.br

Academic Editor: Manal Awad

Purpose. The objective of this study was to evaluate the marginal fit and the flexural resistance of nickel-chromium frameworks welded by different techniques, gas-torch, laser, and tungsten inert gas (TIG), compared with that of frameworks made via one-piece casting. *Methods.* To evaluate the marginal fit, a master model was fabricated simulating four implants. Transfers and replicas were used to transfer the positions of the implants to the model, using a silicone matrix. The bars were waxed up and casted. Three assessments of misfit were performed for each implant using a stereomicroscope before and after welding in two predetermined regions, totaling six readings for each implant. To evaluate the flexural resistance, one group was made casting the specimens in one piece. Other 3 groups using gas-torch, laser, and TIG welding techniques were made after sectioned transversally. The data showed normal distribution and two-way ANOVA for marginal fit and one-way ANOVA for flexural resistance, and Tukey's posttest ($\alpha = 0.05$) was performed. *Results.* For the marginal fit, the three welding methods presented similar results and were different from one-piece casting. For the flexural resistance, significant differences were observed among the studied groups ($p < 0.001$), and the one-piece group presented higher resistance compared to the three welding techniques. *Conclusions.* Within the limits of this study, the three welding techniques yielded similar misfit results, and the laser and TIG techniques presented similar flexural resistance but lower than gas-torch and one-piece casting.

1. Introduction

The success of an oral rehabilitation procedure is associated with the use of techniques and materials that enable a fixed prosthesis supported by teeth or implant a uniform distribution of forces and passive fit [1]. Achieving good adaptation with regard to prosthetic restorations is difficult, especially for extensive or one-piece cast framework [2, 3]. This fact is considered a common cause of fixed prosthesis failure due to alloy shrinkage after solidification or a lack of parallelism between the retainers. In this situation, welding is a method that can provide better adaptation than that achieved via one-piece metal structure [2, 4, 5].

Major advantages associated with welding include the option of using framework segments reducing the likelihood of failures occurring during manufacture, improving the adaptation and distribution of the masticatory forces, and producing structures with lower distortion and better adaptation [5]. A passive fit is essential for maintaining mechanical and biological balance that decreases the loading on the abutments [6]. Engineering advances have contributed to the development of new welding techniques and equipment as an alternative to conventional gas-torch techniques. These new modalities include laser [7] and tungsten inert gas (TIG) welding [8]. These different welding methods have associated advantages and disadvantages. The gas-torch technique causes oxidation, porosity, and overheating that can cause distortion [9] and is contraindicated for cantilever and extensive prostheses. Laser welding is advantageous because it entails the application of concentrated energy in a short time and less distortion; however, it is reportedly associated with variable strength results [10], unlike TIG welding which yields values similar to one-piece casting, with less porosity, and is indicated for sites with high resistance requirements [11].

Given the above-described considerations, investigations aimed at identifying welding processes that result in high-quality prostheses with suitable properties, or at least properties that are within clinically acceptable limits are of fundamental importance. The objective of the current study was to evaluate the marginal misfit and the flexural resistance of different methods of soldering parameters associated with nickel-chromium (Ni-Cr) frameworks welded by gas-torch, laser, and TIG techniques. The null hypothesis was that the welding method has no influence on the vertical misfit and the flexural resistance of Ni-Cr frameworks.

2. Materials and Methods

2.1. Master Model Fabrication. The master model was constructed from a transparent acrylic resin lower jaw model (Nacional Ossos, Jau, SP, Brazil) with four replicas of mini conical abutment (4.1 mm in diameter; Neodent, Curitiba, PR, Brazil), simulating a fixed prosthesis Branemark-type protocol with 4 implants.

2.2. Stone Cast Fabrication. To transfer the position of the mini conical abutment replicas, four square transfers (Neodent, Curitiba, PR, Brazil) were adapted and joined together with dental floss and acrylic resin (Duralay, Reliance, Worth Illinois, USA). After polymerization, the resin and dental floss set were cut between transfers with a #170L carbide bur to compensate for acrylic resin polymerization shrinkage. The sectioned parts were then rejoined with resin (Duralay, Reliance, Worth, Illinois, USA). After acrylic resin polymerization, the splinted transfers were removed from the master model.

The replicas were adapted to the splinted transfers, and the assembly was placed in a silicone matrix (Zetaplus, Dentsply, Petrópolis, RJ, Brazil) that was filled with type IV stone (Durone, Dentsply, Petrópolis, Brazil) and allowed to set on the workbench for 60 min. The model was then removed from the silicone matrix, and splinted transfers were removed from the stone cast and readapted on the master model to verify fit accuracy. The process was repeated to make 30 stone casts, which were subjected to different welding methods: gas-torch ($n = 10$), laser ($n = 10$), and TIG ($n = 10$).

2.3. Wax Pattern Fabrication. Mini conical plastic cylinders (Neodent, Curitiba, PR, Brazil) were adapted onto the models, and wax-ups of the frameworks were made. Twenty wax patterns were cut in the middle of the distance between the plastic cylinders to derive the laser and TIG groups, with a 0.1 mm thick chrome-platinum blade.

2.4. Metal Structure Casting. The wax patterns were invested with high-fusing phosphate bonded investment (Heat Shock, Polidental, Cotia, SP, Brazil) in accordance with the manufacturer's instructions. Samples were cast with a centrifugal machine equipped with a gas oxygen torch (EDG, Sao Carlos, SP, Brazil), using a Ni-Cr alloy (Fit Cast-SB Plus, Talmax, Curitiba, PR, Brazil). Casted samples were finished with airborne-particle abrasion with 100 μm alumina at 90 lib/pol^2. Ten one-piece cast frameworks were adapted in the master model to perform gap measurements between the metal framework and mini conical replica.

2.5. Measurement of One-Piece Cast Framework Discrepancies. Measurements (60x, scale 7.69 μm) were performed using an S8AP0 stereomicroscope (Leica, Leica Microsystems, Wetzlar, Germany) and Leica Application Suite V3 software (Leica Microsystems).

2.6. Gas-Torch Welding Group. After measurement, samples were cut between the retainers with a 1 mm thick carborundum disk, constituting the welding gas-torch group ($n = 10$). Samples were indexed with acrylic resin (Duralay, Reliance, Worth, Illinois, USA) and invested with phosphate investment (Heat Shock, Polidental, Cotia, SP, Brazil). Gas-torch welding was conducted in accordance with the manufacturer's instructions (Dentorium, Labordental, Sao Paulo, SP, Brazil), and the samples were bench cooled at room temperature. The models with the sectioned metal frameworks were randomly divided into laser welding technique ($n = 10$) and TIG welding technique ($n = 10$) groups.

2.7. Laser Welding Group. A desktop laser welder (Dentaurum, Ispringen, Germany) was used to perform the laser welding technique. It was programmed at 310 V, 9.0 ms, and a pulse frequency of 4 focus, so that the welding reached deeper, and 4 welding points were made at anterior, posterior, superior, and inferior areas. Subsequently, the machine configuration was changed to 270 V, 9.0 ms pulse, and 8 focus to facilitate a wider and shallower area of welding to completely fill the sectioned line of the samples.

2.8. TIG Welding Group. A welding machine (NTY 60 model, Kernit, Indaiatuba, SP, Brazil) set to 60 A and a time of 120 ms was used to perform TIG welding. The machine was fitted with a tungsten electrode centered within the ceramic nozzle, following the manufacturer's recommendations. The time for preflow and postflow of argon gas was 2.0 s. Subsequently, the metal frameworks were transferred from the stone cast to the master model to analyze the interface between the frameworks and the mini conical replicas. Frameworks were screwed with a torque of 10 N·cm applied via a manual torque wrench (Neodent).

2.9. Measurement of Metal Framework Discrepancies. All welded groups were analyzed with a stereomicroscope under the same conditions applied to the one-piece cast group. The same operator performed three readings at two different positions (buccal and lingual) for each implant, totaling 6 measurements, and the mean was calculated for each implant. All groups were measured before and after welding.

2.10. Flexural Resistance Test. The cylindrical specimens, 3 mm in diameter and 40 mm in length, were cast in Ni-Cr alloy (Fit Cast-SB Plus, Talmax, Curitiba, PR, Brazil) using one-piece technique. Ten specimens were used as control group or one-piece group, and the other specimens were sectioned in two parts at middle distance and grouped according to the welding techniques in gas-torch, laser, and TIG groups.

The specimens were submitted to the three-point flexural test in the universal testing machine (EMIC DL 2000, São José dos Pinhais, PR, Brazil), where a 500 kg load cell was attached at a speed of 0.5 mm/min. Previously, markings were made that identified the center of the specimen, the weld location, and the location where the test piece should rest. The force, carried by a steel tip of 3.0 mm in diameter, was applied to the welded site until the fracture of the specimen had occurred. The forces necessary to fracture the bars were recorded.

2.11. Statistical Analysis. Statistical analysis was performed with SPSS for windows (SPSS 17.0 statistics software, SPSS Inc., USA), and p values of less than 0.05 were considered significant. A misfit comparison was done using the two-way analysis of variance (ANOVA). A flexural resistance comparison was done using the one-way ANOVA. Tukey's test and Student's t-test were performed to compare the groups.

3. Results

Table 1 shows the mean and standard deviation of the vertical misfit of the one-piece casting framework and different techniques before and after welding. Statistical analysis confirmed a normal distribution. In the two-way ANOVA, there was a statistically significant difference between welding types ($p = 0.004$) and no significant difference for implant position ($p = 0.054$). There was no statistically significant difference for the interaction of variables ($p = 0.153$).

Tukey's posttest was performed to identify differences between welding types. Tukey's test showed similarity between the experimental groups before welding, which differed from the one-piece group. Tukey's test showed that the gas-torch, laser, and TIG groups were similar.

Student's t-test for paired samples was used to compare the results obtained before and after welding, and the gas-torch technique yielded results that were statistically similar before and after welding ($p = 0.56$). This was not the case for the laser group ($p = 0.009$) or the TIG ($p = 0.002$) group, in which there was higher marginal misfit after welding.

Table 2 shows the mean and standard deviation of the flexural resistance (MPa) associated with different types of welding.

For flexural resistance, a significant difference was observed between the groups ($p < 0.001$). After Tukey's test, it was verified that the one-piece group presented greater resistance when compared to the welded groups ($p < 0.001$). Gas-torch group presented higher resistance than the laser ($p = 0.049$) and TIG ($p = 0.026$) groups. And there was no significant difference between the laser and TIG groups ($p = 0.994$).

TABLE 1: Mean and standard deviation of the marginal discrepancy (μm) associated with the different techniques before and after welding.

	Type of welding	Mean (μm)	Standard deviation (μm)	N
Before	One-piece	31.2	12.9	10
	Torch	19.2	7.0	10
	Laser	20.7	2.2	10
	TIG	21.3	3.1	10
After	One-piece	31.2	12.9	10
	Torch	22.3	9.1	10
	Laser	23.7	3.8	10
	TIG	23.8	3.9	10

TABLE 2: Mean and standard deviation of the flexural resistance (MPa) associated with different types of welding.

Type of welding	Mean (MPa)	Standard deviation (MPa)	N
One-piece	1874.7	212.6	10
Torch	1313.5	394.2	10
Laser	987.8	158.8	10
TIG	956.8	253.3	10

4. Discussion

The use of welding is justified by the advantage of working with segments of the prosthesis, reducing possible failures during the design of the metal structure and allowing better adaptation of the framework, uniform distribution of forces and, consequently, minimization of traumas and failures in the prosthesis. However, as several problems related to the welding process have been reported in the literature, considering the type of alloy [5, 9, 11], oxidation of the faces to be joined by the weld, porosity in the joint, and overheating of the bonding site during the welding process [2], welding can still be considered a process that demands more studies and research with materials, techniques, and equipment. In this study, the null hypothesis was partially accepted because the results obtained for the marginal misfit from the gas-torch, laser, and TIG groups did not differ significantly; however, the flexural strength was higher for the gas-torch.

The growth in the use of base alloys and the fact that prosthesis obtained by one-piece casting does not offer desirable adaptation, there is still a concern in welding metal segments, using techniques that do not produce fragile points and be practically and commercially viable. In addition, prosthesis must have the necessary characteristics to resist the chewing force and the high loads coming from bite forces especially the force in the occlusogingival direction.

Despite the impossibility of perfect adaptation between the tooth and metal framework due to various clinical and laboratory procedures [1, 2, 12, 13], the marginal fit of a prosthetic restoration is fundamental for its clinical success in the long term [14], and the presence of microgaps can affect the mechanical performance of the prosthesis [15]. This fact has prompted the elaboration of many studies with the objective to minimize problems associated with marginal discrepancy [14, 16]. In implant-supported prostheses, the lack of passivity of the metal framework on abutments can cause biological complications and prosthetic component failures [13]. Fixed prostheses should have a passive fit with osseointegrated implants because it is very difficult to predict what will happen clinically when a given degree of misfit is present [17]. A prosthesis misfit can cause overload on the adjacent bone and on prosthetic components, resulting in fatigue, screw loosening or fracture, and abutment screw fracture. This may compromise the integrity of the implant bone interface [18]. What does or does not constitute an "accurate" fit with regard to clinical interface relationships has been shown to be difficult to define [19].

Technical improvements have been made in the field of implants to enhance the fit accuracy of the abutment/prosthesis interface [16]. The current study examined the marginal misfit of the Ni-Cr frameworks after different welding procedures, gas-torch (brazing), laser, and TIG methods, and compared the results to those derived from a one-piece cast group. Laser welding has favorable features including heat reduction in the worked area [11] and elimination of the use of solder alloys and investments. The welding process can be performed directly in the plaster model [20] and even directly in the oral cavity [21] resulting in reduced dimensional changes and working times. TIG welding is conducted in an argon gas environment and can join parent metals with or without filling solder. Therefore, corrosion resistance can be increased due to the absence of galvanic effects at the joint. TIG welding is not commonly used in dentistry, but some studies have demonstrated the superiority of the technique over brazing methods in cobalt-chromium and Ni-Cr-based alloys, with similar results to those of laser welding [8, 10, 12]. TIG involves a very rapid cooling process, and all procedures can be performed directly over the definitive cast. The union is obtained via the use of an electric arc with a continuous current within an inert atmosphere (argon) [20].

The highest values of misfit were found in the one-piece group (31.2 ± 12.9 μm) (Table 1), however, within the values considered clinically acceptable and below the average values found in other studies [12, 22–24]. One-piece prosthesis casting is a very sensitive technique, which requires an optimal working protocol and a skilled technician.

Before welding, the experimental groups exhibited similar marginal misfit and the one-piece control group exhibited a statistically significant difference, with average values of major discrepancy, confirming a greater possibility of alterations [13]. After welding, the gas-torch, laser, and TIG groups remained statistically similar to each other, but the gas-torch group differed significantly from the one-piece group. In the current study, after welding, the TIG and laser groups yielded results that did not differ significantly from those of the one-piece group, which was unexpected because it was predicted that the welding process would minimize the negative effects of one-piece casting [13]. These results are concordant with those reported by de Castro et al. [25], who concluded that there was no significant difference between one-piece cast, laser, and TIG welding frameworks.

The results of the current study differ from those of other studies [26–28], in which the authors affirmed that base metal castings do not provide a satisfactory level of fit unless additional refinement treatment is performed. Another study by Barbi [16] showed that TIG welding produced better results than the brazing or laser method. The difference between the one-piece and gas-torch groups in the current study may be related to the need for greater skill and experience of the professional when utilizing the gas-torch welding technique, as it requires standardization and control to achieve consistent and reliable results [2, 4]. Misfits are always present, regardless of the joining procedures used [22].

The gas-torch group presented specimens with excellent resistance values, conferring to this method validity for its use by the laboratories, as an efficient practice. However, the results showed a high standard deviation, indicating that it is a very sensitive technique. This technique is considered as difficult to execute, requiring a skilled professional [2, 9]. Despite the deficiencies, the gas-torch technique continues to be one of the most used by dental laboratories, mainly due to the low cost.

When the equipment is correctly calibrated, the laser and TIG techniques does not require much skill by the operator, compared to gas-torch technique, minimizing the occurrence of unsatisfactory results, as observed by the lower standard deviation of these techniques. Although previous studies, with the TIG technique, were performed with engineering-adapted machines, the results were similar or even superior when compared with other methods [11, 20, 29, 30].

The gas-torch technique produces a large area of the heat-affected zone (HAZ), around 2 mm, whereas the laser energy produces only 0.5 mm of a highly concentrated, localized, and rapid heat source (milliseconds) [7]. The welding performed in the TIG groups presented the same characteristics as the laser technique. This explains the fact that the specimens of the gas-torch group with greater strength always fractured in the region of the heat-affected zone, with complete separation of the two fractured halves and the lower resistance specimens fractured in the welded sites due to the porosities. The TIG and laser groups had their fractures always in the weld sites, but without the complete separation of the halves, showing ductility of the metal provided by minimal structural change and also by the absence of a soldering alloy. The great challenge, in the welding process, is the search for frameworks with the same structural characteristics as the frameworks obtained by one-piece casting with minimal structural changes. The greater the heat-affected zone, the greater the risk of distortions. One can consider that according to these parameters, laser and TIG techniques are more suitable than gas-torch. Since the gas-torch technique uses a third material to effect the welding, which does not occur in the other two techniques, there is improvement in the characteristics of the welded area, both in relation to the strength and to the adhesion of the ceramic to the metal structure.

The results of the misfit and the flexural resistance of this study show that the TIG and laser welding techniques produced good results, and these techniques could be considered as viable as they are easy to perform. The three weld techniques used in this study demonstrated to be able to improve the clinical conditions of a prosthesis by lowering the misfit and producing adequate flexural resistance [31] in spite of lower than the one-piece casting.

One limitation of this study was that the measurements of the misfit were performed in a single plane, not three dimensionally. Future studies should incorporate three-dimensional marginal misfit evaluation.

5. Conclusions

Within the limits of this study, after welding the three techniques, it yielded similar misfit results, and the laser and TIG welding techniques presented similar flexural resistance but lower than the gas-torch and the one-piece casting. Misfits currently remain inevitable regardless of the joining procedures used.

References

[1] S. F. Rosenstiel, M. F. Land, and J. Fujimoto, Contemporary Fixed Prosthodontics, Elsevier, St. Louis, MO, USA, 5th edition, 2016.

[2] G. Byrne, "Soldering in prosthodontics—an overview, part I," *Journal of Prosthodontics*, vol. 20, no. 3, pp. 233–243, 2011.

[3] R. Tiossi, H. B. Falcão-Filho, F. A. de Aguiar Jr., R. C. Rodrigues, M. G. de Mattos, and R. F. Ribeiro, "Prosthetic misfit of implant-supported prosthesis obtained by an alternative section method," *Journal of Advanced Prosthodontics*, vol. 4, no. 2, pp. 89–92, 2012.

[4] K. J. Anusavice, C. Shen, and H. R. Rawls, Phillips' Science of Dental Materials, Saunders, Philadelphia, PA, USA, 12th edition, 2012.

[5] R. Tiossi, H. Falcão-Filho, F. A. Aguiar Junior, R. C. Rodrigues, M. da G. Mattos, and R. F. Ribeiro, "Modified section method for laser-welding of ill-fitting cp Ti and Ni-Cr alloy one-piece cast implant-supported frameworks," *Journal of Oral Rehabilitation*, vol. 37, no. 5, pp. 359–363, 2010.

[6] S. R. BernardeS, C. A. de Araújo, A. J. Neto, P. Simamoto Junior, and F. D. das Neves, "Photoelastic analysis of stress patterns from different implant-abutment interfaces," *Internationsl Journal of Oral Maxillofacial Implants*, vol. 24, no. 5, pp. 781–789, 2009.

[7] T. E. Gordon and D. L. Smith, "Laser welding of prostheses—an initial report," *Journal of Prosthetic Dentistry*, vol. 24, no. 4, pp. 472–476, 1970.

[8] I. C. Matos, I. N. Bastos, M. G. Diniz, and M. S. de Miranda, "Corrosion in artificial saliva of a Ni-Cr-based dental alloy joined by TIG welding and conventional brazing," *Journal of Prosthetic Dentistry*, vol. 114, no. 2, pp. 278–285, 2015.

[9] K. J. Anusavice, T. Okabe, S. E. Galloway, D. J. Hoyt, and P. K. Morse, "Flexure test evaluation of presoldered base metal alloys," *Journal of Prosthetic Dentistry*, vol. 54, no. 4, pp. 507–517, 1985.

[10] C. Bertrand, Y. Le Petitcorps, L. Albingre, and V. Dupuis, "The laser welding technique applied to the non precious dental alloys procedure and result," *British Dental Journal*, vol. 190, no. 5, pp. 255–257, 2001.

[11] R. Rocha, A. L. Pinheiro, and A. B. Villaverde, "Flexural strength of pure Ti, Ni-Cr and Co-Cr alloys submitted to Nd : YAG laser or TIG welding," *Brazilian Dental Journal*, vol. 17, no. 1, pp. 20–23, 2006.

[12] J. W. Mclean and J. A. Von Fraunhofer, "The estimation of cement film thickness by an in vivo technique," *British Dental Journal*, vol. 131, no. 3, pp. 107–111, 1971.

[13] A. G. Wee, S. A. Aquilino, and R. L. Schneider, "Strategies to achieve fit in implant prosthodontics: a review of the literature," *International Journal of Prosthodontics*, vol. 12, no. 2, pp. 167–178, 1999.

[14] D. Y. Kim, J. H. Kim, H. Y. Kim, and W. C. Kim, "Comparison and evaluation of marginal and internal gaps in cobalt-chromium alloy copings fabricated using subtractive and additive manufacturing," *Journal of Prosthodontic Research*, vol. 62, no. 1, pp. 56–64, 2018.

[15] L. M. S. Pereira, M. B. Sordi, R. S. Magini, A. R. Calazans Duarte, and J. C. M. Souza, "Abutment misfit in implant-supported prostheses manufactured by casting technique: an integrative review," *European Journal of Dentistry*, vol. 11, no. 4, pp. 553–558, 2017.

[16] F. C. Barbi, E. T. Camarini, R. S. Silva, E. H. Endo, and J. R. Pereira, "Comparative analysis of different joining techniques to improve the passive fit of cobalt-chromium superstructures," *Journal of Prosthetic Dentistry*, vol. 108, no. 6, pp. 377–385, 2012.

[17] T. Jemt and U. Lekholm, "Measurements of bone and framework deformations induced by misfit of implant superstructures. A pilot study in rabbits," *Clinical Oral Implants Research*, vol. 9, no. 4, pp. 272–280, 1998.

[18] S. Sahin and M. C. Çehreli, "The significance of passive framework fit in implant prosthodontics: current status," *Implant Dentistry*, vol. 10, no. 2, pp. 85–92, 2001.

[19] J. E. Rubenstein and T. Ma, "Comparison of interface relationships between implant components for laser-welded titanium frameworks and standard cast frameworks," *International Journal of Oral Maxillofacial Implants*, vol. 14, no. 4, pp. 491–495, 1999.

[20] R. R. Wang and G. E. Welsch, "Joining titanium materials with tungsten inert gas welding, laser welding, and infrared brazing," *Journal of Prosthetic Dentistry*, vol. 74, no. 5, pp. 521–530, 1995.

[21] M. Degidi, D. Nardi, A. Piattelli, and C. Malevez, "Immediate loading of zygomatic implants using the intraoral welding technique: a 12-month case series," *International Journal of Periodontics and Restorative Dentistry*, vol. 32, no. 5, pp. e154–e161, 2012.

[22] S. Yannikakis and A. Prombonas, "Improving the fit of implant prosthetics," *International Journal of Oral Maxillofacial Implants*, vol. 28, no. 1, pp. 126–134, 2013.

[23] G. M. De Araújo, D. G. B. De França, J. P. S. Neto, and G. A. S. Barbosa, "Passivity of conventional and CAD/CAM fabricated implant frameworks," *Brazilian Dental Journal*, vol. 26, no. 3, pp. 277–283, 2015.

[24] G. A. S. Barbosa, S. R. Bernardes, D. G. B. De França, F. D. Das Neves, M. G. C. Mattos, and R. F. Ribeiro, "Stress over implants of one-piece cast frameworks made with different materials," *The Journal of Craniofacial Surgery*, vol. 27, no. 1, pp. 238–241, 2016.

[25] G. C. de Castro, C. A. de Araujo, M. F. Mesquita, R. L. Consani, and M. A. Nóbilo, "Stress distribution in Co-Cr implant frameworks after laser or TIG welding," *Brazilian Dental Journal*, vol. 24, no. 2, pp. 147–151, 2013.

[26] J. Abduo, K. Lyons, V. Bennani, N. Waddell, and N. Swain, "Fit of screw-retained fixed implant frameworks fabricated by different methods: a systematic review," *International Journal of Prosthodontics*, vol. 24, no. 3, pp. 207–220, 2011.

[27] R. Tiossi, R. C. Rodrigues, M. G. de Mattos, and R. F. Ribeiro, "Comparative analysis of the fit of 3-unit implant-supported frameworks cast in nickel-chromium and cobalt-chromium alloys and commercially pure titanium after casting, laser welding, and simulated porcelain firings," *International Journal of Prosthodontics*, vol. 21, no. 2, pp. 121–123, 2008.

[28] K. A. Lencioni, A. P. Macedo, R. C. Silveira Rodrigues, R. F. Ribeiro, and R. P. Almeida, "Photoelastic comparison of as-cast and laser-welded implant frameworks," *Journal of Prosthetic Dentistry*, vol. 114, no. 5, pp. 652–659, 2015.

[29] C. N. Hart and P. R. Wilson, "Evaluation of welded titanium joints used with cantilevered implant-supported prostheses," *Journal of Prosthetic Dentistry*, vol. 96, no. 1, pp. 25–32, 2006.

[30] P. C. Simanoto Júnior, V. R. Novais, A. R. Machado, C. J. Soares, and L. H. A. Raposo, "Effect of joint design and welding type on flexural strength and weld penetration of Ti-6Al-4V alloy bars," *Journal of Prosthetic Dentistry*, vol. 113, no. 5, pp. 467–474, 2015.

[31] S. Sahin, M. C. Çehreli, and E. Yalçin, "The influence of functional forces on the biomechanics of implant-supported prosthesis – a review," *Journal of Dentistry*, vol. 30, no. 7-8, pp. 271–282, 2002.

Bone Texture Fractal Dimension Analysis of Ultrasound-Treated Bone around Implant Site: A Double-Blind Clinical Trial

Elaf Akram Abdulhameed,[1] **Natheer Hashim Al-Rawi**,[1] **Asmaa Tahseen Uthman**,[2] **and Ab Rani Samsudin**[1]

[1]*College of Dental Medicine, University of Sharjah, Sharjah, UAE*
[2]*College of Dental Medicine, Gulf Medical University, Ajman, UAE*

Correspondence should be addressed to Elaf Akram Abdulhameed; elaf.alzubaidi@gmail.com

Academic Editor: Saso Ivanovski

Objectives. To evaluate the efficacy of bone texture fractal dimension (FD) analysis method in predicting implant stability from intraoral periapical radiographs using two implant protocols. *Materials and Methods.* A double-blind clinical trial was conducted on 22 subjects who needed dental implants. The participants were randomized into two groups, the control group with standard implant protocol treatment and the intervention group with added low-intensity power ultrasound treatment (LIPUS) besides the standard implant protocol. The FD values of bone density were carried out on the mesial and distal sides of the implant on digital intraoral radiographs using the box-counting method. Both resonance frequency (RF) and fractal dimension (FD) were assessed in three time intervals: after surgery and before and after loading. *Results.* FD on both the mesial and distal sides serve as very good-to-excellent tests with high validity (ROC area exceeding 0.8) in predicting high implant stability (ISQ ≥ 70). The mesial side measurements were consistently better than the distal side among the intervention groups. The optimum cutoff value for the FD-mesial side that predicts a highly stable implant (ISQ ≥ 70) is ≥1.505. At this optimum cutoff value, the mesial side FD is associated with a perfect sensitivity (100%) and fairly high specificity (86.5%). *Conclusion.* The FD analysis could be recommended as an adjunctive quantitative method in prediction of the implant stability with very high sensitivity and specificity. This trial is registered with ISRCTN72648040.

1. Introduction

Sufficient bone quality is a prerequisite for a successful dental implant. Proper assessment of the bone quality is a primary objective to determine the osseointegration status. Excessive marginal bone loss after implant or following prosthesis may be seen in the first year [1]. Continuous bone resorption affects function and aesthetic; therefore, there are several ways recommended to restore and regenerate the bone such as advocating bone-grafting procedures, usage of growth factors, low-level laser therapy, and therapeutic ultrasound. Low-intensity pulsed ultrasound (LIPUS) stimulation is a safe noninvasive treatment, and it can accelerate bone regeneration [2]. In dentistry, LIPUS has been found to promote periodontal bone defect healing [3], bone regeneration after oral surgery [4], and osseointegration of an endosseous dental implant [5].

Histological analysis was usually considered the gold-standard method to evaluate successful osseointegration. However, due to the invasiveness of this method and related ethical issues, various imaging modalities have been proposed like intraoral radiographs, panoramic imaging, computed tomography (CT), cone beam computed tomography (CBCT), and micro-CT [6]. Periapical radiographs are traditionally interpreted by measuring peri-implant marginal bone loss. This method has been found with limited diagnostic value for early detection of bone changes [7].

Bone texture analysis provides information about bone structures in a noninvasive manner [8, 9]. Fractal dimension analysis is one of the noninvasive, well-suited methods to analyze the bone texture on a plain radiograph [10]. This method is used to quantify the trabecular bone pattern and bone marrow interface using the box-counting logarithm [11, 12]. The fractal analysis is a statistical analysis of texture based on fractal geometry for describing complex structural patterns recognized and expressed as a ratio termed as the "fractal dimension" FD [13, 14]. The FD method has been used to quantify trabecular bone structures under different conditions, like endodontic treatment [15], periodontitis [16, 17], and implant stability [18, 19]. Jolley et al. [20] showed that the FD can reliably analyze the changes in the alveolar bone density by using the periapical radiographs.

There has been no report to determine the validity of intraoral periapical radiographs to predict the success rate of implant stability. Plethora of reports have tested the bone quality around the dental implants and compared it with the contralateral normal bone, but no study has been conducted to compare bone changes between two implant protocols [18, 19]. The aim of the present study was to evaluate the efficacy of the fractal dimension (FD) method in predicting stability around the dental implants treated with and without LIPUS from an intraoral periapical radiograph.

2. Materials and Methods

This randomized controlled clinical trial (RCT) was conducted on 22 patients attended to the University Dental Hospital Sharjah (UDHS) for dental implant therapy of single missing maxillary, first or second premolars. The age range was between 20 and 40 years (mean 33.13 ± 7.23 years). Patients with smoking habit or patients with any systemic diseases that might affect bone metabolism, or patients with parafunctional habits, and patients with active periodontal diseases or bad oral hygiene were excluded from the study. After explaining the study procedure, informed consent was obtained from all participants. The study participants were allocated randomly and equally divided into two groups; the control group (n = 11) received the standard implant treatment, and the intervention group (n = 11) which received low-intensity pulsed ultrasound (LIPUS) therapy in addition to the standard implant procedure.

All patients underwent 2 stages of implant surgeries. Stage I implant surgery was performed with one SPI dental implant (Thommen Medical SPI Element MC Inicell) bone level type with a length of 9.5 mm, and a diameter of 4 mm was positioned in the maxillary edentulous premolar area in each patient. A stage II implant surgery was carried out after 2 months of implant placement where the dental implant was uncovered and impression was taken for crown placement. All patients received screw-retained porcelain fused to metal crown. The intervention group patients (n = 11) were then subjected to LIPUS exposure two weeks following stage I implant surgery placement. The machine employed was Pulson ®330 Ultrasound Therapy unit (Gymna, Bilzen, Belgium) (Figure 1). According to Kerr et al. [21], the intensity of ultrasound therapy was set at 30 mW/cm^2 with a frequency of 1.5 MHz and temporal average power of 20 mW. LIPUS was delivered intraorally on the buccal part of the implant site for a duration of 20 minutes twice a week started 2 weeks after dental implant placement and lasted for the subsequent 10 weeks.

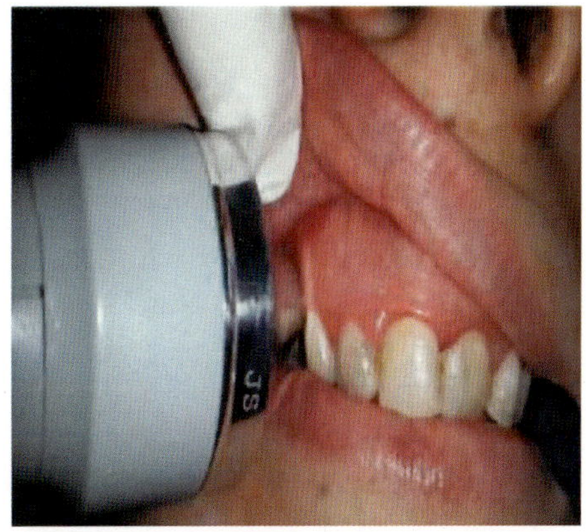

Figure 1: Ultrasound therapy delivered using probe on the buccal aspect of the implant site.

The RF measurements and the FD measurements of bone density were done immediately after surgical dental implant placement and after three and six months, respectively.

For the RF analysis technique, the implant stability is estimated using an Osstell Mentor (Integration Diagnostics, Goteborg, Sweden) and Smart Pegs as described by Isoda et al. [22]. The Smart Pegs were mounted on the implants and tightened with a screw. The RF value was measured in four aspects (mesial, distal, buccal, and lingual) for each implant. The RF values were represented by a quantitative unit called the implant stability quotient (ISQ) on a scale from 1 to 100. High stability means >70 ISQ, between 60 and 69 is medium stability, and <60 ISQ is considered as low stability. The results were expressed in ISQ and averaged for each implant.

The fractal dimension analysis (FD) was made on digital intraoral radiographic images that were taken immediately after the placement of the dental implant and at 3 months and 6 months postoperatively using Image J software (https://imagej.nih.gov/ij/).

The region of interest (ROI) was set to 100 × 200 pixels (1.0 mm wide × 2.0 mm height) at the first macrothread around the mesial and distal aspects of each implant.

The region of interest (ROI) was cropped and was transferred to *Image J version 1.34s* by using the program menu. The saved images were processed using the White and Rudolph method [23]. ROI of duplicated image was blurred with a Gaussian filter (kernel size 35). The blurred image was then subtracted from the original image, and then, the resultant image was converted to binary by threshold at the gray value of 128 so that the segmented objects approximated the bony trabecular pattern. Finally, the image was skeletonized and was used for fractal analysis.

The fractal dimension of the skeletonized image was calculated using the box-counting function method mentioned by Demirbas et al. [24] The resulting numbers of the counted tiles (which refers to the trabecular bone) were plotted against the total number of the tiles in double logarithmic scale, and fractal dimension was calculated from the slope of the line fitted on the data points (Figure 2).

Data were expressed as mean and standard deviation (SD). Differences between groups were analyzed for significance using independent and paired t-test. A simple

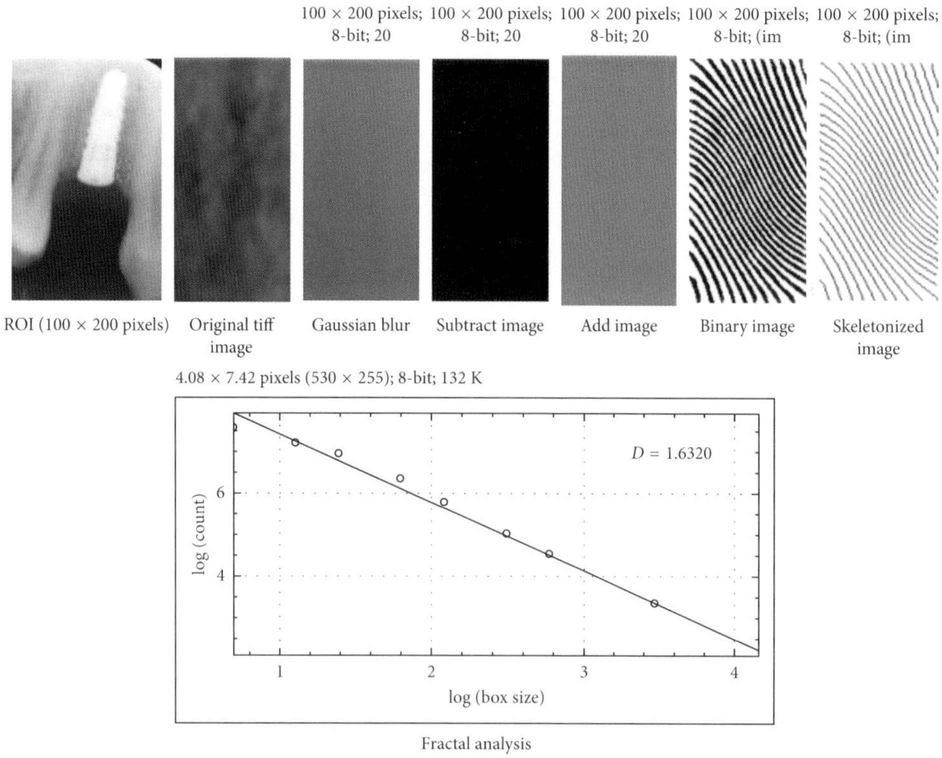

Figure 2: Image-processing procedure.

Table 1: Age and gender comparison between the intervention and control groups.

	Study group				
	Control		Intervention		P
	N	%	N	%	
Age group (years)					0.67 (NS)
21–30	4	36.4	5	45.5	
31–40	7	63.6	6	54.5	
Total	11	100.0	11	100.0	
Gender					1 (NS)
Female	7	63.6	7	63.6	
Male	4	36.4	4	36.4	
Total	11	100.0	11	100.0	

regression model was also used to predict the RF value based on measuring the FD. The statistical significance was defined as $P < 0.05$ using SPSS statistical package (SPSS, Version 24, Chicago, IL, USA).

3. Results

3.1. Reliability and Randomization. FD analyses were done by one investigator (EA), all measurements were repeated by the same investigator after 2 weeks, the intraexaminer reliability test was evaluated, and intraclass correlation coefficient test was measured. The intraclass correlation coefficient was measured first, and it was 0.965 indicating very high internal consistency. There were no obvious or statistically significant differences in age and gender composition between the two comparison groups. This qualifies as an evidence for adequate randomization process (Table 1).

The mean and the standard deviation of RF and FD values for the intervention and control groups are seen in (Table 2).

All the paired measurements of RF and FD values on all study participants (irrespective of their study groups and follow-up time) and all the three time intervals were used in a simple regression model. The model was used to predict the RF value based on measuring the FD.

3.2. Resonance Frequency Analysis. The mean RF measured immediately after surgery showed no important or statistically significant differences between the control and intervention groups (55.3% and 53.2%, resp.). This adds to the evidence for effective randomization process at the design stage (Table 3 and Figure 3).

The outcome of dental implant was assessed after three months and six months of surgery and compared to the immediate postoperative status. The mean change in RF

TABLE 2: The means and standard deviations of RF and FD in the intervention and control groups.

	RF Values (mean ± SD)			FD values (mean ± SD)			FD values (mean ± SD)		
	0 month	3 months	6 months	0 month	3 months Mesial side	6 months	0 month	3 months Distal side	6 months
Control group	55.3 ± 1.90	59.45 ± 4.50	62.09 ± 3.83	1.18 ± 0.19	1.35 ± 0.08	1.44 ± 0.06	1.06 ± 0.16	1.24 ± 0.07	1.36 ± 0.04
Intervention group	53.2 ± 2.99	65.91 ± 6.30	75.45 ± 3.01	1.42 ± 0.10	1.56 ± 0.06	1.68 ± 0.09	1.24 ± 0.07	1.35 ± 0.06	1.49 ± 0.11

RF: resonance frequency; FD: fractal dimension.

TABLE 3: An intervention-control group comparison in mean change in the RF after three and six months of surgery compared to immediate postoperative measurements.

	At baseline	After 3 months	Changes after 3 months compared to immediate	Cohen's *d*	*P* (paired *t*-test)	After 6 months	Changes after 6 months compared to immediate	Cohen's *d*	*P* (paired *t*-test)
Control									
Range	(52 to 58)	(49 to 65)	(−6 to 11)			(54 to 68)	(−1 to 13)		
Mean	55.3	59.5	4.2	1.21	0.009	62.1	6.8	2.25	<0.001
SD	1.9	4.5	4.3			3.8	3.9		
SE	0.57	1.36	1.30			1.16	1.19		
N	11	11	11			11	11		
Intervention									
Range	(49 to 57)	(51 to 75)	(2 to 19)			(70 to 80)	(15 to 28)		
Mean	53.2	65.9	12.7	2.58	<0.001	75.5	22.3	7.42	<0.001
SD	3.0	6.3	4.9			3.0	3.5		
SE	0.90	1.90	1.48			0.91	1.05		
N	11	11	11			11	11		
P (independent samples *t*-test)	0.06 (NS)	0.012	<0.001			<0.001	<0.001		

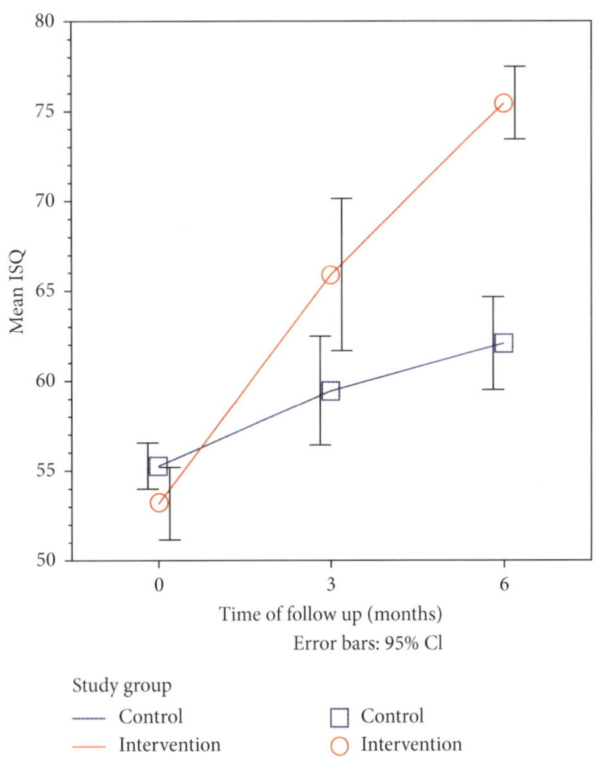

FIGURE 3: Line graph showing the time trend for mean RF values after surgery in the intervention group compared to the control group.

values after these two time intervals was used to assess the magnitude of effect in the healing process in each study group. In addition, Cohen's *d* was used as a standardized measure of effect size to allow fair comparison of effect size between time intervals and between different types of measurements.

As shown in Table 3, after six months of follow-up, the RF values of the control group were significantly increased by a mean of 6.8 units in the control group. This effect was evaluated as a strong effect size (Cohen's $d > 0.8$). On the other hand, the RF values in the intervention group were significantly increased by a mean of 7.4 units after six months. This also translates to a very strong effect size (Cohen's $d > 0.8$). Moreover, the effect size after six months compared to immediate postoperative measurements was much stronger for the intervention group (Cohen's $d = 7.4$) compared to the control group (Cohen's $d = 2.25$). The extra benefit imposed on the intervention group was significantly higher than that on the control group.

3.3. Fractal Dimension Analysis. The mean FD measured immediately after surgery also showed no important or statistically significant differences between the control and intervention groups (1.338 and 1.319, resp.).

After six months of follow-up, the FD-mesial values were significantly increased by a mean of 0.132 units in the control group and 0.342 units in the intervention group which

Table 4: An intervention-control group comparison in mean change in the FD-mesial side after three and six months of surgery compared to immediate postoperative measurements.

	At baseline	After 3 months	Changes after 3 months compared to immediate	Cohen's d	P (paired t-test)	After 6 months	Changes after 6 months composed to immediate	Cohen's d	P (paired t-test)
Control									
Range	(1.229 to 1.393)	(1.293 to 1.498)	(0.018 to 0.124)			(1.377 to 1.568)	(0.06 to 0.26)		
Mean	1.319	1.376	0.056	1.13	<0.001	1.452	0.132	2.64	<0.001
SD	0.044	0.056	0.032			0.052	0.059		
SE	0.013	0.017	0.010			0.016	0.018		
N	11	11	11			11	11		
Intervention									
Range	(1.213 to 1.393)	(1.488 to 1.659)	(0.145 to 0.319)			(1.523 to 1.803)	(0.181 to 0.462)		
Mean	1.338	1.556	0.218	4.35	<0.001	1.680	0.342	4.88	<0.001
SD	0.050	0.058	0.061			0.092	0.097		
SE	0.015	0.018	0.018			0.028	0.029		
N	11	11	11			11	11		
P (independent samples t-test)	0.36 (NS)	<0.001	<0.001			<0.001	<0.001		

reflects a very strong effect size. Moreover, the effect size after six months compared to immediate postoperative measurements was much stronger for the intervention group (Cohen's $d = 4.85$) compared to the control group (Cohen's $d = 2.64$) (Table 4, Figure 4).

Similarly, the FD-distal values were also increased on the distal side of the implant in the intervention group when compared with that of the control group but to a less extent (Table 5, Figure 5).

3.4. Predicting High Implant Stability for FD Measurements. As shown in Figure 6 and Table 6, both FD-mesial and FD-distal sides measurements serve as very good-to-excellent tests with high validity (ROC area exceeding 0.8) for predicting high implant stability (ISQ ≥ 70). The mesial side measurements were consistently better than the distal side in this context.

As shown in Table 7, the optimum cutoff value for the FD-mesial side (associated with highest overall accuracy) that predicts a highly stable implant (ISQ ≥ 70) is ≥1.505. At this optimum cutoff value, the mesial side FD value is associated with a perfect sensitivity (100%) and fairly high specificity (86.5%). The positive predictive value of a positive test result (predicting a real highly stable implant) was calculated at a pretest probability of 50% (equal odds for having high stability versus not having based on chance alone), while that of the negative predictive value of the test (excluding the possibility of having high implant stability) was set at 10% (needing a clinical awareness of high probability of the implant being of low stability).

Having a positive test result for FD-mesial at the optimum cutoff value (FD-mesial measurement of 1.505 or higher) will establish high implant stability with 88.1% confidence level, while testing negative would exclude high implant stability with 100% confidence level. The highest specificity (100%) cutoff value for FD-mesial is ≥1.667. Testing positive at this diagnostic cutoff value (FD-mesial measurement of 1.667 or higher) will establish the diagnosis of high implant stability with 100% confidence, (Table 5).

As shown in Table 8 and Figure 7, for each one-unit increase in FD-mesial side, the RF value is expected to increase by

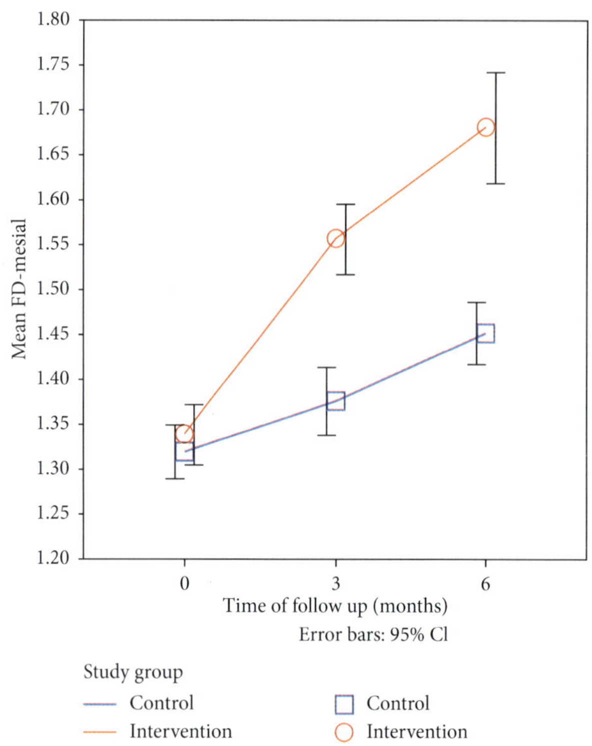

Figure 4: Line graph showing the time trend for mean FD-mesial side after surgery in the intervention group compared to the control group.

TABLE 5: An intervention-control group comparison in mean change in the FD-distal side after three and six months of surgery compared to immediate postoperative measurements.

	At baseline	After 3 months	Changes after 3 months compared to immediate	Cohen's d	P (paired t-test)	After 6 months	Changes after 6 months compared to immediate	Cohen's d	P (paired t-test)
Control									
Range	(1.228 to 1.362)	(1.312 to 1.398)	(0.015 to 0.12)			(1.363 to 1.49)	(0.036 to 0.152)		
Mean	1.308	1.354	0.047	1.55	<0.001	1.398	0.090	2.25	<0.001
SD	0.036	0.031	0.031			0.036	0.038		
SE	0.011	0.009	0.009			0.011	0.011		
N	11	11	11			11	11		
Intervention									
Range	(1.246 to 1.347)	(1.295 to 1.493)	(0.008 to 0.15)			(1.32 to 1.68)	(0.074 to 0.386)		
Mean	1.315	1.370	0.055	1.38	<0.001	1.503	0.188	2.68	<0.001
SD	0.029	0.056	0.037			0.095	0.087		
SE	0.009	0.017	0.011			0.029	0.026		
N	11	11	11			11	11		
P (independent samples t-test)	0.61 (NS)	0.42 (NS)	0.56 (NS)			0.003	0.003		

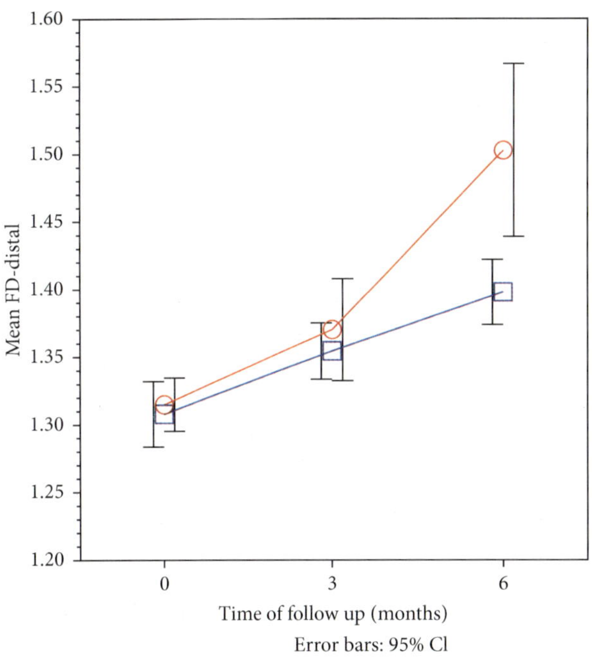

FIGURE 5: Line graph showing the time trend for mean FD-distal side after surgery in the intervention group compared to the control group.

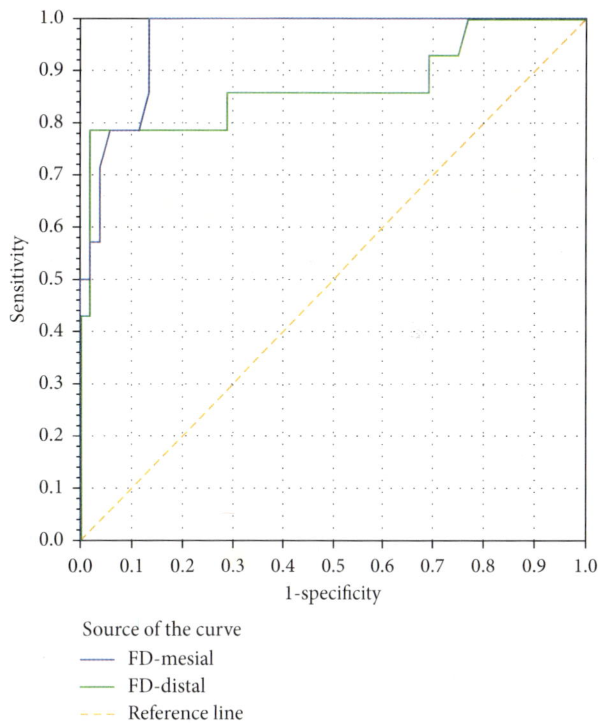

FIGURE 6: ROC curve showing the trade-off between sensitivity (rate of true positive results) and 1-specificity (rate of false positive results) for FD-mesial and FD-distal sides when used as a test to predict high implant stability (RF ≥ 70) in a sample of 66 paired measurements.

47.7 units (for each 0.01-unit increase in measured FD, the RF value is expected to increase by around 0.5). The model is statistically significant and able to explain 66% of observed variation in RF values based on FD-mesial measurements. There was a strong and statistically significant linear correlation between RF values and FD-mesial ($r = 0.81$).

TABLE 6: Area under ROC curve for FD-mesial and FD-distal sides when used as a test to predict high implant stability (ISQ ≥ 70).

	AUROC	P
FD-mesial	0.962	<0.001
FD-distal	0.869	<0.001

Table 7: Validity parameters for FD-mesial and FD-distal sides when used as a test to predict high implant stability (ISQ ≥ 70).

Positive if ≥ cutoff value	k	Specificity	Accuracy	PPV at pretest probability = 50%	NPV at pretest probability = 10%
FD-mesial					
1.505 (highest sensitivity and optimum cutoff value)	100.0	86.5	96.2	88.1	100.0
1.516	92.9	86.5	91.1	87.3	99.1
1.653	50.0	98.1	63.7	96.3	94.6
1.667 (highest specificity)	50.0	100.0	64.3	100.0	94.7
FD-distal					
1.313 (highest sensitivity)	100.0	23.1	78.0	56.5	100.0
1.315	92.9	25.0	73.5	55.3	96.9
1.419	78.6	96.2	83.6	95.3	97.6
1.440 (optimum cutoff value)	78.6	98.1	84.1	97.6	97.6
1.481	42.9	98.1	58.6	95.7	93.9
1.492 (highest specificity)	42.9	100.0	59.2	100.0	94.0

Table 8: Simple linear regression model for FD-mesial side as a predictor variable and RF values as the dependent (outcome) variable.

	Regression coefficient	P
(Constant)	−7.5	0.24 (NS)
FD-mesial	47.7	<0.001

$R^2 = 0.66$, P (model) < 0.001, $r = 0.811$, and $P < 0.001$.

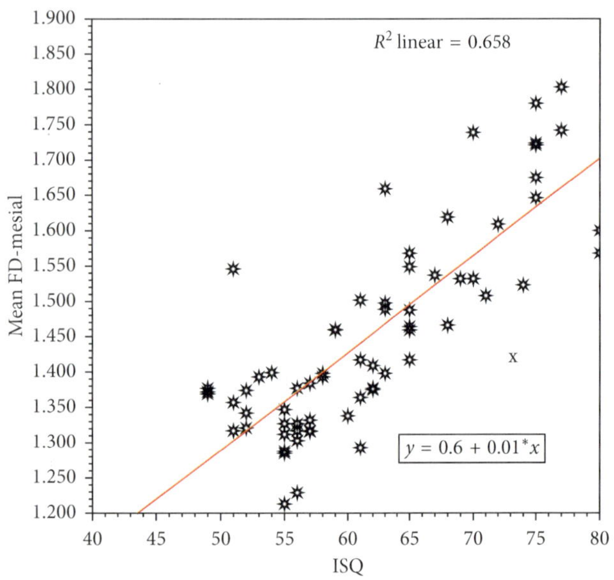

Figure 7: Scatter diagram with fitted regression line describing the linear relation correlation between RF- and FD-mesial side.

As seen in Table 9 and Figure 8, for each one-unit increase in the FD-distal side, the RF value is expected to increase by 68.5 units. The model is statistically significant and able to explain 46% of observed variation in RF values based on FD-distal measurements. There was a statistically significant linear correlation between ISQ and FD-distal ($r = 0.678$), but not as strong as that found in the mesial side.

Table 9: Simple linear regression model for the FD-distal side as a predictor variable and RF as the dependent (outcome) variable.

	Regression coefficient	P
(Constant)	−32.3	0.014
FD-distal	68.5	<0.001

$R^2 = 0.46$, P (*Model*) < 0.001, $r = 0.678$, $P < 0.001$.

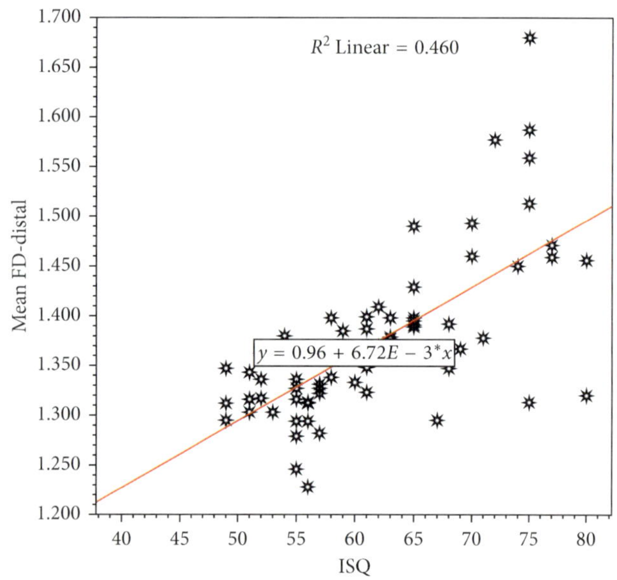

Figure 8: Scatter diagram with fitted regression line describing the linear relation correlation between RF- and FD-distal side.

4. Discussion

Clinically, the implant stability may be assessed either by recording of periotest value, insertion of torque wrench value, or by the use of the resonance frequency analysis. The RF analysis provides valuable clinical objective data of implant stability. It also detects substantial increase or decrease in stability of the implant, giving a clear ability to measure implant-bone contact and makes clinical comparisons during clinical follow-up.

In the present study, all the implant fixtures used had the same surface treatment, implant-abutment interface, and thread characteristics. Regarding the ISQ values obtained from the RF analysis, the effect size after six months was much stronger for the LIPUS-treated intervention group (Cohen's $d = 7.4$) the compared to the control group (Cohen's $d = 2.25$). These findings were in agreement with that of Nedir et al. [25]. However, scarce evidence has been provided so far on Osstell ISQ's reliability [26]. The RF method is influenced by some factors including implant length, implant diameter, implant geometry, implant surface characteristic, and placement position, as well as bone quality and bone quantity [27]. Implant stability quotient (ISQ) is a scale developed by Osstell for implant stability. It converts the resonance frequency values ranging from 3,500 to 8,500 Hz into an ISQ of 0 to 100. A high value indicates greater stability, while a low value indicates instability. Values greater than 65 are recommended as successful implant stability. Even though Osstell is clinically used, there are not much convincing data on the relation between bone-implant interface and ISQ values [28, 29]. RF devices still have some uncertainties because of the observer subjectivity. There has been a search for quantitative methods to control the subjectivity variation in interpretation.

The reliability of fractal dimension calculations from the radiographs was assessed in several studies [15, 30]. Calculation of FD has become a popular method to characterize image textures. In dental radiology, FD calculation can be used to quantify trabecular bone structure for detection of bone changes associated with periodontitis [17], periapical pathology [15], systemic diseases [24, 31], and dental implants [19, 32]. We used standardized digital intraoral radiographs to assess the FD on two implant's protocols. Tolga et al. [32] suggested that fractal analysis could be a useful method for understanding the healing process around implants and implant stability quotient. Onem et al. [33] measured the FD around implants using the box-counting method from the digital panoramic images, and they found that FD values of implant-bearing bone following initial healing was lower than the FD values in the alveolar bone surrounding the contralateral premolar teeth, but the difference was not significant. In the present study, the fractal dimension after 6 months of implant placement had increased significantly ($P < 0.01$) in both groups, suggesting an increase in the amount of bony microstructure around the implant [20]. This increase suggests complete bone healing around implants. Veltri et al. [19] used animal models to investigate the correlations between FA results and insertion torque and RF. A significant correlation was found with final insertion torques, but not with resonance frequencies. Their results also defined a value of 1.83 as the break point of soft bone quality. Veltri et al. [34] measured FD from mesial and distal aspects of implants using the box-counting method on intraoral radiographs, and the mean reported was 1.47 which is close to what was reported in the present study after 6 months of implant placement (1.39–1.45). Lee et al. [18] observed a strong relationship between primary implant stability and FD using digitized panoramic films and the tile-counting method.

In the present study, there was a statistically significant linear correlation between the ISQ values from the RF and the FD values on both sides of the implant with the mesial side of the intervention group being higher than that on the distal side. This could be due to the large surface area of the LIPUS device used in the present study which provides stronger stimulation on the site closer to the probe (the mesial site of the implant); therefore, denser bone formation was expected on this site on a long run. Nevertheless, the FD values on the mesial and distal sides of the implant remains as very good-to-excellent tests with high validity (ROC area exceeding 0.8) for predicting high implant stability (ISQ > 70%). Our results were in agreement with that of Ilhan et al. [35] Lee et al. [18] also suggested that the FD acquired from panoramic radiographs may be a useful predictor of the initial dental implants stability. Therefore, the use of the FD method as a cost-effective one to assess trabecular bone changes around dental implants during follow-up periods is one of the recommendations of this study. No previous studies have been conducted to calculate the optimum cutoff value of FD to predict high implant stability (ISQ > 70%). Using the area under the ROC curve, showed that the optimum cutoff FD value of 1.667 from the mesial side of the implant will establish high implant stability with 100% confidence. Furthermore, for every one-unit increase in the FD-mesial side, the ISQ value from the RF is expected to increase by 47.7 units. Because no other studies have predicted the implant stability from combining the qualitative and quantitative bone at bone-implant interface from digital intraoral radiographs, it is not possible to compare these results with other studies. Onem et al. [33] have used digital panoramic radiographs to quantify the structural changes of mandibular alveolar bone around the dental implants during initial healing. They found that satisfactory bone healing after the implant placement may be monitored by calculating the FD. Lee et al. [18] suggested a unified method to calculate the FD, like proper selection of the area and the size of ROI, methods of FD counting (tile-or box-counting methods), and the type of radiographic image used for the analysis. Although these results may be regarded as preliminary, both ISQ from RF and FD may be reliably recommended for quantitative evaluation of primary and secondary implant stability using digital intraoral radiographic images throughout implant healing and loading periods. Application of the standardized procedures and comparison of the results of these methods with other measures define the bone quality like DEXA, and the value of FD would be more precisely assessed.

5. Conclusion

The fractal dimension analysis as a noninvasive cost-effective method could be helpful in assessing bone trabecular patterns around the implants in different clinical situations. Intraoral digital radiographs could be used to monitor the healing process around the implants. Although these results may be regarded as preliminary, implants with low FD values may indicate a decrease in stability, and this should alert the practitioner to pay more attention through more rigorous follow-up schedules and take further precautions.

References

[1] M. Hof, B. Pommer, N. Zukic, C. Vasak, M. Lorenzoni, and W. Zechner, "Influence of prosthetic parameters on peri-implant bone resorption in the first year of loading: a multi-factorial analysis," *Clinical Implant Dentistry and Related Research*, vol. 17, no. 1, pp. e183–e191, 2015.

[2] X. Q. Gu, Y. M. Li, J. Guo, L. H. Zhang, D. Li, and X. D. Gai, "Effect of low intensity pulsed ultrasound on repairing the periodontal bone of Beagle canines," *Asian Pacific Journal of Tropical Medicine*, vol. 7, no. 4, pp. 325–328, 2014.

[3] R. Shiraishi, C. Masaki, A. Toshinaga et al., "The effects of low-intensity pulsed ultrasound exposure on gingival cells," *Journal of Periodontology*, vol. 82, no. 10, pp. 1498–1503, 2011.

[4] S. H. Kim and K. S. Hong, "Histologic evaluation of low-intensity pulsed ultrasound effects on bone regeneration in sinus lift," *Journal of Periodontal & Implant Science*, vol. 40, no. 6, pp. 271–275, 2010.

[5] S. K. Hsu, W. T. Huang, B. S. Liu, S. M. Li, H. T. Chen, and C.-J. Chang, "Effects of near-field ultrasound stimulation on new bone formation and osseointegration of dental titanium implants in vitro and in vivo," *Ultrasound in Medicine & Biology*, vol. 37, no. 3, pp. 403–416, 2011.

[6] O. Bissinger, F. A. Probst, K. D. Wolf, A. Jeschke, J. Weitz, and A. Kolk, "Comparative 3D micro-CT and 2D histomorphometry analysis of dental implant osseointegration in the maxilla of minipigs," *Journal of Clinical Periodontology*, vol. 44, no. 4, pp. 418–427, 2017.

[7] K. Horner, K. Karayianni, A. Mitsea et al., "The mandibular cortex on radiographs as a tool for osteoporosis risk assessment: the OSTEODENT Project," *Journal of Clinical Densitometry*, vol. 10, no. 2, pp. 138–146, 2007.

[8] W. G. Geraets, P. F. Van der Stelt, C. J. Netelenbos, and P. J. Elders, "A new method for automatic recognition of the radiographic trabecular pattern," *Journal of Bone and Mineral Research*, vol. 5, no. 3, pp. 227–233, 1990.

[9] B. Cortet, P. Dubois, N. Boutry, P. Bourel, A. Cotton, and X. Marchandise, "Image analysis of the distal radius trabecular network using computed tomography," *Osteoporosis International*, vol. 9, no. 5, pp. 410–419, 1999.

[10] N. L. Fazzalari and I. H. Parkinson, "Fractal properties of cancellous bone of the iliac crest in vertebral crush fracture," *Bone*, vol. 23, no. 1, pp. 53–57, 1998.

[11] E. Oczeretko, M. Borowska, I. Szarmach, A. Kitlas, J. Szarmach, and A. Radwański, "Fractal analysis of dental radiographic images in the irregular regions of interest," *Advances in Intelligent and Soft Computing*, vol. 69, pp. 191–199, 2010.

[12] G. M. Tosoni, A. G. Lurie, A. E. Cowan, and J. A. Burleson, "Pixel intensity and fractal analyses: detecting osteoporosis in perimenopausal and postmenopausal women by using digital panoramic images," *Oral Surgery, Oral Medicine, Oral Pathology, Oral Radiology, and Endodontology*, vol. 102, no. 2, pp. 235–241, 2006.

[13] O. Zmeskal, M. Vesely, M. Nezadal, and M. Buchnicek, "Fractal analysis of image structures," *Harmonic and Fractal Image Analysis*, pp. 3–5, 2001.

[14] I. Sánchez and G. Uzcátegui, "Fractals in dentistry," *Journal of Dentistry*, vol. 39, no. 4, pp. 273–292, 2011.

[15] Y. Y. Yu, H. Chen, C. H. Lin et al., "Fractal dimension analysis of periapical reactive bone in response to root canal treatment," *Oral Surgery, Oral Medicine, Oral Pathology, Oral Radiology, and Endodontology*, vol. 107, no. 2, pp. 283–288, 2009.

[16] M. K. Shrout, B. Roberson, B. J. Potter, J. M. Mailhot, and C. F. Hildebolt, "A comparison of 2 patient populations using fractal analysis," *Journal of Periodontology*, vol. 69, no. 1, pp. 9–13, 1998.

[17] S. X. Updike and H. Nowzari, "Fractal analysis of dental radiographs to detect periodontitis-induced trabecular changes," *Journal of Periodontal Research*, vol. 43, no. 6, pp. 658–664, 2008.

[18] D. H. Lee, Y. Ku, I. C. Rhyu et al., "A clinical study of alveolar bone quality using the fractal dimension and the implant stability quotient," *Journal of Periodontal & Implant Science*, vol. 40, no. 1, pp. 19–24, 2010.

[19] M. Veltri, M. Ferrari, and P. Balleri, "Correlation of radiographic fractal analysis with implant insertion torque in a rabbit trabecular bone model," *International Journal of Oral & Maxillofacial Implants*, vol. 26, no. 1, pp. 108–114, 2011.

[20] L. Jolley, S. Majumdar, and S. Kapila, "Technical factors in fractal analysis of periapical radiographs," *Dentomaxillofacial Radiology*, vol. 35, no. 6, pp. 393–397, 2006.

[21] E. N. Kerr, B. L. Mealey, M. E. Noujeim, D. J. Lasho, P. V. Nummikoski, and J. T. Mellonig, "The effect of ultrasound on bone dimensional changes following extraction: a pilot study," *Journal of Periodontology*, vol. 79, no. 2, pp. 283–290, 2008.

[22] K. Isoda, Y. Auykawa, Y. Tsukiyama, M. Sogo, Y. Matsushita, and K. Koyano, "Relationship between the bone density estimated by cone-beam computed tomography and the primary stability of dental implants," *Clinical Oral Implants Research*, vol. 23, no. 7, pp. 832–836, 2012.

[23] S. C. White and D. J. Rudolph, "Alterations of the trabecular pattern of the jaws in patients with osteoporosis," *Oral Surgery, Oral Medicine, Oral Pathology, Oral Radiology, and Endodontology*, vol. 88, no. 5, pp. 628–635, 1999.

[24] A. K. Demirbas, S. Ergun, P. Guneri, B. O. Aktener, and H. Boyacioglu, "Mandibular bone changes in sickle cell anemia: fractal analysis," *Oral Surgery, Oral Medicine, Oral Pathology, Oral Radiology, and Endodontology*, vol. 106, no. 1, pp. e41–e48, 2008.

[25] R. Nedir, M. Bischof, S. Szmukler-Moncler, J. P. Bernard, and J. Samson, "Predicting osseointegration by means of implant primary stability: a resonance frequency analysis study with delayed and immediately loaded ITI SLA implants," *Clinical Oral Implants Research*, vol. 15, no. 5, pp. 520–528, 2004.

[26] M. Herrero-Climent, R. Santos-Garcia, R. Jaramillo-Santos et al., "Assessment of Osstell ISQ's reliability for implant stability measurement: a cross-sectional clinical study," *Medicina Oral Patología Oral y Cirugia Bucal*, vol. 18, no. 6, pp. e877–e882, 2013.

[27] A. H. Muhamed, C. Georges, M. Mustafa, and A. Abdulgani, "Implant stability: methods and recent advances," *IOSR Journal of Dental and Medical Sciences*, vol. 16, no. 8, pp. 13–23, 2017.

[28] N. Meredith, "Assessment of implant stability as a prognostic determinant," *International Journal of Prosthodontics*, vol. 11, pp. 491–501, 1998.

[29] H. M. Huang, C. L. Chiu, C. Y. Yeh, C. T. Lin, L. H. Lin, and S. Y. Lee, "Early detection of implant healing process using resonance frequency analysis," *Clinical Oral Implants Research*, vol. 14, no. 4, pp. 437–443, 2003.

[30] T. E. Southard and K. A. Southard, "Detection of simulated osteoporosis in maxilla using radiographic texture analysis," *IEEE Transactions on Biomedical Engineering*, vol. 43, no. 2, pp. 123–132, 1996.
[31] U. E. Ruttimann, R. L. Webber, and J. B. Hazelrig, "Fractal dimension from radiographs of periodontal alveolar bone: a possible diagnostic indicator of osteoporosis," *Oral Surgery, Oral Medicine, Oral Pathology*, vol. 74, no. 1, pp. 98–110, 1992.
[32] T. Tolga, D. Erhan, and U. Serdar, "Radiographic fractal and clinical resonance frequency analyses of posterior mandibular dental implants: their possible association with mandibular cortical index with 12-month follow up," *Implant Dentistry*, vol. 25, no. 6, pp. 789–795, 2016.
[33] E. Onem, B. G. Baksi, and E. Sogur, "Changes in the fractal dimension, ferret diameter, and lacunarity of mandibular alveolar bone during initial healing of dental implants," *International Journal of Oral & Maxillofacial Implants*, vol. 27, no. 5, pp. 10089–10113, 2012.
[34] M. Veltri, P. Balleri, and M. Ferrari, "Damping factor for monitoring the bone interface at dental implants," *Clinical Oral Implants Research*, vol. 18, no. 6, pp. 738–742, 2007.
[35] B. Ilhan, P. Guneri, A. Saracoglu, H. Koca, and H. Boyacioglu, "A comparison of fractal dimension values of peri-implant bone and healthy contralateral side using panoramic radiographs," *Journal of Oral and Maxillofacial Radiology*, vol. 3, no. 1, pp. 1–6, 2015.

Dental Arch Dimensions in Saudi Adults

Omar Hamad Alkadhi,[1] Sarah Fahad Almahfouz,[2] Hana Abdulmajeed Tokhtah,[3] and Lamia Abdulaziz Binhuwaishel[4]

[1]*Division of Orthodontics, Department of Preventive Dentistry, Riyadh Colleges of Dentistry and Pharmacy, Riyadh, Saudi Arabia*
[2]*Saudi Board of Orthodontics, Department of Orthodontics, King Saud University, Riyadh, Saudi Arabia*
[3]*Orthodontics Residency Program, King Saud University, Riyadh, Saudi Arabia*
[4]*Department of Orthodontics, King Saud Medical City, Riyadh, Saudi Arabia*

Correspondence should be addressed to Omar Hamad Alkadhi; omar.alkadhi@riyadh.edu.sa

Academic Editor: Izzet Yavuz

Objective. The aim of this study was to investigate the arch dimensions (width, length, and depth) in Saudi Arabia. *Materials and Methods.* 169 orthodontic models (73 males and 96 females) made of white stone were selected according to inclusion criteria. Measurement of arch dimensions was taken including width, length, and depth at different reference points. Differences between males and females were tested using independent samples t-test. *Results.* The sample comprised subjects aged 18–33 years old. Most measurements showed higher values for males compared to females. Saudi males showed smaller intercanine widths compared to Caucasians and Southern Chinese but larger widths in females compared to Caucasians and smaller widths compared to Southern Chinese. Saudi males and females showed larger intermolar widths compared to Caucasians but smaller intermolar widths compared to Southern Chinese. For arch length, Saudis showed longer arches compared to Yemenis for both males and females but smaller palatal depths compared to Yemenis. *Conclusions.* Differences in intercanine width, intermolar width, and palatal length and depth were found between Saudis and other nationalities. Male and female participants had differences in most of the measurements.

1. Introduction

Dental arch dimensions are of special interest for dentists and orthodontists in particular. Changes in the arch width, length, and height can result from orthodontic treatment; hence, an understanding of the dental arch dimensions is crucial [1–5]. Dental arches have been investigated using different measurements and reference points, including but not limited to, intercanine, interpremolar, and intermolar widths, either between cusps or fossae, anterior palatal and mandibular lengths, molar vertical distance, total palatal and mandibular lengths, and palatal depth [6–11].

Ward et al. have reported significant changes in maxillary and mandibular intercanine widths in orthodontically treated group compared to untreated group [12]. In patients treated with Frankel II appliance, significant increases in arch width and arch perimeter were found [13].

There are many studies that have been conducted to investigate the dental arch dimensions and relationships in different ethnicities and different geographical areas [14–20]. Few studies have been conducted to investigate arch dimensions in Saudi population [21, 22]. Therefore, the aim of this study was to investigate the arch dimensions (width, length, and depth) in Saudi adults.

2. Materials and Methods

This study was registered at the research center at Riyadh Colleges of Dentistry and Pharmacy with registration number:

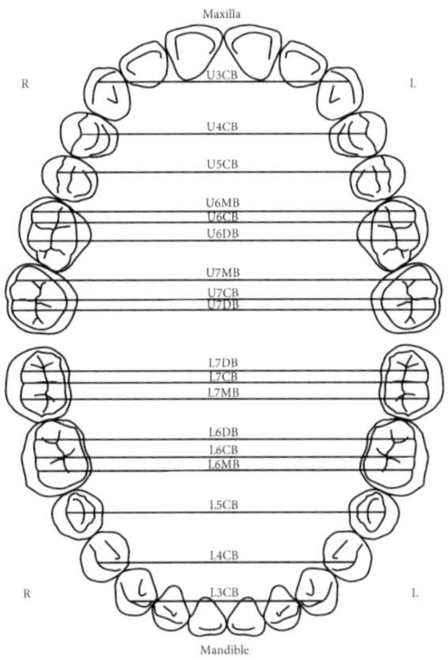

Figure 1: Illustration of the maxillary and mandibular arches' widths as described by Ling and Wong [9]. U3CB: cusp tip of tooth 13 and tooth 23; U4CB: buccal cusp of tooth 14 and tooth 24; U5CB: buccal cusp of tooth 15 and tooth 25; U6MB: mesial buccal cusp of tooth 16 and tooth 26; U6CB: buccal groove at the buccal and occlusal surface interface of tooth 16 and tooth 26; U6DB: distal buccal cusp of tooth 16 and tooth 26; U7MB: mesial buccal cusp of tooth 17 and tooth 27; U7CB: buccal groove at the buccal and occlusal surface interface of tooth 17 and tooth 27; U7DB: distal buccal cusp of tooth 17 and tooth 27; L7DB: distal buccal cusp of tooth 37 and tooth 47; L7CB: buccal groove at the buccal and occlusal surface interface of tooth 37 and tooth 47; L7MB: mesial buccal cusp of tooth 37 and tooth 47; L6DB: distal buccal cusp of tooth 36 and tooth 46; L6CB: buccal groove at the buccal and occlusal surface interface of tooth 36 and tooth 46; L6MB: mesial buccal cusp of tooth 36 and tooth 46; L5CB: buccal cusp of tooth 35 and tooth 45; L4CB: buccal cusp of tooth 34 and tooth 44; L3CB: cusp tip of tooth 33 and tooth 43.

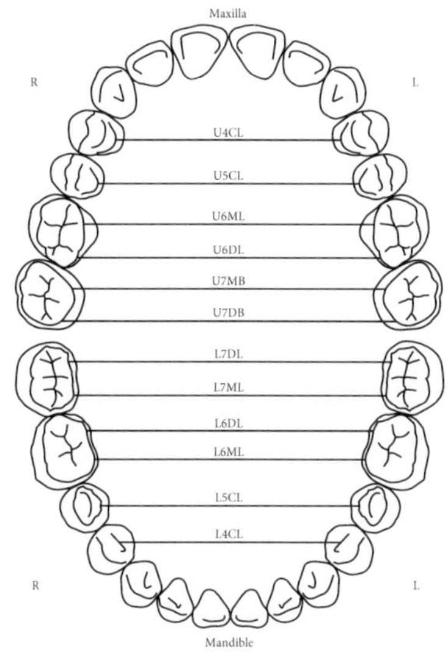

Figure 2: Illustration of the maxillary and mandibular arches' widths as described by Ling and Wong [9]. U4CL: palatal cusp of tooth 14 and tooth 24; U5CL: palatal cusp of tooth 15 and tooth 25; U6ML: mesial palatal cusp of tooth 16 and tooth 26; U6DL: distal palatal cusp of tooth 16 and tooth 26; U7MB: mesial buccal cusp of tooth 17 and tooth 27; U7DB: distal buccal cusp of tooth 17 and tooth 27; L7DL: distal palatal cusp of tooth 37 and tooth 47; L7ML: mesial lingual cusp of tooth 37 and tooth 47; L6DL: distal lingual cusp of tooth 36 and tooth 46; L6ML: mesial lingual cusp of tooth 36 and tooth 46; L5CL: lingual cusp of tooth 35 and tooth 45; L4CL: lingual cusp of tooth 34 and tooth 44.

FRP/2014/73 and IRB approval was obtained. Inclusion criteria were as follows:

(1) Saudi subjects over 18 years of age
(2) Class I canine and molar relationships
(3) Presence of all permanent teeth up to the second molars
(4) No previous orthodontic treatment or facial surgeries
(5) No more than mild crowding or spacing (<3 mm)
(6) No history of parafunctional oral habits
(7) No large restorations or crowns
(8) No tooth anomalies

Orthodontic models ($n = 169$; 73 males and 96 females) made of white stone in the orthodontic clinics were examined; those that satisfied the inclusion criteria were selected. Measurements of arch dimensions of the maxilla and mandible (width, length, and depth) were taken as described by Ling and Wong [9] and Al-Zubair [11]. Definitions and illustrations of all variables are shown in Figures 1–4 and Table 1. Two examiners took the measurements using a digital sliding caliper (Carrera Precision CP9806-TF, Max Tool LLC, Calif., USA).

3. Method Error

For the purpose of calibration, the two examiners took all the measurements on 20 dental models and then their measurements were compared.

3.1. Statistical Analysis. Independent sample t-test was used to determine any statistically significant differences between males and females for each measurement. Interclass correlation coefficient was used to determine interexaminer reliability. SPSS software was used for the statistical analysis (IBM SPSS Statistics for Mac, Version 24.0, IBM Corp., Armonk, NY).

4. Results

The sample consisted of 169 individuals (male: $n = 73$, aged 23.9 years ± 4.5; female: $n = 96$, aged 23.8 years ± 4.3). All results are shown in Tables 2–5. All maxillary and mandibular measurements showed statistically significant greater values for males compared to females (t-test; $P < 0.05$) except for U7ML, U4CB, U3CL, U3CB, U3MC, U2MC, L5CL, L5CG, L4CC, L4CB, L2MC, APL, PL, TPL, AML, ML, and PD (t-test; $P > 0.05$). Interexaminer reliability was high, ranging from 0.88 to 0.92 ($P < 0.05$).

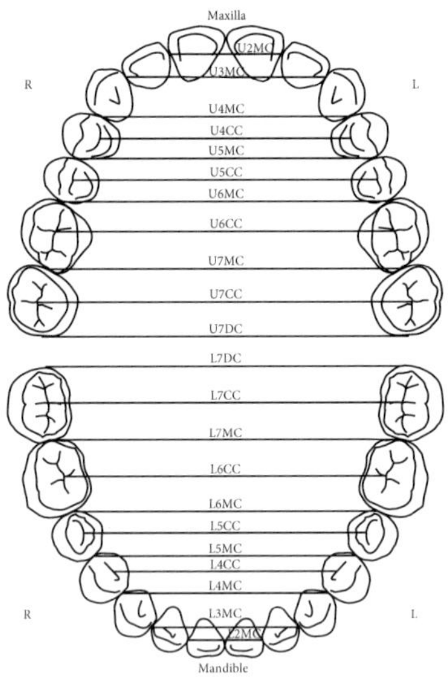

Figure 3: Illustration of the maxillary and mandibular arches' widths as described by Ling and Wong [9]. U2MC: contact points between tooth 11 and tooth 12 and tooth 21 and tooth 22; U3MC: contact points between tooth 12 and tooth 13 and tooth 22 and tooth 23; U4MC: contact points between tooth 13 and tooth 12 and tooth 23 and tooth 22; U4CC: central fossa of tooth 14 and tooth 24; U5MC: contact points between tooth 14 and tooth 15 and tooth 24 and tooth 25; U5CC: central fossa of tooth 15 and tooth 25; U6MC: contact points between tooth 15 and tooth 16 and tooth 25 and tooth 26; U5CC: central fossa of tooth 15 and tooth 25; U7MC: contact points between tooth 16 and tooth 17 and tooth 26 and tooth 27; U7CC: central fossa of tooth 17 and tooth 27; U7DC: estimated distal contact points between tooth 17 and tooth 18 and tooth 27 and tooth 28; L7DC: estimated distal contact points between tooth 37 and tooth 38 and tooth 47 and tooth 48; L7CC: central fossa of tooth 37 and tooth 47; L7MC: contact points between tooth 36 and tooth 37 and tooth 46 and tooth 47; L6CC: central fossa of tooth 36 and tooth 46; L6MC: contact points between tooth 35 and tooth 36 and tooth 45 and tooth 46; L5CC: central fossa of tooth 35 and tooth 45; L5MC: contact points between tooth 34 and tooth 35 and tooth 44 and tooth 45; L4CC: distal fossa of tooth 34 and tooth 44; L4MC: contact points between tooth 33 and tooth 34 and tooth 43 and tooth 44; L3MC: contact points between tooth 33 and tooth 32 and tooth 43 and tooth 44; L2MC: contact points between tooth 32 and tooth 31 and tooth 42 and tooth 41.

5. Discussion

In the present study, an effort was made to establish normal values for some parameters that have never been studied in Saudi. We chose to conduct measurements using many reference points described in the literature to allow for comparison with other populations' measurements [9, 11].

Comparison of intercanine widths among different populations showed small differences in Saudis between the present study and other studies and close measurements compared to Caucasians [20–22], while Southern Chinese showed the largest arch widths in the canine area (Table 6) [9].

Comparisons of the arch widths at the first molar showed a difference of about 1 mm between Saudis in our studies and Saudis in other studies. Southern Chinese were found to have the largest arch width followed by Saudis and then by Caucasians [9, 20] (Tables 7 and 8).

Maxillary arch length was found to be larger in Saudis compared to Yemenis in all measurements, while palatal depth slightly larger in Yemenis compared to Saudis [11] (Table 9).

The measurements established in the present study can serve as a database to which, orthodontic treatment of Saudi adults can be planned. Limitations of this study include a relatively small sample and that the study was confined to Riyadh City.

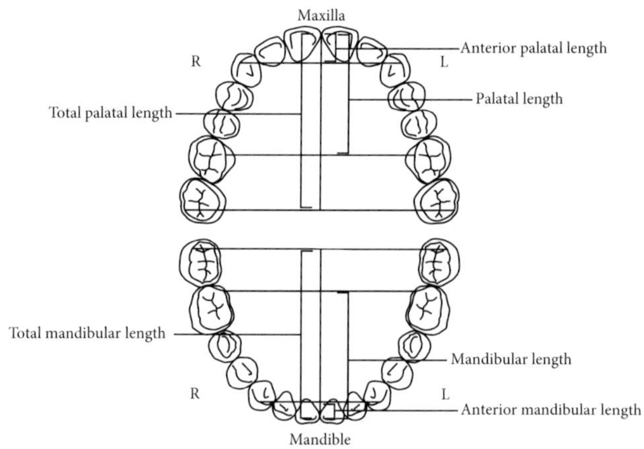

Figure 4: Illustration of the maxillary and mandibular arches' lengths as described by Al-Zubair [11]. Anterior palatal length: the vertical distance from the incisal point to the intercanine distance line; molar vertical distance (palatal length): the vertical distance from the incisal point perpendicular to a line between the mesial lingual cusp tips of the first molars; total palatal length: the vertical distance from the incisal point to the midpoint of a line between the distal buccal cusp tips of the second molars; anterior mandibular length: the vertical distance from the incisal point to the intercanine distance line; molar vertical distance (mandibular length): the vertical distance from the incisal point perpendicular to a line between the mesial lingual cusp tips of the first molar; total mandibular length: the vertical distance from the incisal point to the midpoint of a line between the distal buccal cusp tips of the second molar.

Table 1: Definitions of palatal depth as described by Al-Zubair [11].

Measurement	Definition
Palatal depth	The vertical distance from a point on the palatal width line to the palatal vault in the midline at the mesial palatal cups of 1st molars

6. Conclusions

(i) This study serves the purpose of establishing a database for arch dimensions for Saudi adult population.

(ii) Comparisons between Saudis and other populations showed differences in intercanine width, intermolar width, and palatal length and depth.

(iii) Males and females showed statistically significant differences in most of the measurements where males had larger measured values.

Table 2: Upper and lower molar measurements including independent sample t-tests comparing males to females.

Abbreviation	Gender	n	Mean	Standard error of mean	Standard deviation	Minimum	Maximum	Significance (2-tailed)	Significance	Mean difference	Standard error difference	95% confidence interval of the difference	
												Lower	Upper
Upper molars													
U7CC	M	73	50.69	0.31	2.66	45.81	57.80	0.000	***	1.70	0.42	0.88	2.53
	F	96	48.98	0.28	2.70	44.49	54.71						
U7ML	M	73	44.33	0.71	6.09	5.59	53.17	0.230	NS	1.00	0.83	−0.64	2.64
	F	96	43.33	0.48	4.72	4.87	49.44						
U7MG	M	73	39.98	0.48	4.07	20.93	50.92	0.026	*	1.25	0.56	0.15	2.35
	F	96	38.73	0.32	3.16	30.76	47.38						
U7DL	M	73	46.77	0.41	3.52	40.49	58.30	0.001	**	1.65	0.50	0.66	2.64
	F	96	45.12	0.30	2.98	40.46	52.25						
U7DC	M	73	51.23	0.43	3.69	45.50	64.89	0.000	***	1.86	0.51	0.85	2.86
	F	96	49.38	0.30	2.93	45.05	56.57						
U7DB	M	73	57.98	0.32	2.75	53.12	64.31	0.001	**	1.77	0.51	0.76	2.78
	F	96	56.22	0.37	3.65	51.07	72.79						
U7CB	M	73	57.43	0.33	2.84	52.43	64.54	0.000	***	2.14	0.46	1.24	3.04
	F	96	55.29	0.31	3.01	50.26	62.33						
U7MB	M	73	56.68	0.33	2.80	51.57	63.35	0.000	***	1.63	0.45	0.74	2.52
	F	96	55.05	0.30	2.98	49.46	61.95						
U7MC	M	73	49.16	0.44	3.75	43.97	58.63	0.000	***	2.69	0.53	1.63	3.74
	F	96	46.47	0.32	3.18	38.26	58.10						
U6CC	F	73	45.38	0.34	2.90	39.96	52.32	0.000	***	1.97	0.49	1.00	2.93
	M	96	43.42	0.34	3.32	38.25	53.58						
U6ML	M	73	39.49	0.34	2.87	33.65	46.72	0.000	***	1.91	0.51	0.90	2.92
	F	96	37.58	0.36	3.57	27.81	47.94						
U6MG	M	73	33.80	0.33	2.83	23.12	40.58	0.000	***	1.66	0.46	0.76	2.57
	F	96	32.14	0.31	3.05	27.54	40.58						
U6DL	M	73	41.70	0.35	2.95	36.41	49.31	0.001	**	1.73	0.49	0.76	2.71
	F	96	39.97	0.34	3.35	32.26	53.72						
U6DB	M	73	53.25	0.33	2.80	48.97	61.95	0.000	***	2.02	0.48	1.07	2.97
	F	96	51.23	0.34	3.30	41.35	58.26						
U6CB	M	73	52.10	0.31	2.61	45.87	59.11	0.000	***	2.02	0.44	1.14	2.89
	F	96	50.09	0.31	3.03	42.51	56.82						
U6MB	M	73	51.03	0.36	3.08	36.44	56.78	0.000	***	1.83	0.48	0.88	2.77
	F	96	49.21	0.31	3.06	44.25	56.51						
U6MC	M	73	43.21	0.32	2.75	37.66	49.38	0.000	***	1.75	0.43	0.90	2.60
	F	96	41.45	0.29	2.79	35.96	47.88						

Table 2: Continued.

Abbreviation	Gender	n	Mean	Standard error of mean	Standard deviation	Minimum	Maximum	Significance (2-tailed)	Significance	Mean difference	Standard error difference	95% confidence interval of the difference	
												Lower	Upper
Lower molars													
U6MC	M	73	43.21	0.32	2.75	37.66	49.38	0.000	***	1.75	0.43	0.90	2.60
	F	96	41.45	0.29	2.79	35.96	47.88						
L7CC	M	73	46.82	0.35	2.97	40.78	55.16	0.000	***	2.19	0.44	1.32	3.06
	F	96	44.63	0.28	2.72	39.90	51.71						
L7DL	M	73	43.18	0.37	3.13	36.28	49.91	0.000	***	2.68	0.43	1.83	3.52
	F	96	40.51	0.25	2.44	35.64	45.60						
L7DG	M	73	40.24	0.31	2.63	33.31	45.58	0.000	***	2.34	0.39	1.57	3.11
	F	96	37.90	0.25	2.41	32.95	43.49						
L7ML	M	73	39.87	0.32	2.77	34.60	44.37	0.000	***	1.84	0.40	1.04	2.63
	F	96	38.04	0.25	2.45	33.00	42.89						
L7MC	M	73	44.25	0.32	2.73	39.50	49.42	0.000	***	2.19	0.42	1.37	3.02
	F	96	42.06	0.27	2.64	37.93	48.76						
L7CB	M	73	50.60	0.42	3.56	34.14	56.56	0.000	***	2.44	0.55	1.35	3.52
	F	96	48.17	0.36	3.51	39.37	56.24						
L7DB	M	73	53.32	0.45	3.83	36.10	60.00	0.000	***	2.73	0.58	1.58	3.87
	F	96	50.59	0.38	3.68	40.55	58.40						
L7DC	M	73	49.66	0.39	3.29	42.53	57.21	0.000	***	2.89	0.49	1.92	3.86
	F	96	46.77	0.31	3.05	40.49	53.48						
L6CC	M	73	41.54	0.42	3.61	35.80	53.53	0.000	***	2.03	0.57	0.91	3.14
	F	96	39.51	0.37	3.67	34.75	53.83						
L6ML	M	73	34.72	0.42	3.55	29.52	45.74	0.000	***	2.13	0.50	1.14	3.12
	F	96	32.59	0.30	2.95	28.03	44.83						
L6MG	M	73	32.21	0.32	2.77	27.60	37.79	0.000	***	2.21	0.43	1.36	3.05
	F	96	30.00	0.28	2.75	25.52	37.62						
L6MC	M	73	38.28	0.33	2.82	32.98	43.51	0.025	*	1.07	0.47	0.14	2.00
	F	96	37.21	0.33	3.19	31.49	46.71						
L6MB	M	73	44.81	0.39	3.32	30.14	50.37	0.019	*	1.15	0.48	0.19	2.10
	F	96	43.67	0.30	2.97	38.57	49.81						
L6CB	M	73	46.94	0.29	2.46	42.40	52.24	0.000	***	1.75	0.47	0.81	2.69
	F	96	45.53	0.38	3.69	33.21	51.72						
L6DB	M	73	47.88	0.46	3.92	33.84	54.07	0.000	***	2.34	0.59	1.18	3.51
	F	96	34.44	0.31	3.09	28.62	46.46						

NS: not significant; $^{*}P < 0.05$, $^{**}P < 0.01$, and $^{***}P < 0.001$.

Table 3: Upper and lower premolars' measurements including independent sample t-tests comparing males to females.

Abbreviation	Gender	n	Mean	Standard error of mean	Standard deviation	Minimum	Maximum	Significance (2-tailed)	Significance	Mean difference	Standard error difference	95% confidence interval of the difference	
												Lower	Upper
Upper premolars													
U5CC	M	73	40.53	0.35	2.96	35.43	47.98	0.005	**	1.56	0.55	0.48	2.63
	F	96	38.97	0.40	3.88	32.01	50.58						
U5CL	M	73	35.92	0.40	3.43	29.70	50.04	0.000	***	2.17	0.54	1.11	3.23
	F	96	33.75	0.36	3.48	25.50	40.34						
U5CG	M	73	32.07	0.34	2.93	25.91	38.19	0.005	**	1.59	0.56	0.49	2.69
	F	96	30.48	0.41	4.03	22.86	46.14						
U5CB	M	73	46.41	0.42	3.60	37.85	53.83	0.002	**	1.73	0.55	0.64	2.82
	F	96	44.68	0.36	3.53	37.24	51.11						
U5MC	M	73	38.78	0.34	2.94	32.49	45.35	0.000	***	1.73	0.46	0.83	2.63
	F	96	37.05	0.30	2.95	31.74	43.31						
U4MC	M	73	35.74	0.38	3.21	29.66	43.44	0.003	**	1.46	0.49	0.49	2.42
	F	96	34.28	0.25	3.10	28.94	40.86						
U4CL	M	73	30.99	0.40	3.40	25.77	38.91	0.024	*	1.22	0.53	0.16	2.27
	F	96	29.78	0.35	3.47	23.81	39.89						
U4CG	M	73	27.84	0.37	3.12	20.85	34.27	0.000	***	1.72	0.48	0.78	2.66
	F	96	26.12	0.31	3.02	19.54	32.87						
U4CB	M	73	41.06	0.55	4.72	14.36	49.59	0.278	NS	0.71	0.65	−0.58	1.99
	F	96	40.35	0.38	3.72	27.66	48.53						
U4MC	M	73	34.57	0.35	2.96	26.37	39.45	0.032	*	1.05	0.48	0.09	2.00
	F	96	33.53	0.33	3.23	25.41	40.55						
Lower premolars													
L5CC	M	73	36.08	0.44	3.78	27.98	50.75	0.002	**	1.64	0.53	0.60	2.68
	F	96	34.44	0.31	3.09	28.62	46.46						
L5CL	M	73	31.32	0.34	2.92	26.34	37.48	0.142	NS	0.74	0.50	-0.25	1.74
	F	96	30.58	0.35	3.47	25.62	45.87						
L5CG	M	73	29.74	0.37	3.16	24.87	38.55	0.606	NS	0.57	1.10	-1.61	2.75
	F	96	29.17	0.92	9.00	23.42	87.64						
L5MC	M	73	34.87	0.33	2.81	30.90	43.34	0.028	*	1.00	0.45	0.11	1.90
	F	96	33.86	0.30	2.99	27.51	44.70						
L5CB	M	73	40.05	0.39	3.32	29.80	46.50	0.013	*	1.37	0.54	0.29	2.44
	F	96	38.68	0.37	3.65	30.26	44.74						
L4CC	M	73	31.23	0.29	2.49	24.89	36.53	0.102	NS	0.66	0.40	-0.13	1.46
	F	96	30.57	0.27	2.67	24.82	37.16						
L4MC	M	73	27.87	0.28	2.41	23.33	33.49	0.005	**	1.06	0.37	0.32	1.79
	F	96	26.81	0.24	2.38	21.86	31.37						
L4CG	M	73	26.55	0.36	3.05	22.28	37.35	0.012	*	1.21	0.48	0.26	2.16
	F	96	25.34	0.32	3.10	19.79	35.15						
L4CB	M	73	34.02	0.39	3.34	24.08	41.57	0.629	NS	0.22	0.46	-0.69	1.14
	F	96	33.79	0.27	2.69	25.46	38.68						
L4MC	M	73	29.14	0.33	2.82	20.60	37.62	0.031	*	0.77	0.35	0.07	1.47
	F	96	28.37	0.18	1.77	24.31	31.41						

NS: not significant; $^{*}P < 0.05$, $^{**}P < 0.01$, and $^{***}P < 0.001$.

TABLE 4: Upper and lower anterior teeth measurements including independent sample t-tests comparing males to females.

Abbreviation	Gender	n	Mean	Standard error of mean	Standard deviation	Minimum	Maximum	Significance (2-tailed)	Significance	Mean difference	Standard error difference	95% confidence interval of the difference	
												Lower	Upper
Upper anterior teeth													
U3CL	M	73	25.95	0.29	2.44	21.79	31.23	0.147	NS	0.70	0.48	−0.25	1.65
	F	96	25.25	0.36	3.51	16.23	36.92						
U3CB	M	73	33.88	0.29	2.47	26.76	39.67	0.680	NS	0.17	0.41	−0.64	0.97
	F	96	33.71	0.28	2.74	28.92	41.78						
U3MC	M	73	27.40	0.27	2.31	22.46	34.49	0.649	NS	−0.31	0.67	−1.63	1.02
	F	96	27.70	0.55	5.35	19.94	57.25						
U2MC	M	73	16.81	0.12	1.04	14.55	19.12	0.886	NS	0.05	0.37	−0.68	0.79
	F	96	16.76	0.31	3.05	12.26	42.73						
Lower anterior teeth													
L3CG	M	73	21.76	0.30	2.55	17.02	31.93	0.000	***	1.33	0.34	0.66	2.00
	F	96	26.73	0.26	2.19	22.46	33.15						
L3CB	M	73	26.73	0.26	2.19	22.46	33.15	0.031	*	0.71	0.33	0.06	1.35
	F	96	26.02	0.21	2.03	20.96	29.94						
L3MC	M	73	21.45	0.15	1.32	18.74	25.31	0.007	**	0.59	0.22	0.16	1.01
	F	96	20.86	0.15	1.44	16.47	22.99						
L2MC	M	73	10.81	0.11	0.95	9.18	13.11	0.090	NS	0.23	0.14	−0.04	0.50
	F	96	10.58	0.08	0.81	8.70	12.40						

NS: not significant; $^{*}P < 0.05$, $^{**}P < 0.01$, and $^{***}P < 0.001$.

Table 5: Anterior palatal length (APL), palatal length (PL), total palatal length (TPL), anterior mandibular length (AML), mandibular length (ML), total mandibular length (TML), and palatal depth (PD) measurements including independent sample *t*-tests comparing males to females.

Abbreviation	Gender	n	Mean	Standard error of mean	Standard deviation	Minimum	Maximum	Significance (2-tailed)	Significance	Mean difference	Standard error difference	95% confidence interval of the difference	
												Lower	Upper
APL	M	73	11.10	0.96	8.16	5.95	78.60	0.134	NS	1.28	0.85	−0.40	2.97
	F	96	9.82	0.16	1.59	6.78	14.67						
PL	M	73	31.98	0.56	4.75	2.91	53.11	0.107	NS	0.94	0.58	−0.21	2.08
	F	96	31.04	0.28	2.72	22.91	38.26						
TPL	M	73	44.42	0.63	5.34	5.03	51.73	0.182	NS	0.87	0.65	−0.41	2.16
	F	96	43.55	0.31	3.04	34.31	50.12						
AML	M	73	6.27	0.13	1.14	3.52	8.75	0.276	NS	0.20	0.18	−0.16	0.56
	F	96	6.07	0.12	1.20	3.60	10.52						
ML	M	73	26.10	0.25	2.14	20.95	30.23	0.587	NS	0.22	0.41	−0.58	1.03
	F	96	25.88	0.30	2.95	20.94	48.42						
TML	M	73	40.76	0.64	5.50	4.75	52.60	0.014	*	1.71	0.69	0.35	3.07
	F	96	39.05	0.35	3.44	15.31	47.82						
PD	M	73	20.90	0.24	2.08	15.02	24.21	0.264	NS	0.36	0.32	−0.28	1.00
	F	96	20.54	0.21	2.09	14.72	24.80						

NS: not significant; $^{*}P < 0.05$.

Table 6: Comparison of intercanine (upper canine cusp to cusp) widths between Saudis (different studies), Caucasians, and Southern Chinese.

Population	Males				Females			
	n	Mean	SE	SD	*n*	Mean	SE	SD
Saudis (present study)	73	33.88	0.29	2.47	96	33.71	0.28	2.74
Saudis [22]	60	33.9	—	2.29	60	32.58	—	2.58
Saudis [21]	71	35.43	—	1.6	68	33.69	—	1
Caucasians [20]	60	34.05	—	2.1	83	32.77	—	2.2
Southern Chinese [9]	166	36.92	0.23	2.9	124	35.09	0.32	3.5

n, number; SE, standard error; SD, standard deviation.

Table 7: Comparison of intermolar (upper first molar central fossa to central fossa) widths between Saudis (different studies).

Population	Males				Females			
	n	Mean	SE	SD	*n*	Mean	SE	SD
Saudis (present study)	73	45.38	0.34	2.9	96	43.42	0.34	3.32
Saudis [21]	60	46.38	—	3.24	60	44.29	—	3.03

n, number; SE, standard error; SD, standard deviation.

Table 8: Comparison of intermolar (upper first molar distal buccal cusp to distal buccal cusp) widths between Saudis, Caucasians, and Southern Chinese.

Population	Males				Females			
	n	Mean	SE	SD	*n*	Mean	SE	SD
Saudis (present study)	73	53.25	0.33	2.8	96	51.23	0.34	3.3
Caucasians [20]	56	45.59	—	2.5	77	44.28	—	2.1
Southern Chinese [9]	209	56.17	0.19	2.8	130	54.15	0.22	2.6

n, number; SE, standard error; SD, standard deviation.

Table 9: Comparisons of maxillary arch length and depth between Saudis and Yemenis.

Population	Males				Females			
	n	Mean	SE	SD	*n*	Mean	SE	SD
Anterior palatal length								
Saudis (present study)	73	11.1	0.96	8.16	96	9.82	0.16	1.59
Yemenis [11]	113	8.88	—	1.08	101	8.54	—	1.35
Palatal length								
Saudis (present study)	73	31.98	0.56	4.75	96	31.04	0.28	2.72
Yemenis [11]	113	29.71	—	2.02	113	30.39	—	2.12
Total palatal length								
Saudis (present study)	73	44.42	0.63	5.34	96	43.55	0.31	3.04
Yemenis [11]	113	42.62	—	2.32	101	42.3	—	2.43
Palatal depth								
Saudis (present study)	73	20.90	0.24	2.08	96	20.54	0.21	2.09
Yemenis [11]	113	21.17	—	1.51	101	20.71	—	1.39

n, number; SE, standard error; SD, standard deviation.

References

[1] T. R. Hart, R. R. J. Cousley, L. S. Fishman, and R. H. Tallents, "Dentoskeletal changes following mini-implant molar intrusion in anterior open bite patients," *The Angle Orthodontist*, vol. 85, no. 6, pp. 941–948, 2015.

[2] D. P. Singh, A. K. Garg, S. P. Singh, U. S. Krishna Nayak, and M. Gupta, "Comparison of the dental arch changes in patients with different malocclusions," *Indian Journal of Dental Research*, vol. 25, no. 5, pp. 623–629, 2014.

[3] A. Ugolini, C. Cerruto, L. Di Vece et al., "Dental arch response to Haas-type rapid maxillary expansion anchored to deciduous vs permanent molars: a multicentric randomized controlled trial," *The Angle Orthodontist*, vol. 85, no. 4, pp. 570–576, 2015.

[4] T. U. Taner, S. Ciğer, H. El, D. Germeç, and A. Es, "Evaluation of dental arch width and form changes after orthodontic treatment and retention with a new computerized method," *American Journal of Orthodontics and Dentofacial Orthopedics*, vol. 126, no. 4, pp. 464–475, 2004.

[5] X. Hua, H. Xiong, G. Han, and X. Cheng, "Correction of a dental arch-width asymmetric discrepancy with a slow maxillary contraction appliance," *American Journal of Orthodontics and Dentofacial Orthopedics*, vol. 142, no. 6, pp. 842–853, 2012.

[6] A. Lundstrom, "An investigation of 202 pairs of twins regarding fundamental factors in the aetiology of malocclusion," *The Dental Record*, vol. 69, no. 10, pp. 251–264, 1949.

[7] H. V. Meredith and G. C. Cox, "Widths of the dental arches at the permanent first molars in children 9 years of age," *American Journal of Orthodontics*, vol. 40, no. 2, pp. 134–144, 1954.

[8] G. Heithersay, "Further observations on the dentition of the Australian aborigine at Haast's Bluff," *Australian Dental Journal*, vol. 6, no. 1, pp. 18–28, 1961.

[9] J. Y. K. Ling and R. W. K. Wong, "Dental arch widths of Southern Chinese," *The Angle Orthodontist*, vol. 79, no. 1, pp. 54–63, 2009.

[10] I. A. Aluko, O. O. DaCosta, and M. C. Isiekwe, "Dental arch widths in the early and late permanent dentitions of a Nigerian population," *Nigerian Dental Journal*, vol. 17, no. 1, 2009.

[11] N. M. Al-Zubair, "Determinant factors of Yemeni maxillary arch dimensions," *Saudi Dental Journal*, vol. 27, no. 1, pp. 50–54, 2015.

[12] D. E. Ward, J. Workman, R. Brown, and S. Richmond, "Changes in arch width: a 20-year longitudinal study of orthodontic treatment," *The Angle Orthodontist*, vol. 76, no. 1, pp. 6–13, 2006.

[13] R. A. McWade, A. H. Mamandras, and W. S. Hunter, "The effects of Fränkel II treatment on arch width and arch perimeter," *American Journal of Orthodontics and Dentofacial Orthopedics*, vol. 92, no. 4, pp. 313–320, 1987.

[14] P. J. Mack, "Maxillary arch and central incisor dimensions in a Nigerian and British population sample," *Journal of Dentistry*, vol. 9, no. 1, pp. 67–70, 1981.

[15] E. S. J. Abu Alhaija and M. A. Qudeimat, "Occlusion and tooth/arch dimensions in the primary dentition of preschool Jordanian children," *International Journal of Paediatric Dentistry*, vol. 13, no. 4, pp. 230–239, 2003.

[16] K. Tsujino and Y. Machida, "A longitudinal study of the growth and development of the dental arch width from childhood to adolescence in Japanese," *The Bulletin of Tokyo Dental College*, vol. 39, no. 2, pp. 75–89, 1998.

[17] H. Noroozi and R. Saeeda, "Interrelationships between the width, depth, and perimeter of the dental arch," *The International Journal of Adult Orthodontics and Orthognathic Surgery*, vol. 15, no. 1, pp. 69–71, 2000.

[18] T. M. Walkow and S. Peck, "Dental arch width in Class II Division 2 deep-bite malocclusion," *American Journal of Orthodontics and Dentofacial Orthopedics*, vol. 122, no. 6, pp. 608–613, 2002.

[19] K. Heikinheimo, M. Nystrom, T. Heikinheimo, P. Pirttiniemi, and S. Pirinen, "Dental arch width, overbite, and overjet in a Finnish population with normal occlusion between the ages of 7 and 32 years," *The European Journal of Orthodontics*, vol. 34, no. 4, pp. 418–426, 2012.

[20] F. Van der Linden, H. Boersma, T. Zelders, K. A. Peters, and J. H. Raaben, "Three-dimensional analysis of dental casts by means of the optocom," *Journal of Dental Research*, vol. 51, no. 4, p. 1100, 1972.

[21] H. A. Hashim and S. Al-Ghamdi, "Tooth width and arch dimensions in normal and malocclusion samples: an odontometric study," *The Journal of Contemporary Dental Practice*, vol. 6, no. 2, pp. 36–51, 2005.

[22] S. Abd-el Samad Younes, "Maxillary arch dimensions in Saudi and Egyptian population sample," *American Journal of Orthodontics*, vol. 85, no. 1, pp. 83–88, 1984.

Oral Hygiene Practices among Saudi Arabian Children and Its Relation to Their Dental Caries Status

M. F. A. Quadri,[1] M. A. Shubayr,[2] A. H. Hattan,[2] S. A. Wafi,[2] and A. H. Jafer[3]

[1]*Dental Public Health, Jazan University, Jizan, Saudi Arabia*
[2]*Department of Preventive Dentistry, Jazan University, Jizan, Saudi Arabia*
[3]*Ministry of Health, Riyadh, Saudi Arabia*

Correspondence should be addressed to M. F. A. Quadri; dr.faeq.quadri@gmail.com

Academic Editor: Andrea Scribante

Dental caries is one of the most common preventable diseases occurring among children. The aim here is to survey the oral hygiene practices that are commonly followed by Arab children and to see its relationship with their dental caries status. A cross-sectional study with multistage random sampling technique was conducted. Sociodemographic data and information on oral hygiene practices like use of toothbrush, dental floss, siwak, frequency of brushing along with number of snack between meals per day, and consumption of sugar per day was obtained. Presence of plaque on tooth surfaces was reported using plaque index, which was followed by DMFT index to determine the dental caries status. Among the sample of 500 school children, the mean plaque score in male (mean = 0.69; SD = 0.50) was slightly higher than the female (mean = 0.66; SD = 0.46). Increased frequency of snacks ($P = 0.05$; $ß = 0.08$; CI = −0.00, 0.09) and sugar consumption ($P = 0.01$; $ß = 0.16$; CI = 0.04, 0.27) per day significantly showed higher values of DMFT. Also, the odds of dental caries among the school children who were irregular in brushing their teeth was higher in contrast to the children brushing once ($P = 0.03$; OR = 0.89; CI = 0.70, 1.12) or twice ($P = 0.03$; OR = 0.80; CI = 0.64, 0.93) per day. It is recommended that the dental public health practitioners here should consider the effect of oral hygiene practices on oral health status in order to design the future health promotion interventions.

1. Background

Oral health is linked with general health, and diseases occurring in oral cavity are of major public health importance due to their high prevalence and tremendous social impact [1]. Oral diseases in children are reported to affect their everyday activities both at school and at home. Moreover, the psychosocial impact of these diseases often diminishes their quality of life [2]. Dental caries and periodontal diseases are the most frequently diagnosed oral diseases in young individuals [3]. Good oral hygiene practices are recommended by specialists for preventing these oral diseases [4, 5], and studies conducted earlier have reported poor oral hygiene among children to be associated with the onset of dental caries [6–10]. There are also reports which specifically say that brushing twice daily is important in preventing teeth caries [6]. Apart from brushing, the complete concept of oral hygiene like frequency and duration of brushing; time of brushing; flossing; and so on should be studied and improved among individuals of different age groups and also in different parts of the world [11]. For instance, a study conducted in Nigeria portrayed that immediate teeth cleaning after sweet food or beverage consumption decreases the risk of dental caries [12]. Furthermore, it is also reported that fluoride-containing tooth pastes provide a better check on caries when compared to nonfluoridated tooth pastes [11, 13]. Thus, there are many factors that contribute to oral hygiene practices. Likewise, even for initial plaque formation on the teeth of children, factors such as poor diet, improper brushing, and no flossing contributed actively [14].

In Saudi Arabia, the prevalence of dental caries among children ranges from medium to high as stated in the World Oral Health report [14]. Some region-based studies in Saudi Arabia had also indicated high prevalence of dental caries among school going children [15–17]. We assume that there may be variances in the practices of oral hygiene among the population residing in different sectors of the world specially attributed to their culture and beliefs. One example could be the use of siwak (miswak); which is a name given by Arabs alternatively for chewing stick (*Salvadora persica*) [18]. Knowing about oral hygiene practices of children among Arab regions like that of Saudi Arabia will aid in proper design and implementation of oral health promotion programs, thus reducing the prevalence of oral diseases. Gizan, a province of Saudi Arabia is reported with high prevalence of dental caries among school-aged children [16], but there are very less published researches to explain the contributory risk factors. Due to the scarcity of data in this region, proper prevention programs by the department of dental public health at Jazan University and various other governmental authorities are difficult to implement. Hence, the aim here is to survey the oral hygiene practices that are commonly followed by Arab children residing in Gizan region of Saudi Arabia and to see its relationship with their dental caries status.

2. Materials and Methods

2.1. Ethical Consideration. Permission from the research committee at college of dentistry, Jazan University was obtained. This was followed by the permission from the regional education office to approach the schools. An informed consent was also taken from parents for the participation of their children in the current study.

2.2. Study Setting and Population. The study was conducted in Gizan, which is located at the southern tip of Saudi Arabia bordering Yemen. Six different schools and a dental camp organized at a public place were the sites for data collection. Only Saudi Arabian children aged 12 and 13 years were included to maintain the homogeneity of the study population.

2.3. Study Design and Sample Size. A cross-sectional study with multistage random sampling technique was conducted in the year 2016. Size of the sample was calculated ($N = 500$) with an absolute precision of 0.05, expected proportion of 0.5, and an estimated design effect of 1 [16]. A complete list of schools was obtained from the Ministry of Education, and in the first stage of sampling, out of four districts (Sabya, Jazan city, Abu Arish, and Samtha) in the Gizan region, three were selected (Jazan city, Sabya, and Abu Arish). In the second stage, six schools (three male and three female schools) were randomly selected from the aforementioned areas. The third stage involved simple random selection of high school pupils from both male and female schools using their national identification numbers. To reach the calculated sample size, children attending the annual dental camp were also targeted, and national identification numbers were matched to avoid duplication of the data.

2.4. Variables Assessed

2.4.1. Oral Hygiene Practices. Oral hygiene information was collected using a predesigned and prevalidated questionnaire. This self-reported structured questionnaire included the following variables: (i) use of toothbrush, (ii) dental floss, (iii) siwak (Miswak), (iv) frequency of brushing, (v) number of snack between meals per day, (vi) consumption of sugar, and (vii) number of meals per day. The questionnaire was originally formulated in English and then translated into Arabic, and prior to the survey, pretests took place to control reliability and validity (ICC = 0.77) of the questions. Information on demographic details such as age, gender, parent's education, and parent's employment status were self-reported.

2.4.2. Clinical Examination. Clinical examination was conducted by pretrained and precalibrated (interrater = 0.98 and intrarater = 0.98) fours graduating dentists. Dental caries status of the school children was determined using DMFT and plaque indices [1]. The procedure involved careful quadrant by quadrant examination and recording of the findings. One class room in each school was dedicated for examination, where the child was given an ordinary chair to sit, and the examiner embraced the standing position for diagnosis. Each examiner was provided with an assistant to manually record the findings on dedicated questionnaires. Standard infection control practices were maintained, and disposable diagnostic set of instruments were used under the normal light. As recommended by WHO, a decay in tooth was considered if the cavitation stage has been reached, while teeth extracted for reasons other than caries were not considered as missing.

2.5. Statistical Analysis. Recorded data were checked for missing values and normality distribution. Obtained values were either summarized as means ± SD or percentages. Correlation between oral hygiene practice and oral health status was tested by determining the correlation values. Initially, bivariate analysis and later, multivariate analysis (negative binomial regression) after adjusting for confounders were performed to comment on the relation between the oral hygiene and oral health status. All the data entry and analysis were done using SPSS (IBM, USA) version 24.

3. Results

The study sample comprised of 500 (N) 12- and 13-year-old school going children, in which male and female were of equal proportion (50%). There was no gender difference in the demographic data evaluated in the current study (Table 1). The overall mean plaque score was observed to be on a higher side. With regards to location, there was no statistical variation between the plaque score among school children residing in the urban (mean = 0.66; SD = 0.33) or the rural (mean = 0.67; SD = 0.39) areas. Whereas in terms of gender, the mean plaque score in male school children (mean = 0.69; SD = 0.50) was slightly higher than the female school children (mean = 0.66; SD = 0.46). Also, the plaque score in the 13-year-olds (mean = 0.69; SD = 0.44) was slightly higher than the 12-year-olds (mean = 0.60; SD = 0.36) (Table 2).

Table 1: Gender variation in the demographic characteristics.

Variable*	Gender Male	Gender Female	Total
Age			
12-year-old	137 (49%)	138 (51%)	275 (55%)
13-year-old	112 (49%)	113 (51%)	225 (45%)
Location			
Urban	215 (43.0%)	233 (46.5%)	448 (89.5%)
Rural	15 (3.0%)	38 (7.5%)	53 (10.5%)
Father's education			
No formal schooling	3 (0.5%)	3 (0.5%)	5 (1%)
Primary school	15 (3.0%)	3 (0.5%)	18 (3.5%)
Secondary school	8 (1.5%)	13 (2.5%)	20 (4%)
High school	63 (12.5%)	78 (15.5%)	140 (28%)
University	143 (28.5%)	175 (35.0%)	318 (63.5%)
Mother's education			
No formal schooling	3 (0.5%)	3 (0.5%)	5 (1%)
Primary school	13 (2.5%)	18 (3.5%)	30 (6%)
Secondary school	3 (0.5%)	13 (2.5%)	15 (3%)
High school	40 (8.0%)	60 (12.0%)	100 (20%)
University	173 (34.5%)	178 (35.5%)	350 (70%)
Mother occupation			
Full time	75 (15.0%)	93 (18.5%)	168 (33.5%)
Part time	25 (5.0%)	13 (2.5%)	38 (7.5%)
House maker	130 (26.0%)	165 (33.0%)	295 (59%)

*Gender differentiation was not statistically significant.

Table 2: Mean plaque score (OHI-S), by age, gender, and location.

Variable	N (%)	Plaque mean (SD)
Age		
12-year-old	275 (55)	0.60 (0.36)
13-year-old	225 (45)	0.69 (0.44)
Gender$		
Male	250 (50)	0.69 (0.50)
Female	250 (50)	0.66 (0.46)
Location$		
Urban	338 (67.5)	0.66 (0.33)
Rural	163 (32.5)	0.67 (0.39)

$No significant difference in the mean plaque score.

Bivariate analysis revealed that oral hygiene habits, such as use of miswak (stick), flossing, and brushing, had strong negative relation with plaque formation. It is also observed that the children who brushed once daily (mean = 0.64; $ß = -0.10$; CI = −0.16, −0.04) had higher plaque formation than the children who brushed twice daily (mean = 0.62; $ß = -0.11$; CI = −0.18, −0.04) (Table 3). On analyzing mean DMFT against dietary habits, a strong correlation between frequency of eating, number of snack between meals, and sugar consumption per day was observed. It suggested that increased frequency of snacks ($P = 0.05$; $ß = 0.08$; CI = −0.00, 0.09) and sugar consumption ($P = 0.01$; $ß = 0.16$; CI = 0.04, 0.27) among children per day significantly showed higher values of DMFT (Table 4).

Multivariate analysis was performed to check the effect of various independent variables on plaque and DMFT scores. It revealed that 13-year-old children had higher odds of plaque formation in comparison to 12-year-olds ($P = 0.05$; OR = 0.06; CI = −0.00, 0.12). Also, plaque formation was more in the school children who were irregular in brushing their teeth in comparison to one-time brushers ($P = 0.00$; OR = −0.06; CI = −0.14, 0.00) and two-time brushers ($P = 0.00$; OR = −0.09; CI = −0.17, −0.00) per day (Table 5). Similarly, the odds of dental caries among the school children who were irregular in brushing their teeth were higher in contrast to the children brushing once ($P = 0.03$; OR = 0.89; CI = 0.70, 1.12) or twice ($P = 0.03$; OR = 0.80; CI = 0.64, 0.93) per day (Table 5).

4. Discussion

This cross-sectional study is first to determine the association between oral hygiene practices and oral health status among 12- and 13-year-old school children in Saudi Arabia. Researchers elsewhere have considered oral hygiene as a key factor associated with good oral health [4, 5, 19, 20], and in the current study, it is evident that both frequency of brushing and sugar consumption per day are significantly related to the oral health status of school children in Saudi Arabia.

Fewer gender differences were subject to identification in regards to various demographic items. Moreover, the study indicates that placing both genders at the identical educational level puts them at the same threshold of the oral health issues. Also, there is no considerable difference between boys and girls when it comes to the elements of oral health status. The overall DMFT score among the school children aged 12 and 13 years in Jazan region of Saudi Arabia was observed to be considerably high. This finding is in accordance with a recent systematic review which reported that the mean DMFT of 70% permanent dentition among school going children in Saudi Arabia is 3.5 [21]. In contrast to this, a school-based survey conducted in the neighboring Arab country revealed a mean DMFT of 0.42 among 12-year-olds [22].

The current study also portrayed that a large proportion of children (70%) were from urban areas while a small proportion (30%) were from rural settings. Authors presumed that the use of miswak or chewing stick would be a common practice among the Arab children and would be the only practice by those residing in the rural regions. However, this was not the case with the findings from the current study. Arguably, it could be stated that brushing is common for those children coming from urbanized centers, but this may not be true always as one study conducted among children residing in rural region of southern Saudi Arabia showed that children residing in both the rural as well as urban regions used tooth-brush along with miswak to clean their teeth [23]. It is also seen that a good percentage of children in the current study reported using toothbrush for cleaning their teeth in comparison to miswak, and this shows that there is a general awareness on oral hygiene among children in Jazan region of Saudi Arabia, but another study conducted in Al-Jouf region of Saudi Arabia reported otherwise [24]. However, to confirm the findings, there is a need to ensure that these self-administered reports are confirmed through various objective assessments.

TABLE 3: Mean plaque score and differences in scores by oral hygiene habits.

Oral hygiene habits	N (%)	Mean plaque score (SD)	Difference (95% CI)	P
Miswak	156 (31.2)	0.87 (0.5)	−0.09 (−0.17, −0.01)	0.04*
Flossing	51 (10.1)	0.64 (0.4)	−0.02 (−0.10, 0.05)	0.06
Brushing				
Irregular	135 (27)	0.75 (0.6)	0.00	0.02*
Once	158 (31.5)	0.64 (0.6)	−0.10 (−0.16, −0.04)	
Twice or more	208 (41.5)	0.62 (0.5)	−0.11 (−0.18, −0.04)	

*Significant relation between the mean plaque score and oral hygiene habit.

TABLE 4: Mean DMFT score and differences in scores by dietary habits.

Dietary habits	N (%)	Mean DMFT (SD)	Difference (95% CI)	P
Frequency of eating/day				
1-2 times	77 (15.3)	0.73 (0.9)	0.00	0.05*
3-4 times	326 (65.2)	0.63 (0.4)	−0.09 (−0.18, −0.02)	
More than 4 times	98 (19.5)	0.71 (0.8)	−0.02 (−0.09, 0.06)	
Snack between meals/day				
Once	189 (37.8)	0.62 (0.5)	0.00	0.05*
Twice	200 (40.0)	0.70 (0.5)	0.06 (0.01, 0.11)	
Three or more	111 (22.2)	0.70 (0.7)	0.08 (−0.00, 0.09)	
Sugar consumption level/day				
Low	169 (33.7)	0.58 (0.5)	0.00	0.01*
Moderate	206 (41.2)	0.66 (0.5)	0.07 (0.00, 0.15)	
High	126 (25.1)	0.74 (0.6)	0.16 (0.04, 0.27)	

CI: confidence interval. SD: standard deviation. *Significant relation between the mean DMFT score and dietary habits.

TABLE 5: Multivariate model for the association between decay, missing, filled, and plaque.

Variables	N (%)	Plaque adjusted OR (95% CI)	P	DMFT adjusted OR (95% CI)	P
Age					
12-year-old	275 (55)	0.00	0.05*	1.00	0.18
13-year-old	225 (45)	0.06 (−0.00, 0.12)		1.12 (0.93, 1.35)	
Gender					
Male	250 (50)	0.00	0.28	1.00	
Female	250 (50)	−0.04 (−0.11, 0.12)		0.92 (0.81, 1.06)	
Mothers education					
University	128 (25.6)	0.00	0.77	1.00	0.26
High school	240 (47.9)	−0.02 (−0.11, 0.06)		0.97 (0.80, 1.17)	
Primary school	133 (26.5)	0.01 (−0.10, 0.13)		1.11 (0.92, 1.33)	
Snacks between meals/day					
Once	189 (37.8)	0.00	0.30	1.00	0.01*
Twice	202 (40.4)	0.03 (−0.02, 0.09)		1.06 (0.86, 1.31)	
Three or more	109 (21.8)	0.06 (−0.03, 0.15)		1.25 (1.00, 1.57)	
Sugar consumption level/day					
Low	168 (33.6)	0.00	0.03*	1.00	0.00*
Moderate	207 (41.4)	0.07 (0.00, 0.14)		1.06 (0.86, 1.31)	
High	125 (25.0)	0.13 (0.02, 0.24)		1.25 (1.00, 1.57)	
Frequency of brushing/day					
Irregular	136 (27.1)	0.00	0.00*	1.00	0.03*
Once	159 (31.7)	−0.06 (−0.14, 0.00)		0.89 (0.70, 1.12)	
Twice or more	206 (41.2)	−0.09 (−0.17, −0.00)		0.80 (0.64, 0.93)	

*Significant relation of the assessed independent variables with plaque and DMFT scores.

Core findings of this study revealed that there is a clear association between frequency of tooth brushing and sugar consumption with both: accumulation of plaque and dental caries. One part of this finding, that is, frequency of sugar consumption and its association with dental caries is supported by another study performed in Jazan region [17]. But, there are no previous studies conducted in or around this region among high school children in order to compare the oral hygiene practices with dental caries. However, studies conducted in other developing nations in the Asian continent displayed similar findings [25, 26]. We hope that the current study will aid in initiating future publications to address the oral hygiene issues surrounding oral health status among children in this region.

Strengths of the study are the selection of study participants was random and an appropriate sampling strategy was ensured to obtain a near representative sample, the questionnaire used was prevalidated and in addition, and clinical examination was performed to report oral health status. Also, the study included diverse group of children who attended the annual dental camp. Thus, unlike most previous studies in the kingdom that recruited participants from a specified location, our results can be more generalized to young Saudi population in Jazan. A limitation of this study is its cross-sectional design, and it is recommended that more studies with robust longitudinal design should be performed in future to provide stronger evidences.

To conclude, dental caries status of high school children in Jazan region of Saudi Arabia needs to be improved. The dental public health practitioners here should consider the effect of oral hygiene practices on oral health status in order to design the future health promotion interventions.

Acknowledgments

The authors would like to acknowledge the research committee at Jazan University for their support. The authors would also like to extend their sincere gratitude to the school authorities for their continuous support throughout the project.

References

[1] WHO, *The World Health Report 2003-Shaping the Future*, World Health Organization, Geneva, Switzerland, 2016, http://www.who.int/whr/2003/en/.

[2] F. Ashley, "Role of dental health education in preventive dentistry," in *Prevention of Dental Disease*, J. J. Murray, Ed., pp. 406–414, Oxford University Press, Oxford, UK, 1996.

[3] H. B. A. Bodur, V. Yücesoy, and K. Baloş, "The evaluation of dental caries prevalence and periodontal status in two-different age groups," *GÜ Dişhek Fak Derg*, vol. 21, no. 1, pp. 35–39, 2004.

[4] J. Z. Anaise, "The toothbrush in plaque removal," *Journal of Dentistry for Children*, vol. 42, no. 3, pp. 186–189, 1975.

[5] A. Blinkhorn, D. Gratrix, P. Holloway, Y. Wainwright-Stringer, S. Ward, and H. Worthington, "A cluster randomised, controlled trial of the value of dental health educators in general dental practice," *British Dental Journal*, vol. 195, no. 7, pp. 395–400, 2003.

[6] S. Gibson and S. Williams, "Dental caries in preschool children: associations with social class, toothbrushing habit and consumption of sugars and sugar containing foods," *Caries Research*, vol. 33, no. 2, pp. 101–113, 1999.

[7] R. Harris, A. Nicolli, P. Adair, and C. Pine, "Risk factors for dental caries in young children: a systematic review of the literature," *Community Dental Health*, vol. 21, pp. 71–85, 2004.

[8] L. Oliveira, A. Sheiham, and M. Bonecker, "Exploring the association of dental caries with social factors and nutritional status in Brazilian preschool children," *European Journal of Oral Sciences*, vol. 116, no. 1, pp. 37–43, 2008.

[9] A. Sayegh, E. Dini, R. Holt, and R. Bedi, "Food and drink consumption, sociodemographic factors and dental caries in 4-5 year old children in Amman Jordan," *International Dental Journal*, vol. 52, no. 2, pp. 87–93, 2002.

[10] A. Sowole, E. Sote, and M. Folayan, "Dental caries pattern and predisposing oral hygiene related factors in Nigerian preschool children," *European Archives of Paediatric Dentistry*, vol. 8, no. 4, pp. 206–210, 2007.

[11] G. Winter, "Caries in the preschool child," *Journal of Dentistry*, vol. 18, no. 6, pp. 325-326, 1990.

[12] M. Folayan, A. Sowole, and A. Kola-Jebutu, "Risk factors for caries in children from South-Western Nigeria," *Journal of Clinical Pediatric Dentistry*, vol. 32, no. 2, pp. 171–175, 2007.

[13] E. Newbrun, "Preventing dental caries: breaking the chain of transmission," *Journal of the American Dental Association*, vol. 123, no. 6, pp. 55–59, 1992.

[14] P. Petersen, "The world oral health report 2003: continuous improvement of oral health in the 21st century–the approach of the WHO global oral health programme," *Community Dentistry and Oral Epidemiology*, vol. 31, no. 1, pp. 3–23, 2003.

[15] A. Alzailai, M. Quadri, M. Nayeem, A. Inamdar, and S. Tadakamadla, "Caries status of school children in Jazan city, KSA and its relation with dental literacy of their parents," *Journal of Oral Health Research*, vol. 5, no. 1, pp. 1–5, 2014.

[16] N. N. Al-Hebshi, A. Abdulhaq, M. Quadri, and F. Tobaigy, "Salivary carriage of Candida species in relation to dental caries in a population of Saudi Arabian primary school children," *Saudi Journal for Dental Research*, vol. 6, no. 1, pp. 54–59, 2015.

[17] F. H. Quadri, A. Pramono , and M. Jafer, "Knowledge, attitudes and practices of sweet food and beverage consumption and its association with dental caries among schoolchildren in Jazan, Saudi Arabia," *Eastern Mediterranean Health Journal*, vol. 21, no. 6, pp. 403–411, 2015.

[18] H. S. Halawany, "A review on miswak (*Salvadora persica*) and its effect on various aspects of oral health," *Saudi Dental Journal*, vol. 24, no. 2, pp. 63–69, 2012.

[19] L. Freitas-Fernandes, A. B. Novaes, A. C. R. Feitosa, and A. B. Novaes, "Effectiveness of an oral hygiene program for Brazilian orphans," *Brazilian Dental Journal*, vol. 13, no. 1, pp. 44–48, 2002.

[20] F. García-Godoy, M. Marcushamer, M. Cugini, and P. Warren, "The safety and efficacy of a children's power toothbrush and a manual toothbrush in 6-11 year-olds," *American Journal of Dentistry*, vol. 14, no. 4, pp. 195–199, 2001.

[21] D. E. Al Agili, "A systematic review of population-based dental caries studies among children in Saudi Arabia," *Saudi Dental Journal*, vol. 25, no. 1, pp. 3–11, 2013.

[22] N. M. Nurelhuda, T. A. Trovik, R. W. Ali, and M. F. Ahmed, "Oral health status of 12-year-old school children in Khartoum state, the Sudan; a school-based survey," *BMC Oral Health*, vol. 9, p. 15, 2009.

35

Diagnosis of Oral Hairy Leukoplakia: The Importance of EBV In Situ Hybridization

Luana L. Martins,[1] José Henrique F. Rosseto,[1] Natália Silva Andrade,[1] Juliana Bertoldi Franco,[1] Paulo Henrique Braz-Silva,[2,3] and Karem L. Ortega[1]

[1]*Special Care Dentistry Center, Division of Oral and Maxillofacial Pathology, Department of Stomatology, School of Dentistry, University of Sao Paulo, Sao Paulo, SP, Brazil*
[2]*Division of General Pathology, Department of Stomatology, School of Dentistry, University of Sao Paulo, Sao Paulo, SP, Brazil*
[3]*Laboratory of Virology, Institute of Tropical Medicine of Sao Paulo, University of Sao Paulo, Sao Paulo, SP, Brazil*

Correspondence should be addressed to Karem L. Ortega; klortega@usp.br

Academic Editor: Tommaso Lombardi

Oral hairy leukoplakia (OHL) is caused by the Epstein-Barr virus (EBV), which has been related to HIV infection. In situ hybridization (ISH) is the gold-standard diagnosis of OHL, but some authors believe in the possibility of performing the diagnosis based on clinical basis. The aim of this study is diagnose incipient lesions of OHL by EBV ISH of HIV-infected patients and the possible correlations with clinical characteristics of the patients. Ninety-four patients were examined and those presenting with clinical lesions compatible to OHL were submitted to biopsy prior to EBV ISH. Twenty-eight patients had lesions clinically compatible to the diagnosis of OHL, but only 20 lesions were confirmed by EBV ISH. The patients with OHL had a mean age of 41.9 years and were HIV-infected for 11.2 years, on average, including CD4 count of 504.7 cells/mm^3 and $\log_{10}$ viral load = 1.1. Among the quantitative variables, there was a statistically significant correlation with age only ($P = 0.030$). In conclusion, the presence of OHL in patients with HIV/AIDS results in changes in the epidemiological characteristics of the disease, and this fact allied with subtle clinical-morphological features makes clinical diagnosis very difficult. Therefore, EBV ISH is important for a definitive diagnosis of OHL.

1. Introduction

Approximately 60 percent of the HIV-infected individuals and 80 percent of those with acquired immunodeficiency syndrome (AIDS) present oral manifestations such as oral candidiasis (erythematous and pseudomembranous), oral hairy leukoplakia (OHL), Kaposi's sarcoma, non-Hodgkin's lymphoma, linear gingival erythema, necrotizing ulcerative gingivitis, and necrotizing ulcerative periodontitis [1, 2].

The presence of oral candidiasis and OHL within the oral cavity not only suggests HIV infection, but is possibly one of the first signs of development into AIDS in the HIV-infected individual [3, 4].

OHL represents an opportunistic infection related to the Epstein-Barr virus (EBV), being particularly present in patients infected by HIV [3, 5, 6]. Clinically, OHL is a white plaque with corrugated surface, painless, and not removable by scraping. According to Greenspan et al. "Puzzled by these findings, we tentatively applied to this lesion the name *oral hairy leukoplakia* (HL) because of the white color and corrugated or shaggy appearance of the lateral tongue seen many cases" [2]. This lesion is commonly found in the lateral border of the tongue. The histopathological characteristics are not exclusive to this lesion, which may include hyperkeratosis, epithelial hyperplasia, ballooning degeneration, and discrete or even absent inflammatory mononuclear cells infiltrate. For this reason, the criteria used for the final diagnosis of OHL have been always discussed [2, 7]. Previous study published by our group showed that among 36 cases of OHL diagnosed in clinical and histopathological basis, only 80.55% were EBV positive, confirming the previous diagnosis [8].

EBV can be detected by several techniques, such as polymerase chain reaction (PCR), immunohistochemistry, electron microscopy, and in situ hybridization (ISH), with the latter being considered the gold-standard exam [2, 8–13].

Therefore, the objective of this work is to diagnose incipience lesions of OHL by using in situ hybridization for identification of EBV within the oral mucosa of HIV-infected patients and to verify whether there is a relationship between the presence of OHL and clinical characteristics of the patients.

2. Materials and Methods

The present study was performed after approval by the ethics committee of the University of Sao Paulo Faculty of Dentistry, Sao Paulo, Brazil. The informed consent document was signed by all participants of the study, as dictated by the Declaration of Helsinki.

HIV-seropositive male and female patients older than 18 years attending the Special Care Dentistry Center (CAPE), School of Dentistry, University of Sao Paulo (FOUSP), were included in the present study, regardless of the use of antiretroviral therapy. CAPE is an outpatient dental clinic inside FOUSP facilities. All patients of CAPE were covered by the Brazilian public health system (SUS: Sistema Único de Saude). The patients having cognitive impairment (which does not allow the understanding of anamnesis and informed consent form), undergoing oncological treatments, or taking antiviral drugs (for herpes virus) in the past three months prior to evaluation were excluded from the study.

To calculate the sample size, we used the estimation of HIV-seropositive patients in CAPE-FOUSP in 2009 (1,867 patients). OHL prevalence considered was equal to 13.4 percent, which was previously reported in Brazilian study [14]. With a confidence interval of 90 percent, a power of sample of 80 percent, and a possible loss of 10 percent estimated for cross-sectional studies, the ideal sample size consisted of 97 patients. The sample size calculation was performed using the EpiInfo™ software (version 3.5.2; Centers for Disease Control and Prevention, Atlanta, GA, USA). The sample was consecutive; all patients that met the inclusion criteria and returned for routine visits from May 2010 to October 2010 were examined.

The patients were submitted to complete clinical examination, consisting of anamnesis and physical exam. Data on age, gender, smoking habits (cigarettes), ethnic group, HIV-exposure category, morbidities or chronic systemic diseases, duration of HIV-seropositivity, type and time of antiretroviral therapy, CD4 count, and viral load were collected. Physical exam was performed in a dental outpatient setting under artificial light and the patients were submitted to oral mucosa examination for identification and clinical diagnosis of oral manifestations related to HIV infection.

Biopsy was performed when there was clinical hypothesis of OHL. The biopsied material was fixed in 10% buffered formaldehyde solution before being sent to the Surgical Pathology Laboratory of the Oral Pathology Department of the University of Sao Paulo Faculty of Dentistry. Histological sections were blocked into paraffin and stained with Hematoxylin and Eosin (H&E) according to standard laboratory procedure, and in situ hybridization was performed for identification of EBV according our previous published work [8].

The histological diagnoses of all lesions were performed by an expert oral pathologist and the characteristics considered to diagnose OHL were the same as those described by Greenspan et al. (2016), Khammissa et al. (2016), and Braz-Silva et al. (2008) [2, 6, 8].

The data were analyzed using the EpiInfo software (Centers for Disease Control and Prevention, Atlanta, GA, USA). Descriptive statistics were used for univariate analysis. In bivariate analysis, qualitative variables [e.g., gender, CDC classification, and smoking habits (cigarettes)] were assessed by using Fisher's exact test. To compare the quantitative variables (age, time of infection, lowest CD4 count, current CD4 count, HIV-viral load, duration of ARVT, and current duration of ARVT) and the presence of OHL, we applied the nonparametric Mann–Whitney U test, because these variables showed a nonnormal distribution by the Kolmogorov-Smirnov test. In all analyses, the significance level was fixed as alpha = 5%. This analysis was used to reveal potential associations between clinical characteristics of the patient and the presence of OHL.

3. Results

A total of 94 HIV-seropositive patients were included in the present study representing 96.9% of the ideal sample, in which 68 (72.3%) were males and 26 (27.7%) females, with mean age of 45.2 years. With regard to skin color, 53 (56.4%) were classified as white, 23 (24.5%) as black, and 18 (19.1%) as mulatto. Evaluation of deleterious oral habits revealed that 29.8% of the patients were current smokers, 24.5% were former smokers, and 20.2% drank alcoholic beverages regularly. The patients were also classified according to the HIV-exposure category reported: three patients (3.2%) contracted HIV by using injectable drugs, 42 (44.7%) by heterosexual relation, 39 (41.5%) by homosexual relation, and two (2.1%) by vertical transmission and eight (8.5%) did not know about the probable route of contamination. The mean duration of HIV infection was 12.4 years, with 63.8% developing AIDS (36.2% were in category B2 and 63.8% were in category C3 of the 1993 Revised Classification System for HIV Infection and Expanded Surveillance Case Definition for AIDS Among Adolescents and Adults). All patients were on antiretroviral therapy.

Medical history revealed that 68 patients had been suffering from morbidities [systemic arterial hypertension (18), diabetes mellitus type 2 (8), anemia (23), viral hepatitis (24), and hypercholesterolemia (4)] and 73 from systemic opportunistic infections [toxoplasmosis (9), leishmaniasis (1), pneumonia (36), tuberculosis (27), meningitis (7), syphilis (23), and gonorrhea (10)] during the clinical course of the HIV disease. Eighty-eight patients (89.7%) were using antiretroviral therapy for 9.4 years, on average, whereas the current therapeutic regimen lasted 3.8 years, on average.

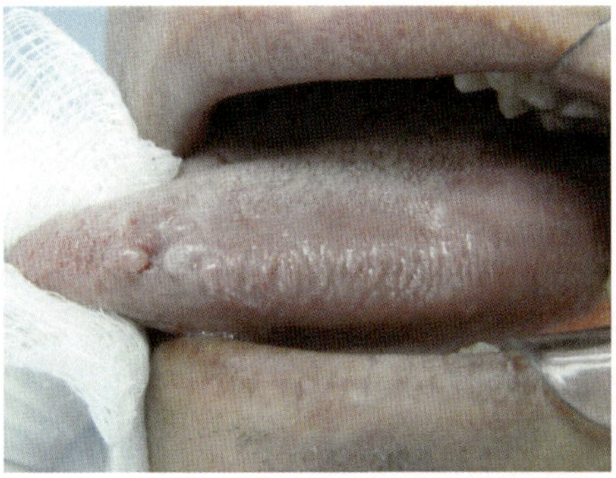

FIGURE 1: Clinical aspect of the oral hairy leukoplakia.

On the intraoral clinical examination, patients were diagnosed with oral manifestations of HIV infection such as candidiasis (n = 5), herpes labialis (n = 1), aphthous ulcers (n = 1), necrotizing gingivitis (n = 1), and angular cheilitis (n = 1).

Twenty-eight patients were clinically suspected of having OHL and underwent biopsy for confirmation of diagnosis. Clinically, none of the lesions showed expressive increase in the epithelial keratinization or significant elevation of the affected mucosa (Figure 1). The histological characteristics taken into consideration were the following: acanthosis, epithelial hyperplasia, cells resembling koilocytes, cells with ground glass nuclei and perinuclear halo, and absent or discrete inflammatory infiltrate in the surrounding connective tissue. The lamina propria consisted of dense connective tissue, in some cases with both presence and absence of a few inflammatory mononuclear cells.

Both histological examination and in situ hybridization confirmed the clinical diagnosis in 20 patients (71.42% of the clinically diagnosed patients), with the lateral border of the tongue being the only site where these lesions were found (Figure 2). Cohen's kappa coefficient between clinical examination and in situ hybridization was 0.78.

The white lesions in eight EBV negative lesions were diagnosed as irritative hyperkeratosis.

The qualitative variables (i.e., gender, CDC classification, and smoking) were assessed by using the Fisher's exact test and no statistically significant correlation was found between the variables and presence of OHL. With regard to quantitative variables, statistically significant association was found only between patient age and presence of OHL (P = 0.030), with the mean age of patients with OHL being lower than that of those without it (Table 1). The age of patients with OHL ranged from 19 to 51 and the age of HIV patients without OHL lesions ranged from 18 to 69 years.

4. Discussion

By analyzing the 2015 HIV/AIDS Epidemiological Bulletin, it was found that in Brazil there are 830,000 people living with HIV and 44,000 new cases were registered only in 2015. The highest prevalence is observed in male individuals, with an increase among homosexual men. Another important observation is the increase in cases of AIDS in the age groups of 15–19 and 20–24 years [15, 16].

In our study group, the high incidence of opportunistic systemic infections linked to the immunosuppression caused by HIV reflects the clinical staging of the disease, thus contributing to the diagnosis for these patients [17]. On the other hand, the systemic morbidities presented by HIV+ patients on this study may be reflecting the adverse effect of the long-term use of medication, since the patients had been taking it for more than nine years, on average. Although the highly active antiretroviral therapy (HAART) has extraordinarily contributed to increasing the life expectancy and to improving the quality of life of HIV/AIDS patients, today it is known that this treatment has also accounted for the emergence of several adverse reactions in these patients like hematological, gastrointestinal, hepatic, and metabolic effects, among others. In addition, these patients present symptoms involving nausea, diarrhea, hyperlipidemia, dyslipidemia, neuropathy, allergic reactions, myocardial infarction, diabetes, myalgia, lactic acidosis, nephropathies, osteoporosis, and osteopenia [18].

We believe that the current therapeutic regimen of the studied patients was demonstrated to be effective as the patients showed suitable virological and immunological responses (CD4 count > 500 and CV log < 1). According to the literature, low viral loads and high CD4 counts reflect clinically the decreased amount of opportunistic oral lesions [19] found in the patients. Our results confirm the literature data. In a previous study published by our group, the prevalence of oral manifestations was 53.29% in patients with mean CD4 count of 160 cells/mm^3. In the present study, the prevalence of patients with oral lesions dropped to 22.34% [14, 20].

Lesions of OHL were identified in 21.27% of the patients evaluated. This figure does not reflect the decrease reported by other studies on prevalence after use of HAART [21, 22], all indicating a marked drop in the prevalence of OHL. Despite the reduced incidence, OHL was found to be the most refractory lesion in the antiretroviral therapy as although the number of occurrences decreased over the years, it was not gradual and constant as in the case of candidiasis and SK [14]. In our study, we have observed that the clinical characteristics of OHL were different compared to the historical pattern found in our outpatient unit: from an ample, flower-shaped lesion occupying a large area of the lateral border of the tongue to a much more discrete lesion with clinical characteristics less exacerbated than those found at the beginning of the epidemics. However, because many lesions have not been diagnosed, it is necessary to perform both biopsy and in situ hybridization for a correct diagnosis. Gold-standard laboratory exams should also be performed for the diagnosis of OHL, which became clear in our work. Some recently published studies have showed the usefulness of the cytopathology to diagnosis of the OHL, always associated with molecular tools to EBV detection, opening a new perspective to use less invasive diagnostic methods for this condition [23, 24].

Some researchers also state that the presence of this lesion could indicate a therapeutic failure or serve as a marker of

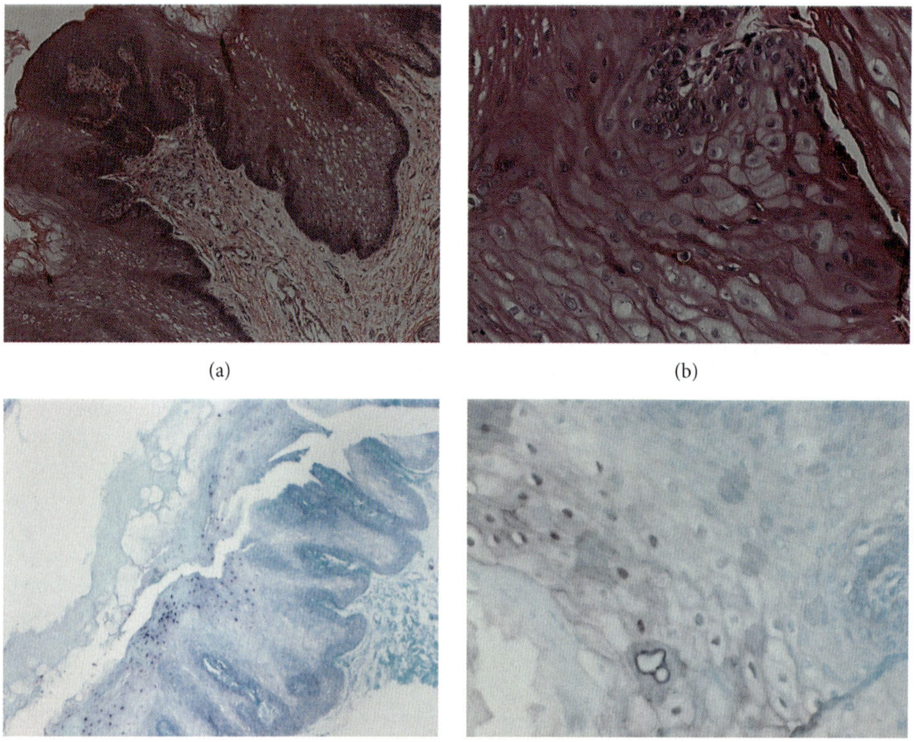

Figure 2: Histological characteristics of OHL and in situ hybridization reaction. (a) Histopathological section, stained with H&E, showing stratified squamous epithelium, acanthosis, epithelial hyperplasia, cells resembling koilocytes, cells with opaque nucleus, and perinuclear halo (100x magnification). (b) Section stained with H&E showing cells resembling koilocytes (400x magnification). (c) In situ hybridization reaction with positivity for EBV (100x magnification). (d) In situ hybridization reaction with positivity for EBV (400x magnification).

Table 1: Comparison between presence of oral hairy leukoplakia and quantitative variables of the patients.

Variable	Oral hairy leukoplakia	n	Mean	SD	Median	U	P^*
Age (years)	Yes	20	41.9	6.8	42.5	505	**0.030**
	No	74	46.1	10.7	47.0		
Time of infection (years)	Yes	20	11.2	5.5	11.0	613	0.239
	No	74	12.8	4.9	13.0		
Lowest CD4 count (cells/mm^3)	Yes	20	197.4	200.8	150.0	648.5	0.446
	No	73	212.4	168.4	200.0		
Current CD4 count (cells/mm^3)	Yes	20	504.7	243.1	507.0	692.5	0.726
	No	73	544.5	301.4	500.0		
HIV-viral load (log copies/ml)	Yes	20	1.1	1.9	0.0	625	0.155
	No	73	0.6	1.4	0.0		
Duration of ARVT (years)	Yes	20	8.8	5.0	8.5	606	0.360
	No	70	9.6	4.6	10.0		
Current duration of ARVT (years)	Yes	20	2.9	2.7	2.0	554	0.154
	No	70	4.1	3.6	3.5		

*Mann-Whitney U test. SD: standard deviation; ARVT: antiretroviral therapy.

AIDS progression [4, 7, 9, 25]. In our case, it was not possible to correlate the presence of OHL with an occasional failure of the treatment because patients with OHL had a viral load of 1.1 log ($P = 0.155$), on average, or consider the lesion as a marker of AIDS progression because the correlation between presence of OHL and disease staging was not statistically significant ($P = 0.301$). The high CD4 count in patients with OHL (mean value of 504.7 cells/mm^3) was very close to the mean value of patients without OHL (504.7 cells/mm^3) ($P = 0.726$) and also differed from the literature, which always correlated the lesion with low TCD4 counts [14, 20, 25]. It was not possible to correlate the presence of OHL with either the use of tobacco ($P = 1.000$), time of HIV infection ($P = 0.239$), or duration of antiretroviral therapy ($P = 0.36$).

5. Conclusion

The clinical aspects of OHL in patients with HIV/AIDS have been changed in the past years, making the diagnosis based only on clinical basis very difficult. The use of in situ hybridization for EBV detection has been fundamental for achieving a definitive diagnosis of OHL, mainly in patients with oral lesions out of the classic patterns.

Ethical Approval

This study was approved by the Research Ethics Committee of the School of Dentistry of the University of Sao Paulo, Brazil.

Disclosure

Data from the patients included in this study were treated anonymously.

Authors' Contributions

Luana L. Martins, José Henrique F. Rosseto, and Juliana Bertoldi Franco performed all the clinical aspects of this study. Natália Silva Andrade performed the statistical analysis. Paulo Henrique Braz-Silva performed all the histopathological and molecular analysis. Karem L. Ortega performed the study design and the clinical supervision. All authors participated in preparation of the manuscript.

References

[1] P. G. Robinson, "The oral manifestations of HIV infection," *International Journal of STD and AIDS*, vol. 8, no. 11, pp. 668–674, 1997.

[2] J. S. Greenspan, D. Greenspan, and J. Webster-Cyriaque, "Hairy leukoplakia; lessons learned: 30-plus years," *Oral Diseases*, vol. 22, supplement 1, pp. 120–127, 2016.

[3] L. L. Patton, R. G. McKaig, J. Eron J.J., H. P. Lawrence, and R. P. Strauss, "Oral hairy leukoplakia and oral candidiasis as predictors of HIV viral load," *AIDS*, vol. 13, no. 15, pp. 2174–2176, 1999.

[4] A. Chattopadhyay, D. J. Caplan, G. D. Slade, D. C. Shugars, H.-C. Tien, and L. L. Patton, "Risk indicators for oral candidiasis and oral hairy leukoplakia in HIV-infected adults," *Community Dentistry and Oral Epidemiology*, vol. 33, no. 1, pp. 35–44, 2005.

[5] M. D. G. Moura, S. D. M. C. Grossmann, L. M. D. S. Fonseca, M. I. B. Senna, and R. A. Mesquita, "Risk factors for oral hairy leukoplakia in HIV-infected adults of Brazil," *Journal of Oral Pathology and Medicine*, vol. 35, no. 6, pp. 321–326, 2006.

[6] R. A. G. Khammissa, J. Fourie, R. Chandran, J. Lemmer, and L. Feller, "Epstein-Barr virus and its association with oral hairy leukoplakia: a short review," *International Journal of Dentistry*, vol. 2016, Article ID 4941783, 6 pages, 2016.

[7] D. A. Vale, F. M. Martins, P. H. Silva, and K. L. Ortega, "Retrospective analysis of the clinical behavior of oral hairy leukoplakia in 215 HIV-seropositive patients," *Brazilian Oral Research*, vol. 30, no. 1, 2016.

[8] P. H. Braz-Silva, N. P. M. de Rezende, K. L. Ortega, R. T. de Macedo Santos, and M. H. C. G. de Magalhães, "Detection of the Epstein-Barr virus (EBV) by in situ hybridization as definitive diagnosis of hairy leukoplakia," *Head and Neck Pathology*, vol. 2, no. 1, pp. 19–24, 2008.

[9] A. S. Batavia, R. Secours, P. Espinosa et al., "Diagnosis of HIV-Associated oral lesions in relation to early versus delayed antiretroviral therapy: Results from the CIPRA HT001 Trial," *PLoS ONE*, vol. 11, no. 3, article e0150656, 2016.

[10] D. M. Walling, C. M. Flaitz, F. G. Hosein, M. Montes-Walters, and C. M. Nichols, "Effect of Epstein-Barr virus replication on langerhans cells in pathogenesis of oral hairy leukoplakia," *Journal of Infectious Diseases*, vol. 189, no. 9, pp. 1656–1663, 2004.

[11] M. Loughrey, M. Trivett, S. Lade, W. Murray, H. Turner, and P. Waring, "Diagnostic application of Epstein-Barr virus-encoded RNA in situ hybridisation," *Pathology*, vol. 36, no. 4, pp. 301–308, 2004.

[12] J. S. Greenspan, Y. G. De Souza, J. A. Regezi et al., "Comparison of cytopathic changes in oral hairy leukoplakia with in situ hybridization for EBV DNA," *Oral Diseases*, vol. 4, no. 2, pp. 95–99, 1998.

[13] C. A. Migliorati, A. C. Jones, and P. A. Baughman, "Use of exfoliative cytology in the diagnosis of oral hairy leukoplakia," *Oral Surgery, Oral Medicine, Oral Pathology*, vol. 76, no. 6, pp. 704–710, 1993.

[14] K. L. Ortega, D. A. Vale, and M. H. C. G. Magalhães, "Impact of PI and NNRTI HAART-based therapy on oral lesions of brazilian HIV-infected patients," *Journal of Oral Pathology and Medicine*, vol. 38, no. 6, pp. 489–494, 2009.

[15] Boletim epidemiológico HIV e AIDS. Ministério da Saúde. Secretaria de Vigilância Sanitária. Departamento de DST, AIDS e hepatites virais. Ano IV, n^{0}1. Brasília. Brasil, 2015.

[16] Boletim Epidemiológico de Aids - HIV/DST e Hepatites B e C do Município de São Paulo. Boletim Epidemiológico de AIDS do Município de São Paulo; 2010;XIV (13):12-91.

[17] Center for Disease Control and Prevention (CDC). Revised surveillance case definition for HIV infection-United States, 2014. MMWR Recomm Rep. 2014;63(RR-03):1-10.

[18] F. Vidal, F. Gutiérrez, M. Gutiérrez et al., "Pharmacogenetics of adverse effects due to antiretroviral drugs," *AIDS Reviews*, vol. 12, no. 1, pp. 15–30, 2010.

[19] J. D. Eyeson, M. Tenant-Flowers, D. J. Cooper, N. W. Johnson, and K. A. A. S. Warnakulasuriya, "Oral manifestations of an HIV positive cohort in the era of highly active anti-retroviral therapy (HAART) in South London," *Journal of Oral Pathology and Medicine*, vol. 31, no. 3, pp. 169–174, 2002.

[20] A. Berberi and Z. Noujeim, "Epidemiology and relationships between CD4+ counts and oral lesions among 50 patients infected with human immunodeficiency virus," *Journal of International Oral Health*, vol. 7, no. 1, pp. 18–21, 2015.

[21] A. Pinheiro, W. Marcenes, J. M. Zakrzewska, and P. G. Robinson, "Dental and oral lesions in HIV infected patients: A study in Brazil," *International Dental Journal*, vol. 54, no. 3, pp. 131–137, 2004.

[22] C. H. Shiboski, J. F. Hilton, J. M. Neuhaus, A. Canchola, and D. Greenspan, "Human immunodeficiency virus-related oral manifestations and gender: A longitudinal analysis," *Archives of Internal Medicine*, vol. 156, no. 19, pp. 2249–2254, 1996.

[23] P. H. Braz-Silva, R. T. M. Santos, J. L. Schussel, and M. Gallottini, "Oral hairy leukoplakia diagnosis by Epstein-Barr virus in situ hybridization in liquid-based cytology," *Cytopathology*, vol. 25, no. 1, pp. 21–26, 2014.

[24] P. H. Braz-Silva, M. H. C. G. Magalhães, V. Hofman et al., "Usefulness of oral cytopathology in the diagnosis of infectious diseases," *Cytopathology*, vol. 21, no. 5, pp. 285–299, 2010.

[25] W. Birnbaum, T. A. Hodgson, P. A. Reichart, W. Sherson, S. W. Nittayannanta, and T. E. Axell, "Prognostic significance of HIV-associated oral lesions and their relation to therapy," *Oral Diseases*, vol. 8, no. 2, pp. 110–114, 2002.

Prevalence of TMJ Disorders among the Patients Attending the Dental Clinic of Ajman University of Science and Technology–Fujairah Campus, UAE

Kashef K. AlShaban [1] and Zainab Gul Abdul Waheed [2]

[1] *Faculty of Medical and Health Sciences, Emirates College of Technology, Abu Dhabi, UAE*
[2] *Mint Dental Care LLC., Dubai, UAE*

Correspondence should be addressed to Kashef K. AlShaban; kashefjo@yahoo.co.uk

Academic Editor: Li Wu Zheng

The objective of this study was to determine the prevalence of temporomandibular joint (TMJ) disorders (if any) among the patients attending the dental clinic (for routine dental treatment) of Ajman University of Science and Technology (AUST)–Fujairah campus, UAE, and its possible causes. A sample of 100 adult patients attending the dental clinic of AUST for different types of dental treatment were collected; the routine examination of the TMJ and possible disorders such as clicking, crepitation, limitation or deviation during mouth opening, or tenderness reveals that 41% of the sample experience varying degrees of disorders in the TMJ. Radiographs were taken if needed (panoramic radiograph). The information was collected and recorded for each patient through questionnaires.

1. Introduction

The proper function of (TMJ) depends upon the harmony of the different structures of the TMJ (including mandibular condyles, meniscus, glenoid fossa, ligaments, and muscles) that is well documented [1–4].

The TMJ continues in its function as usual until it is disturbed by external influences that affect the function of the joint, such as mechanical, psychological, occupational, and habits [5, 6].

The human body continues to try to repair its aggression; but if this continues, the body loses the ability to repair its aggression and the signs & symptoms begin to appear.

The signs and symptoms of TMD involve orofacial and preauricular pain, as well as limitation of mouth opening, TMJ bruit during function and displacement of articular disc [7].

Disorders of the (TMJ), and how people respond to them, vary widely and fall into three main categories:

(1) Myofascial pain dysfunction syndrome involves tenderness or pain in the muscles that control jaw function.

(2) Internal derangement of the TMJ involves anterior displacement of the meniscus with or without auto reduction, dislocated jaw, or injury to the condyle.

(3) Arthritis refers to a group of degenerative/inflammatory joint disorders [8].

2. Materials and Methods

A random sample of 100 patients that attended the dental clinic for dental treatment underwent the routine examination of the TMJ, such as clicking, crepitation, limitation or deviation during mouth opening, and pain. 41% of these patients had varying degrees of TMD and were not aware of these disorders.

In the preliminary examination of the TMJ, we relied on the principles based on International RDC/TMD and the amendments thereto (version: 20 Jan 2014) [9].

This was done by individually examining each patient, taking a thorough history, and filling out a questionnaire for each patient, respectively.

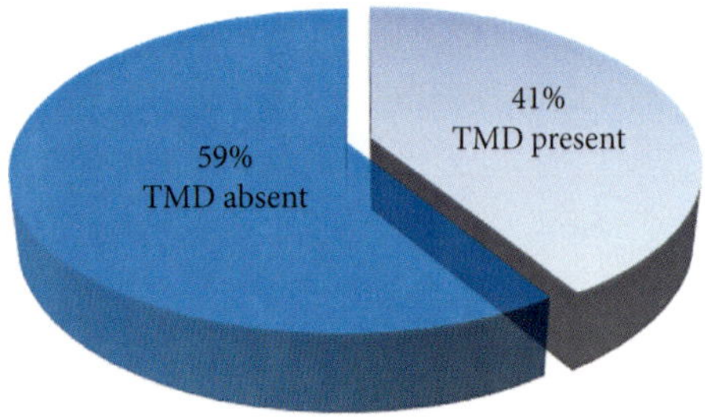

Figure 1: Pie chart demonstrating the presence and absence of TMD among the collected sample.

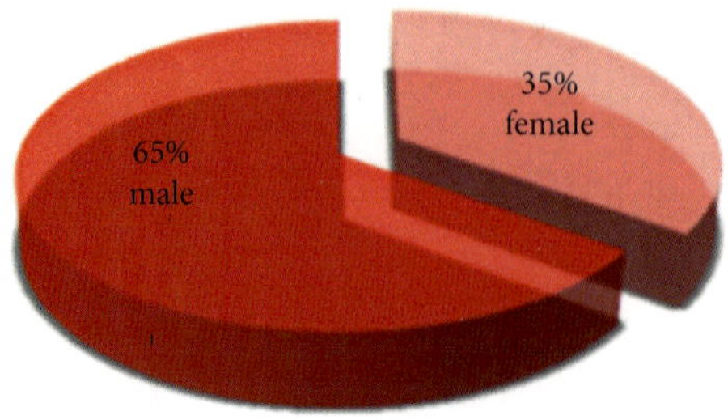

Figure 2: Pie chart demonstrating the percentages of male and female patients among the collected sample.

Physical examination of the collected sample was done in two ways:

(1) Lateral position: assessment of mandibular condylar movement by direct palpation over the joint while the patient opens and closes the mandible, at the preauricular area;

(2) Posterior position: assessment of mandibular condylar movement by direct palpation of the mandibular condyle while the patient opens and closes the mandible, through the external auditory meatus.

A mandibular opening less than 35 mm (the distance between the edges of upper and lower incisors) is considered in our study as restriction of mouth opening.

A thorough history was collected from the samples on any history of previous trauma to the head and neck region, any previous long dental appointments that could be the reason for any of the TMJ disorders, or any habits or any occupation-related habits that could precipitate a TMD.

Along with the clinical examination of the patient, the aid of radiographs (if necessary) was also taken.

3. Results

Among the randomly collected sample of a 100 patients, 41% (Figure 1) of the patient showed to have TMJ disorders out of which 65% were male patients and 35% were female patients (Figure 2).

Maximum percentage of patients (58%) was between the age ranges of 19–29 and the minimum (1%) were between the age ranges of 60–69 (Figure 3).

Patients were further categorized based on their occupation for evaluation of any occupation-related habits affecting the TMJ (Figure 4). The maximum numbers of patients were firm employees (30%), whereas the minimum numbers of patients were tailors and teachers (2%) among the total sample of 100 patients.

Among the 41% of the patients having the TMJ disorder, only 5% (Figure 5) of the patients had an occupation-related habit that could be a precipitating factor of the TMJ disorders.

The 41% of subjects that had the TMJ disorder were examined of various TMJ pathologies such as clicking, crepitation, limitation, deviation, and tenderness.

As a result of the examination, most percentage of subjects presented to have clicking (89%), and least percentage had crepitation (12%) (Figure 6).

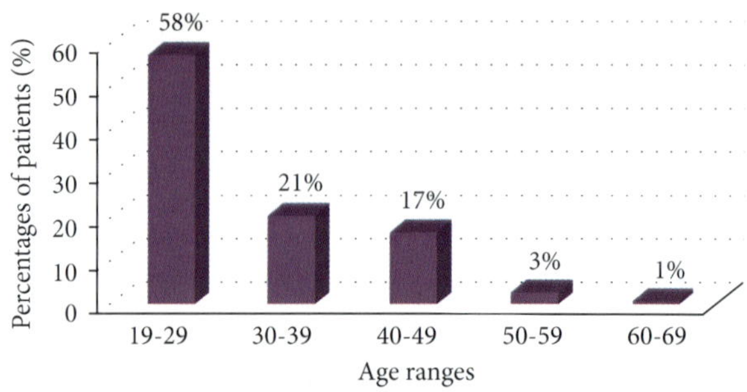

Figure 3: Bar graph showing the percentages of the collected sample of 100 patients and their respective age ranges.

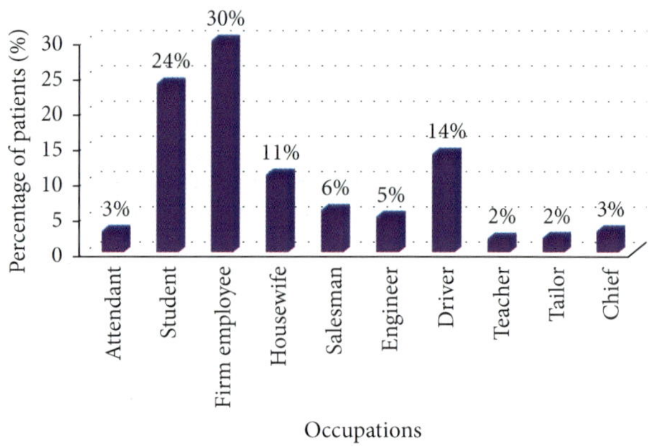

Figure 4: Bar graph representing the percentages of the collected sample of 100 patients with their respective occupations.

The involvement in TMJ Pathologies among the 41% of the patients either involved one side (unilateral) or both sides (bilateral) (Figures 7, 8, 9, 10, and 11).

The 41% of subjects were further inquired about five different criteria in order to achieve a conclusion of the possible causative factors of the TMJ disorders (Figure 12).

The subjects were inquired about the type of diet they consume and how it may affect the TMJ (Figure 13).

Figure 14 represents the percentages of patients and their respective habits.

4. Discussion

The research concluded that among the 41% of patients who had TMJ disorders, the most common TMJ pathology was clicking which was 89%, and most patients had either bilateral

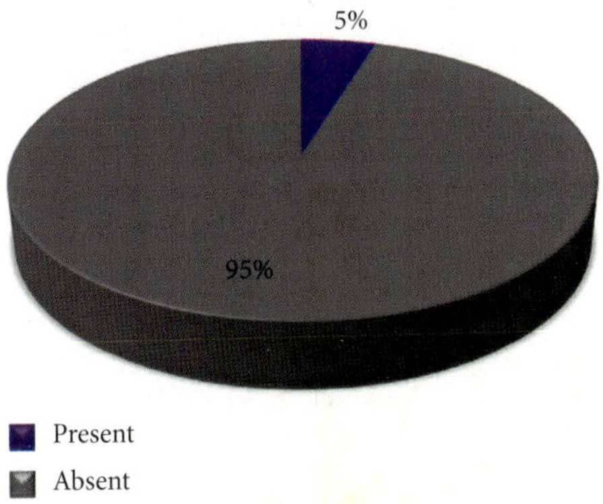

FIGURE 5: Pie chart representing the percentages of presence or absence of occupational habits in patients with TMJ disorders.

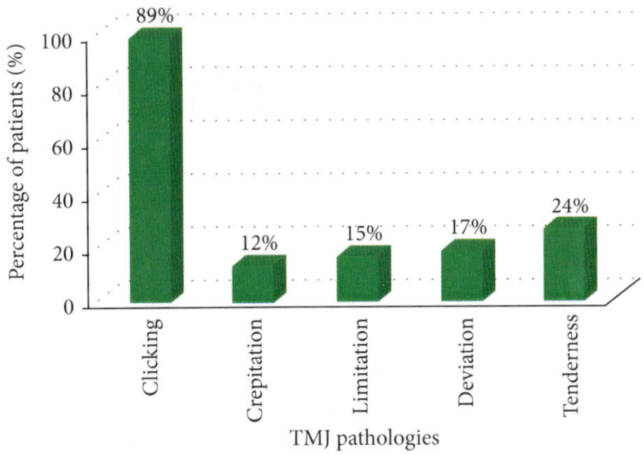

FIGURE 6: Bar graph showing the percentages of the patients having the different TMJ pathologies.

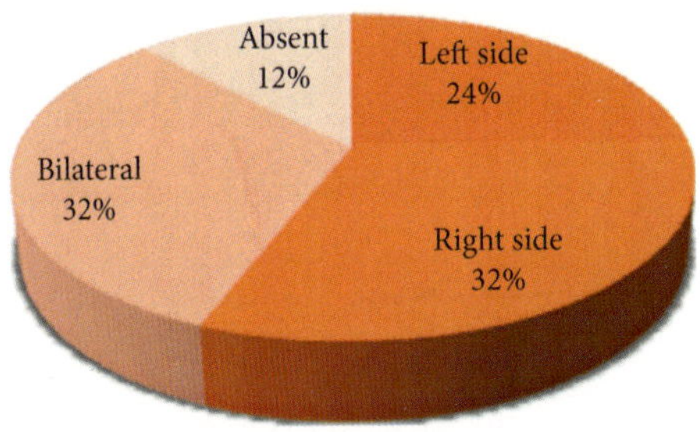

FIGURE 7: Pie chart demonstrating the percentages of patients with presence or absence of clicking on either side.

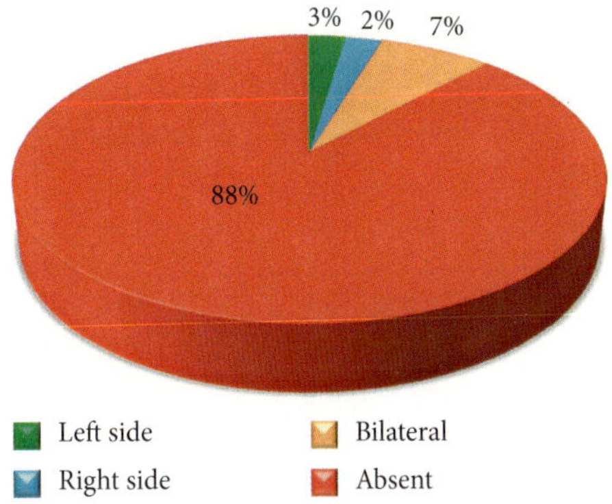

FIGURE 8: Pie chart demonstrating the percentages of patients with presence and absence of crepitation on either side.

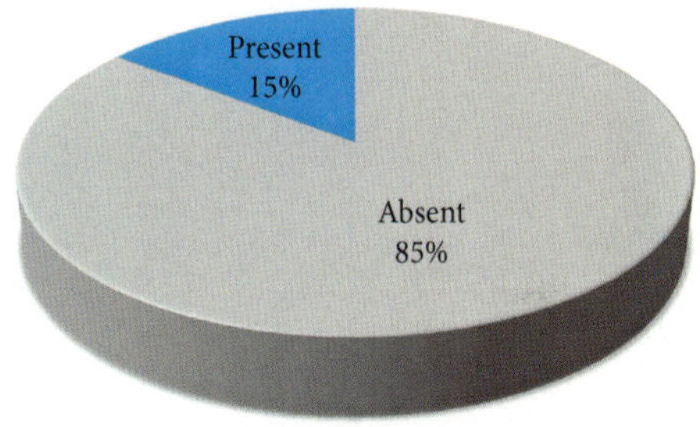

FIGURE 9: Pie chart representing the percentages of subjects with presence or absence of limitation during mouth opening.

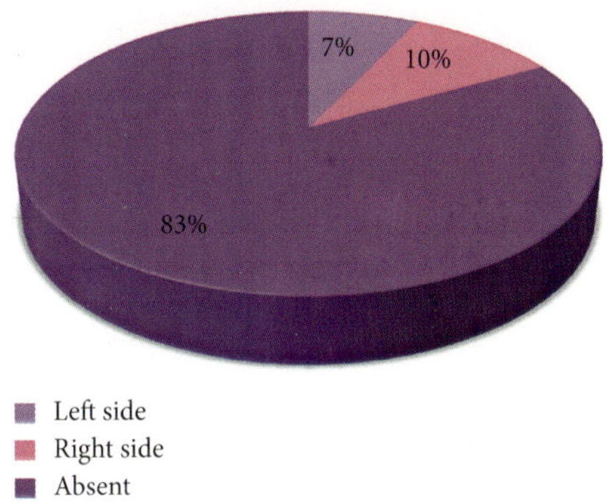

FIGURE 10: Pie chart demonstrating the percentages of patients representing presence or absence of deviation during mouth opening on either side.

clicking (32%) or clicking on the right side (32%), followed by tenderness (24%), deviation (17%), limitation (15%), and crepitation (12%), as shown in related studies [6, 10, 11].

Further, the patients were questioned on different criteria with the goal of identifying the causative factors of the disorder:

(i) The gravest cause concluded from the research was habits (32%). Most patients had associated habits that resulted in TMJ disorders. Patients had habits like chewing gum (75%), nail or lip biting (18%), and bruxism (7%). Most patients were not aware of the severity of the habits on the TMJ, as shown in related studies [12–17].

(ii) The second most common cause concluded was previous dental treatments (29%), specifying to a history of long dental appointments or previous orthodontic treatment [18].

(iii) Patients were inquired about having any history of trauma to the head and neck area that may have had an impact on the TMJ. The results concluded that 17% of the patient had a history of trauma, as shown in related studies [19, 20].

(iv) 10% of the patients had rheumatoid arthritis, as shown in related studies [21, 22].

(v) The lowest percentage was with occupational habits (5%). They were noticed in two patients, one was

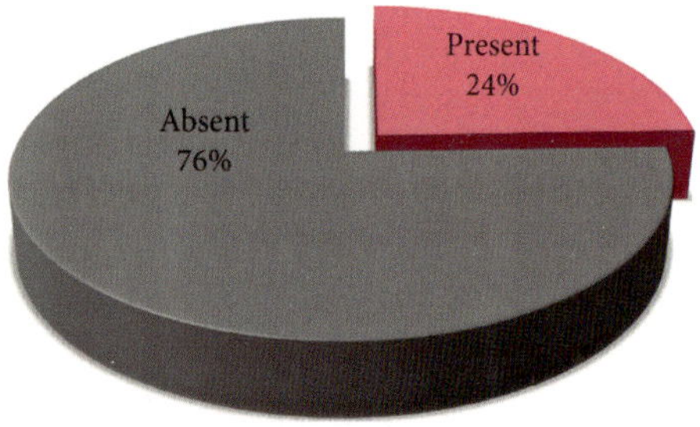

Figure 11: Pie chart representing the percentages of presence and absence of tenderness.

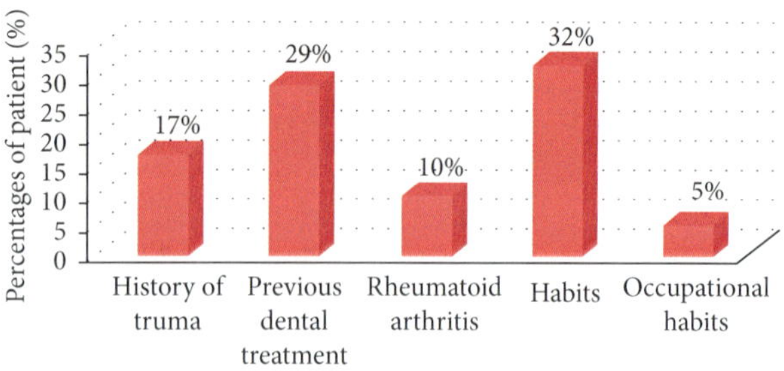

Figure 12: Bar graph representing the percentages of patients having different criteria.

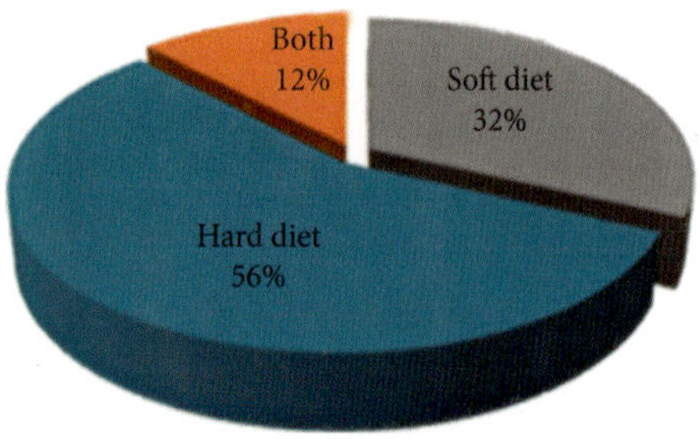

Figure 13: Pie charts demonstrating the percentages of patients whose diets are soft, hard, or both.

a teacher who had a history of clenching her jaws at the time of stress while teaching, and the other patient was a tailor having a history of biting off threads with his teeth.

(vi) Patients were also inquired on the type of diet they consumed to access any possible relationship between the type of diet and TMJ disorder:

The results stated that most patients had a hard diet (56%) which could be a contributing factor in causing the disorders, as shown in related studies [23, 24]. Long-term consumption of hard diet has a direct impact on the TMJ; hence, the patients should be educated and motivated to discontinue the habit.

(i) In our study, the percentage of male patients who show TMJ disorders (65%) was higher than that of female patients (35%):

Lee et al. [6] reported in their study, the predominance of the male with TMJ disorders; Another study [10] concluded that no significant relationship between females and males

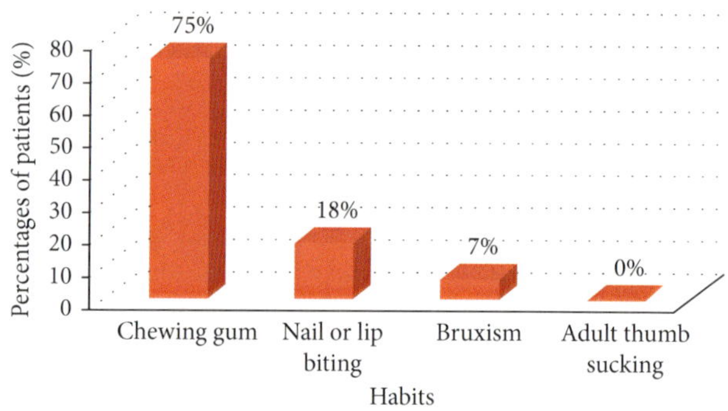

Figure 14: Bar graph representing the percentages of patients and their respective habits.

regarding TMJ disorders; Some studies [11, 12, 17, 25] have shown clearly the predominance of the female with TMJ disorders; Hirsch et al. [26] reported in their study, the predominance of the female with TMJ disorders during pubertal development, but the diagnosis remains unknown.

More research is needed to try to elucidate the relationship between female hormones and TMJ disorders (cause and effect).

(i) Finally, the psychological pressure (state-anxiety) and disorders play a role in TMJ disorders [5, 6, 18, 27] (it is not included in our study). Most probably, the psychological stress results in bruxism (bite force) that increases the load on the masticatory system which is manifested by TMJ dysfunction.

While conducting the research, it was observed that majority of the patients had lack of awareness of having a TMJ disorder and the adverse effects they could experience in the future. Therefore, patient education is an important factor in the treatment of the disorder, and grave importance should be given to this subject in order to reduce the incidence of the disorders.

Patients who had habits should be educated and enlightened about the severe effects they are on to the TMJ and the further possible severities to the TMJ if the habits are not discontinued.

4.1. Treatment. This analysis demonstrated that most of the patients from the collected sample needed a nonsurgical approach towards the treatment (95%) such as splint therapy [28], physiotherapy [29], and transcutaneous electrical nerve stimulation [30]. The patients should be reassured and well informed regarding the at-home practices to relieve the symptoms.

Only 5% of the patient with long-term chronic conditions may need a surgical approach.

5. Conclusions

The research concluded that the incidence of TMJ Disorders is not uncommon among the patients attending the dental clinic of AUST–Fujairah campus.

TMD is a complex symptom, caused by multiple factors that are poorly understood. It affects people between 20 and 40 years old.

About 20% to 40% of the adult population is affected to some degree.

The harmony and balance between the masticatory system and the function are crucial to keep the TMJ complex healthy. If anything that disrupts this equation, the body tries to correct it but to a certain limit; when the abnormal functions continue, at that time the signs and symptoms appear.

So, we can conclude (according to our research) that the main etiology of the TMD is the abnormal functions of TMJ due to incorrect habits and practices, as demonstrated by our study.

Hence, more importance should be given towards educating the patient on how to avoid behaviors that are abusive to the TMJ as patient education is also a key to successful TMJ rehabilitation.

References

[1] M. Bath-Balogh and M. Fehrenbach, *Illustrated Dental Embryology, Histology, and Anatomy*, Elsevier Saunders, St. Louis, MO, USA, 2011.

[2] M. Fehrenbach and S. Herring, *Illustrated Anatomy of the Head and Neck*, Elsevier, St. Louis, MO, USA, 2012.

[3] L. Moss-Salentijn, *Biology of Mineralized Tissues: Prenatal Skull Development*, Columbia University College of Dental Medicine Post-Graduate Dental Lecture Series, New York, NY, USA, 2007.

[4] M. L. Moss, "The non-existent hinge axis," *American Institute of Oral Biology*, pp. 59–66, 1972.

[5] G. D. Slade, R. Ohrbach, J. D. Greenspan et al., "Painful temporomandibular disorder: decade of discovery from OPPERA studies," *Journal of Dental Research*, vol. 95, no. 10, pp. 1084–1092, 2016.

[6] J.-Y. Lee, Y.-K. Kim, S.-G. Kim, and P.-Y. Yun, "Evaluation of Korean teenagers with temporomandibular joint disorders," *Journal of the Korean Association of Oral and Maxillofacial Surgeons*, vol. 39, no. 5, pp. 231–237, 2013.

[7] T. List and R. H. Jensen, "Temporomandibular disorders: old ideas and new concepts," *Cephalalgia*, vol. 37, no. 7, pp. 692–704, 2017.

[8] V. Tsai, *Temporomandibular Joint Syndrome*, February 2010.

[9] R. Ohrback, Ed., *Diagnostic Criteria for Temporomandibular Disorders; Clinical Protocol and Assessment Instruments*, International RDC/TMD Consortium Network, 2014, http://www.rdc-tmdinternational.org.

[10] P. Modi, S. S. Shaikh, and A. Munde, "A cross sectional study of prevalence of temporomandibular disorders in university students," *International Journal of Scientific and Research Publications*, vol. 2, no. 9, 2012.

[11] M. Ebrahimi, H. Dashti, M. Mehrabkhani, M. Arghavani, and A. Daneshvar-Mozafari, "Temporomandibular disorders and related factors in a group of iranian adolescents: a cross-sectional survey," *Journal of Dental Research, Dental Clinics, Dental Prospects*, vol. 5, no. 4, pp. 123–127, 2011.

[12] G. Fernandes, A. L. Franco-Micheloni, J. T. T. Siqueira, D. A. G. Gonçalves, and C. M. Camparis, "Parafunctional habits are associated cumulatively to painful temporomandibular disorders in adolescents," *Brazilian Oral Research*, vol. 30, no. 1, 2016.

[13] L. Pereira, T. Pereira-Cenci, A. A. Del Bel Cury et al., "Risk indicators of temporomandibular disorder incidences in early adolescence," *Pediatric Dentistry*, vol. 32, no. 4, pp. 324–328, 2010.

[14] B. E. Cairns, "The influence of gender and sex steroids on craniofacial nociception," *Headache*, vol. 47, no. 2, pp. 319–324, 2007.

[15] V. Motghare, J. Kumar, S. Kamate et al., "Association between harmful oral habits and sign and symptoms of temporomandibular joint disorders among adolescents," *Journal of Clinical and Diagnostic Research*, vol. 9, no. 8, pp. ZC45–ZC48, 2015.

[16] L. J. Motta, "Association between parafunctional habits and signs and symptoms of temporomandibular dysfunction among adolescents," *Oral Health and Preventive Dentistry*, vol. 11, no. 1, pp. 3–7, 2013.

[17] B. Murad, N. G. Sepah, B. Rehman, and T. Ahmad, "Parafunctional habits among undergraduate clinical students and house officers at Khyber College of Dentistry," *Journal of Khyber College of Dentistry*, vol. 6, no. 2, 2016.

[18] S. R. Habiba, M. Q. Al Rifaiy, K. H. Awan, A. Alsaif, A. Alshalan, and Y. Altokais, "Prevalence and severity of temporomandibular disorders among university students in Riyadh," *The Saudi Dental Journal*, vol. 27, no. 3, pp. 125–130, 2015.

[19] N. Pham Dang, E. Hugonnet-Boby, I. Barthelemy, and J. Shi, "Zygomatic arch fracture extended to the glenoid fossa: a cause of TMJ pain," *Revue de Stomatologie, de Chirurgie Maxillo-faciale et de Chirurgie Orale*, vol. 115, no. 2, pp. 121–123, 2014.

[20] G. L. Xiang, X. Long, M. H. Deng, Q. C. Han, Q. G. Meng, and B. Li, "A retrospective study of temporomandibular joint ankylosis secondary to surgical treatment of mandibular condylar fractures," *British Journal of Oral and Maxillofacial Surgery*, vol. 52, no. 3, pp. 270–274, 2014.

[21] S. Witulski, T. J. Vogl, S. Rehart, and P. Ottl, "Evaluation of the TMJ by means of clinical TMD examination and MRI diagnostics in patients with rheumatoid arthritis," *BioMed Research International*, vol. 2014, Article ID 328560, 9 pages, 2014.

[22] L. M. Zwir, M. T. Terreri, S. A. Sousa, A. R. Fernandes, A. S Guimarães, and M. O. Hilário, "Are temporomandibular joint signs and symptoms associated with magnetic resonance imaging findings in juvenile idiopathic arthritis patients? A longitudinal study," *Clinical Rheumatology*, vol. 34, no. 12, pp. 2057–2063, 2015.

[23] E. M. Kogawa, P. S. Calderon, J. R. Lauris, C. R. Araujo, and P. C. Conti, "Evaluation of maximal bite force in temporomandibular disorders patients," *Journal of Oral Rehabilitation*, vol. 33, no. 8, pp. 559–565, 2006.

[24] B. I. Kim, S. H. Jeong, K. H. Chung, Y. K. Cho, H. K. Kwon, and C. H. Choi, "Subjective food intake ability in relation to maximal bite force among Korean adults," *Journal of Oral Rehabilitation*, vol. 36, no. 3, pp. 168–175, 2009.

[25] F. Bahrani, P. Ghadiri, and M. Vojdani, "Comparison of temporomandibular disorders in Iranian dental and non-dental students," *Journal of Dental Contemporary Practice*, vol. 13, no. 2, pp. 173–177, 2012.

[26] C. Hirsch, J. Hoffmann, and J. C. Türp, "Are temporomandibular disorder symptoms and diagnoses associated with pubertal development in adolescents? An epidemiological study," *Journal of Orofacial Orthopedics/Fortschritte der Kieferorthopädie*, vol. 73, no. 1, pp. 6–18, 2012.

[27] A. A. Pesqueira, P. R. Zuim, D. R. Monteiro, P. Ribeiro Pdo, and A. R. Garcia, "Relationship between psychological factors and symptoms of TMD in university undergraduate stu-

dents," *Acta Odontologica Latinoamericana (AOL)*, vol. 23, no. 3, pp. 182–187, 2010.

[28] N. N. Giannakopoulos, E. N. Katsikogianni, D. Hellmann et al., "Comparison of three different options for immediate treatment of painful temporomandibular disorders: a randomized, controlled pilot trial," *Acta Odontologica Scandinavica*, vol. 74, no. 6, pp. 480–486, 2016.

[29] J. M. Pho Duc, S. V. Hüning, and M. L. Grossi, "The effectiveness of physiotherapy in the management of temporomandibular disorders: a systematic review and meta-analysis," *International Journal of Prosthodontics*, vol. 29, no. 4, pp. 340–350, 2016.

[30] A. P. Ferreira, D. R. Costa, A. I. Oliveira et al., "Short-term transcutaneous electrical nerve stimulation reduces pain and improves the masticatory muscle activity in temporomandibular disorder patients: a randomized controlled trial," *Journal of Applied Oral Science*, vol. 25, no. 2, pp. 112–120, 2017.

Permissions

All chapters in this book were first published in IJD, by Hindawi Publishing Corporation; hereby published with permission under the Creative Commons Attribution License or equivalent. Every chapter published in this book has been scrutinized by our experts. Their significance has been extensively debated. The topics covered herein carry significant findings which will fuel the growth of the discipline. They may even be implemented as practical applications or may be referred to as a beginning point for another development.

The contributors of this book come from diverse backgrounds, making this book a truly international effort. This book will bring forth new frontiers with its revolutionizing research information and detailed analysis of the nascent developments around the world.

We would like to thank all the contributing authors for lending their expertise to make the book truly unique. They have played a crucial role in the development of this book. Without their invaluable contributions this book wouldn't have been possible. They have made vital efforts to compile up to date information on the varied aspects of this subject to make this book a valuable addition to the collection of many professionals and students.

This book was conceptualized with the vision of imparting up-to-date information and advanced data in this field. To ensure the same, a matchless editorial board was set up. Every individual on the board went through rigorous rounds of assessment to prove their worth. After which they invested a large part of their time researching and compiling the most relevant data for our readers.

The editorial board has been involved in producing this book since its inception. They have spent rigorous hours researching and exploring the diverse topics which have resulted in the successful publishing of this book. They have passed on their knowledge of decades through this book. To expedite this challenging task, the publisher supported the team at every step. A small team of assistant editors was also appointed to further simplify the editing procedure and attain best results for the readers.

Apart from the editorial board, the designing team has also invested a significant amount of their time in understanding the subject and creating the most relevant covers. They scrutinized every image to scout for the most suitable representation of the subject and create an appropriate cover for the book.

The publishing team has been an ardent support to the editorial, designing and production team. Their endless efforts to recruit the best for this project, has resulted in the accomplishment of this book. They are a veteran in the field of academics and their pool of knowledge is as vast as their experience in printing. Their expertise and guidance has proved useful at every step. Their uncompromising quality standards have made this book an exceptional effort. Their encouragement from time to time has been an inspiration for everyone.

The publisher and the editorial board hope that this book will prove to be a valuable piece of knowledge for researchers, students, practitioners and scholars across the globe.

List of Contributors

Manal A. Awad, Mariam Malalla, Zainab Maklai, Aisha Tariq, Badria Al-Ali and Hisham El Batawi
Department of Preventive and Restorative Dentistry, College of Dental Medicine, University of Sharjah, Sharjah, UAE

Eman AlHammadi
Dubai Health Authority, Dubai, UAE

Alaa Al Jameel
Princess Nourah Bint Abdulrahman University, Riyadh, Saudi Arabia

Anahita Punj, Santhosh Shenoy, N. and Priyanka Pampani
Department of Periodontics, A.B. Shetty Memorial Institute of Dental Sciences, Nitte University, Deralakatte, Mangalore, Karnataka 575018, India

Suchetha Kumari
Department of Biochemistry, K.S. HegdeMedical Academy, NitteUniversity, Deralakatte, Mangalore, Karnataka 575018, India

Basma Abdelaleem Elsaadany
Faculty of Dentistry, Cairo University, Giza, Egypt

Eman Magdy Ahmed
Faculty of Oral and Dental Medicine, Beni Suef University, Beni Suef, Egypt

Sana Maher Hasan Aghbary
Faculty of Dentistry, Aden University, Aden, Yemen

Ryuichi Ishikawa, Maiko Kawasaki, Akane Yamada, Supaluk Trakanant, Fumiya Meguro, Atsushi Kitamura, Takehisa Kudo and Atsushi Ohazama
Division of Oral Anatomy, Department of Oral Life Science, Niigata University Graduate School of Medical and Dental Sciences, Niigata, Japan

Katsushige Kawasaki
Division of Oral Anatomy, Department of Oral Life Science, Niigata University Graduate School of Medical and Dental Sciences, Niigata, Japan
Research Center for Advanced Oral Science, Department of Oral Life Science, Niigata University Graduate School of Medical and Dental Sciences, Niigata, Japan

Takeyasu Maeda
Research Center for Advanced Oral Science, Department of Oral Life Science, Niigata University Graduate School of Medical and Dental Sciences, Niigata, Japan

Alaa Gamaleldin Sulieman and Elhadi Mohieldin Awooda
Department of Endodontics, Faculty of Dentistry, University of Medical Sciences and Technology, Khartoum, Sudan

Leyla Sadighpour, Vanya Rasaei
Department of Prosthodontics, Faculty of Dentistry, Tehran University of Medical Sciences, Tehran, Iran

Farideh Geramipanah
Dental Implant Research Center, Faculty of Dentistry, Tehran University of Medical Sciences, Tehran, Iran

Mohammad J. Kharazi Fard
Dental Research Center, Faculty of Dentistry, Tehran University of Medical Sciences, Tehran, Iran

André Göhler and Ivo Steinmetz
Friedrich Loeffler Institute of Medical Microbiology, University Medicine Greifswald, Greifswald, Germany
Institute for Hygiene, Microbiology and Environmental Medicine, Medical University of Graz, Graz, Austria

Stefanie Samietz
Department of Prosthodontics, Gerostomatology and Biomaterials, University Medicine Greifswald, Greifswald, Germany

Carsten Oliver Schmidt
SHIP-Clinical-Epidemiological Research, Institute for Community Medicine, University Medicine Greifswald,Greifswald, Germany

Thomas Kocher and Birte Holtfreter
Department of Restorative Dentistry, Periodontology, Endodontology, and Preventive and Pediatric Dentistry, University Medicine Greifswald, Greifswald, Germany

Kaoutar Laslami, Sara Dhoum and Iman Benkiran
Department of Conservative Dentistry and Endodontics, School of Dentistry of Casablanca, Casablanca, Morocco

Amine El Harchi
Private Practice, Casablanca, Morocco

Yoshiaki Nomura and Ayako Okada
Department of Translational Research, School of Dental Medicine, Tsurumi University, 2-1-3 Tsurumi, Tsurumi-ku, Yokohama 230-8501, Japan

Yoh Tamaki
Department of Health and Welfare Services, National Institute of Public Health, 2-3-6 Minami, Wako-shi, Saitama 351-0197, Japan

Svetlana Razumova, Anzhela Brago, Lamara Khaskhanova, Ammar Howijieh, Haydar Barakat and Ashot Manvelyan
Peoples' Friendship University of Russia (RUDN University), 6 Miklukho-Maklaya Street, Moscow 117198, Russia

John K. Drisdale III, Monica G. Thornhill and Alexandre R. Vieira
Department of Oral Biology, University of Pittsburgh School of Dental Medicine, Pittsburgh, PA, USA

Danilo Bacchiocchi
Private Practice, Castelfidardo, 60022 Ancona, Italy

Andrea Guida
Fundacao Universitaria Vida Crista (FUNVIC), 12400-010 Pindamonhangaba, SP, Brazil

Natheer H. Al-Rawi
College of Dental Medicine, University of Sharjah, Sharjah, UAE

Ahmed S. Alnuaimi
College of Medicine, University of Baghdad, Baghdad, Iraq

Asmaa T. Uthman
College of Dental Medicine, Gulf Medical University, Ajman, UAE

Yoshimune Hiratsuka
Department of Health and Welfare Services, National Institute of Public Health, 2-3-6 Minami, Wako, Saitama 351-0197, Japan
Department of Ophthalmology, Juntendo University School of Medicine, 3-1-3, Hongo, Bunkyo-ku, Tokyo 113-8431, Japan

Toshiro Kumakawa
Department of Health and Welfare Services, National Institute of Public Health, 2-3-6 Minami, Wako, Saitama 351-0197, Japan
The University of Fukuchiyama, 3370, Aza Hori, Fukuchiyama-shi, Kyoto 620-0886, Japan

Hiroko Miura
Department of International Health and Collaboration, National Institute of Public Health, 2-3-6 Minami, Wako-shi, Saitama 351-0197, Japan

Jouko Kallio and Lasse Suominen
1Social and Health Services of Espoo, City of Espoo, Finland

Timo Kauppila
Department of General Practice and Primary Healthcare, Institute of Clinical Medicine, University of Helsinki, Helsinki, Finland

Anna Maria Heikkinen
Department of Oral and Maxillofacial Diseases and Surgery, Head and Neck Center, Helsinki University Hospital, HUS, Helsinki, Finland
Department of Oral and Maxillofacial Diseases, University of Helsinki and Helsinki University Hospital, Helsinki, Finland

Sabrina Gonçalves Riatto
Faculty of Dentistry, IESP, Joao Pessoa, PB, Brazil
Department of Stomatology, University of Seville, Seville, Spain

Antonio Castaño-Séiquer and David Ribas Pérez
Department of Stomatology, University of Seville, Seville, Spain

Javier Montero and Abraham Dib
Department of Surgery, University of Salamanca, Salamanca, Spain

Ebtissam M. Al-Madi
Department of Restorative Dentistry, College of Dentistry, King Saud University, Riyadh 11545, Saudi Arabia
Department of Clinical Dental Sciences, College of Dentistry, Princess Nourah bint AbdulRahman University, Riyadh 11671, Saudi Arabia

SamarA. Al Saleh, Sundus M. Bukhary and Maha M. Al-Ghofaily
Department of Prosthetic Dental Sciences, College of Dentistry, King Saud University, Riyadh 11545, Saudi Arabia

Naji Ziad Arandi
Department of Conservative Dentistry and Prosthodontics, Faculty of Dentistry, Arab American University, Jenin, State of Palestine

Tarek Rabi
Department of Conservative Dentistry, Al-Quds University, Jerusalem, State of Palestine

Helder H. M. Menezes
Department of Periodontology and Implant Dentistry, HD Post Graduation Dental School, Uberl^andia 38408-394, Brazil

Marina M. Naves, Jéssica A. Ferreira and Denildo Magalhães
School of Dentistry, Federal University of Uberlandia, Uberl^andia 38405-320, Brazil

Henara L. Costa
School of Mechanical Engineering, Federal University of Uberlandia, Uberlandia 38400-901, Brazil
School of Engineering, Federal University of Rio Grande, Rio Grande 96203-900, Brazil

Tarsis P. Barbosa
School of Mechanical Engineering, Federal University of Uberlandia, Uberlandia 38400-901, Brazil
Department of Telecommunications and Mechatronics, Federal University of Sao Joao Del-Rei, Ouro Branco 36420-000, Brazil

Elizabeth F. Martinez
Department of Cellular and Mollecular Biology, São Leopoldo Mandic Research, Campinas 13045-755, Brazil

Faezeh Eslamipour
Torabinejad Dental Research Center, Department of Oral Public Health, School of Dentistry,
Isfahan University of Medical Sciences, Isfahan, Iran

Arash Najimi
Department of Medical Education, Medical Education Research Center, Isfahan University of Medical Sciences, Isfahan, Iran

Azade Tadayonfard
Department of Prosthodontics, School of Dentistry, Shahid Beheshti University of Medical Sciences, Tehran, Iran

Zeinab Azamian
Department of Orthodontics, School of Dentistry, Isfahan University of Medical Sciences, Isfahan, Iran

Heba Ashi
Department of Cariology, Institute of Odontology, Sahlgrenska Academy, University of Gothenburg, Gothenburg, Sweden
Department of Preventive Dentistry, Faculty of Dentistry, King Abdulaziz University, Jeddah, Saudi Arabia

Peter Lingström
Department of Cariology, Institute of Odontology, Sahlgrenska Academy, University of Gothenburg, Gothenburg, Sweden
WHO Collaborating Center for Epidemiology and Preventive Dentistry, Milan, Italy

Guglielmo Campus
Department of Surgery, Microsurgery and Medicine, School of Dentistry, University of Sassari, Sassari, Italy
WHO Collaborating Center for Epidemiology and Preventive Dentistry, Milan, Italy

Heléne Bertéus Forslund
Department of Internal Medicine and Clinical Nutrition, Institute of Medicine, Sahlgrenska Academy, University of Gothenburg, Gothenburg, Sweden

Waleed Hafiz
Department of Prosthodontics, North Jeddah Speciality Dental Center, Jeddah, Saudi Arabia

Neveen Ahmed
Department of Pedodontics, Jeddah Speciality Dental Center, Jeddah, Saudi Arabia

Chai Kit Lu, Margaret Chia Soo Yee, Spoorthi Banavar Ravi and Rohit Pandurangappa
School of Dentistry, International Medical University, 126/Jalan 19/155B, Bukit Jalil, 57000 Kuala Lumpur, Malaysia

Luljeta Zajmi
Lipjan Correctional Center, Family Medicine Center Prishtina, Prishtina, Kosovo

Agim Begzati and Lumnije Krasniqi
Department of Pediatric and Preventive Dentistry, University Dentistry Clinical Center of Kosovo, Prishtina, Kosovo

Milaim Sejdini and Nora Berisha
Department of Orthodontics, University Dentistry Clinical Center of Kosovo, Prishtina, Kosovo

Marco Tallarico
Implantology and Prosthetic Aspects, Master of Science in Dentistry Program, Aldent University, Tirana, Albania
Private Practice, Rome, Italy

Luigi Canullo
Private Practice, Rome, Italy

Marco Caneva
ARDEC Academy, Ariminum Odontologica Srl, Rimini, Italy

Yuki Omori
ARDEC Academy, Ariminum Odontologica Srl, Rimini, Italy
Department of Oral Implantology, Osaka Dental University, Hirakata, Osaka, Japan

Silvio Mario Meloni
Dentistry Unit, University Hospital of Sassari, Sassari, Italy

Erta Xhanari
Private Practice, Tirana, Albania

John Michael Nyorobi
Dental Unit, Misungwi District Hospital Misungwi, Mwanza, Tanzania

Lorna Celia Carneiro
Department of Restorative Dentistry, Muhimbili University of Health and Allied Sciences, Dar es Salaam,Tanzania

Msafiri Nicodemus Kabulwa
Oral Health Section, Ministry of Health, Community Development, Gender, Elderly and Children, Dodoma, Tanzania

Priscilla Naiff
Ph.D. Student, Faculty of Health Sciences, University of Brasilia, Distrito Federal, Brazil

Valéria Carneiro and Maria do Carmo Guimarães
Ph.D. Professor at Periodontics Division, University of Brasilia, Distrito Federal, Brazil

Giorgio Lombardo, Jacopo Pighi, Giovanni Corrocher and Pier Francesco Nocini
School of Dentistry, Department of Surgery, Dentistry, Paediatrics and Gynaecology (DIPSCOMI), University of Verona, Verona, Italy

Mauro Marincola
Dental Implant Unit, University of Cartagena, Cartagena, Colombia

Miguel Simancas-Pallares
Dental Implant Unit, University of Cartagena, Cartagena, Colombia
Research Department, Faculty of Dentistry, University of Cartagena, Cartagena, Colombia

Gabriella Balli, Andreas Ioannou, Nikola Angelov and Nikolaos Soldatos
Department of Periodontics and Dental Hygiene, School of Dentistry, University of Texas Health Science Center at Houston,Houston, TX, USA

Charles A. Powell
Department of Surgical Dentistry, Division of Periodontics, School of Dental Medicine, University of Colorado,Anschutz Medical Campus, Aurora, CO, USA

Georgios E. Romanos
Department of Periodontology, Stony Brook University School of Dental Medicine, Stony Brook, NY, USA
Department of Oral Surgery and Implant Dentistry, Johann Wolfgang Goethe University of Frankfurt, Frankfurt, Germany

Gisele Pavão Spaulonci, Ricardo Salgado de Souza, Vanessa Gallego Arias Pecorari and Luciano Lauria Dib
Paulista University (UNIP), Indian´opolis, SP, Brazil

Ruchanee Salingcarnboriboon Ampornaramveth and Jesita Lertnukkhid
Research Unit on Oral Microbiology and Immunology, Department of Microbiology, Faculty of Dentistry, Chulalongkorn University, Bangkok, Thailand

Nilada Akeatichod
Research Unit on Oral Microbiology and Immunology, Department of Microbiology, Faculty of Dentistry, Chulalongkorn University, Bangkok, Thailand
Pakhum Hospital, Buriram, Thailand

Nichakorn Songsang
Research Unit on Oral Microbiology and Immunology, Department of Microbiology, Faculty of Dentistry, Chulalongkorn University, Bangkok, Thailand Trat Hospital, Trat, Thailand

Wilson Matsumoto, Rossana Pereira de Almeida, Ana Paula Macedo, Beatriz Roque Kubata and Takami Hirono Hotta
Department of Dental Materials and Prosthodontics, Dental School of Ribeirão Preto, University of São Paulo, Ribeirão Preto 14040-904, Brazil

Paula Pastana Beraldo
Private Practice, Ribeirão Preto 14025-010, Brazil

Elaf Akram Abdulhameed, Natheer Hashim Al-Rawi and Ab Rani Samsudin
College of Dental Medicine, University of Sharjah, Sharjah, UAE

Asmaa Tahseen Uthman
College of Dental Medicine, Gulf Medical University, Ajman, UAE

Omar Hamad Alkadhi
Division of Orthodontics, Department of Preventive Dentistry, Riyadh Colleges of Dentistry and Pharmacy, Riyadh, Saudi Arabia

Sarah Fahad Almahfouz
Saudi Board of Orthodontics, Department of Orthodontics, King Saud University, Riyadh, Saudi Arabia

Hana Abdulmajeed Tokhtah
Orthodontics Residency Program, King Saud University, Riyadh, Saudi Arabia

Lamia Abdulaziz Binhuwaishel
Department of Orthodontics, King Saud Medical City, Riyadh, Saudi Arabia

M. F. A. Quadri
Dental Public Health, Jazan University, Jizan, Saudi Arabia

M. A. Shubayr, A. H. Hattan and S. A. Wafi
Department of Preventive Dentistry, Jazan University, Jizan, Saudi Arabia

A. H. Jafer
Ministry of Health, Riyadh, Saudi Arabia

Luana L. Martins, José Henrique F. Rosseto, Natália Silva Andrade, Juliana Bertoldi Franco and Karem L. Ortega
1Special Care Dentistry Center, Division of Oral and Maxillofacial Pathology, Department of Stomatology, School of Dentistry, University of Sao Paulo, Sao Paulo, SP, Brazil

Paulo Henrique Braz-Silva
Division of General Pathology, Department of Stomatology, School of Dentistry, University of Sao Paulo, Sao Paulo, SP, Brazil
Laboratory of Virology, Institute of Tropical Medicine of Sao Paulo, University of Sao Paulo, Sao Paulo, SP, Brazil

Kashef K. AlShaban
Faculty of Medical and Health Sciences, Emirates College of Technology, Abu Dhabi, UAE

Zainab Gul Abdul Waheed
Mint Dental Care LLC., Dubai, UAE

Index